Positive Psychology in the Middle East/North Africa

Louise Lambert · Nausheen Pasha-Zaidi
Editors

Positive Psychology in the Middle East/North Africa

Research, Policy, and Practise

Springer

Editors
Louise Lambert
Editor in Chief
Middle East Journal of Positive Psychology
Dubai, United Arab Emirates

Nausheen Pasha-Zaidi
Department of Social Science
Houston Community College
University of Houston-Downtown
Houston, TX, USA

ISBN 978-3-030-13920-9 ISBN 978-3-030-13921-6 (eBook)
https://doi.org/10.1007/978-3-030-13921-6

Library of Congress Control Number: 2019932598

This Springer imprint is published by the registered company Springer Nature Switzerland AG
The registered company address is: Gewerbestrasse 11, 6330 Cham, Switzerland

Acknowledgements

This book could not have been completed without the help of numerous individuals who have contributed their thoughts and expertise. We are particularly grateful to each of the authors who were exceedingly patient with rewrites, suggestions and questions as we navigated this process. We would also like to thank Silvia King, Positive Psychology coach, for proofreading and providing another set of eyes in the editing of the manuscript.

Disclaimer

The information provided in this book is designed to provide helpful information on the subjects discussed. This book is not meant to be used, nor should it be used, to diagnose or treat any psychological, medical or health condition. For diagnosis or treatment of any medical problem, consult a qualified professional.

The views and opinions expressed in this book are those of the author(s) and do not necessarily reflect the views and opinions of the editors, their academic institutions, sponsors or publisher. Therefore, the publisher, editors, individual authors and their organisations are not liable for any damages or negative consequences from any treatment, action, application or preparation, to any person reading or following the information in this book. Any sponsors of the textbook are also exempt from any liability. References are provided for informational purposes only and do not constitute endorsement of any particular sources. Readers should be aware that the websites listed in this book may change.

While best efforts have been used in preparing this book, period updates and changes to the information may produce inconsistencies therein. In this event, every attempt shall be made by the editors to update the information in consequent publications.

Contents

Editors and Contributors

About the Editors

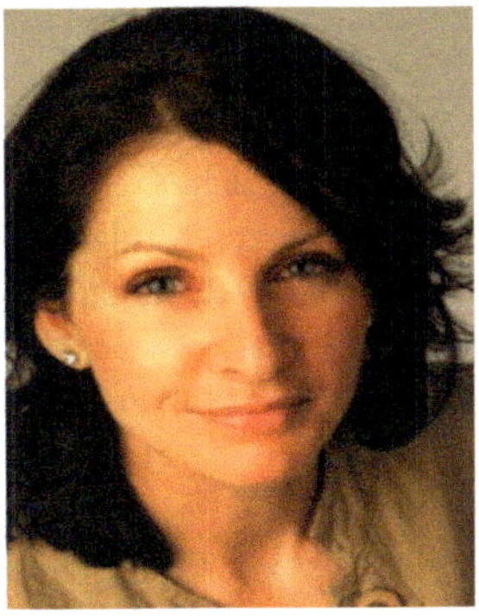

Dr. Louise Lambert, Ph.D. is a Registered Psychologist (#2659, College of Alberta Psychologists, Canada) and Professor with almost 20 years experience in counselling, mental health, not-for-profit organisations, higher education and research, and primary healthcare. She has lived in the UAE for 9 years and is currently working with the United Arab Emirates University's (UAEU) Emirates Center for Happiness Research. She has established three evidence-based positive psychology intervention programmes. Her 'Happiness 101' programme is used in clinical settings and has shown 6-month post-treatment effectiveness (Lambert D'raven, Moliver, & Thompson, 2015), while her workplace character strengths programme for teens, young adults and entry-level employees is currently being trialled in Saudi Arabia (Lambert, Budhraja, Mullan, & Gupta, 2018). Finally, her university intervention programme showed sustainable gains in well-being at 3-month post-intervention relative to a control group, as well as significant decreases in the fear of happiness (Lambert, Passmore, & Joshanloo, 2018). She also developed AlNowair's Bareec positivity school programme (Lambert, Passmore, Al-Sabah, Hussain, & Scull, 2018), now adopted by the Kuwait Ministry of

Education for use in government schools and higher education institutions. She is well published and also the Founder and Editor-in-Chief of the *Middle East Journal of Positive Psychology*, a journal dedicated to uncovering human excellence in the region.

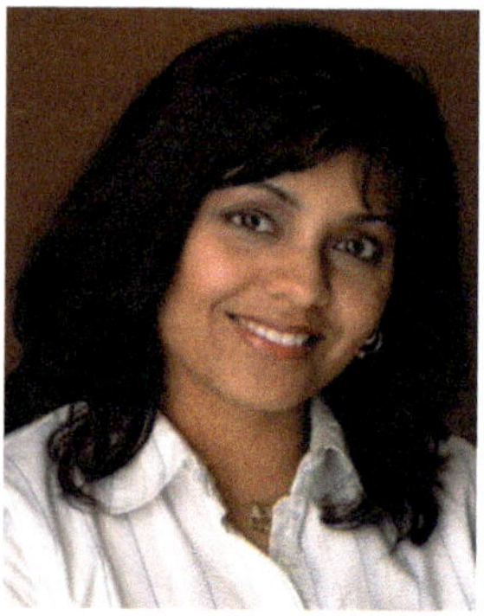

Dr. Nausheen Pasha-Zaidi, Ph.D. has degrees in Communications, Education and Psychology. She has worked as an international educator for almost 20 years focusing on language development and cultural studies with an emphasis on Muslim populations. Her articles have appeared in a number of professional journals including the *Middle East Journal of Positive Psychology, Ethnicities* and *The Journal of International Women's Studies*. She is the author of *The Colour of Mehndi*, a novel that explores acculturation, family values and mental illness within the Pakistani-American community and the lead editor of *Mirror on the Veil: A Collection of Personal Narratives on Hijab and Veiling*. After working in the UAE for almost 8 years as a K-12 ESL teacher, teacher trainer and Assistant Professor of General Studies in Engineering Communication, she recently moved back to the United States in 2016 and currently teaches psychology at Houston Community College and the University of Houston-Downtown. She also serves on the Board of Trustees for the Chicago School of Professional Psychology and is a founding member and Editor with the *Middle East Journal of Positive Psychology*. She continues to do international research through collaborations in the United States, Turkey and the UAE.

Contributors

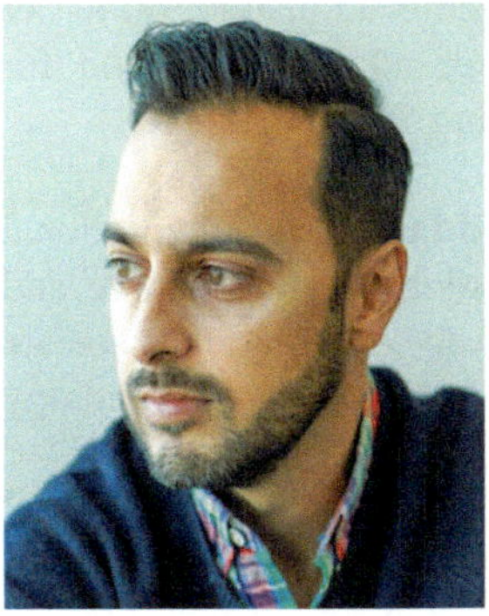

Dr. Rehman Abdulrehman, Ph.D., C.Psych. is a clinical psychologist and consultant, working with individual clients and organisations. He is the Director of Clinic Psychology Manitoba and Assistant Professor with the Department of Clinical Health Psychology in the Max Rady College of Medicine, Faculty of Health Sciences at the University of Manitoba (Canada). He works locally and abroad; he has been a visiting professor at three universities in Tanzania, currently working out of the State University of Zanzibar, where he teaches and consults on programme development in low-resource settings. His other work is focused on his LeadWithDiversity.com initiative, where he helps professionals and organisations understand psychological aspects of diversity and actionable steps to improving workplace inclusion. He has training and experience in cognitive behavioural therapy, focusing on anxiety disorders and PTSD. He is the former president of the Manitoba Psychological Society and past chair of the Committee on International Relations in Psychology for the American Psychological Association. *Photo Credit* Daniel Crump.

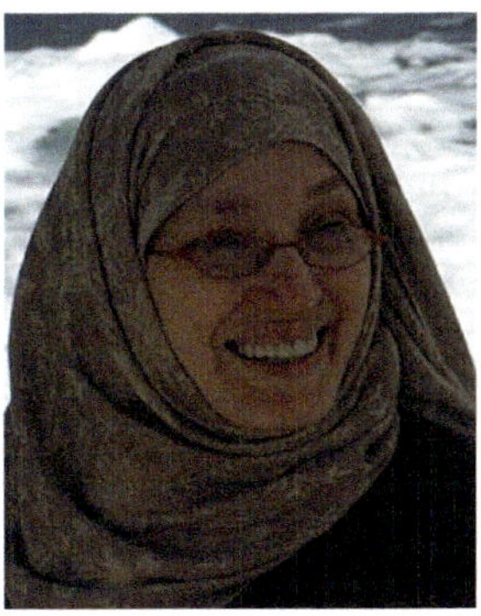

Dr. Saddiga Jaber Al-Ghalib is Assistant Professor at the Psychology Department at Effat University (Saudi Arabia) and the founder and director of the Positive Psychology and Wellbeing Research Lab. She received her Ph.D. in Educational Psychology from the Southern Illinois University Carbondale (USA). She has been active in the fields of educational psychology, leadership, learning styles, mindfulness, positive psychology and well-being. She formerly served at Effat University as the first Dean of Graduate Studies and Scientific Research, Director of the Research and Consultancy Institute, Director of the Center of Excellence in Teaching and Learning and Chair of the Psychology Department. She is an experienced instructor, data analyst and statistical consultant. She has attended conferences and forums all over the world, both as a speaker and guest. She is a life-long learner, always finding new ways to bring healing to people and making life easier for them. She is an inspiration to her students and peers due to her relentless passion for knowledge, learning and having fun.

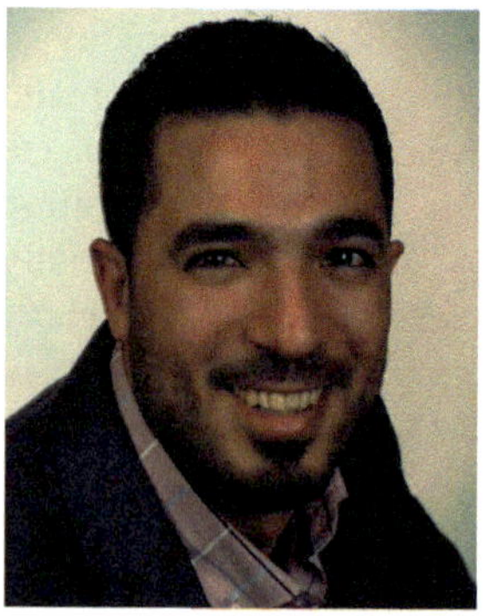

Mohammed K. Al-Haj Baddar is an International Positive Education Network global representative and International Positive Psychology Association associate and has a Master's degree in educational psychology from Al Balqaa University, Jordan. His thesis described the relationship between self-regulated learning and rational thoughts among students in Amman and was awarded Best Thesis in education and psychology in 2014. As a positive psychology specialist at the Jannati Clinic, Jordan, he uses positive psychology interventions with groups, individuals and schools. An appreciation of beauty and excellence and love of learning are his strengths, leading him to take dozens of online courses on psychology and positive psychology since 2013. This past year, in collaboration with CARE International, he conducted seven positive psychosocial support programmes with 22 Syrian refugee groups in Mafraq and Azraq. He is now writing an Arabic-language practice guide in positive psychology to spread the message of positivity called نفسي الإيجابية (My Positive Psych).

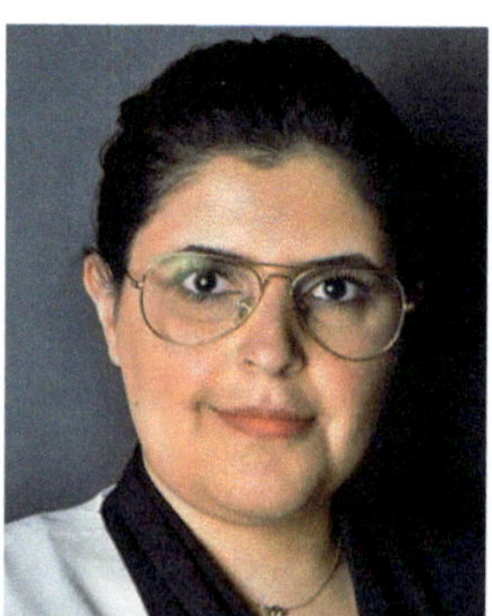

Shaden Abdul-Hakeem Al-Khalifah is a psychology graduate from Effat University (Jeddah, Saudi Arabia) and co-founder of the Positive Psychology & Wellbeing Research Lab. She formerly worked as a Research Assistant at the Infant Language and Learning Lab at Carnegie Mellon University, USA. She is interested in studying spirituality and religiosity and their clinical application within a Middle Eastern population. She has also worked as a psychologist assistant at a number of public and private psychiatric facilities in the kingdom of Saudi Arabia.

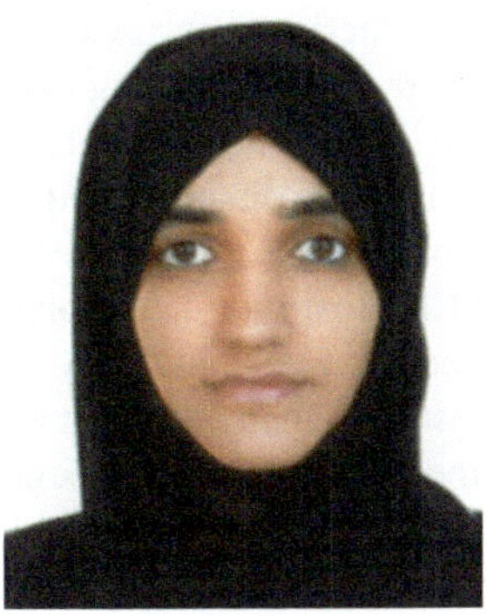

Aamna Al-Shehhi is a Post-doctoral Fellow at the Khalifa University of Science Technology and Research in Abu Dhabi, United Arab Emirates (UAE). She received her Ph.D. in Electrical Engineering and Computer Science Department in 2017 from Masdar Institute of Science and Technology in Abu Dhabi, UAE. Her present domains of interests are big data, data analytics, machine learning, as well as argumentation and time series analysis.

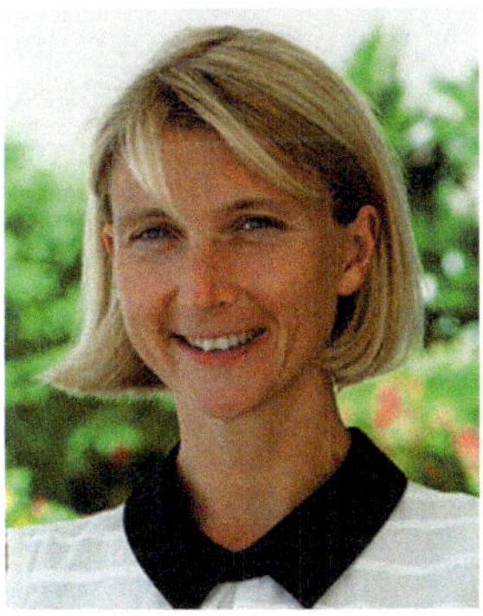

Dr. Annie E. Crookes, M.Sc., Ph.D., PGCertHE has been in Dubai, UAE for 11 years as a lecturer and department leader in Psychology for two British institutions. She is now Academic Head of Psychology for Heriot-Watt University (Dubai campus), developing and managing the psychology programmes at B.Sc. and M. Sc. levels and overseeing student support. She works with professional psychologists in the UAE and helps organise the annual International Psychology Conference Dubai (IPCD; www.psych-me.com). Her main areas of teaching are cognitive psychology (memory, learning and perception), biopsychology and advanced courses in consciousness and mental health studies. Following a recent sabbatical year in which she gained an M.Sc. in International Addiction Studies, she has a research interest in substance use among young people based in Dubai.

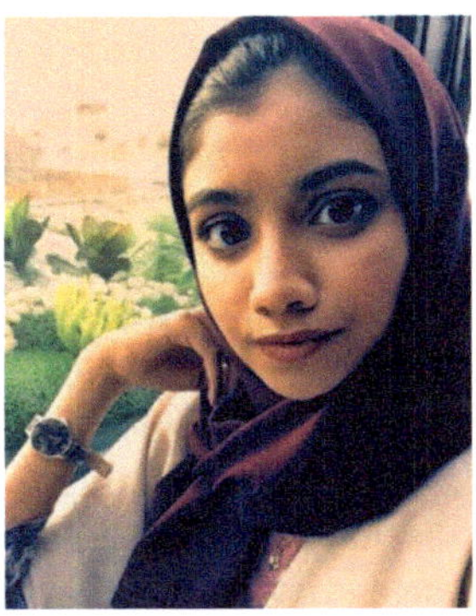

Rana Abdulrahman Hafed Dahlawi holds a Bachelor of Science in Psychology degree from Effat University, Jeddah, Saudi Arabia. She is also one of the Co-Founders of the 'Positive Psychology & Wellbeing Research Lab' at Effat University and is currently working as a Research Assistant under the Research Lab. She is hoping to pursue a career as a Clinical Psychologist in the Kingdom and is interested in studying mental illnesses, genetics, resilience and cognition and how they can apply to various clinical and non-clinical settings in the Middle Eastern society.

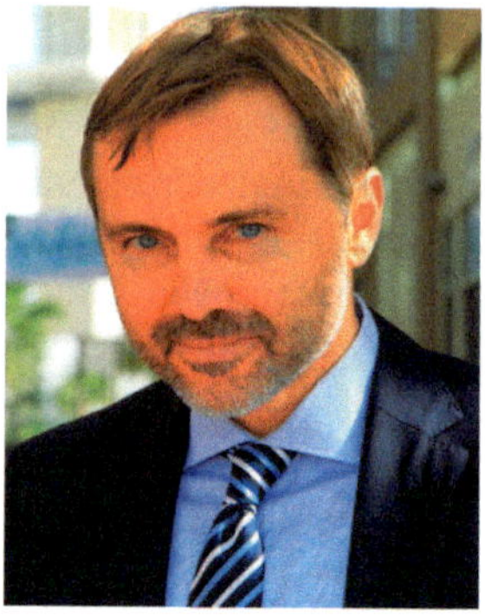

Karim El-Jisr has 20 years of experience in resource management, climate change and urban planning. He visited The Sustainable City in January 2014, during the initial construction phase, and immediately decided to relocate there to promote sustainable living. He is currently establishing the SEE Institute—a global platform for advancing knowledge in sustainability in the built environment. The Institute manages several multi-year research programmes, implements special projects with industry partners and is deploying a modular training programme for professionals in the built environment. He holds a Bachelor of Science and a Bachelor of Engineering in Agriculture, and a Master of Science in Ecosystem Management from the American University of Beirut. He also holds a course certificate in Business Sustainability Management from the University of Cambridge Institute for Sustainability Leadership (CISL). A seasoned speaker, he is fluent in Arabic, English, French and Danish.

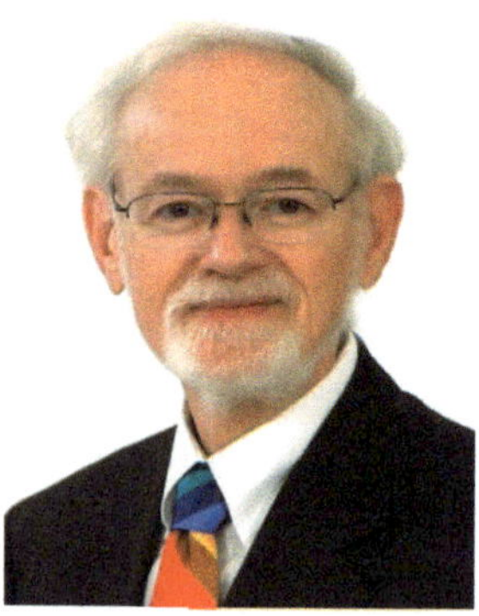

Dr. Richard J. Estes is Professor Emeritus of Social Welfare of the School of Social Policy and Practice with the University of Pennsylvania in Philadelphia, USA. He holds graduate degrees in social work (University of Pennsylvania, Master of Social Work; University of California at Berkeley, Doctor of Social Welfare), as well as a post-master's Certificate in Psychiatric Social Work. He has worked throughout the world and garnered professional awards for his work on social development and nation-building. In recent years, he has focused on patterns of social development and progress in societies that are predominately Islamic. He has authored many articles and his recent books include *Advances in wellbeing: Toward a better world for all* (2018, with M. J. Sirgy); *The pursuit of human wellbeing: The untold global history* (2018, with M. J. Sirgy), and *Social progress in Islamic societies: Social, political, economic, and ideological challenges* (2016, with H. Tiliouine) among earlier volumes on a variety of topics. He has a special interest in the origins of Jihadist terrorism and for the formulation of more peaceful ways of settling legitimate grievances between Western and Islamic countries.

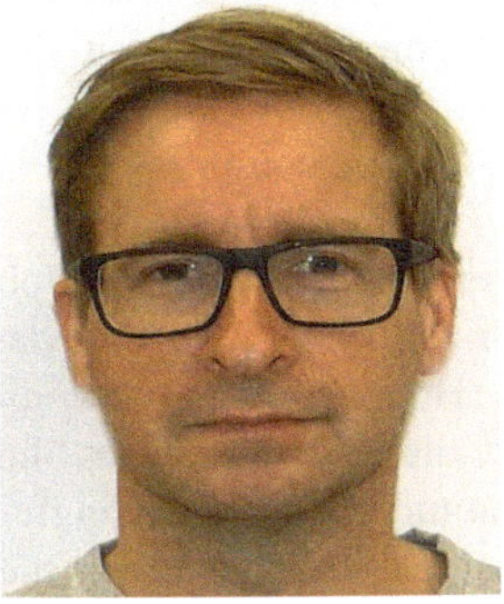

Dr. Ian Grey holds a Ph.D. from the National University of Ireland and a D.Clin.Psych. from Trinity College Dublin, Ireland. He holds additional postgraduate qualifications in Applied Behaviour Analysis and in Forensic Psychology. He worked as a clinical psychologist for almost 20 years and previously specialised in the application of assessment and intervention methodology to the remediation of behavioural disorders in children and adolescents with neurodevelopmental disorders. He has more recently worked in forensic psychology settings specialising in psychometric assessment in legal settings. He has also worked as an applied practitioner and research simultaneously over his career. In addition to being Director of Services for a centre for children and adolescents with neurodevelopmental disorders and published over 40 book chapters and journal articles, he has held numerous grants. He is currently transitioning from his position as co-founder of the Culture, Cognition and Psychological Wellbeing unit within Zayed University, Abu Dhabi (UAE), to the Lebanese American University in Beirut, Lebanon.

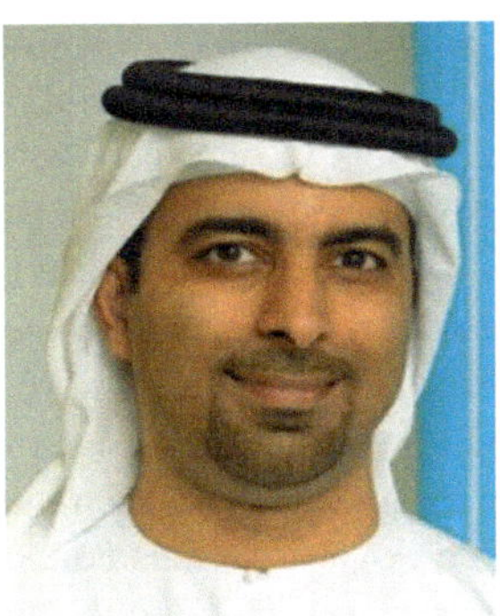

Dr. Mansoor Anwar Habib is a Family Medicine and Occupational Health Consultant with *du*. Joining in 2009, he established two staff clinics and a wellness department where he treats patients, tackles occupational health complaints, manages chronic disease and implements prevention strategies. He restructured du's entire wellness department and launched a dedicated executive wellness programme that set wellness KPIs for company executives. He was recognised with the 'Idea Arabia' award by the Dubai Quality Group and in 2016, the national agenda for happiness and positivity was assigned to his department. Since 2012, he has been the Regional Chair of the International Association of Worksite Health Promotion, and Chair of the Workplace Wellness Taskforce Group with the Dubai Chamber. In 2017, he was nominated as the company's happiness champion and graduated from the UAE government executive leadership programme in collaboration with Oxford University and Wharton University's private sector happiness and positivity programme. He writes regularly about wellness in newspapers and magazines around the country.

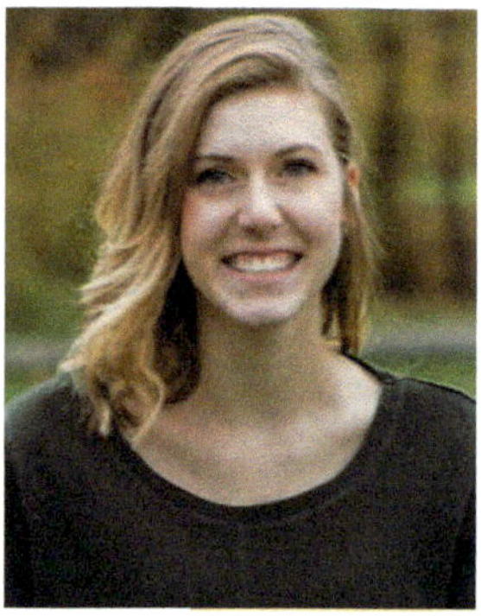

Lauren Hotchkiss is a Research Assistant and Job Coach at the University of British Columbia, Canada. She has a Bachelor of Science (Honours) in Psychology from the University of British Columbia Okanagan. She has conducted research on gratitude, hope, meaningful work and well-being. For her Honour's Thesis, she investigated how virtual communication and helping others influenced job meaningfulness and well-being. She continues to work with researchers around the world on well-being projects.

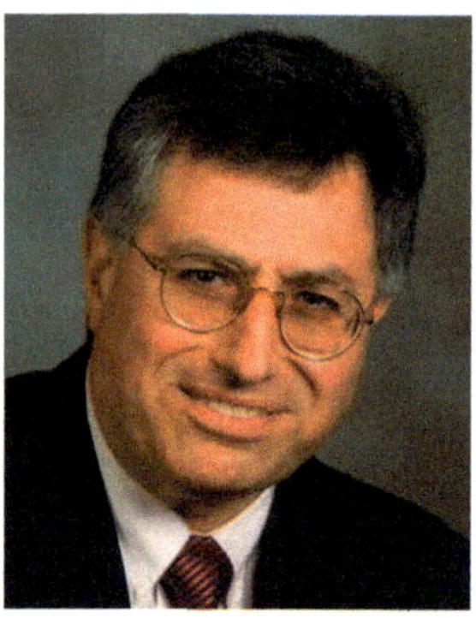

Dr. M. Joseph Sirgy is a Management Psychologist and Virginia Tech Real Estate Professor of Marketing at Virginia Polytechnic Institute and State University (USA). He spent his early years in Cairo and Beirut, with his parents being of Lebanese and Syrian descent. He is well published in well-being and quality-of-life (QOL) research and is the author/editor of many books. He co-founded the International Society for Quality-of-Life Studies (ISQOLS) in 1995 as well as its official journal, *Applied research in quality of life* (2005), where he continues to serve as editor. In those years, he received the Distinguished Research Fellow Award, Distinguished QOL Researcher Award and a record of lifetime achievement. In 2012, he was further given the EuroMed Management Research Award. He has edited the ISQOLS/Springer book series on *Handbooks in quality-of-life research and community quality-of-life indicators (best practices)* and his recent book includes *The pursuit of wellbeing: The untold global history* (2017). He is now serving as Springer's book series co-editor for *Human wellbeing and policy-making*.

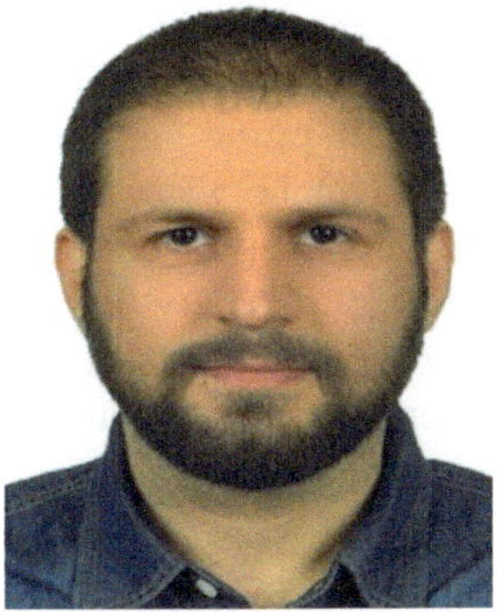

Dr. Mohsen Joshanloo is an Assistant Professor of Psychology at Keimyung University, South Korea. He has completed his Ph.D. in 2013 at Victoria University of Wellington, New Zealand. His research is focused on mental well-being, personality and research methodology. He has extensively published on mental well-being in non-western cultures with a particular focus on the Muslim world. He advocates culturally inclusive research into well-being and works with a vast network of international colleagues from a broad range of nations, including the UAE.

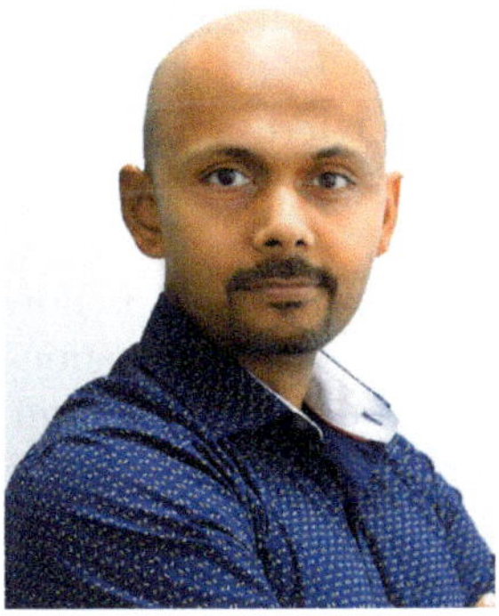

Amol Kadam is the co-founder of RBBI, the region's first User Experience (UX) and usability consultancy established in Dubai in 2011. He is an expert in User Experience, Usability, User Research, Strategy and CX and has written for leading publications within the region and participated as a speaker in international conferences. For more than 22 years, he has conceptualised, designed and managed significant projects for a wide range of clients involving digital transformation, CX, UX and strategy and usability. He is a certified usability professional and a registered member of Usability Professionals Association Worldwide. He holds a Bachelor of Fine Arts in Applied Design from Sir J.J. Institute of Applied Arts, Mumbai University (India) and Master's Certificate in Human–Computer Interaction from Washington University (USA).

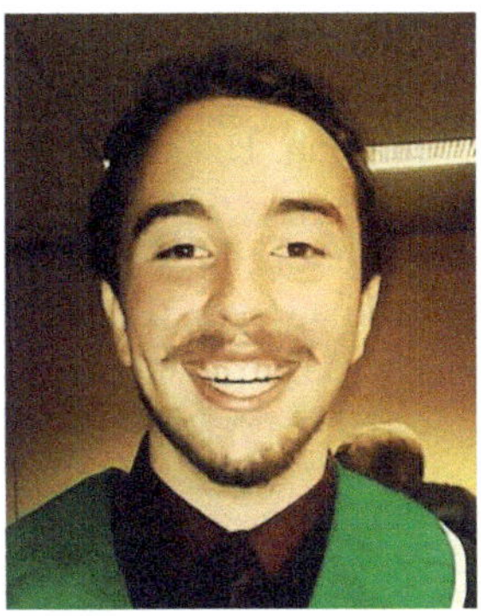

Paul K. Lutz is a third-year undergraduate student currently pursuing a Bachelor of Arts (Honours) in Psychology at the University of British Columbia Okanagan (Canada). His primary research interests fall at the intersection of moral and positive psychology. Specifically, he has conducted research on moral emotions, well-being, meaning in life and moral identity under the supervision of Holli-Anne Passmore (Ph.D. Candidate) and Dr. Derrick Wirtz. He is also currently serving as a Research Assistant for the Enduring Happiness and Continued Self-Enhancement (ENHANCE) trials, a comprehensive intervention programme helmed by world-renowned researcher Dr. Ed Diener and colleagues, that aims to promote various aspects of well-being.

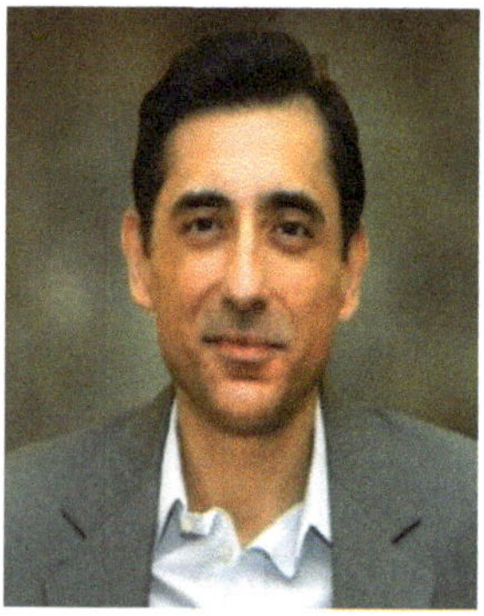

Cameron Mirza is a skilled education leader with both international experience, and within the UK and Middle East including working with two UK prime ministers. At the Department for Education (UK), he was responsible for the establishment of the young apprenticeship programme and led the review of diversity in the curriculum with Sir Keith Ajegbo. He was appointed Director for Strategy for Higher Education Council, Bahrain from December 2011 to May 2016 where he co-authored a national higher education strategy and the nation's first industry-led graduate skills guide. In 2016, he was appointed Head of Transformation at the University of Bahrain, authoring the transformation plan of the national university. He is a board member of BETT Middle East and a fellow of Oxfords Gulf Talent advisory board.

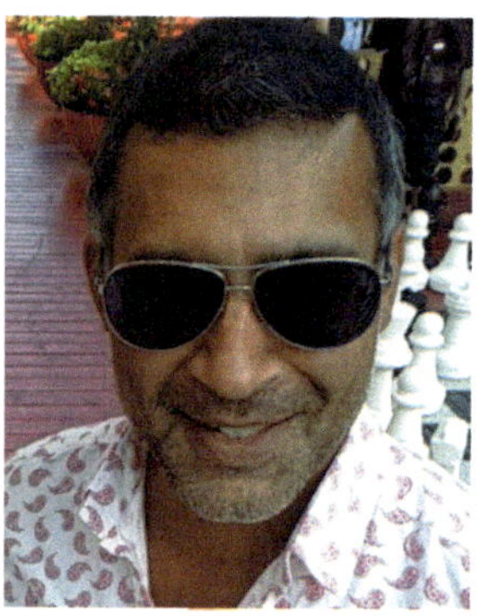

Aziz Mulay-Shah former Canadian diplomat, is now the Managing Director of Global Communications Agency (GCA), a well-being policy advisory firm, specialising in commercial happiness audits across the UAE and GCC region. GCA also develops social impact investment strategies as a component of Corporate Social Responsibility projects for clients in the Gulf, Canada and MENASA region. He is a leader in developing strategic ideas, policy prescriptions and leading teams to implement them. He favours a holistic approach when advising his clients in which he combines policy planning, implementation and evaluation to address challenges relating to international assistance and humanitarian aid, strategic political communications, and coalition building. His goal is to create new civic models and enhanced communities, whether local, regional or international. He holds advanced graduate degrees in International Relations, public policy and music.

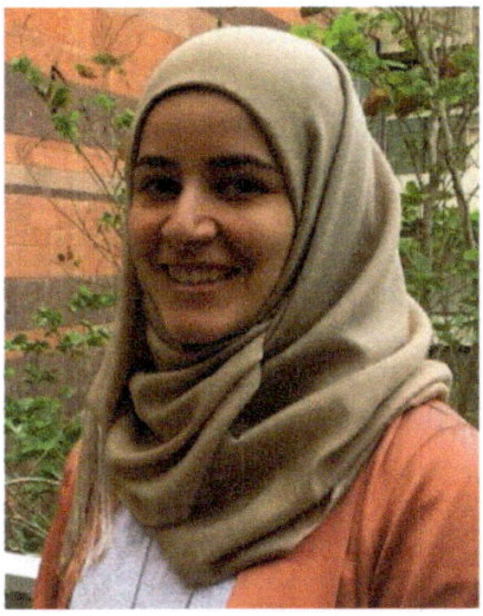

Muna Odeh is a Palestinian Jordanian now living in Dubai (UAE) and a graduate of the American University of Sharjah (Sharjah, UAE). She received her Bachelor's degree in International Studies with a minor in Psychology and currently works in media content analysis. Her interests are positive psychology, media psychology, identity development and creative writing. She takes great interest in considering how a positive Islamic identity can be developed, by young adults in particular, given contemporary media portrayals.

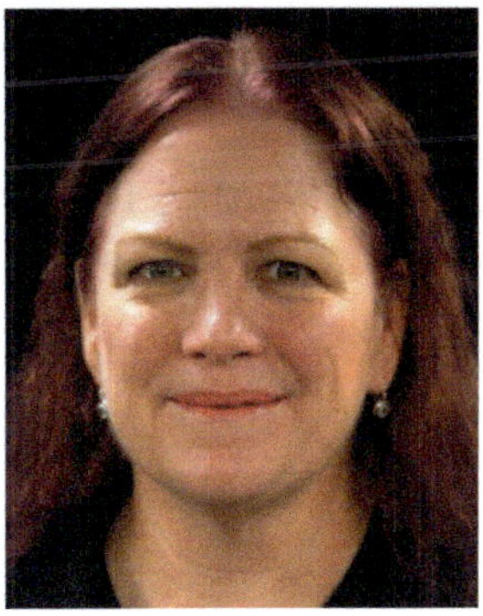

Dr. Lily O'Hara is Associate Professor of Public Health at Qatar University. She is a public health and health promotion academic and practitioner with extensive experience in Australia, United Arab Emirates and Qatar in community, workplace, university and school-based programmes. Her research focuses on assessing health and well-being status at the community and organisational level, and developing setting-based critical health promotion initiatives. She is actively engaged in critiquing public health approaches to body weight and developing ethical and evidence-based public health initiatives using the Health at Every Size approach. Her research is also focused on developing the competencies of the health promotion workforce. She is the co-author of the Red Lotus Health Promotion Model, a model for holistic, salutogenic and ecological health promotion.

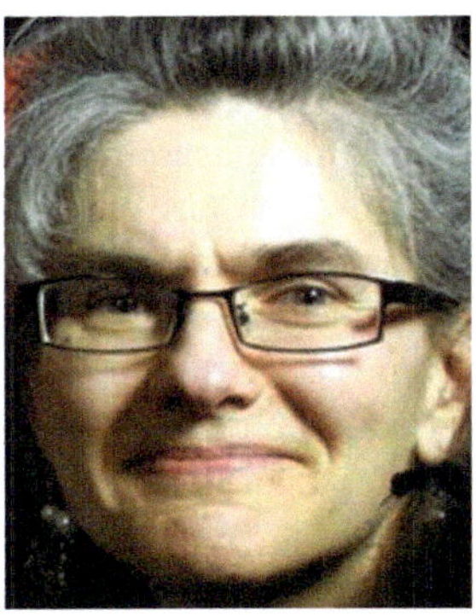

Holli-Anne Passmore (ABD) is a positive psychology researcher focusing on the connection of nature to well-being, meaning in life and the sense and experience of being alive. Her work has been published in many academic journals (e.g. Journal of Positive Psychology, Journal of Happiness Studies and International Journal of Wellbeing) and books (e.g. International Contributions to the Study of Positive Mental Health, Positive Psychology among Children and Adolescents). She has presented her work at many conferences including the past four World Congresses on Positive Psychology, Canadian Positive Psychology Association and International Network on Personal Meaning conferences. She was awarded (2017) the

University of British Columbia's (Canada) Provost's Award for Teaching Assistance Excellence and received over $200,000 in grants and scholarship funding for her research. She is currently collaborating with researchers in the UAE, China, Germany, Japan, Korea and Russia.

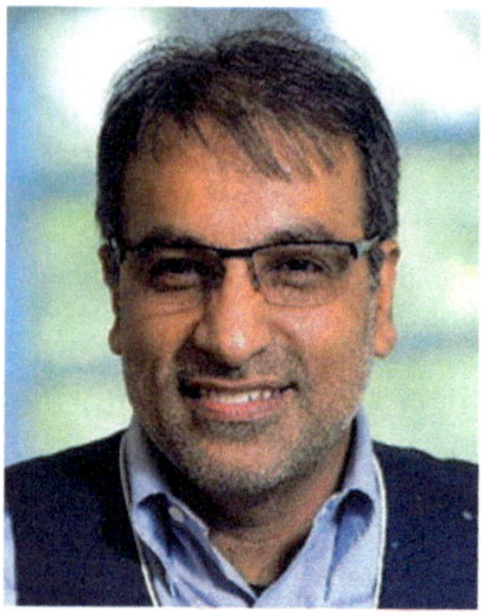

Dr. Tayyab Rashid is a Therapist by heart and Researcher by head at the Health & Wellness Centre, University of Toronto Scarborough Canada (UTSC) who tries to integrate symptoms with strengths, resources with risks, weaknesses with values and hope with regrets. He has worked with 9/11 families and survivors of Asian tsunamis as examples of his clientele. He is best known for the development of a positive clinical psychology and protocol for a positive strength-based psychotherapy (Rashid, 2014). He has shared his insights from these connections through training at diverse settings including Kings College, UK, University of Maastricht, U of Paris, Princeton University, Wellington College, UK, and the Geelong Grammar School, Australia. Many of these insights were published in several peer-reviewed journals, book chapters and caught the attention of Wall Street Journal, Psychology Today, Toronto Star, The Globe and Mail, and Canadian Broadcasting Corporation (CBC).

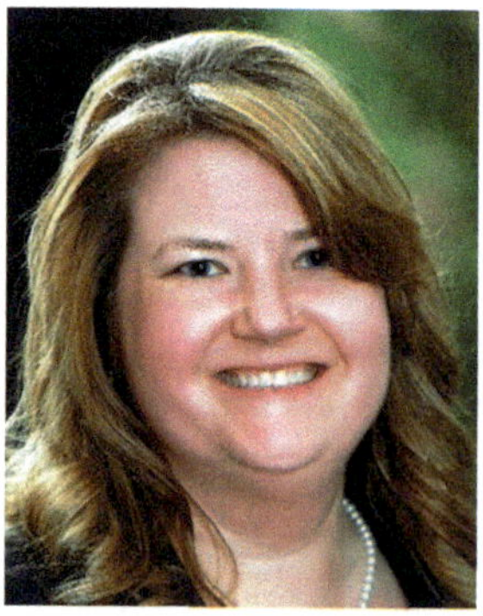

Aubrilyn Reeder supports United World Infrastructure's (UWI) Urban Ecology initiatives, including Happier Cities. She has presented this work at international conferences, such as the International Gross National Happiness Conference in Bhutan and the FIABCI International Real-Estate Congress in Dubai. She was a judge for the Happiest Communities designation at the most recent Gulf Real Estate Awards. She has over 15 years of experience working with communities to improve educational and livelihood opportunities including designing and managing training programmes for the Supreme Education Council of Qatar, leading curriculum and leadership training development programmes for over 1000 schools in India, and working with migrant farm workers in the United States. She began her career with

Teach for America, working with children in under-resourced public school systems. She earned a Bachelor of Arts in Cognitive Science from the University of Virginia (USA) and a Master of Education from Harvard University (USA).

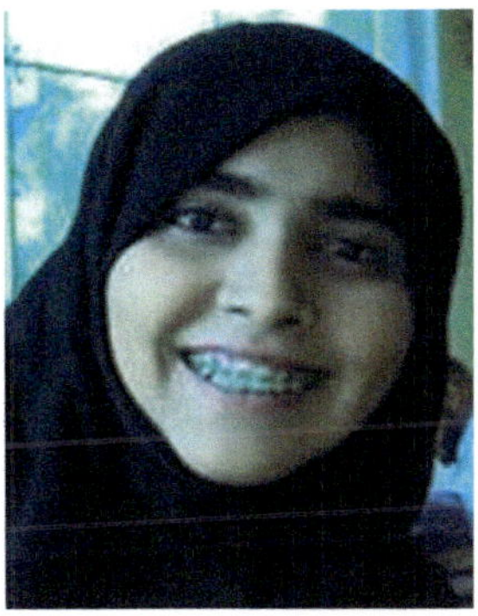

Afeefah Y. Salim is a highly motivated individual who graduated from Effat University (Jeddah, Saudi Arabia) with a Bachelor of Science in Psychology with First Honors. Her dissertation was an experiment on a mindfulness intervention for university students, discussed in her chapter. Her interests lay in the subjects of well-being, positive psychology, mindfulness, spirituality, as well as mental health. Her love for conducting research in general is the reason she helped co-found Saudi Arabia's first Positive Psychology and Wellbeing Lab.

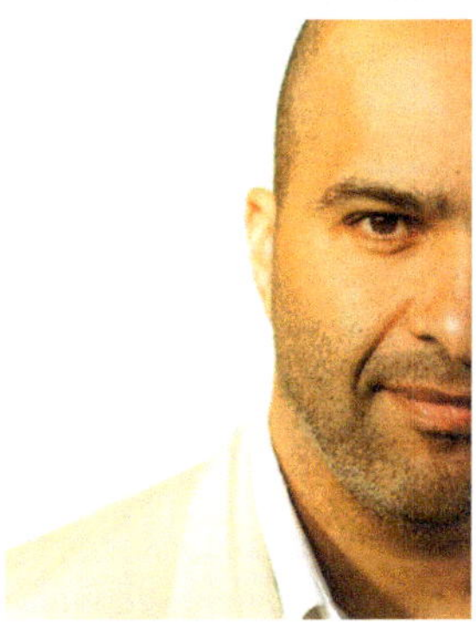

Dr. Justin Thomas earned his Ph.D. in experimental psychology from the University of Manchester, UK, and has professional postgraduate qualifications in health psychology and cognitive therapy. He is a Chartered Health Psychologist with the British Psychological Society and Professor of Psychology at Zayed University in Abu Dhabi (UAE). There, he directs the Research Cluster for Culture, Cognition and Wellbeing. He also publishes extensively on topics related to culture and psychological well-being, as well as psychopathology. His most recent book is *Psychological wellbeing in the Gulf states: The new Arabia Felix* (2015). He also believes in promoting a public understanding of science and writes for the popular press, like *The National* (UAE), and makes regular media appearances and gives public lectures and workshops on a variety of psychology topics.

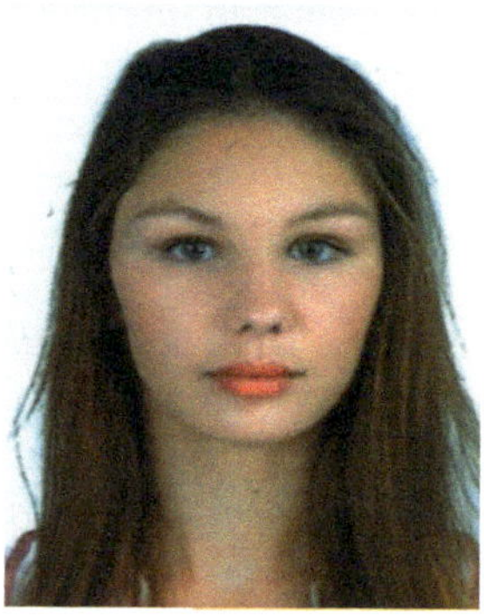

Elizabeth Topolskaya is working in Dubai (UAE) as an instructional designer with Pearson Education, the world's largest educational company. Much like the company's slogan, 'always learning', she pursues her passion in research and has published works on online learning in the GCC, emerging HR trends and public health awareness initiatives on male cancer. She has a background in public health and has worked in an HR consultancy firm, which allowed her to understand the nuances of the HR practices across the GCC region. Following her passion for research and learning, she strives to ensure that science becomes easily available to professionals and that the most progressive research is implemented across industries by visionary management.

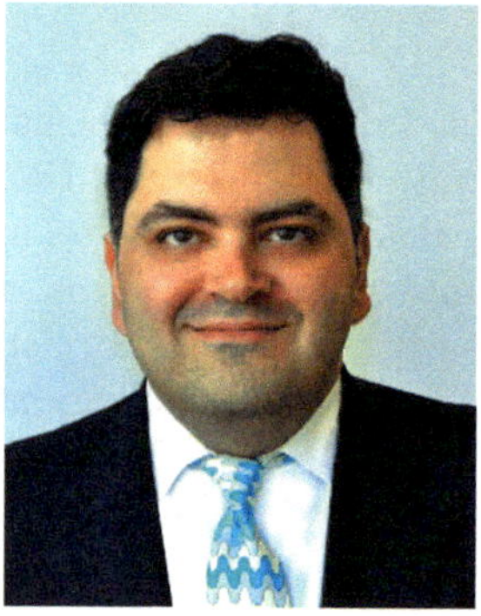

Vafa Valapour is the Co-Founder/Principal of United World Infrastructure (UWI) and leads its strategic investments in real estate and infrastructure assets, and guides new business initiatives. He has worked extensively with multinational organisations, banks and government-linked agencies to develop strategic infrastructure systems that encourage economic integration and technology transfer. He has overseen multibillion-dollar transnational investments across the Americas, Asia, the Middle East and North Africa. Serving in different positions in The Executive Office of Dubai, including Chief Investment Officer in the real estate and infrastructure group, he managed the financial planning and development of large-scale real estate assets. He earned his Bachelor of Arts in Economics and History from the University of Pennsylvania (USA).

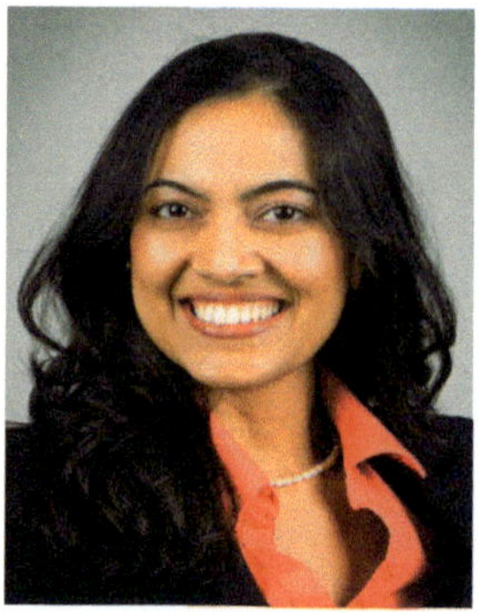

Dr. Meg A. Warren is Assistant Professor of Management at Western Washington University, USA. She is the Past-President of the Work & Organizations Division of the International Positive Psychology Association (IPPA), and Co-Founder and Associate Director of the Western Positive Psychology Association (WPPA). Her research includes positive approaches to diversity and inclusion, empowering work relationships and organisational virtuousness. She has a strong interest in cultural influences on well-being and actively works with collaborators in Africa, the Middle East and South

America. She is the lead editor of two 2017 volumes, *Scientific Advances in Positive Psychology* and *Toward a Positive Psychology of Relationships: New Directions in Theory and Research*. She has published articles in many peer-reviewed journals, including the *Middle East Journal of Positive Psychology, Journal of Positive Psychology, International Journal of Wellbeing, Journal of Wellbeing Assessment*, as well as *Canadian Psychology*. She holds two graduate degrees in business and a Ph.D. in psychology.

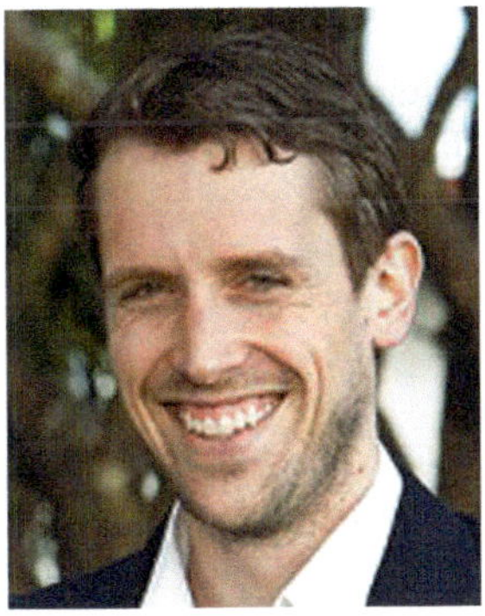

Dr. Dan Weijers was formally Assistant Professor at California State University Sacramento (USA) and is now a Philosophy Lecturer in the School of Social Sciences at the University of Waikato (New Zealand). Although primarily a philosopher, most of his research is on interdisciplinary happiness and well-being studies. He has published in a range of disciplines, including philosophy, psychology, economics, politics and public policy. He has also promoted research on interdisciplinary happiness and well-being studies by co-founding and co-editing the *International Journal of Wellbeing*, an interdisciplinary open access academic journal, and co-organising a series of international conferences on well-being and public policy.

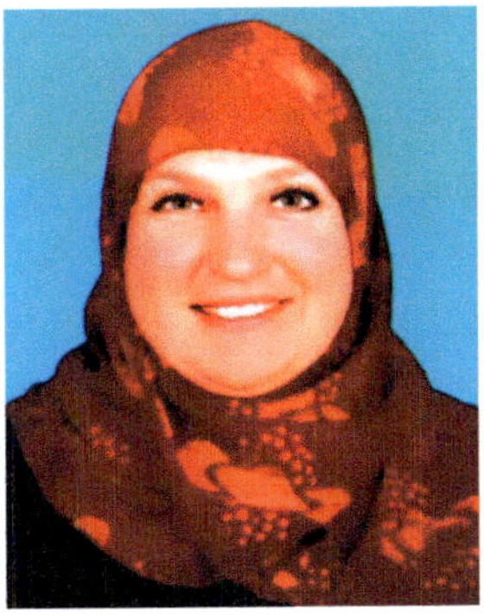

Dr. Bronwyn P. Wood has a consulting, research and teaching background in consumer research, especially consumer values, and with a special interest in Islamic Marketing. She serves as Associate Editor of the *International Journal of Islamic Marketing and Branding*, and on the Senior Editorial Advisory Board of the *Journal of Islamic Marketing*. Her research has been published in the Journal of Business Research, Marketing Intelligence and Planning and the International Journal of Tourism Management, among others. She has taught in her native New Zealand, Saudi Arabia, Oman, and has lived in Japan. She is currently in the Business Administration Department at the United Arab Emirates University in Al Ain (UAE).

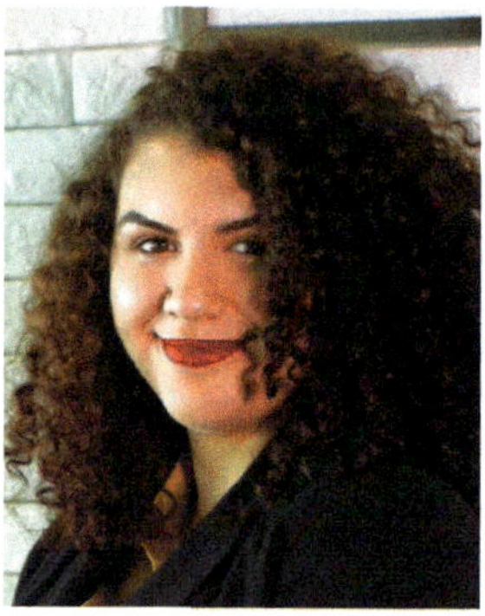

Yara Younis though born and raised in Dubai (UAE), nonetheless feels detached from her 'home' in the Gaza Strip of Palestine. Now, having spent years contemplating traditional Arab society, she considers the meaning of modern Arab identity, as well as how and whether policy decisions can have an impact on such questions. She graduated from the Canadian University Dubai with a B.A. (hons) in media and communication studies, with a focus on advertising. She joined the Delma Institute in Abu Dhabi as a MENA research analyst and is currently working as the Deputy Advisor and Project Coordinator for the UAE Minister of Culture and Knowledge Development. She recently received a full international Master's level scholarship to study in Canada and is preparing for an illustrious career in International Studies.

Chapter 1
Introduction: Musings on a Regional Positive Psychology

Louise Lambert and Nausheen Pasha-Zaidi

Abstract In 2015, we launched the first issue of the *Middle East Journal of Positive Psychology* with the intent of developing an indigenous positive psychology across the Middle East/North Africa (MENA) region. We felt it was imperative to do so, not only to counter the indiscriminate use of Western positive psychological models and interventions in the region, but equally, to encourage the growth of this new science of wellbeing by offering a platform for regional research to be showcased. As our work grew, it became clear that more was needed to help the field prosper; in particular, a focus on science was missing with many consultants speaking louder than academics and setting the dominant tone for the field by focusing on the "positive", but overlooking the "psychology". This book grew out of those concerns. In it, we offer a variety of chapters across the many growing domains of positive psychology, such as positive education, positive organizational development, positive clinical psychology and positive health. We also take a look at a number of growing themes in the field, such as the use of Big Data, the building of happy cities, and the use of happiness research to inform national policy to name a few. In this manner, we explore what makes life meaningful, worth living and what leads to conditions of social, national and individual flourishing.

In our 2015 inaugural issue of the Middle East Journal of Positive Psychology, we launched a call for the development of an indigenous positive psychology across the United Arab Emirates (UAE) and Middle East/North Africa (MENA) region (Lambert, Pasha-Zaidi, Passmore, & York Al-Karam, 2015). The reasons for that call remain valid today and we hope to have captured many of those issues in the writing of this book. For example, we felt it was critical to counter Western models, theories and notions of wellbeing that are presently being adopted indiscriminately in the region. There is nothing inherently wrong with these models; it is that we cannot assume

L. Lambert (✉)
United Arab Emirates University, Al Ain, UAE
e-mail: ltlamber@yahoo.com

N. Pasha-Zaidi
Houston Community College, University of Houston-Downtown, Houston, TX, USA
e-mail: nausheenpasha@outlook.com

L. Lambert and N. Pasha-Zaidi (eds.), *Positive Psychology in the Middle East/North Africa*, https://doi.org/10.1007/978-3-030-13921-6_1

that they always work here, nor do we know how they work, on whom, and what long-term effects they may have on individuals and societies in general. Even if they are congruent with regional cultural contexts, there is still plenty of scope to develop and identify models and concepts that might work better and reflect local cultural and religious landscapes, as well as the multicultural diversity which has now become the norm across the Gulf Cooperation Council (GCC) nations of Saudi Arabia, UAE, Oman, Bahrain, Kuwait, and Qatar. In the absence of such research, the void is presently being filled by importing Western concepts and understandings of optimal functioning which are then used as the basis for what individuals and communities should aspire to become. This bias not only impoverishes an understanding of the region; it removes its ability to understand itself and take steps towards greater growth on its own terms. It also undermines the field of positive psychology overall as the normative assumptions of what constitute wellbeing are never challenged, nor corrected. The importation of such knowledge further diminishes the need to understand regional views around the world. Thus, in order to develop a positive psychology that reflects a regional view of what makes life meaningful and worth living and which helps to understand the factors that lead to conditions of growth, as well as how quality of life is understood, defined and measured, this book was brought to life.

Second, we chose to write this book because we felt a focus on illbeing is still the dominant psychological view in the region and the potential for positive psychology to help lead individuals, families, and communities toward better lives remains an overlooked asset. The region gets a lot of negative press about terrorism, youth unemployment, corruption, and a lack of human rights; yet, that same view on illbeing obscures the fact that the region is also progressing, developing, accomplishing and superseding standards and expectations in every direction. It has massive potential, which needs to be fostered and channeled through wellbeing practises, research and policies. We wanted most importantly to change people's minds about themselves and move away from a position of victimhood to taking charge of one's destiny and actualizing one's self and nation towards what it can be. It is not enough to merely point at problems and remove them; we must also identify opportunities and build upon them. If our readers feel a sense of optimism and are inspired to pull out a pen and paper while reading this book and take on ideas for their workplaces, schools, and communities, we will have accomplished our goal.

Third, we felt it was critical to write such a book to temper the field's popularity. Given its reputation and association with smiley yellow faces, we felt that a focus on its science was essential. The fact that there are more happiness consultants in the UAE than in any other nation on earth might be positive on the one hand as it means wellbeing is on everyone's mind. But on the other, it also means there are a lot of people professing to understand positive psychology and who stand to make a tremendous amount of money from peddling hula hoop parties in the name of science. The smiley face needs to go. In exchange, it must be replaced by sound evidence-based practises and we hope to have captured much of that science in this volume.

Accordingly, as the field is still new, there is an opportunity to set it on the right path by developing a policy, practise and research agenda for the future. But, what is the right path? How should the field proceed? What opportunities and issues need inquiry? These questions need to address, uncover and explore non-Western views of wellbeing and consider how these findings can be applied across education, organizations, policy, governance and other domains of life. This is where the role of social scientists working under the umbrella of positive psychology can put their research skills to good use by defining regional or local wellbeing, proposing theories and models, implementing findings, collecting data to support interventions, as well as advocate and participate at a national, community, and individual level. Yet, this has not been the case. Diener and Diener (2017), in discussing their trip to the UAE's World Government Summit, expressed confusion at the lack of participation by researchers and psychologists in particular. We share their confusion. Positive psychologists and researchers have not been asked to sit at the decision-making tables and yet, they are eager to participate in continued nation building with an eye on wellbeing and indeed, have the necessary skills to do so.

We are perplexed by the attitudes of some of our colleagues too, as they maintain rigid notions of positive psychology and fail to accept it as science. Ironically, they are versed in models like learned helplessness (Seligman, 1972, 1975), but fail to credit that same researcher with positive psychology (Seligman & Csikszentmihalyi, 2000). Just as we study very seriously all that goes wrong in life like depression, anxiety, anger, divorce, ill health, conduct disorders, etc., positive psychology merely studies the other half of human experience, like satisfaction with life, flow, awe, hardiness, peak experiences, cardiovascular fitness, and good workplaces with as much scientific rigour. Perhaps resistant psychologists feel there is less money to be made in studying the positive. Yet, given the small numbers of individuals who are struggling with mental health issues compared to those who are languishing, the choice is clear, especially when positive psychology interventions address the positive as well as the negative (i.e., depression, symptoms of schizophrenia, diabetes management, etc.) and as effectively (Bolier et al., 2013; Hone, Jarden, & Schofield, 2015; Huffman, DuBois, Millstein, Celano, & Wexler, 2015; Johnson et al., 2009, 2011; Poppe, 2017; Seligman, Steen, Park, & Peterson, 2005; Sin & Lyubomirsky, 2009; Weiss, Westerhof, & Bohlmeijer, 2016). We thus challenge researchers, theorists, practitioners, policymakers, governments, as well as students to read through the chapters and familiarize themselves with this new sub-field of psychology, which is taking a permanent position in many regional organizations and institutions. It cannot be ignored. We offer to this effect in Table 1.1, research ideas for some of the major areas in positive psychology as inspiration.

In this book, we introduce a range of chapters across multiple routes in positive psychology and provide a brief overview of our chapters here. In Part I, we begin our journey into wellbeing by taking a bird's eye view of the role governments can play in the development of national wellbeing. We begin with a broad look, considering how national policy development can and should include wellbeing concerns. We propose various ideas for national initiatives across a number of government sectors using an evidence-based scientific view, while identifying caveats for their implementation

Table 1.1 Research questions of interest in positive psychology

Stream and scope	Examples of research questions/activity
Positive Clinical Psychology focuses on the determinants of flourishing states of mental health, and strategies to remediate negative states of functioning.	• What role do positive psychology interventions play in increasing wellbeing in the elderly? • How can positive emotions remediate and prevent mental illness? • How are positive psychology interventions mediated by culture and religion?
Positive Health promotes the physical and psychological strengths that prolong life, promote better disease prognosis and predict health outcomes.	• What role does optimism play in the treatment of cardiovascular disease? • Does religiosity influence the remission of cancer? • What effect does mindfulness have on blood pressure? • Can researchers partner with healthcare institutions to develop interventions with both patients and healthy individuals?
Positive Media aims to facilitate, depict, and promote aspects of wellbeing by creating a positive outcome or process in viewers, as well as investigate the effects of positive media on societies.	• How can media promote prosocial behavior in children, or positive relationships in adults? • Can video games promote character strengths? • Can researchers be useful in developing television series, cartoons, or video games to boost wellbeing? • Can media promote and build peace in areas with civil strife?
Positive Planning aims to inform the building of cities, offices, neighborhoods, and other public spaces for greater human and ecological wellbeing.	• Can architects, urban planners and municipalities integrate wellbeing into city planning to build social trust, physical and mental health, and a better relationship with nature? • What role do green spaces, pedestrian zones, and affordable housing play in creating a sense of belonging, attachment, or engagement?
Positive Community Development focuses on what allows people to feel included and work towards shared goals. What are features of 'good' communities?	• Can reconciliation programs increase peace in post-war societies? • What role does sport play in the unification of divided nations? • Can community engagement boost microenterprise, gender equality, or school attendance? • What role do the arts, culture, food and music play in strengthening social cohesion?

(continued)

Table 1.1 (continued)

Stream and scope	Examples of research questions/activity
Positive Education aims to deliver academics along with the skills to promote wellbeing in students, staff, and parents.	• How can character strengths and positive psychology interventions be embedded into curriculums? • Can positive parenting be a pillar of positive education? • How can school administrations champion positivity for teachers and management through HR policies?
Positive Organizational Psychology seeks to increase productivity and innovation, as well as create virtuous organizations that contribute to a common good.	• Can positive psychology interventions boost organizational citizenship behavior? • What leadership qualities contribute to virtuous organizations? • What leads to employee engagement? • How can resilience mitigate the stress of economic downturns?

(Mulay-Shah, Lambert, Warren, & Younis). Along these same lines, we explore a chapter on commercial life, the missing component across the wellbeing pillars. We make the case that commercial life, the interactions individuals have with commercial entities, whether as consumers, employees, or users of products and services, plays a critical, yet overlooked role in wellbeing. Thus, we urge a rethink by governments in their inclusion to that effect (Mulay-Shah, Lambert, Younis, & Wood). We end our segment by taking a look at the role of infrastructure—again, implicating the role of governments, as well as municipalities, builders and planners, in literally, building wellbeing. We explore a number of examples of good infrastructure design with the aim of seeing what is in fact possible to do on a large scale (Reeder, Lambert, & Pasha-Zaidi with contributions from Karim El-Jisr, Amol Kadam, and Vafa Valapour).

We move into our next segment, Part II, thinking about how smaller entities like schools and workplaces can conceptualize and implement wellbeing. We explore the field of positive education and the development of positive universities, offering practical strategies for implementing character strengths programming to equip young adults with the skills they need to transform the region into socially progressive, prosperous, and economically viable nations (Lambert, Abdulrehman, & Mirza). To bring this theory alive, our next chapter explores the development of a positive university at Saudi Arabia's Effat University and takes a look at their nation's first positive psychology lab and the research emerging from it (Al-Ghalib, Al-Khalifah, Salim, & Dahlawi). We end this section with a chapter by Lambert, Topolskaya, Warren and Habib, where we explore why wellbeing is of interest to workplaces and what interventions are available. We also include cautions about how these should be applied lest they backfire for both organizations and their employees. This chapter also includes an example of local telecommunications company *du*'s wellbeing practises for its employees.

In Part III, we explore measurement, data, as well as research trends and challenges across the region beginning with a chapter by Al-Shehhi, Grey and Thomas on the usefulness of Big Data in understanding and tracking wellbeing in the UAE. Their ongoing studies offer insight as to how Facebook and Twitter feeds, for example, can shed light on when and how wellbeing might be affected and in what ways it may differ from other parts of the world. We also take a deep dive into the world of publishing and hope this chapter is of interest to anyone who conducts or consumes research as we explore a variety of publication biases, inherent inequalities and why it is more difficult to get published in certain journals over others, especially when originating from the region (Lambert, Pasha-Zaidi, & Crookes). We end the segment by looking at measurement issues (Lambert, Hotchkiss, & Passmore), describing why wellbeing should be measured and how, offering several existing scale examples that are free to use by researchers.

Part IV moves into culture, identity and history, where we explore how Islam underlies existing views of wellbeing and a sense of identity. Joshanloo and Weijers take us on an exploration of how wellbeing is construed from a religious perspective, as well as a philosophical exploration of the concept. Pasha-Zaidi and Odeh build on these notions and prompt the question: How can a positive Islamic identity evolve when negative media connotations suggest an Islamic identity is not a positive construct? The authors consider how existing identity development models can be used to help young people in particular see themselves as contributing, worthy individuals. Finally, Estes and Sirgy take a historical tour of wellbeing, exploring statistical social trends over time up to today across the MENA region, accentuating the positives and identifying where work is still needed.

Finally, in Part V, we focus on health and clinical psychology and explore a qualitative study (Lambert & O'Hara) conducted in the UAE on a number of Emirati athletes in a bid to explore the field of positive health. That chapter offers the views of healthy individuals (versus those who are merely not ill) to counter the negative health lens still in force across many public health institutions, and consider why a positive lens may be of greater benefit. In the chapter by Rashid and Al-Haj Baddar, we explore the field of positive clinical psychology, a critical read for practitioners treating depression and states of languishing. A variety of supporting studies—both international and regional—are reviewed as evidence for the efficacy of a positive psychotherapy (PPT) approach in clinical populations. At last, and perhaps paradoxically, Lutz and Passmore suggest that happiness itself should not be a goal, but rather a by-product of a life well lived. This last chapter is a must-read for anyone thinking of improving their own wellbeing and feeling social pressure to do so.

We hope you enjoy reading this book as much as we have enjoyed writing it and working with all of our collaborators in bringing it to life over the many months. We also hope to get to work soon on our next edition and bring you more evidence and stories of the good research being conducted in positive psychology across the region. But, until then, don't be shy to send us your comments and views. Happy reading and thanks for supporting a regional positive psychology.

References

Bolier, L., Haverman, M., Westerhof, G. J., Riper, H., Smit, F., & Bohlmeijer, E. (2013). Positive psychology interventions: A meta-analysis of randomized controlled studies. *BMC Public Health, 13,* 119.

Diener, E., & Diener, C. (2017, March 31). Governments testing wellbeing initiatives: A call for psychological scientists to get involved. *APS Observer.* Retrieved from https://www.psychologicalscience.org/observer/governments-testing-wellbeing-initiatives.

Hone, L. C., Jarden, A., & Schofield, G. M. (2015). An evaluation of positive psychology intervention effectiveness trials using the re-aim framework: A practice-friendly review. *The Journal of Positive Psychology, 10*(4), 303–322.

Huffman, J. C., DuBois, C. M., Millstein, R. A., Celano, C. M., & Wexler, D. (2015). Positive psychological interventions for patients with type 2 diabetes: Rationale, theoretical model, and intervention development. *Journal of Diabetes Research,* 428349.

Johnson, D. P., Penn, D. L., Fredrickson, B. L., Kring, A. M., Meyer, P. S., Catalino, L. I., & Brantley, M. (2011). A pilot study of loving-kindness meditation for the negative symptoms of schizophrenia. *Schizophrenia Research, 129,* 137–140.

Johnson, D. P., Penn, D. L., Fredrickson, B. L., Meyer, P. S., Kring, A. M., & Brantley, M. (2009). Loving-kindness meditation to enhance recovery from negative symptoms of schizophrenia. *Journal of Clinical Psychology, 65,* 499–509.

Lambert, L., Pasha-Zaidi, N., Passmore, H.-A., & York Al-Karam, C. (2015). Developing an indigenous positive psychology in the United Arab Emirates. *Middle East Journal of Positive Psychology, 1*(1), 1–23.

Poppe, G. M. (2017, September 13). *Positive psychological interventions in the treatment of schizophrenia: A systematic review of the effects of positive psychology on wellbeing and symptoms of people with schizophrenia.* University of Twente, Netherlands. Retrieved from https://pdfs.semanticscholar.org/5132/74adae6c93cd874a17313f56cefb933265cd.pdf.

Seligman, M. E. P. (1972). Learned helplessness. *Annual Review of Medicine, 23*(1), 407–412.

Seligman, M. E. P. (1975). *Helplessness: On depression, development, and death.* San Francisco, CA: W. H. Freeman.

Seligman, M. E. P., & Csikszentmihalyi, M. (2000). Positive psychology: An introduction. *American Psychologist, 55*(1), 5–14.

Seligman, M. E. P., Steen, T., Park, N., & Peterson, C. (2005). Positive psychology progress: Empirical validation of interventions. *American Psychologist, 60*(5), 410–421.

Sin, N., & Lyubomirsky, S. (2009). Enhancing wellbeing and alleviating depressive symptoms with positive psychology interventions: A practice-friendly meta-analysis. *Journal of Clinical Psychology, 65,* 467–487.

Weiss, L. A., Westerhof, G. J., & Bohlmeijer, E. T. (2016). Can we increase psychological wellbeing? The effects of interventions on psychological wellbeing: A meta-analysis of randomized controlled trials. *PLoS ONE, 11*(6), e0158092.

Part I
Government and Policy

Chapter 2
The Pursuit of National Wellbeing Policies Across the GCC: The What, How, and Why?

Louise Lambert, Aziz Mulay-Shah, Meg. A. Warren and Yara Younis

Abstract Social scientists working under the umbrella of positive psychology are putting their research to good use by helping to define wellbeing, propose theories and models, implement their findings, collect and provide data to support interventions, and propose policy ideas and frameworks at national and community levels. These players, including the populace who will benefit from and live under wellbeing policies and activities, are foundational to achieving individual and social prosperity as they collaborate under an expansive vision to develop a repertoire of practises that can be emulated around the globe. As a team of social scientists representing expertise in policy and psychology, we briefly visit the distinction between happiness and wellbeing, the inadequacies of using GDP as a measure of prosperity and consider why wellbeing is of interest to governments. We further outline potential steps to developing a national wellbeing framework with governments at the helm and propose policy ideas as future pathways for Gulf Cooperation Council (GCC) nations in particular, but with relevance to other Middle East nations as well, to consider as they embark on their national pathways towards wellbeing.

L. Lambert (✉)
United Arab Emirates University, Al Ain, UAE
e-mail: ltamber@yahoo.com

A. Mulay-Shah
Global Communications Agency, Dubai, UAE
e-mail: aziz@gc.agency

M. A. Warren
Western Washington University, Bellingham, WA, USA
e-mail: meg@megwarren.com

Y. Younis
UAE Ministry of Culture and Knowledge Development, Abu Dhabi, UAE
e-mail: yarayounis96@gmail.com

L. Lambert and N. Pasha-Zaidi (eds.), *Positive Psychology in the Middle East/North Africa*, https://doi.org/10.1007/978-3-030-13921-6_2

2.1 Introduction

The global attention paid to wellbeing and happiness in public policy has recently grown. From Bhutan, the first country to establish wellbeing indicators as a benchmark for social progress, to the recent announcement of a Minister of Happiness in the United Arab Emirates (UAE) in 2016, the move towards greater wellbeing is on its way to meeting the goal set by the initiator of the positive psychology movement: 50% of the world's population flourishing by the year 2050 (Seligman, 2009). No small challenge, the amount of work undertaken by international organizations and governments attests to the commitment towards this policy goal (Pykett & Cromby, 2017). For instance, the Organisation for Economic Co-operation and Development (OECD) places human wellbeing on its agenda and helps governments of its 35 member states to foster social and economic prosperity by providing data, resources, recommendations, support in the establishment of formal agreements by countries, and offers the assistance of between-country peer reviews to improve accountability. The United Kingdom government, a leader in the wellbeing movement, also developed an arm called the What Works Centre for Wellbeing (https://www.whatworkswellbeing.org/) that feeds research directly into policy and mandates that all government ministries and departments regularly account for how their policies improve wellbeing. Commissioned reports such as the Stiglitz, Sen and Fitoussi (2009) document endorsed by then President Sarkozy of France, questioned the continued use of income as an indicator of social progress and proposed a focus on wellbeing, which now serves as a reference point for many governments. Independent organizations like the New Economics Foundation (London, UK; http://neweconomics.org/) further engage the grassroots in campaigns and events on issues like Brexit, climate change, inequality, and migration to facilitate change towards greater social prosperity.

Organizations and cities are also joining the action. The HappyCity group (Bristol, UK) improves wellbeing through campaigns and participatory development training sessions whereby citizens are engaged in the process of public inquiry to determine what is working to improve social prosperity (http://www.happycity.org.uk/). Events include filmmaking, intercultural discussions about happiness, and the creation of HappyLists to honor residents who make a difference. Vancouver's (Canada) Happy City initiative (www.thehappycity.com) also works to influence the planning and development of urban spaces, homes, streets, and buildings for greater health, livability, altruism, and wellbeing by consulting with planners, municipalities, and builders around the world. Similarly, since 2013, the Alnowair group in Kuwait (www.alnowair.com), a socially progressive non-profit group dedicated to spreading national positivity, holds campaigns and activities designed to improve individual positivity and boost social cohesion, like movie nights, summer camps, gratitude activities, yellow car parades for kinder driving, photography competitions, and initiatives like the installation of 30 yellow benches strategically placed to encourage Kuwaitis to see metropolitan beauty. Other groups focus on the development of green spaces, volunteerism and civic participation, as well as physical and mental health initiatives to improve wellbeing. These developments reflect the commonalities humans need to enjoy greater wellbeing as well as the cultural uniqueness of political systems, geographies, economies, and environments worldwide.

Towards this aim, social scientists working under the umbrella of positive psychology are putting their research to good use by helping to define wellbeing, propose theories and models, implement their findings, collect and provide data to support interventions, and propose policy ideas and frameworks at national and community levels (Diener & Diener, 2011; Seligman & Csikszentmihalyi, 2000). These players, including the populace who will benefit from and live under wellbeing policies and activities, are foundational to achieving individual and social prosperity as they collaborate under an expansive vision to develop a repertoire of best practises that can be emulated around the globe (Diener & Diener, 2011). Thus, as a team of social scientists representing expertise in policy and psychology, we visit the distinction between happiness and wellbeing, the inadequacies of using GDP as a measure of prosperity and consider why wellbeing is of interest to governments. We also consider the steps to developing a national wellbeing framework with governments at the helm and propose policy ideas as future pathways for the GCC nations of Saudi Arabia, Kuwait, Oman, Qatar, Bahrain, and the UAE to consider as they embark on their national trajectories towards wellbeing.

The GCC region is facing a great demographic shift whereby half of its population comprises of young people under the age of 30 who are graduating from universities in unprecedented numbers and paradoxically, have glaring rates of unemployment (World Economic Forum, 2014). These rates are high as a result of young people waiting for well paid jobs in oversaturated government sectors and a surplus of cheap expatriate labour in the private sector (Al-Waqfi & Forstenlechner, 2012). Managing the expectations that stem from unsustainable welfare state entitlements, the realities of low oil prices and the desire of governments to become more competitive will need careful management due to the potential for social and political instability (Forstenlechner & Baruch, 2013). Further, a focus on regional wellbeing is timely as studies reveal a growing trend towards a lack of concern for injustice and inequality (Oxford Strategic Consulting, 2014), high levels of self-entitlement (Al-Gergawi, 2008; Eide & Rösler, 2014; World Economic Forum, 2014), and materialism (Arthur, Sherman, Al Hameli, & Al Marzooqi, 2017; Forstenlechner & Rutledge, 2011). Given the high GDPs in the region, the prioritization of monetary goals and potential overconsumption of goods is ill advised as these are known to undermine wellbeing at high levels (Dittmar, Bond, Hurst, & Kasser, 2014; Kasser et al., 2014). Finally, in the face of religious extremism in areas of the region, never before has a need for policies around the development of sustainable wellbeing been more acute and timely.

2.2 Defining Happiness and Wellbeing

Not officially used in the scientific literature as it carries no standard definition, the layman's term "happiness" often denotes the experience of having more immediate positive emotion than negative (Diener, 2000). Yet, a narrow focus on happiness can lead to the development of activities that have high entertainment value and low returns beyond what is experienced in a music festival for example, and may trivialize the real work of improving wellbeing in the domains of health, the environment, education, labour, and employment as the remit is too narrow to be of value (Lelkes, 2013). Thus, we make a distinction between the positive emotions capitalized upon by the happiness industry and the public policy concern over wellbeing for its own sake (Pykett & Cromby, 2017). Accordingly, rather than rely on empty words, terms like satisfaction with life, flourishing, flow, meaning, engagement, or other empirically derived proxies are utilized instead (Csikszentmihalyi, 1990; Hart & Sasso, 2011; Joseph & Wood, 2010; Kashdan, Biswas-Diener, & King, 2008; Keyes, 2005; Norrish & Vella-Brodrick, 2008). More commonly used to determine individual happiness is the term subjective wellbeing (SWB) (Diener, 1984), which includes the balance of positive and negative emotions, and a favourable cognitive perception of satisfaction with one's life. Determined solely by the individual, the term does not however distinguish between the moral causes of wellbeing, such that SWB might be derived by a life of deceit and crime or from volunteerism and devotion to worthy causes (Carlisle, Henderson, & Hanlon, 2009; Kern, Waters, Adler, & White, 2015; Nikolova, 2016).

As such, we use the more general term of "wellbeing", an umbrella categorization that includes many domains of influence such as trust in government institutions, neighbors or police, the freedom to pursue one's dreams, the availability of time and space to enjoy family, work, and leisure, satisfaction with one's choices, and future optimism (Diener, Scollon, & Lucas, 2003). It is the preferred conceptualization for policy development as it is comprehensive in its purview and avoids placing the responsibility of happiness solely on the individual, acknowledging the influence of activities, work, organizations, the natural and built environment, other people and government actions. To consider wellbeing beyond the limits of the individual is critical as studies show for instance, that the further down one is in the socio-economic scale, the more wellbeing is impacted by contextual factors versus psychological ones (Lomas, 2015). Thus, it has been stated that the social costs of unhappiness which stem from systemic factors like poverty, unemployment, social isolation, crime, mental health issues, and religious or ethnic minority status have larger effects than those gained from wellbeing efforts, and as such the targets of wellbeing policies should equally aim to minimize or prevent avoidable unhappiness caused by such conditions (Clark, Flèche, Layard, Powdthavee, & Ward, 2017; Lelkes, 2013).

Nonetheless, a focus on reducing illbeing can also lead policymakers to overlook opportunities. Policymakers have almost exclusively taken a removal approach to wellbeing, i.e., reducing poverty, decreasing crime, or minimizing illness to lower social costs. These have had positive results, yet a true wellbeing approach implies adding a positive condition or state (White, 2010) and using it as the measure of progress such as, individuals engaging in entrepreneurship will be increased by 10%, volunteering boosted by 20%, health assets like cardiorespiratory fitness will be strengthened, or the number of individuals reporting close friendships, stable marriages, or membership in recreational groups will double. The focus of wellbeing policies consequently is not only on needs but on capabilities. By strengthening social and political institutions as well as the structures in place to support the determinants of wellbeing, policymakers can affect changes to increase wellbeing and not only reduce misery.

It should be noted that while positive psychology has explored the determinants of both social and individual wellbeing, its interventions for increasing wellbeing have largely targeted the psychological makeup of individuals, many of which have been imported into the GCC region from the West (Lambert, Pasha-Zaidi, Passmore, & York Al-Karam, 2015). This has had the effect of overlooking cultural, social, political, religious, and economic contexts that influence the effectiveness of such interventions. While academics are still examining the relevance and usefulness of interventions, their inappropriate practise and popularity, not to mention the profits to be made from them, are quickly outpacing their available evidence and giving rise to moral dilemmas around the impact of their use in sociocultural contexts for which they were not designed. As social and individual definitions of happiness are strongly influenced by culture (Senik, 2011), copying others' interventions or policy models is not advised as the fit is often not appropriate, can have harmful consequences and undermines the ability of communities to determine what is important for them (Lambert et al., 2015; Layous, Lee, Choi, & Lyubomirsky, 2013; Layous & Lyubomirsky, 2014; Pykett & Cromby, 2017).

As the indicators and definitions of wellbeing continue to vary and the research provides few definite parameters around the scope of government intervention so far, seeking consensus among researchers and policy developers continues (Canaviri, 2016; OECD, 2013; Tay, Chan, & Diener, 2014). In response, many governments are developing personalized accounts of their nation's wellbeing instead. For example, Bhutan, the first country to introduce its own measures and collect data towards this aim, defines wellbeing in its composite measure of Gross National Happiness (GNH; http://media.gnhcentrebhutan.org/four-pillars-9-domains/). It has as its pillars, physical, mental and spiritual health; time-balance; community and cultural vitality; education; living standards; good governance; and environmental health. Several organizations and governments alike have adopted the GNH, while others have developed measures to fit their own social context, like the Canadian Index of Wellbeing (https://uwaterloo.ca/canadian-index-wellbeing/), which involves democratic engagement, community vitality, as well as leisure and culture, or more inclusive indices like the global Social Progress Index (http://www.socialprogressimperative.org/global-index/) that focuses on basic needs, personal rights, as well as tolerance and freedom and which can be used as a tool to develop scorecards and rankings of entire nations through to city neighborhoods. Broader conceptualizations include an environmental component and propose that a state of planetary health must ensure that human health gains (physical health, wellbeing and equity) are not attained at the cost of the natural systems (food, shelter, fuel, and water) that allowed those gains to be achieved and on which the sustainability of human life depends (Whitmee et al., 2015).

2.3 What's Wrong with the GDP?

While income is an indicator of national prosperity, the inadequacy of measuring social progress via the GDP is gaining recognition (Adler & Seligman, 2016; Forgeard, Jayawickreme, Kern, & Seligman, 2011; Nikolova, 2016; Stiglitz et al., 2009; Whitmee et al., 2015). For instance, only measuring the market values of goods and services produced by a nation's economy does not tell us whether people feel safe, loved, intellectually stimulated, or who is reaping the benefits of a high GDP (Stiglitz et al., 2009). It also fails to capture costs to the environment or human health (Whitmee et al., 2015). A sole pursuit of GDP can also jeopardize ethical standards and create a society where the less privileged lose their place in the economy, or worse, their dignity (Helliwell, Layard, & Sachs, 2012). Further, although GDP and life satisfaction are linked, this relationship only holds true for low-income countries and low-income individuals within it (Easterlin, 1995, 2013). This has been a point of contention in the research literature; Stevenson and Wolfers (2008) argue that for each doubling in per capita GDP, there is a corresponding increase in life satisfaction. Yet, Easterlin (2015) maintains that within countries, higher income generates greater life satisfaction but, as countries overall become wealthier, corresponding increases in life satisfaction do not materialize.

Examples of this discrepancy are frequently identified. For instance, the Eurofound organization (2013) observed that Denmark consistently scores high on SWB across Europe, yet it has a GDP lower than Ireland suggesting that something else contributing to wellbeing is not being captured by traditional measures. Likewise, Senik (2011) investigated French nationals who consistently rank high on GDP and simultaneously express high dissatisfaction, depressiveness and low levels of social and institutional trust. It would appear that while national circumstances matter, so do mentalities. As discussed by Senik, the contradiction between France's focus on equality yet existing aristocratic hierarchy and one's chances of finding employment in that context are not captured by existing measures, yet salient in influencing perceptions of wellbeing and an example of where cultural narratives are influential.

Another reason why GDP is not an accurate measure can be explained by the diminishing returns of wealth. Beyond the point at which basic needs are met, the effects of happiness become less pronounced and produce fewer returns due to adaptation, the fact that individuals habituate to levels of wealth and return to wellbeing set points over time (Headey, 2008) (with exceptions for unemployment, disability, and widowhood; Diener, Lucas, & Scollon, 2006). As a result, governments of wealthy nations intent on boosting wellbeing via increases to the GDP may be misguided, especially since the contribution of income to the variance in life satisfaction has been shown to be less than 5% (Flèche & Layard, 2017). Instead, what makes the biggest difference to wellbeing is not absolute but relative income, how individuals evaluate their positions compared to others (Clark, Frijters, & Shields, 2008; Easterlin, 2013; Mayraz, Wagner, & Schupp, 2009); thus, attention to social equality and the equal distribution of and access to opportunities that generate wealth like education and financial credit are better options in which to invest.

Finally, Easterbrook's (2004) progress paradox, where increasing levels of personal affluence are matched by corresponding levels of unhappiness, has become a feature of many highly developed countries focused on the pursuit of goods over subjective intangibles. Gasper (2007) as well as Schwartz and Ward (2004) explain that progress brings about much material choice. This overload results in frustration and confusion as a greater number of goods to buy creates knowledge of what exists and suggests that if it is to buy, it is desirable to have. This increases expectations about what one should possess and what should make one happy, invariably giving rise to social comparisons, a known detractor from wellbeing (Lyubomirsky, Tucker, & Kasri, 2001; White, Langer, Yariv, & Welch, 2006). The pursuit of goods also crowds out other values, like achievements or engagement with sports and the arts, and can activate the hedonic treadmill (Lyubomirsky, 2011), chasing, with weakening returns, the newest product, updating goods due to planned obsolescence, or changing preferences to conform to what is considered "hot" yet not especially valuable. The pressure to keep up causes individuals to not appreciate what they have and lose control over their own values. Such paradoxes suggest that pursuing subjective avenues to wellbeing, like sports, the arts or relationships, may be better given findings which indicate that interpersonal relationships at any income level matter more to wellbeing than income itself, as the latter does not protect individuals from divorce, drug abuse or illness, nor does it necessarily promote a virtuous life (Helliwell & Barrington-Leigh, 2010).

Further, evidence that paying attention to emotions as a predictor of social and political stability is gaining traction. For example, Ward's (2015) study showed that a nation's overall level of SWB accounted for greater variance in elections than the usual macroeconomic variables and could predict to a more accurate degree, what economists, political scientists and leaders themselves often miss. An overreliance on monetary data led to the exclusion of subjective measures, which would have helped predict the onset of the Euromaidan Revolution in Ukraine and the Brexit vote. Despite economic progress, a decrease in daily positive emotion due to rising aspirations and corresponding crushed hopes for one's economy and failed leadership in delivering quality jobs, fairness in accessing those jobs, and social equality has been termed the "unhappy development paradox" (Arampatzi, Burger, Ianchovichina, Röhricht, & Veenhoven, 2015). Had SWB been more carefully noted in Syria, Egypt, Iraq, Tunisia and Yemen, Arampatzi et al. (2015) contend that the Arab Spring could have been foreseen as rankings had been dropping steadily and were among some of the lowest in the world by then. They propose that subjective measures be taken more seriously and the degree to which people are satisfied with their nation's political systems also be considered to a larger extent than at present.

Topic Box: Global Emotions Report

Daily emotions in 142 countries are now tracked by Gallup's Global Emotions Report (2017). It highlights which nations have thriving, positive populations despite slow growth. For instance, nations like El Salvador, Latvia, Liberia, Honduras and Tajikistan almost tripled their nations' percentages of citizens reporting their lives to be quite positive, falling into the "thriving" condition between 2007 and 2017. To be considered in the thriving condition, respondents score 7 and higher on positive views of their present life situation, 8 and above on their positive views of the next five years, and report fewer health issues, sick days, less stress, worry, sadness, anger, and more happiness, interest, respect and enjoyment. El Salvador in particular made significant changes to levels of poverty and public safety with respect to street gangs. Kosovo, Benin, the Ivory Coast and Ghana record the largest thriving increases between 2014 and 2017. Nations like Greece, Russia, Spain, Egypt, and India on the other hand, are showing the opposite trends. For example, only 3% of Indians rated their lives positively enough to be considered thriving. Several of these nations will be holding elections in the near future with pollsters interested in how well subjective measures will predict electoral outcomes. Negative emotions are also tracked with nations like Yemen, Turkey, Iraq, and Iran scoring among the highest negativity nations (anger, worry, sadness, stress, and physical pain) in the world. Iraq in particular has been number one in the report five times, reflecting much of its nation's current difficulties

Such paradoxes serve as lessons for policymakers who believe that merely observing GDP and other objective measures offers a full picture of development. Individuals want to reach their goals, have a sense of equality with their colleagues, feel optimistic with good reason, as well as trust their neighbors. Failures to achieve these forms of progress are done at a nation's peril. GDP may provide the means to a good life, but not necessarily the will, personal ability, or social circumstance in which to create it. Additional aspects of social development and its measures are needed (Biswas-Diener, Diener, & Lyubchik, 2015).

2.4 Why Does Wellbeing Matter?

The objective effects of greater wellbeing are infrequently reported as this line of inquiry typically focuses on the contributors to wellbeing versus its outcomes. Yet, a review by Lyubomirsky, King and Diener (2005) of over 200 studies showed validity to the argument that resources, such as money, relationships, health, and employment led to greater SWB. However, they also showed that SWB brought about these same resources to individuals and confirmed wellbeing as a causal factor. We review that evidence here.

More likely to economize, be financially responsible and save money as well as control expenditures by consuming less and considering the long-term implications of choices are such results of greater initial wellbeing on finances (Guven, 2012). Individuals with greater SWB, or positive emotionality, were also likely to show more empathy and compassion, and engage in greater perspective taking towards groups that did not share the same cultural background (Nelson, 2009). Similarly, they showed less racial bias and took part in more pro-social cooperative actions (Johnson & Fredrickson, 2005; Rand, Kraft-Todd, & Gruber, 2015). They were more sociably engaged, had more frequent contact with family and friends, talked more to others and had more substantive conversations when they did (Mehl, Vazire, Holleran, & Clark, 2010; Richards & Huppert, 2011). Greater SWB also resulted in a greater likelihood of investing more volunteer hours and extending service to causes like the donation of money, blood, or organizing food bank donations (Priller & Shupp, 2011; Son & Wilson, 2012; Thoits & Hewitt, 2001). Those higher in SWB in a study of over 300,000 Americans were less likely to engage in risky behaviors, instead wearing seatbelts, being mindful of others on roads or in public spaces and less likely to be in car accidents (Goudie, Mukherjee, De Neve, Oswald, & Wu, 2012). They were also more likely to make more ethical and honest decisions (James & Chymis, 2004). Higher SWB scores even predicted higher grade point averages a year later and fewer school absences (Howell, 2009; Suldo, Thalji, & Ferron, 2011).

Health-wise, individuals with higher SWB took more direct action in improving their health by being more physically active, smoking less, and using sun protection (Grant, Wardle, & Steptoe, 2009; Huang & Humphreys, 2012). They had stronger immune systems (Fredrickson et al., 2013) and were able to withstand the psychological and physiological effects of stress more astutely (Folkman, 2008; Fredrickson, Mancuso, Branigan, & Tugade, 2000). Greater positivity was also negatively correlated with the incidence of cardiovascular disease (Boehm & Kubzansky, 2012; Sin, 2016), reports of chronic pain (Finan & Garland, 2015), and increased resilience in the face of physical pain, enabling patients to return to better functioning quickly (Lambert D'raven, Moliver, & Thompson, 2015; Zautra, Johnson, & Davis, 2005). More positive affectivity also resulted in greater life expectancy (Danner, Snowdon, & Friesen, 2001; Diener & Chan, 2011; Wiest, Schüz, Webster, & Wurm, 2011; Xu & Roberts, 2010).

Workplace benefits also emerged. Boehm and Lyubomirsky's (2008) review showed that greater SWB also preceded greater earnings, higher performance, as well as the deployment of coping skills, while other studies showed positive relationships with engagement attitudes and organizational citizenship (pro-social activity in an organization), and negative relationships with deviance and cynicism (Avey, Wernsing, & Luthans, 2008; Chi, Chung, & Tsai, 2011). Organizations with more positive employees have shown up to a 12% increase in productivity, a 6% value-added measure per hours worked and an increase in profit and future stock-market performance (Bockerman & Ilmakunnas, 2012; Edmans, 2012; Ford, Cerasoli, Higgins, & Decesare, 2011; Oswald, Proto, & Sgroi, 2012), while absenteeism, sick time, and turnover were reduced (Erdogan, Bauer, Truxillo, & Mansfield, 2012). A study conducted among unemployed Germans showed that initial greater SWB was correlated with higher re-employment one year later (Krause, 2013).

Greater wellbeing may be the strongest tool within the realm of policy making to reduce the occurrence of debt, social isolation, perceptions of safety and crime, long-term unemployment and ill-health, and increase social capital, workplace engagement, productivity, and health and learning outcomes that add to a nation's productive years, while lessening the burden of care and long-term costs on governments, all of which are indicators the GCC states aim to improve.

2.5 Developing National Wellbeing Policies

Policy science or public policy analysis is concerned with the decision-making processes taken in the interest of public order. DeLeon and Vogenbeck (2007) suggest that the analysis and development of policy is also defined by a focus on the practical resolution of problems and determination of solutions to public policy challenges; as such, inquiry for the sake of inquiry is antithetical to the field and a "so, what?" question is always required. Policy science further includes many disciplines from the social sciences and is consequently value oriented, rejecting objectivism as it must take into account diverse and competing values as well as biases inherent to the realities of the social and political contexts in which policy is developed. Finally, as governments and stakeholders form complex relationships in which policy agendas and their design, implementation, and evaluation aim to improve the quality of life for people, the process can create externalities, unforeseen and often unintended challenges, such as environmental degradation as a result of generating greater electric outputs in urban areas for instance. Consequently, dealing with unanticipated consequences is part of the policy analysis process (Whitmee et al., 2015).

In this section, we examine the possibility of creating a wellbeing policy framework with the recognition of two challenges in mind: namely, how to develop a comprehensive framework that can be readily used within existing GCC governmental fiscal and organizational realities and, how to balance ministerial and sectoral agendas and priorities as well as competing bureaucratic disagreements that exist under and within one overarching strategy. To overcome these, a "whole of government" approach (Treasury Board of Canada, 2015) to policy planning and analysis is advised in contrast to traditional means of operating by which government departments ordinarily operate in silos, where costs and responsibilities are divided between them. Further, to meet the named challenges, there is a need to create a mechanism by which the implementation of policy is applied holistically; that is, an authoritative body is necessary to ensure that policy assessment and evaluation is made part of the implementation process. Creating a policy planning unit within the highest levels of government with enough authority to mandate line departments to incorporate wellbeing policies into existing policy frameworks is also required.

The model that applies to most policy design is what is known as the five essentials of a policy cycle framework (Sabatier, 1999); namely, agenda setting, policy formulation, decision-making, implementation, and evaluation, while some models include a sixth termination stage. Agenda setting refers to how policymakers define problems, rank them by order of importance, and prioritise them. Policies are then formulated and must pass the analysis of government decision-makers, and in the case of democracies, public stakeholders as well. They are then implemented and evaluated by both the implementing authorities and the public. If the policy proves successful, it is repeated and if not, it is terminated. These stages have nonetheless been criticized as being prescriptive, inflexible and perhaps not a true reflection of how policy making and implementation occurs. Yet, despite these limitations (Jann & Weigrich, 2007), the policy stage model remains, since the 1940s, a central model of policy analysis.

2.6 Policy Development in the GCC Nations

In the GCC nations, the process differs. For example, the policy stage process and policy cycle model are influenced by the political dynamics involved in the constitutions of the societies in which policies are created, whereby policy cycles are influenced by the interaction between the federal and emirate levels of governments as well as by tribal, sectoral, and family political influences. As a result, policy formulation in the GCC countries offers less transparency and evidence for the public to understand how policy formulations occurred. Political systems theory and analysis (Easton, 1979) explains policy formulation as a series of inputs made by interest groups that are evaluated, analysed, and developed into policy by government, which then implements policy as a series of outputs. This process has become an accepted theory of policy making processes in liberal democracies where policy ideas must withstand the scrutiny of public interest groups, parliaments, the bureaucracy, and ultimately, the executive branch in order to be implemented. However, in the GCC nations, policy ideas come from leaders and elites close to them, where power is most often concentrated (Al Marzouqi & Forster, 2011).

Another avenue of policy formulation in the GCC often comes from the use of expert consultants and external advisors who are not always familiar with the region's sociocultural context. These consultants are sometimes used to propose previously agreed-upon but, as yet unapproved ideas by management to upper echelons in a way that controls for political risk should the idea or its implementation fail (Al-Ubaydli & Mirza, 2017). Either due to a lack of capacity from which to formulate policy within the ranks of governments or from a desire to align themselves with world class standards and practices, public stakeholder needs and views are typically not included in this process like they are in democratic countries where policy failures can have negative effects on the political chances of re-election. As a result, decision-making, as is the case with policy formulation, is often much faster, more agile, and possibly more efficient in the GCC nations because of the lack of political actors involved, fewer inputs to consider from other governing bodies and less need for lengthy and time-consuming consultation. From here, councils are summoned to review drafted policies and decrees issued. While public engagement is uncommon, efforts are nonetheless being made to improve with the development of consultative bodies such as the Federal National Council in the UAE and the Shura Council in Saudi Arabia, both of which were created to debate public concerns (Yaghi & Antwi-Boateng, 2015).

Consequently, the policy approval process is less complicated in the GCC nations where decision making on a policy idea undergoes consultation within the executive branch to the exclusion of the public and often occurs behind closed doors. Yet, this same process can run the risk of decision makers not understanding the concerns of those the policy will address; a pertinent concern given that up to 85% of the workforce in the GCC nations are migrant workers who live and work in these nations for several months up to decades at a time (Al-Ubaydli & Mirza, 2017). This form of policy making may make it challenging to develop an effective wellbeing framework that responds adequately to the needs of those it will ultimately serve as existing policy development models are designed for democratic systems where public engagement is a given and where labour structures are more stable (Kinninmont, 2015).

2.7 Creating a Policy Framework

Raising the profile of wellbeing is not about making people happy, but about creating the conditions, as well as the built and natural environments conducive for wellbeing across society, while developing the skills and receptiveness of people to use those conditions effectively (Frey & Gallus, 2012, 2013; Whitmee et al., 2015). Thus, a policy framework towards these aims guides and supports the work of public service and provides for business and civil society alike to reach the highest levels of wellbeing possible. We reiterate the steps identified as necessary in facilitating the development of such a framework proposed by Northern Ireland's Carnegie Roundtable on Measuring Wellbeing (Carnegie Trust, 2016), and urge governments not to short circuit the policy making process by outsourcing it to external consultants or to develop it behind cabinet doors, but to include the participation and voices of those (temporary or otherwise) the framework will affect. This democratic consultation is not antithetical to the GCC governing traditions as consultative mechanisms such as the open majlis system or councils held by local leaders through which citizens can express their concerns already exist (Katzman, 2017).

The first step in the development of wellbeing policy is to integrate the concept of wellbeing as a purpose of all ministry mission statements ranging from education, health, defense and security, religious affairs, to economic development. The messaging involved in these initiatives should be framed along the lines of existing cultural norms and not merely pay lip service to an empty term, but involve lengthy discussions, facilitated workshops and awareness seminars of what wellbeing is composed and how its contributors can be amplified throughout each ministry. The output of these ministry activities will include recommendations that can be incorporated into the development of the framework alongside the views, desires and goals of other groups as well.

Public consultations are next; given that broad changes are the targets of wellbeing initiatives, the buy-in, sense of ownership and participation of the public is of absolute necessity, if for no other reason than to boost wellbeing rankings (Hall & Rickard, 2013). But conversations about wellbeing and how individuals would like it to be expressed in their communities can also help the public reflect, self-monitor, prioritize and make better decisions as well as build capacity, especially when done communally (Hall & Rickard, 2013; White, 2010). Collaborative efforts may emerge from these conversations that would not otherwise as well as more personal responsibility taken by residents who see a role to play in their communities' wellbeing instead of relying on governments to take the lead. An engaged public is also more patient as discussions about wellbeing reveal the hard realities of making social progress (O'Donnell, 2013). Costing little, engaging the public is a way for governments to show transparency, build trust and legitimacy, and show that their goals are not mere PR exercises (Biswas-Diener et al., 2015; Dolan, 2011; Helliwell, Huang, & Wang, 2015).

Thus, the aim of society-wide conversations is to generate the goals and priorities, i.e., the content of wellbeing, which will be fed back into the development of a national framework and guide the selection and administration of wellbeing measures in order to begin collecting wellbeing data. Here, "society" does not mean those with the most influence, like the ministries from step 1, nor cities and municipalities (who can have their own feedback sessions), but small businesses, non-profit organizations who work in fulfilling social prosperity needs on a daily basis, educational institutions, religious groups, and neighborhoods, sporting, volunteer and recreational groups, families, and individuals of working age, as well as youth, the retired, unemployed, incarcerated, and ill. The latter groups, too often neglected in these activities, must be sought out as these are the people who experience the lowest SWB and drag scores down (Lelkes, 2013). Thus, not only for moral reasons but on purely instrumental grounds, those at the lower end of the socio-economic scale must be included.

There are many ways this can occur. Televised or radio examples (in Arabic, English and other languages) of groups led by a community leader or neighborhood ambassador trained by community engagement specialists following an official script of pre-selected questions devised by the framework advisory group can inquire about what currently leads people to feel secure, loved, respected, interested, engaged, and optimistic, as well as what does not. Their responses can offer clues as to what areas policy should strengthen. Emirati radio channel "Emarat FM" allows citizens to call in with concerns and, as an example, could be used to introduce wellbeing themes and effectively reflect the commitment of government in responding to national concerns. Roundtable talks with non-profit and community groups or kitchen conversations in family rooms, while relying on downloadable questions from a dedicated website for this purpose, can also work. Using social media can attract people to this process whereby they can upload photos, videos, or audio recordings of themselves having the "wellbeing talk" with others across the nation doing the same. The results of these conversations across neighborhoods, cities, and regions can be uploaded to a sanctioned website for inclusion in the list of priorities to be considered for the framework. Using Apps, mobile data collection stations, or other online means can increase engagement and facilitate the task.

Governments may well be worried about what will emerge in listening to people's needs. Yet, we advocate for this act of courage and demonstration of leadership for varied reasons. Whether the concerns are voiced or not, they nonetheless exist and simply being heard can de-escalate grievances and buy significant goodwill and mutual respect. Further, asking for concerns can also include a request for solutions. In fact, there are no better people to ask for constructive solutions than those suffering with the issue. Finally, much like in organizations or relationships, the danger occurs when people stop complaining. As long as people care enough about their wellbeing and the circumstances in which they live, their complaints offer leadership a necessary gift as the absence of feedback signals indifference and a lack of civic engagement—states not conducive to the development of social prosperity.

In conjunction with the priorities and needs set out by the ministerial and community consultations, policymakers can then include the best practises of high scoring countries such as Denmark, Switzerland, Iceland, and Norway (Helliwell, Layard, & Sachs, 2016). The factors that put them at the top of the wellbeing index and which account for almost 75% of the differences between nations include a strong GDP, healthy life expectancy, social support, trust, perceived freedom to make decisions, and generosity (Helliwell, Layard, & Sachs, 2015). Diener, Oishi and Lucas' (2015) extensive review also included economic development, strong rule of law and human rights, low corruption, efficient government, progressive taxation, social safety nets (i.e., pension, maternity, disability support), political freedom to associate, write and speak, unemployment policies, health services/coverage, and environmental policies and actions. The Danish Happiness Research Institute (2014) also adds quality work and working conditions where employees can exit jobs without penalty, enjoy work from home options and experience egalitarian working relationships. Good governance exemplified by democratic processes, and strong civil society characterized by volunteer work, civic action, community relationships, and a decentralization of decision-making permitting communities to act on their own behalf are further involved. The time to enjoy life through progressive work conditions like the ability to work shorter hours or enjoy flex-time, both options known to boost productivity and retention (Pencavel, 2014; Smeaton, Ray, & Knight, 2014) also help.

GCC governments interested in boosting their wellbeing scores may want to see what can be done in these areas and in ways that reflect and support their social and politico-cultural contexts. The triangulation of data from the ministerial recommendations, community feedback processes and the research literature can be used to define policy objectives that meet local needs and views of wellbeing, as well as international best practises to actualize social prosperity and progress. The reforms required to implement such practises as well as budget recommendations with the relevant ministries also need to be identified, and once objectives are defined, a process for their operationalization and implementation, and by whom, is needed. We offer examples of policy actions from around the world in Table 2.1 below.

Table 2.1 Policy ideas

Area	Policy action, intervention, proposition
Mental and physical health	• As poor mental health undermines wellbeing more than poverty, unemployment, and physical illness (Flèche & Layard, 2017), offer free mental health services in primary healthcare centers for individuals of all ages • Introduce cigarette sales tax (Leicester & Levell, 2016); public smoking bans • Encourage volunteer work by establishing platforms for citizens to give time, which benefits the less happy and social issues (Binder & Freytag, 2013)
Family and marital supports	• Provide culturally appropriate parenting courses for mothers and fathers of infants, children, and teens, as well as marital supports through counselling, enrichment, divorce and mediation services (Clarke, Younas, & Family Kids, & Youth, 2017; Layard & Hagell, 2015; Scourfield, Cheung, & Macdonald, 2014) • Offer maternity and paternity leave of adequate duration to support families (Borrell et al., 2013; Hewitt, Strazdins, & Martin, 2017)
Wellbeing education	• Fund independent research into local aspects of wellbeing • Share best practise resources in positive psychology for schools, universities, communities, organizations (Shillabeer et al., 2015) and prisons (Adler & Seligman, 2016), as well as how-to guides for neighborhoods who want to develop and organize happiness councils • Facilitate with members of the general public and non-governmental organizations an inclusive "Citizens Happiness Conference" targeted to and for communities versus international experts, to build social capital and civic participation in the development of community wellbeing initiatives
Built and natural environment	• Limit outdoor construction, worksite activity, and airport traffic hours to reduce noise/light pollution and improve sleep (Kahneman & Krueger, 2006; Lawton & Fujiwara, 2016) • Offer adult play areas (outdoor gyms, mobile libraries, outdoor public game areas) to increase social connection, physical activity, creativity, better use of time, and sense of neighborliness (Proyer, 2013) • Alter zoning laws for the development of green/natural spaces; use grey spaces until developed as public parks, community gardens, exercise/game areas, urban art spaces, theatre and music locales (Mensah, Andres, Perera & Roji, 2016) • Line boulevards with shade and fruit trees and/or community gardens rather than annual flowers or shrubs (Mensah et al., 2016) • Enforce no-honking/idling zones to reduce noise/air pollution (Schwela, 2017) • Offer communal or co-housing alternatives for group living with shared spaces to reduce social isolation and support parenting families (see Anderson, 2015) • Expand/improve public transportation, bike/walking lanes, and/or offer organized carpool services to improve commute times known to decrease wellbeing (Kahneman & Krueger, 2006; Stutzer & Frey, 2008); promote public transport across high and low socio-economic classes • Align social and economic policies to stronger environmental policies to support health, human wellbeing and sustainability (Whitmee et al., 2015)

(continued)

Table 2.1 (continued)

Area	Policy action, intervention, proposition
Labour	• Introduce minimum wage (Krassa & Radcliffe, 2014; Ritzen, 2015), language and education requirements to boost worker wellbeing and reduce labour issues • Offer confidential hotlines to report labour law abuses in many languages • Offer free psychological support in labour camps via Ministry of Health/Labour
Policy/mandates	• Introduce mandatory happiness tax (e.g., 0.5% for small to medium size enterprise, 1% for corporations) to offset or contribute to community initiatives • Introduce mandatory corporate social responsibility programs for large corporations with guidelines on evidence-based programming • Introduce regulation requiring large corporations to outline how employee wellbeing is achieved and disclose expenditure on non-financial employee wellbeing (Shillabeer et al., 2015); offer annual prize for entities that comply

A dedicated team can develop training and capacity building programs to help ministers and civil society implement objectives. To help democratize the process (Pykett & Cromby, 2017; Shillabeer, Cartwright, Engel, & Barnes, 2015) as well as empower and engage people, local wellbeing councils, such as the Emirates Youth Council, can be established at the municipal level (akin to town councillors who operate on a volunteer or nominally paid basis for a specific term). This can further serve a double function; in light of the value-added tax being introduced across the GCC nations starting in 2018 and a corresponding absence of political representation, councils can offer one means for the populace to be heard. These councils take responsibility for nominating or electing interested citizens or residents of all ages and socio-economic status, as well as liaise with organizations or municipal departments like libraries, parks, museums, or cultural organizations to operate in specific neighborhoods or jurisdictions so as not to concentrate efforts in one area, neglecting others and creating further inequality. Natural supports can also be sourced via university social work, sociology, or policy program internships, socially productive community projects for unemployed job seekers to develop additional skills, or the equivalent of a gap year for young adults during which they can contribute time in these councils. Wellbeing councils work with local governments and municipalities to implement and monitor activities as well as update and communicate successes, opportunities, and challenges to solicit ideas, support, as well as celebrate the coming together of so many players with a positive effect. This communication further enhances the transparency of policies and activities and builds social trust not only between citizens and residents, but with governments too. Finally, the advisory group leading the development of the framework produces an annual report with proposals to reassess measures and objectives according to the data collected.

2.8 Final Thoughts

Many governments are fearful of including citizen and resident feedback in the participatory process; yet, their inclusion is critical not only for buy-in, but for the provision of content (goals, needs, and priorities) as well as for their efforts in tackling well-being later on alleviating a great deal of responsibility and burden on governments themselves. Further, this process builds social capital (Putnam, 2000), the networks of shared norms, values and understandings that allow cooperation between and within groups of individuals, and acts as a resource in building further wellbeing (DeNeve, Diener, Tay, & Xuereb, 2013; Keltner, Kogan, Piff, & Saturn, 2014). Social capital can be an especially productive asset in mobilizing for opportunities like Expo 2020 or the 2022 FIFA World Cup for instance, or buffer the effects of negative circumstances like the 2008 economic crisis where countries that had greater social capital during the crisis fared much better and were less affected compared to nations with weaker social capital that fragmented further and developed more problems (i.e. crime, social isolation, mental health issues) as a result (Helliwell, Huang, & Wang, 2014). The process of working from the bottom up, that is *from* consultation *towards* the identification and creation of policy and goals, is admittedly antithetical to what most regional governments do; yet, it is what progressive governments do as it pays off over time. The process just described is not representative, it is participatory; that is, it is not done in isolation or to people, but in partnership with them.

Finally, developing greater wellbeing should not be considered a competition despite governments and media proposing that it become so with claims to become the happiest nation in the world by a certain date. It has been suggested that once governments adopt happiness and wellbeing as its official goals for government policy, there is an incentive to manipulate or distort scores out of political interest (Frey & Gallus, 2012, 2013; Frey & Stutzer, 2007). In these situations, individuals have an incentive to help or punish governments by mispresenting their wellbeing scores accordingly when it is known that there is a score to achieve or surpass. When governments announce they are close to achieving or surpassing previous scores just prior to releasing the annual data collection survey among its people, respondents are often inclined to help scores along via their boosted optimism and desire for the nation to be globally recognized, undermining local efforts to obtain true representations of local opportunities, growth and remaining challenges. These concerns apply in particular to governments who use one measure, often of their own creation, rather than a range of measures already in existence and developed expressly for these reasons. Established measures are developed through consensus and based on valid, empirical evidence provided by the international community, which are standardized and confirmed to be valid and reliable tools and involve several complex indices comprised of multiple assessments that are difficult to influence.

Governments can further manipulate scores by including tourists or visitors in their measures (who presumably feel positive towards the country by virtue of choosing it as a destination and who neither avail themselves of government services nor live under its auspices) or excluding certain groups that could decrease wellbeing scores like those with low socio-economic status, or non-citizens. An example is the UAE in 2016, which saw its position drop to 28 from a previous 14 (in 2013) as the sampling was changed to include not only national citizens and Arab expatriates, but non-Arab expatriate residents in the polling for the first time (Helliwell et al., 2016, p. 23 for details). Media can also boost rankings by releasing news that is premature, inflated or not subject to fact-checking, i.e. news that a record number of jobs are being created giving people a sense of hope, even without details of what those jobs may be or if they will be available to them or be outsourced elsewhere. Governments can also distort objective data by manipulating unemployment rates, for example by removing long-term job seekers versus new seekers from the past 12 months, or more commonly, outsource public debt to bodies unrelated to governments for the short-term.

It is for this reason that we recommend that wellbeing ministries develop dedicated, allied, yet independent research units to oversee the collection of wellbeing data, report it "as is" and provide the necessary feedback to government for policy inclusion as governments are subject to bias and strongly motivated to prevent a slip in rankings to gain international esteem. In sum, they must consider wellbeing a public good just like health, education, or security (Pykett & Cromby, 2017). But the biggest reason to do so is to maintain the integrity of the wellbeing mandate and activities that stem from it as a legitimate goal not designed to win popularity contests but to impact the lives of men, women, children, and families who seek and deserve a better life in these GCC nations and beyond.

References

Adler, A., & Seligman, M. E. P. (2016). Using wellbeing for public policy: Theory, measurement, and recommendations. *International Journal of Wellbeing, 6*(1), 1–35.

Al-Gergawi, M. (2008, September 12). *Emiratisation and the curse of entitlement*. Retrieved from http://www.zawya.com/blogs/mishaal/080912081800/

Al Marzouqi, A. H., & Forster, N. (2011). An exploratory study of the under-representation of Emirati women in the United Arab Emirates' information technology sector. *Equality, Diversity and Inclusion, 30*(7), 544–562.

Al-Ubaydli, O., & Mirza, C. (2017). *Making the best use of consultants in the GCC*. London School of Economics and Political Science, Middle East Centre Blog. Retrieved from http://blogs.lse.ac.uk/mec/2017/02/17/making-the-best-use-of-consultants-in-the-gcc/

Al-Waqfi, M., & Forstenlechner, I. (2012). Of private sector fear and prejudice. *Personnel Review, 41*(5), 609–629.

Anderson, J. (2015). "Living in a communal garden" associated with wellbeing while reducing urban sprawl by 40%: A mixed-methods cross-sectional study. *Frontiers in Public Health, 20*(3), 173.

Arampatzi, E., Burger, M. J., Ianchovichina, E., Röhricht, T., & Veenhoven, R. (2015). *Unhappy development: Dissatisfaction with life on the eve of the Arab spring*. World Bank Policy Research Working Paper No. 7488. Retrieved from https://ssrn.com/abstract=2690017

Arthur, D., Sherman, C., Al Hameli, N. S., & Al Marzooqi, S. Y. (2017). Materialism and UAE nationals (working paper). Retrieved from Zayed University (UAE) https://www.zu.ac.ae/main/en/research/publications/_documents/Materialism%20and%20UAE%20Nationals%20-%20Working%20Paper.pdf

Avey, J., Wernsing, T. S., & Luthans, F. (2008). *Can positive employees help positive organizational change? Impact of psychological capital and emotions on relevant attitudes and behaviors*. Management Department Faculty Publications, Paper 32. Retrieved from http://digitalcommons.unl.edu/managementfacpub/32

Binder, M., & Freytag, A. (2013). Volunteering, subjective wellbeing and public policy. *Journal of Economic Psychology, 34*(C), 97–119.

Biswas-Diener, R., Diener, E., & Lyubchik, N. (2015). Wellbeing in Bhutan. *International Journal of Wellbeing, 5*(2), 1–13.

Bockerman, P., & Ilmakunnas, P. (2012). The job-satisfaction-productivity nexus: A study using matched survey and register data. *Industrial and Labor Relations Review, 65,* 244–262.

Boehm, J. K., & Kubzansky, L. D. (2012). The heart's content: The association between positive psychological wellbeing and cardiovascular health. *Psychological Bulletin, 138*(4), 655–691.

Boehm, J. K., & Lyubomirsky, S. (2008). Does happiness promote career success? *Journal of Career Assessment, 16*(1), 101–116.

Borrell, C., Palencia, L., Muntaner, C., Urquia, M., Malmusi, D., & O'Campo, P. (2013). Influence of macrosocial policies on women's health and gender inequalities in health. *Epidemiologic Reviews, 36*(1), 31–38.

Canaviri, J. A. (2016). Measuring the concept of "wellbeing": A first approach for Bolivia. *International Journal of Wellbeing, 6*(1), 36–80.

Carlisle, S., Henderson, G., & Hanlon, P. (2009). 'Wellbeing': A collateral casualty of modernity? *Social Science and Medicine, 69,* 1556–1560.

Carnegie Trust. (2016). *Towards a wellbeing framework: Background report prepared for the Roundtable on Measuring Wellbeing in Northern Ireland*. Retrieved from http://www.carnegieuktrust.org.uk/carnegieuktrust/wp-content/uploads/sites/64/2016/02/pub1455011422.pdf

Chi, N., Chung, Y., & Tsai, T. (2011). How do happy leaders enhance team success? The mediating roles of transformational leadership, group affective tone, and team processes. *Journal of Applied Social Psychology, 41,* 1421–1454.

Clark, A. E., Flèche, S., Layard, R., Powdthavee, N., & Ward, G. (2017). *The key determinants of happiness and misery.* CEP Discussion Papers, CEPDP1485. Centre for Economic Performance, London School of Economics and Political Science, London, UK. Retrieved from http://eprints.lse.ac.uk/83622/

Clark, A. E., Frijters, P., & Shields, M. A. (2008). Relative income, happiness, and utility: An explanation for the Easterlin paradox and other puzzles. *Journal of Economic Literature, 46*(1), 95–144.

Clarke, B., Younas, F., & Family, Kids & Youth. (2017). *Helping parents to parent.* Published by the Social Mobility Commission, UK. Retrieved from https://www.gov.uk/government/news/helping-parents-to-parent

Csikszentmihalyi, M. (1990). *Flow: The psychology of optimal experience*. New York, NY: Harper & Row.

Danner, D. D., Snowdon, D. A., & Friesen, W. V. (2001). Positive emotions in early life and longevity: Findings from the nun study. *Journal of Personality and Social Psychology, 80*(5), 804–813.

DeLeon, P., & Vogenbeck, D. M. (2007). The policy sciences at the crossroads. In F. Fischer, G. J. Miller, & M. S. Sidney (Eds.), *Handbook of public policy analysis: Theory, politics, and methods* (pp. 3–14). Boca Raton, FL (USA): CRC Press/Taylor & Francis Group.

DeNeve, J- E., Diener, E., Tay, L., & Xuereb, C. (2013). The objective benefits of subjective wellbeing. In J. F. Helliwell, R. Layard, & J. Sachs (Eds.), *World happiness report 2013* (pp. 54–79). New York: UN Sustainable Network Development Solutions Network.

Diener, E. (1984). Subjective wellbeing. *Psychological Bulletin, 95,* 542–575.

Diener, E. (2000). Subjective wellbeing: The science of happiness, and a proposal for a national index. *American Psychologist, 55,* 34–43.

Diener, E., & Chan, M. Y. (2011). Happy people live longer: Subjective wellbeing contributes to health and longevity. *Applied Psychology: Health and Wellbeing, 3*(1), 1–43.

Diener, E., & Diener, C. (2011). Monitoring psychosocial prosperity for social change. In R. Biswas-Diener (Ed.), *Positive psychology for social change* (pp. 55–72). Dordrecht: Springer.

Diener, E., Oishi, S., & Lucas, R. E. (2015). National accounts of subjective wellbeing. *American Psychologist, 70*(3), 234–242.

Diener, E., Scollon, C. N., & Lucas, R. E. (2003). The evolving concept of subjective wellbeing: The multifaceted nature of happiness. In P. T. Costa & I. C. Siegler (Eds.), *The psychology of aging* (pp. 187–219). New York, NY: Elsevier Science.

Diener, E., Lucas, R. E., & Scollon, C. N. (2006). Beyond the hedonic treadmill: Revising the adaptation theory of wellbeing. *American Psychologist, 61,* 305–314.

Dittmar, H., Bond, R., Hurst, M., & Kasser, T. (2014). The relationship between materialism and personal wellbeing: A meta-analysis. *Journal of Personality and Social Psychology, 107*(5), 879–924.

Dolan, P. (2011). Happiness questions and government responses: A pilot study of what the general public makes of it all. *Revue d'economie politique, 121*(1), 3–15.

Easterbrook, G. (2004). *The Progress Paradox*. New York: Random House.

Easterlin, R. A. (1995). Will raising the incomes of all increase the happiness of all? *Journal of Economic Behavior & Organization, 27,* 35–47.

Easterlin, R. A. (2013). Happiness, growth, and public policy. *Economic Inquiry, 51*(1), 1–15.

Easterlin, R. A. (2015). Happiness and economic growth: The evidence. In W. Glatzer, L. Camfield, V. Møller, & M. Rojas (Eds.), *Global handbook of quality of life: Exploration of wellbeing of nations and continents* (pp. 283–299). New York, NY: Springer.

Easton, D. (1979). *A framework for political analysis*. Chicago, IL (USA): University of Chicago Press.

Edmans, A. (2012). The link between job satisfaction and firm value, with implications for corporate social responsibility. *Academy of Management Perspectives, 26*(4), 1–19.

Eide, E. P., & Rösler, P. (2014, October). *Rethinking Arab employment: A systemic approach for resource-endowed economies*. Report by the World Economic Forum (REF220814). Retrieved from http://reports.weforum.org/rethinking-arab-employment/

Erdogan, B., Bauer, T. N., Truxillo, D. M., & Mansfield, L. R. (2012). Whistle while you work: A review of the life satisfaction literature. *Journal of Management, 38,* 1038–1083.

Eurofound. (2013). *Third European quality of life survey – Quality of life in Europe: Subjective wellbeing*. Publications Office of the European Union, Luxembourg. Retrieved from http://www.eurofound.europa.eu/publications/report/2013/quality-of-life-social-policies/quality-of-life-in-europe-subjective-wellbeing

Finan, P. H., & Garland, E. L. (2015). The role of positive affect in pain and its treatment. *The Clinical Journal of Pain, 31*(2), 177–187.

Flèche, S., & Layard, R. (2017). Do more of those in misery suffer from poverty, unemployment or mental illness? *Kyklos, 70*(1), 27–41.

Folkman, S. (2008). The case for positive emotions in the stress process. *Anxiety Stress and Coping, 21*(1), 3–14.

Ford, M. T., Cerasoli, C. P., Higgins, J. A., & Decesare, A. L. (2011). Relationships between psychological, physical, and behavioural health and work performance: A review and meta-analysis. *Work and Stress: An International Journal of Work, Health and Organisations, 25*(3), 185–204.

Forgeard, M. J. C., Jayawickreme, E., Kern, M., & Seligman, M. E. P. (2011). Doing the right thing: Measuring wellbeing for public policy. *International Journal of Wellbeing, 1*(1), 79–106.
Forstenlechner, I., & Baruch, Y. (2013). Contemporary career concepts and their fit for the Arabian Gulf context: A sector level analysis of psychological contract breach. *Career Development International, 18*(6), 629–648.
Forstenlechner, I., & Rutledge, E. J. (2011). The GCC's "Demographic Imbalance": Perceptions, realities and policy options. *Middle East Policy, 18*(4), 25–43.
Fredrickson, B. L., Grewen, K. M., Coffey, K. A., Algoe, S. B., Firestine, A. M., Arevalo, J. M. G., … Cole, S. M. (2013). A functional genomic perspective on human wellbeing. *Proceedings of the National Academy of Sciences, 110,* 13684–13689.
Fredrickson, B. L., Mancuso, R. A., Branigan, C., & Tugade, M. M. (2000). The undoing effect of positive emotions. *Motivation and Emotion, 24,* 237–258.
Frey, B. S., & Gallus, J. (2012). Happiness policy and economic development. *International Journal of Happiness and Development, 1*(1), 102–111.
Frey, B. S., & Gallus, J. (2013). Subjective wellbeing and policy. *Topoi, 32*(2), 207–212.
Frey, B. S., & Stutzer, A. (2007). *Should national happiness be maximized?* Zurich IEER Working Paper No. 306. Retrieved from http://econpapers.repec.org/paper/crawpaper/2006-26.htm
Gallup. (2017). *Gallup 2017 Global emotions report.* Retrieved from http://news.gallup.com/reports/212648/gallup-global-emotions-report-2017.aspx
Gasper, D. (2007). Uncounted or illusory blessings? Competing responses to the Easterlin, Easterbrook and Schwartz paradoxes of wellbeing. *Journal of International Development, 19*(4), 473–492.
Goudie, R., Mukherjee, S., De Neve, J.-E., Oswald, A. J., & Wu, S. (2012). *Happiness as a driver of risk-avoiding behavior.* The Centre for Economic Performance, Discussion Paper No. 1126. Retrieved from http://cep.lse.ac.uk/pubs/download/dp1126.pdf
Grant, N., Wardle, J., & Steptoe, A. (2009). The relationship between life satisfaction and health behavior: A cross-cultural analysis of young adults. *International Journal of Behavioral Medicine, 16,* 259–268.
Guven, C. (2012). Reversing the question: Does happiness affect consumption and savings behavior? *Journal of Economic Psychology, 33*(4), 701–717.
Hall, J., & Rickard, L. (2013). *People, progress and participation: How initiatives measuring social progress yield benefits beyond better metrics.* Gütersloh: Bertelsmann Stiftung.
Hart, K. E., & Sasso, T. (2011). Mapping the contours of contemporary positive psychology. *Canadian Psychology, 52*(2), 82–92.
Headey, B. (2008). The set-point theory of wellbeing: Negative results and consequent revisions. *Social Indicators Research, 85*(3), 389–403.
Helliwell, J. F., & Barrington-Leigh, C. P. (2010). Measuring and understanding subjective wellbeing. *Canadian Journal of Economics, 43*(3), 729–753.
Helliwell, J. F., Huang, H., & Wang, S. (2014). Social capital and wellbeing in time of crisis. *Journal of Happiness Studies, 15,* 145–162.
Helliwell, J. F., Huang, H., & Wang, S. (2015a). The geography of happiness. In J. F. Helliwell, R. Layard, & J. Sachs (Eds.), *World Happiness Report 2015* (pp. 12–41). New York, NY: Sustainable Development Solutions Network.
Helliwell, J. F., Layard, R., & Sachs, J. (2012). Some policy implications. In J. F. Helliwell, R. Layard, & J. Sachs (Eds.), *World Happiness Report 2012* (pp. 90–107). New York, NY: The Earth Institute, Columbia University.
Helliwell, J. F., Layard, R., & Sachs, J. (2015b). Setting the stage. In J. F. Helliwell, R. Layard, & J. Sachs (Eds.), *World Happiness Report 2015* (pp. 2–11). New York, NY: Sustainable Development Solutions Network.
Helliwell, J., Layard, R., & Sachs, J. (2016). *World Happiness Report 2016, Update* (Vol. I). New York, NY: Sustainable Development Solutions Network. Retrieved from http://worldhappiness.report/download/

Hewitt, B., Strazdins, L., & Martin, B. (2017). The benefits of paid maternity leave for mothers' post-partum health and wellbeing: Evidence from an Australian evaluation. *Social Science and Medicine, 182,* 97–105.

Howell, A. J. (2009). Flourishing: Achievement-related correlates of students' wellbeing. *Journal of Positive Psychology, 4,* 1–13.

Huang, H., & Humphreys, B. R. (2012). Sports participation and happiness: Evidence from US microdata. *Journal of Economic Psychology, 33*(4), 776–793.

James H. S. Jr., & Chymis A. G. (2004). *Are happy people ethical people? Evidence from North America and Europe* (Working Paper No. AEWP 2004-08). Department of Agricultural Economics. Retrieved from http://ageconsearch.umn.edu/bitstream/26034/1/wp040008.pdf

Jann, W., & Weigrich, K. (2007). Theories of the policy cycle. In F. Fischer, G. J. Miller, & M. S. Sidney (Eds.), *Handbook of public policy analysis: Theory, politics, and methods* (pp. 43–62). Boca Raton, FL (USA): CRC Press/Taylor & Francis Group.

Johnson, K. J., & Fredrickson, B. L. (2005). "We all look the same to me": Positive emotions eliminate the own-race bias in face recognition. *Psychological Science, 16,* 875–881.

Joseph, S., & Wood, A. (2010). Assessment of positive functioning in clinical psychology: Theoretical and practical issues. *Clinical Psychology Review, 30,* 830–838.

Kahneman, D., & Krueger, A. B. (2006). Developments in the measurement of subjective wellbeing. *Journal of Economic Perspectives, 20*(1), 3–24.

Kashdan, T., Biswas-Diener, R., & King, L. (2008). Reconsidering happiness: The costs of distinguishing between hedonics and eudaimonia. *Journal of Positive Psychology, 3*(4), 219–233.

Kasser, T., Dungan, N., Rosenblum, K. L., Sameroff, A. J., Deci, E. L., Niemiec, C. P., … Dittmar, H. (2014). Changes in materialism, changes in psychological wellbeing: Evidence from three longitudinal studies and an intervention experiment. *Motivation and Emotion, 38,* 1–22.

Katzman, K. (2017, June 28). *The United Arab Emirates (UAE): Issues for U.S. policy.* Retrieved from the Federation of American Scientists website, https://fas.org/sgp/crs/mideast/RS21852.pdf

Keltner, D., Kogan, A., Piff, P. K., & Saturn, S. R. (2014). The sociocultural appraisals, values, and emotions (SAVE) framework of prosociality: Core processes from gene to meme. *Annual Review of Psychology, 65,* 425–460.

Kern, M. L., Waters, L. E., Adler, A., & White, M. A. (2015). A multidimensional approach to measuring wellbeing in students: Application of the PERMA framework. *Journal of Positive Psychology, 10*(3), 262–271.

Keyes, C. L. M. (2005). Mental illness and/or mental health? Investigating axioms of the complete state model of health. *Journal of Consulting and Clinical Psychology, 73,* 539–548.

Kinninmont, J. (2015, February). *Future trends in the Gulf.* London, UK: Chatham House, The Royal Institute of International Affairs. Retrieved from: https://www.chathamhouse.org/sites/files/chathamhouse/field/field_document/20150218FutureTrendsGCCKinninmont.pdf

Krassa, M. A., & Radcliffe, B. (2014, November). *Evidence that higher minimum wages improve economic wellbeing.* Retrieved from Scholars Strategy Network, http://www.scholarsstrategynetwork.org/brief/evidence-higher-minimum-wages-improve-economic-wellbeing

Krause, A. (2013). Don't worry, be happy? Happiness and reemployment. *Journal of Economic Behavior & Organization, 96*(C), 1–20.

Lambert, L., Pasha-Zaidi, N., Passmore, H.-A., & York Al-Karam, C. (2015). Developing an indigenous positive psychology in the United Arab Emirates. *Middle East Journal of Positive Psychology, 1*(1), 1–23.

Lambert D'raven, L., Moliver, N., & Thompson, D. (2015). Happiness intervention decreases pain and depression and boosts happiness among primary care patients. *Primary Health Care Research & Development, 16*(2), 114–126.

Lawton, R., & Fujiwara, D. (2016). Living with aircraft noise: Airport proximity, aviation noise and subjective wellbeing in England. *Transportation Research Part D: Transport and Environment, 42,* 104–118.

Layard, R., & Hagell, A. (2015). Healthy young minds: Transforming the mental health of children. In J. F. Helliwell, R. Layard, & J. Sachs (Eds.), *2015 World Happiness Report* (pp. 106–130). New York, NY: Sustainable Development Solutions Network.
Layous, K., Lee, H., Choi, I., & Lyubomirsky, S. (2013). Culture matters when designing a successful happiness-increasing activity: A comparison of the United States and South Korea. *Journal of Cross-Cultural Psychology, 44,* 1294–1303.
Layous, K., & Lyubomirsky, S. (2014). The how, why, what, when, and who of happiness: Mechanisms underlying the success of positive interventions. In J. Gruber & J. Moscowitz (Eds.), *Positive emotion: Integrating the light sides and dark sides* (pp. 473–495). New York: Oxford University Press.
Leicester, A., & Levell, P. (2016). Anti-smoking policies and smoker wellbeing: Evidence from Britain. *Fiscal Studies, 37*(2), 224–257.
Lelkes, O. (2013). Minimising misery: A new strategy for public policies instead of maximising happiness? *Social Indicators Research, 114*(1), 121–137.
Lomas, T. (2015). Positive social psychology: A multilevel inquiry into socio-cultural wellbeing initiatives. *Psychology, Public Policy, and Law, 21*(3), 338–347.
Lyubomirsky, S. (2011). Hedonic adaptation to positive and negative experiences. In S. Folkman (Ed.), *Oxford handbook of stress, health, and coping* (pp. 200–224). New York, NY: Oxford University Press.
Lyubomirsky, S., King, L., & Diener, E. (2005). The benefits of frequent positive affect: Does happiness lead to success? *Psychological Bulletin, 131,* 803–855.
Lyubomirsky, S., Tucker, K. L., & Kasri, F. (2001). Responses to hedonically conflicting social comparisons: Comparing happy and unhappy people. *European Journal of Social Psychology, 31,* 511–535.
Mayraz, G., Wagner, G., & Schupp, J. (2009). *Life satisfaction and relative income: Perceptions and evidence* (CEP Discussion Paper, No. 938). Centre for Economic Performance, London School of Economics and Political Science, London, UK. Retrieved from http://eprints.lse.ac.uk/28606/
Mehl, M. R., Vazire, S., Holleran, S. E., & Clark, C. S. (2010). Eavesdropping on happiness: Wellbeing is related to having less small talk and more substantive conversations. *Psychological Science, 21*(4), 539–541.
Mensah, C. A., Andres, L., Perera, U., & Roji, A. (2016). Enhancing quality of life through the lens of green spaces: A systematic review approach. *International Journal of Wellbeing, 6*(1), 142–163.
Nelson, D. (2009). Feeling good and open-minded: The impact of positive affect on cross cultural empathic responding. *Journal of Positive Psychology, 4,* 53–63.
Nikolova, M. (2016). *Happiness and development.* IZA Discussion Paper No. 10088. Retrieved from https://ssrn.com/abstract=2819369
Norrish, J., & Vella-Brodrick, D. (2008). Is the study of happiness a worth scientific pursuit? *Social Indicators Research, 87*(3), 393–407.
O'Donnell, G. (2013). Using wellbeing as a guide to policy. In J. Helliwell, R. Layard and J. Sachs (eds.), *World Happiness Report 2013* (pp. 98–111). Retrieved from http://unsdsn.org/wp-content/uploads/2014/02/WorldHappinessReport2013_online.pdf
Organisation for Economic Co-operation and Development (OECD). (2013). *OECD Guidelines on measuring subjective wellbeing.* Paris, France: Organisation for Economic Co-operation and Development. Retrieved from http://www.oecd.org/statistics/oecd-guidelines-on-measuring-subjective-wellbeing-9789264191655-en.htm
Oswald, A. J., Proto, E., & Sgroi, D. (2012). *Happiness and productivity.* University of Warwick. Retrieved from http://www.andrewoswald.com/docs/6MayOsProtoSgroi2012.pdf
Oxford Strategic Consulting. (2014, November 9). *GCC nationals are not after 'Status' or an 'Easy life' finds Oxford survey.* Retrieved from http://www.oxfordstrategicconsulting.com/gccnationals-status-easy-life-finds-oxford-survey/
Pencavel, J. (2014). *The productivity of working hours.* IZA Discussion Paper No. 8129. Bonn, Germany: IZA (Institute for the Study of Labor). Retrieved from ftp.iza.org/dp8129.pdf

Priller, E., & Schupp, J. (2011). Social and economic characteristics of financial and blood donors in Germany. *DIW Economic Bulletin, 6,* 23–30.

Proyer, R. T. (2013). The wellbeing of playful adults: Adult playfulness, subjective wellbeing, physical wellbeing, and the pursuit of enjoyable activities. *European Journal of Humour Research, 1*(1), 84–98.

Putnam, R. (2000). *Bowling alone: The collapse and revival of American community*. New York, NY: Simon & Schuster.

Pykett, J., & Cromby, J. (2017). Mapping happiness, managing urban emotions. In V. Higgins & W. Larner (Eds.), *Assembling neoliberalism: Expertise, practices, subjects* (pp. 195–216). Palgrave MacMillan US.

Rand, D. G., Kraft-Todd, G., & Gruber, J. (2015). The collective benefits of feeling good and letting go: Positive emotion and (dis)inhibition interact to predict cooperative behavior. *PLoS ONE, 10*(1), e0117426.

Richards, M., & Huppert, F. A. (2011). Do positive children become positive adults? Evidence from a longitudinal birth cohort study. *The Journal of Positive Psychology, 6*(1), 75–87.

Ritzen, J. (2015). Happiness as a guide to labor market policy. *IZA World of Labor, 149.* Retrieved from https://wol.iza.org/articles/happiness-as-guide-to-labor-market-policy/long.

Sabatier, P. (1999). The need for better theories. In P. A. Sabatier (Ed.), *Theories of the policy process* (pp. 3–17). Boulder, CO: Westview.

Schwartz, B., & Ward, A. (2004). Doing better but feeling worse: The paradox of choice. In P. A. Linley & S. Joseph (Eds.), *Positive psychology in practice* (pp. 86–104). Hoboken, N.J.: John Wiley and Sons.

Schwela, D. (2017). *Review of environmental noise policies and economics in 2014–2016.* Paper presented at the 12th ICBEN Congress on Noise as a Public Health Problem. Retrieved from www.icben.org/2017/ICBEN%202017%20Papers/SubjectArea07_Schwela_0701_3611.pdf

Scourfield, J., Cheung, S. Y., & Macdonald, G. (2014). Working with fathers to improve childen's wellbeing: Results of a survey exploring service provision and intervention approach in the UK. *Children and Youth Services Review, 43,* 40–50.

Seligman, M. E. P. (2009, June 18–21). *Positive psychology and positive education.* International Positive Psychology Association first world congress on Positive Psychology, Philadelphia.

Seligman, M. E. P., & Csikszentmihalyi, M. (2000). Positive psychology: An introduction. *American Psychologist, 55,* 5–14.

Senik, C. (2011). *The French unhappiness puzzle: The cultural dimension of happiness* (Discussion paper no. 6175). The Institute for the Study of Labor (IZA), Bonn, Germany. Retrieved from ftp.iza.org/dp6175.pdf

Shillabeer, O., Cartwright, D., Engel, K., & Barnes, W. (2015). *The implications of wellbeing research on government policy.* Hertford Business and Economics Society: Hertford College, University of Oxford. Retrieved from https://ssrn.com/abstract=2711708

Sin, N. L. (2016). The protective role of positive wellbeing in cardiovascular disease: Review of current evidence, mechanisms, and clinical implications. *Current Cardiology Reports, 11*(18), 106.

Smeaton, D., Ray, K., & Knight, G. (2014). *Costs and benefits to business of adopting work life balance working practices: A literature review.* Department for Business, Innovation and Skills. Retrieved from http://www.psi.org.uk/site/publication_detail/1760

Son, J., & Wilson, J. (2012). Volunteer work and hedonic, eudemonic, and social wellbeing. *Sociological Forum, 27*(3), 658–681.

Stiglitz, J., Sen, A., & Fitoussi, J.-P. (2009). *The measurement of economic performance and social progress revisited.* Commission on the Measurement of Economic Performance and Social Progress, Paris. Retrieved from http://www.ofce.sciences-po.fr/pdf/dtravail/WP2009-33.pdf

Stevenson, B., & Wolfers, J. (2008). Economic growth and subjective wellbeing: Reassessing the Easterlin paradox. *Brookings Papers on Economic Activity, 1,* 1–87.

Stutzer, A., & Frey, B. S. (2008). Stress that doesn't pay: The commuting paradox. *Scandinavian Journal of Economics, 110*(2), 339–366.

Suldo, S. M., Thalji, A., & Ferron, J. (2011). Longitudinal academic outcomes predicted by early adolescents' subjective wellbeing, psychopathology, and mental health status yielded from a dual-factor model. *Journal of Positive Psychology, 6*(1), 17–30.

Tay, L., Chan, D., & Diener, E. (2014). The metrics of societal happiness. *Social Indicators Research, 117,* 577–600.

The Happiness Research Institute. (2014). *The happy Danes: Exploring the reasons behind the high levels of happiness in Denmark.* Copenhagen, Denmark: The Happiness Research Institute. Retrieved from www.happinessresearchinstitute.com/publications/4579836749

Thoits, P. A., & Hewitt, L. N. (2001). Volunteer work and wellbeing. *Journal of Health and Social Behavior, 42,* 115–131.

Treasury Board of Canada. (2015). *Whole-of-government framework.* Retrieved from the Government of Canada website, www.tbs-sct.gc.ca/ppg-cpr/frame-cadre-eng.aspx

Ward, G. (2015). *Is happiness a predictor of election results?* CEP Discussion Papers, CEPDP1343. London, UK: Centre for Economic Performance, London School of Economics and Political Science. Retrieved from http://eprints.lse.ac.uk/61698/

White, E. J., Langer, L., Yariv, I. V., & Welch, J. C. (2006). Frequent social comparisons and destructive emotions and behaviors: The dark side of social comparisons. *Journal of Adult Development, 13*(1), 36–44.

White, S. C. (2010). Analysing wellbeing: A framework for development practice. *Development in Practise, 20*(2), 158–172.

Whitmee, S., Haines, A., Beyrer, C., Boltz, F., Capon, A. G., de Souza Dias, B. F., …Yach, D. (2015). Safeguarding human health in the Anthropocene epoch: Report of The Rockefeller Foundation–Lancet Commission on planetary health. *The Lancet, 386*(10007), 1973–2028.

Wiest, M., Schüz, B., Webster, N., & Wurm, S. (2011). Subjective wellbeing and mortality revisited: Differential effects of cognitive and emotional facets of wellbeing on mortality. *Health Psychology, 30*(6), 728–735.

World Economic Forum. (2014). *Rethinking Arab employment: A systemic approach for resource-endowed economies.* Retrieved from http://reports.weforum.org/rethinking-arab-employment/

Xu, J., & Roberts, R. E. (2010). The power of positive emotions: It's a matter of life or death—Subjective wellbeing and longevity over 28 years in a general population. *Health Psychology, 29*(1), 9–19.

Yaghi, A., & Antwi-Boateng, O. (2015). Determinants of UAE voters' preferences for Federal National Council candidates. *Digest of Middle East Studies, 24*(2), 213–235.

Zautra, A. J., Johnson, L. M., & Davis, M. C. (2005). Positive affect as a source of resilience for women in chronic pain. *Journal of Consulting and Clinical Psychology, 73*(2), 212–220.

Chapter 3
Commercial Life: The Private Sector's Contribution to Wellbeing

Aziz Mulay-Shah, Louise Lambert, Yara Younis and Bronwyn P. Wood

Abstract The global attention paid to wellbeing and happiness shows no signs of abating. From Bhutan, the first country to establish wellbeing indicators as a benchmark for social progress, to the announcement of a Minister of Happiness and Wellbeing in the United Arab Emirates in 2016, the move towards establishing policies, practices, and programs to support that which makes life worthwhile and contributes to the development of stronger, more vibrant nations is becoming accepted policy practice. The World Happiness Report has been a contributor to this development by highlighting the need for, and possibility of measuring wellbeing at a national level by GDP, life expectancy, social support, generosity, freedom and perceptions of corruption. While chosen for their impact on wellbeing, we highlight a missing facet; that is, Commercial Life and its related social interactions, emotional experiences and long-term psychosocial outcomes, and propose that it be included as a measure of a nation's wellbeing. Thus, we highlight the importance of the consumer experience, employee wellbeing, and product/service innovation possibilities that can contribute to greater social, environmental, and individual wellbeing and draw upon various theories in positive psychology to inform our approach.

A. Mulay-Shah (✉)
Global Communications Agency, Dubai, UAE
e-mail: aziz@gc.agency

L. Lambert · B. P. Wood
United Arab Emirates University, Al Ain, UAE
e-mail: ltlamber@yahoo.com

B. P. Wood
e-mail: bwood@uaeu.ac.ae

Y. Younis
UAE Ministry of Culture and Knowledge Development, Al Ain, UAE
e-mail: yarayounis96@gmail.com

L. Lambert and N. Pasha-Zaidi (eds.), *Positive Psychology in the Middle East/North Africa*, https://doi.org/10.1007/978-3-030-13921-6_3

3.1 Commercial Life: The Missing Component for Greater Wellbeing

As global policy-making initiatives increasingly accept wellbeing as a framework for solving national development and prosperity challenges, there is a need to reflect on existing analytic frameworks, such as the one tabled by the World Happiness Report (WHR). Among many frameworks, the WHR has attracted significant positive international attention for its ease of understanding and simplicity. That nations can be ranked in this manner suggests that wellbeing can and should be measured, and that wellbeing thus matters not only to individuals, but to communities and national development as well. The WHR ranks nations based on a single question called the *Cantril's Ladder of Life*, asking respondents to rank their quality of life on a scale from zero to ten at that point in time, with zero representing the worst and ten the best possible life. It offers a retrospective explanation based on six indicators. These indicators include Gross Domestic Product (GDP); Life Expectancy; Freedom to Live one's Life; Trust in Institutions; Generosity; and Social Support. The data for the six pillars themselves are not included in the WHR but taken from Gallup and other reports.

Yet, the WHR has garnered criticism. For example, van Dijk, Spencer and Ramirez (2014) suggest it is limited in scope and the data it provides offers little in the way for policy development. While it may satisfy policymakers need for quick results, the aggregation of individual scores into a single one is problematic as it overlooks cultural diversity, as well as immigration and labour market issues as is the case in many Arabian Gulf nations where more than half (up to 90%) of the population is composed of expatriate labour. It is impossible to know what individuals are thinking of or referring to for the basis of their responses. Linking one score to specific factors or policies is difficult and while subjective data is a progressive step beyond objective data alone, in this case, a single score upon which the ranking is devised puts too much emphasis on the individual and not enough on public and private sector efforts. Attempts to increase this score often result in closing the door on more meaningful and useful measurement tools, at least as far as public policy is concerned. While a methodological critique is beyond the purview of this chapter and despite the utility of the data produced by the WHR through the examination of the six indicators, the satisfaction individuals experience across their daily interactions with the bodies that matter most—commercial and business entities, is overlooked. This omission is glaring given that material wellbeing has been identified as the single most important contributor to subjective wellbeing beyond domains of physical health, social support, altruism, etc., in over 150 nations and 10 geopolitical regions comparing over 60 variables from the Gallup World Poll (Diego-Rosell, Tortora, & Bird, 2018).

Given the first WHR's (Helliwell, Layard, & Sachs, 2012) suggestion that "material life must be harnessed to meet these human needs, most importantly to promote the end of suffering, social justice, and the attainment of happiness" (p. 3), we propose that governments such as the United Arab Emirates (UAE), in addition to the six pillars objectively measured by Gallup and other organizations, include commercial life as a means to positively influence wellbeing. In fact, the latest WHR (Sachs,

2019) stated that happiness and wellbeing as a lens through which organizations can thrive and prosper, has not been used enough or taken seriously. Their inclusion is not meant to create additional government interventions to regulate the private sector, but instead is a mechanism through which governments can capture the impact of private sector entities on wellbeing. This will require a government championed re-ordering of private sector commercial activity to address prevailing social inequalities, social status anxieties, loss of social trust, and materialism, as well as environmental degradation of proportions threatening to human life. In short, commercial life should not be overlooked in the global march to greater wellbeing. The inclusion of commercial life as an area for intervention may go some way in re-centering commercial activity as a contender to building wellbeing instead of undermining it. We propose how steps in this direction may be taken and offer this chapter as food for thought towards reshaping commercial life towards better ends, and challenge governments to take on prosperity, growth, and innovation with wellbeing at its core.

3.2 What is Commercial Life?

"Commercial Life" refers to the interactions individuals have on a daily basis with business entities, either in the purchase of a product, good, or service. These interactions engender an emotional response; consider the embarrassment of being snubbed by a sales person in a high-end store. Equally, consider the experience when a waiter is funny, welcoming and leaves you feeling like you've made a new friend. Beyond the immediate emotional response is also the longer-term impact of that transaction, which in the case of a service or product, can limit or facilitate one's ability to live a positive life and produce spill-over effects to greater wellbeing, such that a pleasant evening in a restaurant spills over to warm feelings towards one's spouse, which impacts productivity at work the next day. It is not only that a good dinner was had; it is also the positive emotions that were generated and shared with others, as well the goals attained over time that matter. Our view on commercial life differs from traditional wellbeing products such as yoga mats and vitamins, or the standard customer service focus, which takes into account consumer satisfaction insofar as it adds to profit and brand loyalty. Instead, construing commercial life as a serious factor in wellbeing can inspire entities to consider in what ways their offerings contribute to individual, social and environmental prosperity and spawn product and service innovations towards that end. As such, the consideration of commercial life will have implications for products and profits, as well as policy prescriptions for governments.

Yet, commercial activity is often considered a necessary evil from which individuals and societies cannot escape. On one hand, it is necessary for the economic growth of nations and while well meaning, consumption is often promoted by governments to ensure such security. Yet, on the other, overconsumption can turn to materialism, which not only undermines wellbeing (Sirgy et al., 2013), but is unsustainable, with household consumption alone being responsible for over 60% of worldwide emissions and 80% of water, land and material use (Ivanova et al., 2016). Thus, a proposal for the inclusion of a commercial life as a pillar of wellbeing must not be confused with an encouragement to simply produce or consume more. Commercial life and its contribution to wellbeing invites critical reflection on materialistic values, ethics, as well as environmental harm due to overconsumption (Brown & Vergragt, 2016; Brown, Kasser, Ryan, & Konow, 2016; Dittmar, Bond, Hurst, & Kasser, 2014; Kasser, 2018; Kasser et al., 2014; Whitmee et al., 2015). Coupled with these concerns is the growing recognition that money, beyond a certain threshold, does not promote wellbeing (Kahneman & Deaton, 2010). As other sectors of society are making strides towards reorienting their activities towards wellbeing, the time has come for commercial life to also become a vehicle towards a more conscious form of consumption that positively contributes to social development.

3.3 Commercial Life: A Theoretical Model for Wellbeing

To illustrate the commercial life components, we offer a framework that includes attention to positive emotion, eudaimonic goal strivings, and social connections (Botella et al., 2012; Gaggioli, Riva, Peters, & Calvo, 2017), with much supporting evidence showing that wellbeing improves as these needs are fulfilled and attended to (Kim, Kim, & Kim, 2017; Ryan & Deci, 2000). Research further shows that of the three components, social connections have the greatest influence on wellbeing and should be the main targets of any workplace intervention (Helliwell & Wang, 2012; Krekel, Ward, & De Neve, 2019) and as such, it bears noting as policymakers consider new policies to enhance wellbeing across societies as a whole. We also include the built and natural environment, as the latter is increasingly in peril and responsible for human health and wellbeing. Accordingly, in the sections that follow, we outline what is meant by hedonic, eudaimonic and social wellbeing and explore how each can be expressed across the consumer, employee/organizational and product/service experience.

3.3.1 Hedonic Happiness: The Experiencing Self

Hedonic happiness is the concern for how things feel in terms of their emotional value. Individuals seek to increase positive emotions through activities, products, and relationships. There are over 25 positive emotions (Desmet, 2012), examples of which include relief, inspiration, interest, courage, and desire. The Broaden and Build Theory (Fredrickson, 2006) posits that under the influence of such emotions, individuals experience immediate "broadening", which "builds" long-term resources. Broadening refers to the expanded visual ranges and resulting perception, focus, and attention that positively impact thought and behaviour (De Neve, Diener, Tay, & Xuereb, 2013; Johnson, Waugh, & Fredrickson, 2010; Schmitz, De Rosa,

& Anderson, 2009). Flexible broad thinking and resulting actions help build health, social, cognitive, and psychological assets and undo the impact of negative emotions (Fredrickson, Mancuso, Branigan, & Tugade, 2000). Positive emotions are vital to both short and long-term wellbeing as their experience contributes to longevity (Pressman & Cohen, 2012; Wiest, Schüz, Webster, & Wurm, 2011) and resiliency (Cohn, Fredrickson, Brown, Mikels, & Conway, 2009); they also influence likeability (Boehm & Lyubomirsky, 2008), ease cooperation (Barsade, 2002; Carnevale, 2008), improve interpersonal trust (Lount, 2010), and facilitate altruism and compassion (Aknin, Dunn, & Norton, 2012; Shin, Choi, Suh, & Koo, 2013).

3.3.2 Eudaimonic Happiness: The Striving Self

Eudaimonia is a way of life that does not always entail pleasant emotion, but activity, effort, and failure (Steger, Kashdan, & Oishi, 2008). This philosophy leads to greater life satisfaction, meaning, positive affect, and activity engagement (Higgins, 2006; Huta & Ryan, 2010; Seligman, Parks, & Steen, 2005; Waterman, Schwartz, & Conti, 2008). Examples of eudaimonic activity include starting a business, running a race, or mastering the piano, all of which can lead to flow (Csikszentmihalyi, 2006), a feeling of personal control, intense and focused concentration, time distortion, and a loss of self-consciousness, along with anticipation, and the experience of activity being rewarding. People who experience flow report greater subjective wellbeing (Hefferon & Ollis, 2006; Tsaur, Yen, & Hsiao, 2013). Self-determination theory (Ryan, Huta, & Deci, 2008) posits three values which comprise a eudaimonic lifestyle, namely competence, autonomy, and relatedness. Competence relates to feelings of effectiveness and efficiency in task completion. Relatedness refers to the feeling of belonging, while autonomy includes the perception of choice and control over the regulation of one's goal-driven activity. As individuals meet these needs, wellbeing accrues. Eudaimonia and hedonia overlap and are two types of happiness (Disabato, Goodman, Kashdan, Short, & Jarden, 2016).

3.3.3 Social Connection: The Relating Self

The social facet has often been considered a mere externality in economics research (Bruni, 2010), but is commanding more respect in light of increasing rates of loneliness (Holt-Lunstad, Robles, & Sbarra, 2017) and the fact that when it comes to wellbeing, social connections reign (Helliwell & Wang, 2012). Whether through professional networks, non-profit/volunteer groups, religious organizations, or friends, all connections count and are a suggested route for workplace intervention (Krekel et al., 2019). Interacting with others, generating acts of kindness, charity, concern, empathy, and cooperation generate wellbeing (Dillard, Schiavone, & Brown, 2008; Pressman, Kraft, & Cross, 2015; Schreier, Schonert-Reichl, & Chen, 2013; Yeung,

Zhang, & Kim, 2018) and build social capital and connections (Helliwell, Huang, & Wang, 2014). These connections are estimated to be the equivalent of £85,000 a year in terms of life satisfaction (Powdthavee, 2008). The relating self also includes community engagement, actions designed to address opportunities of public concern which help individuals develop skills and knowledge, work together, and trust others in the community. Sharing interests offers a sense of collective efficacy, cultural continuity and identity, greater health outcomes and life satisfaction (Albanesi, Cicognani, & Zani, 2007; Goth & Småland, 2014; Viswanath, Steele, & Finnegan, 2006).

3.3.4 *Built and Living Environments: The Functioning Self*

Gaining traction in architectural design is biophilia (Beatley, 2016; Kellert & Wilson, 1993), the notion that humans not only thrive in nature, but need it to flourish. As modern humans recently moved indoors, our disconnection with nature is blamed for many health issues (Kellert & Calabrese, 2015). Yet, when exposed to natural elements, benefits to physical and psychological health materialize, including greater hedonic and eudaimonic wellbeing, as well as increases in positive emotion (Capaldi, Passmore, Nisbet, Zelenski, & Dopko, 2015; McMahan, 2018; McMahan & Estes, 2015). Spending time in and being exposed to nature in the built environment also boosts sociability and prosocial acts (Guéguen, Meineri, & Stefan, 2012; Guéguen & Stefan, 2016; Joye & Bolderdijk, 2014; Weinstein, Przybylski, & Ryan, 2009; Zelenski, Dopko, & Capaldi, 2015). Yet, it is not only the buildings in which work occurs; it is also about the processes that take place there that are critical. Sustainability involves cutting waste, becoming resource efficient, improving relationships with suppliers, developing new markets and innovations, as well as valuing and prioritizing the environment (Table 3.1).

The framework of hedonic, eudaimonic and social wellbeing, including attention to the built and natural environment, provides the structure to analyze three aspects of commercial life. These aspects include the employee and workplace experience, the consumer retail experience, as well as the product and service design process.

3.4 The Work Experience

The latest WHR (Krekel et al., 2019) estimated that addressing wellbeing in the workaplce in a sustainable manner generated increases in productivity of approximately 10% and greater firm level performance. As commercial life is built upon organizations composed of employees who have relationships with consumers, other employees, the living and built environment, and the community, in each exists the real possibility of experiencing positive emotion, realizing personal goals, developing relationships, and having a positive impact. Organizations can fulfill their roles as positive institutions (Seligman & Csikszentmihalyi, 2000) and become

Table 3.1 Commercial life theoretical framework

Component	Descriptor	Impact
Hedonic life	Positive emotions are highly valued. The Broaden and Build Theory posits that positive emotions contribute to immediate benefits conducive to daily functioning as well as longer-term development of health, social, cognitive, and psychological assets.	The employee, consumer, and product/service design processes are impacted by all aspects of wellbeing.
Eudaimonic life	Higher order values, like meaning, striving and purpose are vital to human development. Self-determination theory posits that growth is possible when autonomy, competence and relatedness are exercised.	
Social life	Social relationships of all sorts matter to human flourishing, whereby connections provide a source of support, emotional resonance, the feeling of being understood, as well as fun, altruism and kindness.	
Natural and built environment	The natural and physical contexts in which humans function and interact on a daily basis impact their wellbeing. Whether through the natural elements of light, air or sound, or via the protection and promotion of environmental values expressed through one's organization, this sector of wellbeing is increasing in importance.	

a force for good. The concept of a "Positive Business" as proposed by the University of Michigan, https://www.positivebusinessproject.com), includes environmental and community stewardship, as well as employee empowerment, which leads to positive social, workplace and environmental changes, as well as profit. In their quest to produce social, environmental and economic prosperity, positive businesses address the processes and structures that give rise to such issues. They not only remediate them, but constructively build positive cultures which prevent disharmony from taking root. (Readers will notice that attention to gender, inclusion, and diversity is omitted. We take as a given that these are addressed in positive workplaces).

Topic Box: Health—A Given in Wellbeing

One contributor to workplace stress is long hours. Data from 2000 to 2016 across most OECD countries shows the average number of weekly hours worked is declining below 40 h. Long hours increase fatigue, depression, obesity, and heart disease, including workplace accidents and errors, and result in more absenteeism, turnover, and healthcare costs. Add to long days, time commuting, cooking, shopping, and parenting, little is left for sleep, exercise, or socializing. Pencavel (2014) suggests that businesses undermine their returns by trying to get more hours worked per employee, especially when fewer hours lower costs and yield equal outputs (Lorentzon, 2015; von Thiele & Hasson, 2011). The latest WHR identified work life balance as a significant route to promoting the wellbeing of employees (Krekel et al., 2019).

Another area is sitting disease or sedentariness, stemming from desk work, television, or commuting (Owen, Healy, Matthews, & Dunstan, 2010). A Canadian study showed the worst "sitters" to be university educated, employed men who do little exercise and are obese (Gebel et al., 2017), problematic especially for those who lead sedentary lifestyles outside work. The relationship between depression and a lack of physical activity is also worrisome (Biddle, Mutrie, & Gorely, 2015; Ekkekakis, 2015). Yet, physical activity contributes to physical and psychological health (see Lambert, D'Cruz, Schlatter, & Barron, 2016) in ways equal to antidepressant medication, but is far under-prescribed (Pinto Pereira, Geoffroy, & Power, 2014; Wegner et al., 2014).

Organizations can also do more against smoking. In the US, smokers are absent six extra days and make six additional doctor visits (Ekpu & Brown, 2015). Smokers are less productive about 76 h a year (Baker, Flores, Zou, Bruno, & Harrison, 2017; Suwa et al., 2017). Smoking cessation services may generate cost savings and productivity gains (Ong & Glantz, 2004).

3.4.1 Hedonic Work Experiences

Frequent positive and infrequent negative emotions signal a good work environment and boost job satisfaction (Turban & Yan, 2016). Employees who experience positive emotion show greater task performance (Knight & Eisenkraft, 2015), better decision-making (Chuang, 2007), and originality of group ideas and consensus seeking behavior (Grawitch, Munz, Elliott, & Mathis, 2003). They are less prone to burnout (Walkiewicz, Tartas, Majkowicz, & Budzinski, 2012) and are more committed (Herrbach, 2006; Mignonac & Herrbach, 2004). Another reason organizations have in prioritizing positive emotion is its influence on prosocial organizational action (Crede, Chernyshenko, Stark, Dalal, & Bashshur, 2007; Dalal, Baysinger, Brummel, & Lebreton, 2012; Ilies, Scott, & Judge, 2006). Hope, resilience, and optimism correlate positively with engagement attitudes and voluntary actions that benefit one's organization, and negatively with deviance and cynicism (Avey, Wernsing, & Luthans, 2008; Chi, Chung, & Tsai, 2011). Positive emotions are resources organizations can leverage (Klarner, By, & Deifenbach, 2011) and generate through fun events, or collegial, relaxed workplace atmospheres where playfulness, gratitude, and kindness are the norm. Yet, organizations still need pessimism, even conflict (Todorova, Bear, & Weingart, 2014), or neutral affect, which can signal concentration, absorption, focus and a state of flow (Csikszentmihalyi, 2006) that contribute to job satisfaction and positive affect (Ceja & Navarro, 2011; Fullagar & Helloway, 2009; Ilies et al., 2017). This is especially true for those with an achievement orientation (Eisenberger, Jones, Stinglhamber, Shanock, & Randall, 2005), suggesting that satisfaction is possible from work itself.

3.4.2 Eudaimonic Work Experiences

A eudaimonic view involves fulfilling career potential while using one's character strengths, the traits reflected in thoughts, feelings, and behaviors which lead to good outcomes for the self and others (Niemiec, 2013). A total of 24 strengths exist (Peterson & Seligman, 2004), examples of which include integrity, persistence, and self-regulation. Fairness is one of the top strengths demanded in the workplace (Money, Hillenbrand, & Camara, 2009) and when employees perceive they are treated so, satisfaction, workplace relationships, productivity, and organizational commitment rise (Castro Solano & Cosentino, 2016; Gillet, Colombat, Michinov, Pronost, & Fouquereau, 2013; St-Pierre & Holmes, 2010). Even humour is related to satisfaction (Peterson, Stephens, Park, Lee, & Seligman, 2010), with a positive impact on productivity, interpersonal relationships and group effectiveness (Romero & Pescosolido, 2008). Leadership programs now include character development to limit potential unethical behaviors (Money et al., 2009). Using one's strengths adds to workplace satisfaction and greater earnings (Duckworth, Kirby, Tsukayama, Berstein, & Ericsson, 2010; Lindqvist & Vestman, 2011). Organizations manage talent recognizing that continued learning opportunities, as well as managerial support can help to capitalize on the desire for eudaimonic growth in employees (Hone, Jarden, Duncan, & Schofiled, 2015). From doing what one is good at, meaning emerges and is linked to engagement, career development, performance and fulfillment (Rosso, Dekas, & Wrzesniewski, 2010; Steger & Dik, 2010). Work can also fulfill spiritual concerns, build a sense of national identity, and become a means to express the self or master one's craft. Employees develop meaning by considering what contribution their work has beyond its present function. For some, a corporate social responsibility program, done because it is the right thing to do, may help, while others may be impacted by what the organizational values stand for (Casey & Sieber, 2016; Pratt, Pradies, & Lepisto, 2013).

3.4.3 Social Resources at Work

While positive emotions help in developing social resources through greater openness, they also help employees establish connections, develop teamwork, dialogue and emotional attachments that serve as workplace support and a reason to stay in one's job. In fact, workplace friendships boost engagement by a factor of seven

(Gallup, 2012). Also of interest are what are called high-quality connections (HQCs; Stephens, Heaphy, & Dutton, 2011), the short-term, micro interactions experienced as enlivening and which entail a mutual feeling of "feeling felt". Examples include hallway chats, private texts sent during meetings, and momentary "I get you" looks of support between colleagues that build workplace capital and positive workplace cultures. Finding ways to create HQCs through task sharing, supportive onboarding relationships, or social activities can result in greater cognitive performance, stress resilience, perceptions of support and belonging, and workplace attachment. Such connections contribute to job satisfaction, performance, involvement, team cohesion, and organizational commitment (Berman, West, & Richeter, 2002; Chiaburu & Harrison, 2008; Dickson-Swift, Fox, Marshall, Welch, & Willis, 2014; Fliaster & Schloderer, 2010). They also influence behavior and attitudes. Job satisfaction and discretionary effort may be prone to contagion, and employees high on these behaviors and feelings may benefit organizations when being strategically placed to influence others (Chancellor, Layous, Margolis, & Lyubomirsky, 2017). Chancellor, Margolis, and Lyubomirsky (2018) even found that employees who witnessed kind acts done by others in the office reported more team connection and satisfaction with life.

3.4.4 Environmental Health at Work

In the 1980s, Sick Building Syndrome was identified as harmful to health, centering mostly on ventilation. Since, attention has moved to green architecture and biophilic design, the elements of which involve sound, air, light and movement, and its attention restoring qualities (Browning, Ryan, & Clancy, 2014; Kaplan, 1995). Examples include integrating natural light to improve sleep and physical activity (Boubekri, Cheung, Reid, Wang, & Zee, 2014), introducing noise controls like the sound of nature to reduce fatigue, memory distractions and low motivation found in open plan offices (Jahncke, Hygge, Halin, Green, & Dimberg, 2011). Positioning desks with a view on nature or scenes of it to increase positive affect and reduce stress and blood pressure are other examples, as asphalt views do the opposite (Barton & Pretty, 2010; Brengman, Willems, & Joye, 2012; Brown, Barton & Gladwell, 2013; Velarde, Fry, & Tveit, 2007). Changes need not be onerous; Heschong Mahone Group (2003) reported the costs of rearranging workstations with views of nature at about $1000 per employee, and recouped in four months.

Environmental sustainability programs continue to grow. Yet, a lack of employee engagement upon which sustainability efforts rest, awareness about how these programs help communities and the workplace, and a lack of measurement and demonstrated progress make them fail (Delmas & Pekovic, 2018). Further, many companies claim to be sustainable, i.e., "greenwashing", yet their products, service delivery and practises are not. This undermines the companies who are serious and deflates customer enthusiasm. Beyond the benefits and cost savings of sustainability, the impact on employees is clear. Employee engagement and meaning can be enhanced through sustainability efforts and provide a sense of purpose and means to retain and recruit talent (Cantor, Morrow, & Montabon, 2012; Casey & Sieber, 2016; Elci & Alpkan, 2009; Greening & Turban, 2000). In fact, employees prefer to work for organizations that prioritize the environment and have a pro-social orientation that mirrors their own (Highhouse, Hoffman, Greve, & Collins, 2002; Jones, Willness, & Heller, 2016), and experience a drop in wellbeing when organizational values do not meet the standards they claim (Singhapakdi, Lee, Sirgy, & Senasu, 2015). Further, a study of over 5000 French firms found productivity to be one standard deviation higher where environmental standards were adopted along with other practises (Delmas & Pekovic, 2013, 2018). As employee involvement drives organizational outcomes, this is not trivial. Gallup reported workplace engagement to be a mere 13% worldwide (Harter, 2017). Might sustainability be one thing employees care about and for which they engage with work?

Topic Box: Improve Wellbeing in Your Organization

Create spaces that offer people options to socialize, strategize, and plan as a group. Soundproof spaces in which to talk, debate, and engage in a little healthy conflict and laughter are indispensable for productivity. Yet, take care to not undermine sociability by mandating it. Offer opportunities for connection and reasons to work together where people choose their workmates.

Employees are interrupted every 11 min and open plan offices are famous for a lack of privacy to make a phone call or visual privacy to review confidential data. While such offices are thought to increase collaboration, they merely produce annoyance and greater coffee consumption elsewhere! Consider continuous, low-level ambient background noise to create quiet spaces in which employees can do quality work, on time, and with satisfaction. Employers would also be well-served holding short, regularly scheduled feedback sessions where wellbeing is always a topic. Asking employees for "one small thing" to improve the day would save the expense of many unwanted team building activities. Employees may opt to leave 15 min early, sit next to a window, or participate in projects as an alternative. Management is often fixated on showing how they spend money towards wellbeing; they should seek employee input instead.

Many people have unused skills, or rely on strengths that do not come naturally to them. Thus, job crafting (Wrzesniewski, LoBuglio, Dutton, & Berg, 2013), transforming the work one has into work one likes, is an effective means of developing greater wellbeing and engagement, and aims to ensure an appropriate fit with work and its development towards being more interesting. Employees may swap tasks that rely on their less developed strengths for others that use their top strengths. Or they could start the day with activities involving their lower strengths before moving on to those playing to their higher strengths. It can also involve additional training. Job crafting requires a perspective of employee strengths instead of a typical view of limitations only.

3.5 The Consumer Experience

It has been more than a decade since Mick (2006) called for a serious look at the consumer's wellbeing, with past research taking a largely economic view. Since, the notion of consumer wellbeing has taken many forms (see Pancer & Handelman, 2012; Sirgy, Lee, & Rahtz, 2007). With the growth of positive psychology and multi-disciplinary collaboration, research in the area has focused on the effects of consumption on physical, psychological, economic, and social needs (Burroughs & Rindfleish, 2011), extending to its emotional, spiritual, environmental and political impacts as well (Mick, Pettigrew, Pechmann, & Ozanne, 2011). Developments have also addressed the role of commercial interactions in the determination of shopping "illbeing" and "wellbeing" (Ekici, Sirgy, Lee, Yu, & Bosnjak, 2018), determined by the fulfillment of functional needs, hedonic needs and spill-over effects into other life domains. Many of these models overlap with our theoretical categories (Fig. 3.1).

3.5.1 *Hedonic Consumer Experiences*

Many brands and organizations have already shifted their marketing and customer service experiences towards the generation of positive emotion and states of happiness. This is not without cause as inducing positive emotional experiences influences levels of consumer satisfaction (Biscaia, Correia, Rosado, Marôco, & Ross, 2012; Pedragosa, Biscaia, & Correia, 2015), purchasing behavior (Parboteeah, Valacich, & Wells, 2009; Yuan & Dennis, 2014), quality of user experience (Fokkinga &

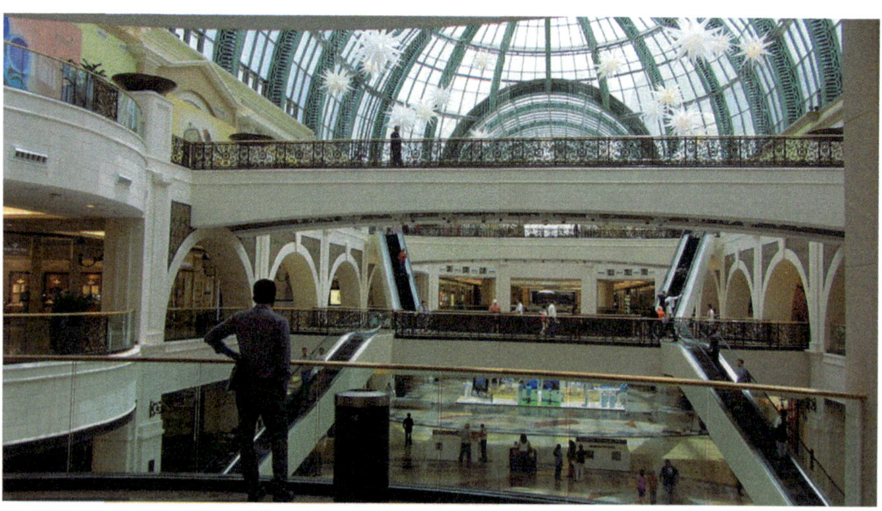

Fig. 3.1 The mall experience in Dubai. *Photo credit* Pixabay

Desmet, 2012), brand loyalty (Chitturi, 2009), and attachment to products (Mugge, Schoormans, & Schifferstein, 2005). Studies also show that shopping in itself can have positive effects on mood (Headey, Muffels, & Wooden, 2008; Kim & Rucker, 2012; Pierceall & Keim, 2007). Indeed, consumption activity is often described as a holiday, treat, or entertainment and does bring joy, albeit short-lived (Backstrom, 2006; Jin & Sternquist, 2004; Richins, 2013). The hedonic perspective posits that positive emotional experiences not only underlie consumer behavior (Alba & Williams, 2013), but serve as feedback for companies to improve services and can be leveraged for greater organizational wellbeing, especially when the positives (i.e., compliments, gratitude and positive consumer experiences) are examined (Nasr, Burton, Gruber, & Kitshoff, 2014).

Topic Box: Warning!

Materialism, the value placed on attaining money and possessions, and the resulting overconsumption to convey it, is known to undermine wellbeing (Sirgy et al., 2013). It is associated with lower self-esteem, life satisfaction and positive affect, a more negative self-image, anxiety, compulsive buying, debt, poor money management, smoking, drinking, depression, treating others less empathically, and holding less sustainable environmental attitudes and behaviors (Brown & Vergragt, 2016; Brown et al., 2016; Dittmar et al., 2014; Donnelly, Iyer, & Howell, 2012; Hurst, Dittmar, Bond, & Kasser, 2013; Kasser, 2018; Kasser et al., 2014; Nepomuceno & Laroche, 2015). Kasser et al. (2014) showed that while highly materialistic consumers experienced a rise in positive emotion at the point of buying, they also experienced stronger post-purchase unpleasant emotion. In contrast, high subjective wellbeing consumers prefer more frequent, low-cost, everyday purchases for sociability and self-improvement over expensive indulgences regardless of wealth (Zhong & Mitchell, 2012).

What contributes to hedonic responses varies. Lim (2014) suggests that hedonic responses in the hospitality industry result from five factors. Service quality involves the level of customer expectation versus its delivery, while the service-scape, the feel of the physical environment in which transactions occur, such as scent (Leenders, Smidts, & El Haji, 2016) and sound (Morrison, Gan, Dubelaar, & Oppewal, 2011) are also involved. The level of exclusivity and distinctiveness consumers feel in relation to others (Teimourpour & Hanzaee, 2011), the brand's reputation offering a sense of familiarity, pride, belonging, and self-confidence, and finally, the degree of personalization, that is, how well needs and habits are catered for, are other contributors. These allow positive emotions to arise, which increase satisfaction and perceived value for money, boosting return intentions. In the tourism industry, hedonic experiences depend on weather, other tourists, political situations, abilities and interest, and overlap with eudaimonic experiences too. Travelers report their best holidays to be those with positive and negative emotion as well as meaningful experience, such that pleasure can be had from a good meal or concert, but a grueling alpine ascent can also be transformative and make a trip memorable (Knobloch, Robertson, & Aitken, 2017).

The difficulty in separating hedonic from eudaimonic motives has been noted, given that life experiences contain both; nonetheless, Alba and Williams' (2013) review posits that hedonic experiences can emerge from many areas. Namely, product aesthetics (how something looks, feels and works; Jordan, 2000; Norman, 2004), interaction with the product (versus merely having it), the meaning attached to products and services (e.g., Newman, Diesendruck, & Bloom, 2011), giving or spending money on others (Geenen, Hohelüchter, Langholf, & Walther, 2014) and having expectations met (Lee, Frederick, & Ariely, 2006). The desire to savor or create nostalgia and positive memories for later (Keinan, & Kivetz, 2011; Zauberman, Ratner, & Kim, 2008) and developing a sense of expertise (LaTour & LaTour, 2010) from product engagement are other sources. Yet, as with all things pleasurable, too much, too often and in the same way diminishes the value of hedonic experiences. As such, introducing variety into service and product experiences can slow adaptation (Percival Carter & Williams, 2014; Wang, Novemsky, & Dhar, 2009) and maximize the effects of positive emotional experiences over time.

3.5.2 Eudaimonic Consumer Experiences

While it is difficult to parse products and services into hedonic and eudaimonic categories, types of consumer experience help frame a eudaimonic view (Carter & Gilovich, 2012; Van Boven & Gilovich, 2003). Consumers can buy objects like shoes, watches or television sets or experiences, such as a ski trip or hot air balloon ride, with the difference being that objects are to have, use and be seen with, whereas experiences are about feeling and meaning making. When experiences are good, consumers tend to rate them higher on satisfaction than they do products (Nicolao, Irwin, & Goodman, 2009). They also derive more satisfaction from them as experiences facilitate social connection (Chan & Mogilner, 2017; Kumar & Gilovich, 2015; Kumar, Mann, & Gilovich, 2014) and foster a sense of appreciation and gratitude, with individuals engaging in more prosocial behavior and generosity thereafter as well (Walker, Kumar & Gilovich, 2016). Bastos (2012) even found that individuals buying experiences were perceived as more worthy of respect than individuals focusing on material objects alone. Focusing on experiential aspects of consumption contributes to a person's sense of self and identity (Carter & Gilovich, 2012; Kumar et al., 2014) and allows individuals to fulfill roles, as well as the identities they desire for themselves (Sirgy et al., 2016). The stories they derive from lifestyle experiences maintain a positive self-view and create a sense of wellbeing (Carter & Gilovich, 2012). Finally, experiential purchases are likely to fulfill one's psychological needs posited by self-determination theory (Ryan et al., 2008) of autonomy, connection, and competency, which also lead to subjective wellbeing (Howell, Pchelin, & Iyer, 2012).

3.5.3 Social Connections and Consumerism

The literature points to two areas in this domain: the connections made during and after a consumer experience, as well as the connections made around it. In the first instance, we point to the experiential aspects of consumption which are often consumed as social events, i.e., a movie and dinner, while physical objects are often consumed individually, i.e., socks and toothpaste (Caprariello & Reis, 2013). In the second, consumers talk about and connect around their experiences to a larger degree than with objects. Experiences create meaningful life events that outlive the importance of material objects in memory. For example, a weekend in Paris may be recounted and spoken of years later, while a shirt, no matter how expensive, is fast forgotten (Kumar & Gilovich, 2015). Experiences encourage social connections not only at the time of consumption but strengthen relationships longer-term through recounting or storytelling. Experiential sharing helps facilitate others' understanding of, kinship with, and desire to connect with the teller. For instance, recounting one's trip provides insight into one's personality in a way that objects cannot (Carter & Gilovich, 2012; Kumar, Mann, & Gilovich, 2014).

Also facilitating sociability are brand communities, where brands connect with consumers and consumers with one another on social media. These communities provide a new set of tools for marketers towards empowering consumers to become active avenues for information (i.e., "How do I change my camera lens?"), and providing a sense of meaning, pleasure, belonging, self-disclosure, mutual trust and identity creation (i.e., "I'm a Dior girl!") (Diffley, Kearns, Bennett, & Kawalek, 2011; Morandin, Bagozzi, & Bergami, 2013; Veloutsou & Moutinho, 2009). S-commerce, the interactions and commerce that occur through social media channels, lead to consumer loyalty, satisfaction, and greater purchase intentions as consumers conform and seek peer approval (Bianchi, Andrews, Wiese, & Fazal-E-Hasan, 2017; Hajli, 2015; Wang, Yu, & Wei, 2012; Yadav, de Valck, Hennig-Thurau, Hoffman, & Spann, 2013). But what is of most value to organizations and consumers is the creation of weak ties, increasingly larger networks of people who would not ordinarily come together that provide support, product referral, and conviviality adding brand value and elements of sociability traditional shopping does not do (Rassega et al., 2015).

3.5.4 Consumerism and the Natural/Built Environment

A sustainable lifestyle is often perceived as sacrificial work. Yet, such choices are correlated with high levels of life satisfaction and wellbeing (Kasser & Sheldon, 2002; Xiao & Li, 2011). Venhoeven, Bolderdijk, and Steg (2013) nonetheless explain that sustainable choices may lower hedonic wellbeing, but increase eudaimonic wellbeing. Individuals who place value on eudaimonic pursuits (i.e., strivings, relationships, learning) and universalist values (appreciating and protecting people and nature), tend to engage in ethical, sustainable consumption behavior (Ganglmair-

Wooliscroft & Wooliscroft, 2017; Thomas & Sharpe, 2013). Increasingly, consumers also feel businesses have a responsibility to do more around social problems, wanting brands to declare their values and take a stand. They are willing to punish brands who fail to act on their values (Edelman, 2017; SproutSocial, 2018). They also believe business has a responsibility to produce socially responsible products and expect ethical considerations to extend throughout the supply chain and attend to issues of child labour, fair trade, and the provision of living wages as examples. Alternative values to curb consumption and to have softer impacts on the environment may be needed as marketing efforts have inadvertently framed environmentalism as a feminine value, with such products seen as unmanly (Brough, Wilkie, Ma, Isaac, & Gal, 2016). Yet, studies show it takes little to sensitize consumers to greener choices (Penz, Hofmann, & Hartl, 2017).

Topic Box: Is Green Going Mainstream?

The opportunity for companies to have less of an impact on the environment is ripe for exploitation. Neither companies nor governments need to wait for consumer demands to dictate better design and stronger regulation. For example, Saltwater Brewery (USA) switched to making their 6-pack plastic holders into biodegradable, edible food for sea turtles. The holders decompose in landfills, but if they make their way into oceans, they serve as a source of food for sea life. North Face, maker of high quality outdoor gear, has started a line called *Renewed*, made up of their own cleaned, refurbished, previously owned garments. Swedish furniture maker, IKEA also recently pledged to use only renewable and recycled materials in its products by 2030, while Hugo Boss even developed a line of shoes made solely from Piñatex, leather derived from pineapple leaf fibers. Most recently, the government of Chile banned the use of plastic bags in a bid to protect its coastline, with regional Oman declaring the same. It is possible to capitalize on this wave of responsible innovation and leadership that moves the development of environmentally sustainable products and practises away from the fringe and into the mainstream so that green options simply become the norm.

The built environment also affects consumers. The traditional focus on atmospherics (i.e., music, color and other variables to explain consumer behavior) is limiting and developers are moving towards the creation of experiences instead (Petermans, Janssens, & Van Cleempoel, 2013). The trend of turning malls into mixed-use open facilities with non-shopping activity (i.e., gym, play areas, hotel, cinema, art gallery, cooking station, entertainment stage, etc.), greenery and nature (i.e., birds, fish), and interaction spaces (i.e., co-working spaces, comfortable seating, open space to people watch) is growing (Yan & Eckman, 2009). Consumers prefer and feel less stressed in these spaces (Brengman et al., 2012; Joye, Willems, Brengmen, & Wolf, 2010; Mower, Kim, & Childs, 2012; Rosenbaum, Ramírez, & Camino, 2018; Rosenbaum, Otalora, & Ramirez, 2016; Tifferet & Vilnai-Yavetz,

2017), spend more time there and in some, are willing to pay more for such products and services (Gwozdz, Steensen Nielsen, & Müller, 2017; Morrison & Beer, 2017; Wolf, 2005). This is explained by Attention Restoration Theory (ART; Kaplan, 1995), which posits that nature helps restore and regenerate attention which, once tired through over-stimuli, limits the ability to focus and regulate negative emotion and behavior (i.e., impatience, stress). ART incorporates elements that allow consumers to take a break from fatigue and duty, move with ease in large spaces, and meet autonomous goals in settings that capture their attention (Felsten, 2009; Rosenbaum & Massiah, 2011; Rosenbaum, Ramírez, & Camino, 2018). Reinventing malls may contribute to social wellbeing (Anderson et al., 2013; Rosenbaum et al., 2016; Söderlund & Newman, 2015) through experiences of socializing, walking, and learning, especially in light of growing loneliness (Holt-Lunstad et al., 2017; Kim, Kang, & Kim, 2005). Building developers will see a role for the creation of such spaces which, along with environmental sustainability, prioritize wellbeing.

3.6 The Product and Service Experience

To date, the design approach has focused on productivity, speed, performance and safety, and perhaps by accident, wellbeing. Yet, there is growing interest in how technology, computing, user experience and design can increase the quality of human experience and wellbeing (Botella et al., 2012; Calvo & Peters, 2014; Desmet & Podshlmeyer, 2013; Gaggioli et al., 2017; Jimenez, Pohlmeyer, & Desmet, 2015). As such, the domains of positive technology, positive computing and positive design overlap, sharing the goal of user wellbeing through the innovation of new products and services or re-engineered ones. These fields developed in response to evidence around the harmful effects of contemporary design and technology, such as young people using video games to replace outdoor play, or adults avoiding sleep and exercise to scroll through social media at night and neglect their partners by day. The harms of technology and/or products are often not foreseen until after they enter the market. Thus, an explicit wellbeing focus in the design of products and services is required and made possible when approached from the integration of positive emotion, goal strivings, sociability and sustainability by product and service design teams (Yoon, Pohlmeyer, & Desmet, 2016).

Positive design is not a smiley campaign to flog new products, nor an algorithm to determine consumer likes. Instead, it is a philosophy behind design. Pavliscak's (2015) Positive Design Manifesto for example, contends its essentials include a product that entails freedom of choice, is intuitive to use, and involves a sense of control. It creates autonomous mastery, supports creativity, builds trust and connectivity, and enables meaning. Pohlmeyer's (2012) Design Wellbeing Matrix proposes that products can be the direct source of happiness (i.e., chocolate), or allow the user to attain happiness indirectly (i.e., running shoes allow for marathon training that brings satisfaction over time). Products can have symbolic value and represent an ideal, value or memory, while products like pedometers, sleep apps or other wearables support users towards wellbeing goals by developing self-knowledge, autonomy, and self-efficacy to track improvement across food consumption, physical activity, emotions, and other areas destined for change (Suh & Cheung, 2017).

Sääksjärvi and Hellén (2013) similarly propose that wellbeing design offers a serious value proposition to businesses. This design includes sociability aspects such as sharing (co-sharing a car, home, or garden), altruism (buying gifts for others, or making donations), supporting others (commenting on other's exercise goals on a running shoe brand website), co-usage such that a product/service requires the help of others to be used (i.e., two-seated bicycle or swing), interactions (i.e., reducing noise levels, offering group seating, and board games for strangers to interact) and a sense of belonging (focusing on aspects of group identity and commonalities and offering group activity like Harley Davidson group rides). They propose that wellbeing designs aim for purpose and meaning, which can include helping consumers rally around a social or environmental issue or choose personal goals and strive to attain these, like an app designed to track financial savings and reinforce one's values at the same time. Designing for wellbeing also includes providing for a sense of doing which facilitates flow and learning, versus only having.

Alternatively, Desmet and Pohlmeyer's (2013) design model includes pleasure (positive emotion and experience), significance (meaning and strivings), and attention to virtue (goodness, character strength and moral action). The hedonic features of a service or product are pleasant to use, interesting, awe-inducing, inspiring, or evoke gratitude, fascination, confidence, or pride as examples (Desmet, 2012). Negative emotions like frustration, boredom, confusion, or anxiety are avoided, yet, not all are bad; video gamers remain interested through goals, the use of skills and effort, as well as the right amount of frustration and challenge (Fokkinga & Desmet, 2012). "Good" negative emotional experiences can lead to flow (Csikszentmihalyi, 2006). Positive design also allows users to do the right thing through the elicitation of strengths (i.e., persistence, integrity, self-control, tolerance, benevolence) (Peterson & Seligman, 2004) aimed at the self, others or the environment, whereby products and services nudge users to do good. An example would be an online checkout prompt, stating: "82% of our customers donate to causes – will you be next?" Virtues extend to philanthropy, honesty (i.e., reporting crime), selflessness (i.e., giving blood), or environmentalism (i.e., accepting store credit to forgo packaging).

Desmet and Pohlmeyer (2013) also suggest that products should be possibility-driven. It is not enough to *remove* the bad like current problem-driven design, it must *add* something positive (Desmet & Hassenzahl, 2012; Jimenez, Pohlmeyer, Desmet, & Huzen, 2014). To illustrate this point: Most design approaches solve problems, i.e., lawnmowers cut unruly grass, high-speed trains cut commute times, and lamps illuminate the dark. But a possibility-driven approach considers what is possible, such that in cutting grass, a mower might also sow flower seeds. Positive product design strives for balance and does not undermine other aspects of wellbeing either. For example, athletes take nutrient replacements for energy, but these should not increase cholesterol as well. The activity, service or product must be customizable (Fritz & Lyubomirsky, 2018) and attend to timing, variety, size, color, branding options, and users' needs. Products should also facilitate an active involvement. Too much automa-

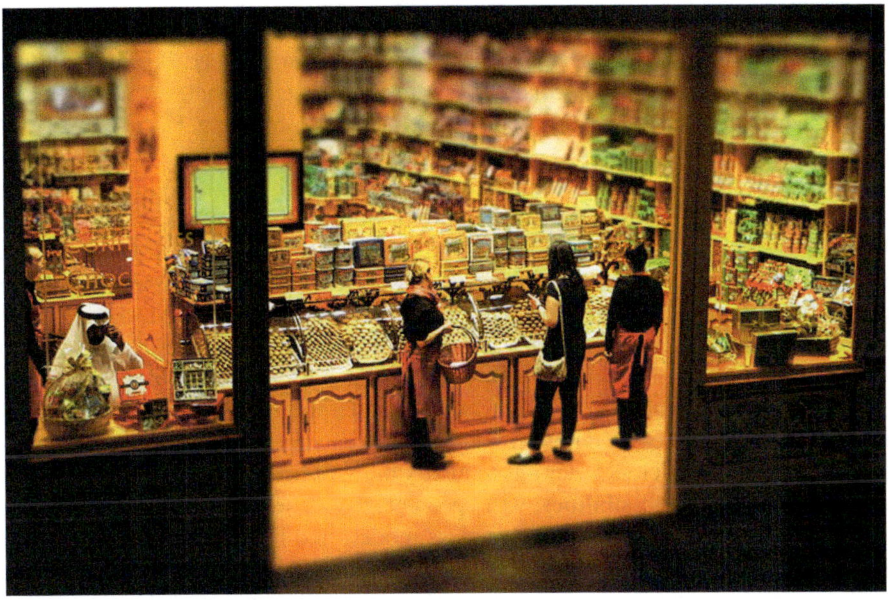

Fig. 3.2 Product and service experience in the UAE. *Photo credit* Pixabay

tion reduces a sense of competence and autonomy. For example, photographers prefer to master apertures versus automating them. Positive design finally creates a long-term impact on the user implicating personal development and involvement through which consumers develop loyal, meaningful and durable relationships that support their aspirations and self-perceptions (Casais, Mugge & Desmet, 2015; Mugge et al., 2005), and address sustainability concerns. To this effect, Sohn and Nam (2015) add that wellbeing design also requires better feedback (i.e., energy indicators, dashboards) to help consumers immediately see their environmental impact as this is usually divorced from use, giving consumers a false sense of confidence (Fig. 3.2).

Designing for wellbeing necessarily involves attention to marketing, which bears a responsibility for whether and how products and services are consumed. The marketer's dilemma is not new: how to make consumers happy so they buy, but not so much that they destroy their own wellbeing or that of society. Early marketing efforts focused on ethical marketing strategies to enhance consumer wellbeing (Sirgy & Lee, 2008) via the product life cycle and in a manner that was safe for the consumer, community, and environment. But, today's focus has moved to positive marketing (Lerman & Shefrin, 2015), leveraging positive emotions, exercising character strengths, facilitating accomplishments and doing good by way of one's community and environment. The approach aims to help consumers feel good about their purchases and understand why. It differs from standard practises aimed at the remediation of failure for which a product or service is offered. In fact, when consumers are exposed to messaging suggesting that wealth and possessions are valued, levels of materialism, competitiveness and negative affect rise (Bauer, Wilkie, Kim, & Bodenhausen, 2012; Brown et al., 2016; Kasser et al., 2014). Positive marketing strategies and guidelines that focus on positive emotional, social and goal driven aspects of experience or products are needed (Lerman & Kachersky, 2012) (Table 3.2).

In sum, designing and marketing for greater wellbeing is still in its infancy and work is needed around translating the science of wellbeing into products and services. User experiences need to be translated into meaningful feedback for designers and marketers, who together as a team must align wellbeing aims. A clear understanding of wellbeing is needed to do so as many designers simply revert to developing next-generation designs, instead of truly designing for wellbeing. As consumers often buy for the purpose of becoming happy and in line with their identities and values, there is great opportunity for designers to broaden their scope and include all of the categories specified to date. Moving away from superficial value propositions, like decorative and useless functions to justify higher prices, towards more authentic ones, like wellbeing possibilities, will open design and service territories as well as market share, invariably changing business models and industries towards smarter, less environmentally impactful, and more experience-oriented consumption to make societies feel, be, and do good over time (Desmet & Pohlmeyer, 2013; Sääksjärvi, & Hellén, 2013). By taking advantage of the wellbeing concept, product and service designers, as well as organizations, from which corporate social responsibility programs can be driven (Koo, 2016), may fulfill their obligations to elevate the status of those who make, buy, sell, and are affected by commercial activity.

3.7 Implications for the UAE

We have put forward an initial scheme for the prioritization and operationalization of the commercial life components which include the consumer, employee and product/service experiences underscored by the hedonic, eudaimonic, social, and environmental paths to greater wellbeing. These categories are consistent with the observations made in the WHR (Helliwell et al., 2012) that happiness is contingent upon sustainability, social life and everyday joys as well as meaningful moments. It is also consistent with the recent WHR mandate for organizations to more seriously attend to happiness and wellbeing in the workplace (Sachs, 2019). While covering only a smattering of evidence, we readily acknowledge that this scheme has far reaching implications. Rethinking commercial life will demand labour reforms, workplace legislation, greater access to innovation funds and spaces for idea incubation, and a reconsideration of marketing guidelines around product advertising, especially to children, to better withstand the pressures of overconsumption, are only the beginning.

Objective standards to guide the development of goods, products and services that directly aim to increase wellbeing and do so sustainably and ethically are also needed, which include government-directed means to measure and certify such processes. A commercial code of wellbeing conduct and other standards are also needed where

Table 3.2 Commercial life pillars

Pillar	Hedonic	Eudaimonic	Social	Environment	
				Built	Natural
Work life	Positive emotions from one's work, colleagues, and interactions with customers, and/or external vendors result in cognitive, health, social and psychological resources that strengthen job performance.	Feeling valued, understanding how decisions are made, and achieving autonomy, competence, and relatedness lead to eudaimonic wellbeing. Effort, character, and purpose matter.	Workplace connections lead to greater support, performance, involvement, retention, and engagement by fostering a sense of belonging and pride.	Work spaces affect employee wellbeing, safety and productivity. Natural light, greenery and open spaces reduce stress, illness; boosts prosocial acts.	Organizational commitments to positively impact the natural environment can improve employee productivity and make recruitment of new personnel easier.
Consumer	Consumption of objects, services, or the serviscapes in which they occur impact satisfaction. Short-lived joys fuel purchase behavior, user experience, satisfaction, brand loyalty, and product attachment.	Consumers defeat challenges via self-improving experiences which boost social ties, gratitude, generosity, competency and autonomy.	Consumption activities provide the impetus for relationship building that creates/sustains social ties and boosts identity.	Consumers prefer to spend time and money in retail settings that are green, airy, open, and have natural lighting; such spaces make them feel more social, relaxed, autonomous, and refreshed.	Consumers care about ethical/environmental issues and respect organizations that truthfully protect/promote such issues; They feel more satisfied by consuming in line with their values.
Product/Service	Product/services build positive emotional experiences, and promote states and emotions like awe, interest, gratitude, benevolence, love, tolerance to create impact.	Products/ services provide opportunities to accomplish goals and have meaningful, flow-inducing moments that lead to growth and subjective wellbeing.	Products/ services are used by multiple individuals, strengthening social capital, building trust among consumers and promoting altruism.	Products/services that integrate nature with the built world are needed to offset the loss of natural environments. Offerings add possibilities as well as solve issues.	Goods/services that protect/promote the natural world are needed for human survival. Actions to help people rally for issues and see environmental impact creates meaning and purpose.

setting defaults are preselected with green options as an example, such that photocopy makers defaults are set to double-sided photocopying, or air conditioning units are pre-set at 23°. More can be done for entities to become green but government regulators are often more fearful than businesses themselves to support such issues. Yet, it is wanted by consumers (Simões, 2016; Vringer, Heijden, Soest, Vollebergh, & Dietz, 2017). A rethink must also consider the definition of and incentivization of good customer service. Commercial entities can also reorganize existing wellbeing teams to not only focus on employee wellbeing, but include on this team key people who consider the consumer, environmental, social, infrastructure, and product/service determinants of wellbeing.

Efforts will also need to convince people that having money is not the problem, but how it is valued, pursued, spent and at what consequence for intangibles. This may go against a liberal market system where freedom of choice is prized. Yet research shows that investing in experiences that generate positive emotions, facilitate goal strivings and deepen relationships should be the priority (Van Boven & Gilovich, 2003) as opposed to objects which are subject to planned obsolescence, social comparisons (Carter & Gilovich, 2010), environmental harm (Ivanova et al., 2016) and to which we easily adapt (Lyubomirsky, 2011). Less consumption does not have to come at the cost of less happiness (Venhoeven et al., 2013), but how to reconcile wellbeing research with a "citizen as consumer" model and the need for economic prosperity will be a hurdle for policymakers, governments and researchers alike (Barr, Shaw, & Coles, 2011).

The WHR (Helliwell et al., 2012) argued for a comprehensive review of all government decision-making and policy design to embed wellbeing as a starting point for policy-making while ensuring that decision-makers move beyond current conceptions of economic progress. As such, governments must adopt consultative policy-making processes with the supply and demand side and find ways to incorporate new measurement and evaluation models. Holistic policy development must re-evaluate what entails a good life. A new paradigm, built on human progress, enlightenment, and eudaimonic growth must take primacy. Governments interested in leading the way globally and who have wellbeing at heart will step up to this consumer, employee and product/service challenge. While some may shudder at the ethical implications of implementing design and service recommendations for greater wellbeing, the implications of doing so are no greater than governments mandating seatbelts, no smoking zones, and immunizations. Good governments support the wellbeing of citizens all the time.

The UAE, whom we nominate to adopt the challenge, already assumes a global leadership role in implementing wellbeing principles as the foundation for public policy and aligns government services to have a wellbeing component within its core activities. It has also created happiness and wellbeing officers in line ministries tasked with championing new ways of thinking about policy design and implementation. The Dubai government has also, to an extent, focused on consumer happiness through its feedback system in all municipal departments, measuring the quality of its services. As such, we believe the UAE is best placed to champion wellbeing-based public policy and governance through the commercial life pillars, given its pioneering spirit, the foresight of its leadership, and the desire of its citizens and residents to become transformative forces with respect to human development.

References

Aknin, L. B., Dunn, E. W., & Norton, M. I. (2012). Happiness runs in a circular motion: Evidence for a positive feedback loop between prosocial spending and happiness. *Journal of Happiness Studies, 13,* 347–355.

Alba, J. W., & Williams, E. F. (2013). Pleasure principles: A review of research on hedonic consumption. *Journal of Consumer Psychology, 23*(1), 2–18.

Albanesi, C., Cicognani, E., & Zani, B. (2007). Sense of community, civic engagement and social well-being in Italian adolescents. *Journal of Community & Applied Social Psychology, 17*(5), 387–406.

Anderson, L., Ostrom, A. L., Corus, C., Fisk, R. P., Gallan, A. S., Giraldo, M., & Shirahada, K. (2013). Transformative service research: An agenda for the future. *Journal of Business Research, 66*(8), 1203–1210.

Avey, J., Wernsing, T. S., & Luthans, F. (2008). Can positive employees help positive organizational change? Impact of psychological capital and emotions on relevant attitudes and behaviors. *The Journal of Applied Behavioral Science, 44*(1), 48–70.

Backstrom, K. (2006). Understanding recreational shopping: A new approach. *The International Review of Retail, Distribution and Consumer Research, 16*(2), 143–158.

Baker, C. L., Flores, N. M., Zou, K. H., Bruno, M., & Harrison, V. J. (2017). Benefits of quitting smoking on work productivity and activity impairment in the United States, the European Union and China. *International Journal of Clinical Practice, 71*(1), e12900.

Barr, S., Shaw, G., & Coles, T. (2011). Times for (un)sustainability? Challenges and opportunities for developing behaviour change policy. A case-study of consumers at home and away. *Global Environmental Change, 21,* 1234–1244.

Barsade, S. (2002). The ripple effect: Emotional contagion and its influence on group behavior. *Administrative Science Quarterly, 47,* 644–675.

Barton, J., & Pretty, J. (2010). What is the best dose of nature and green exercise for improving mental health. *Environmental Science and Technology, 44,* 3947–3955.

Bastos, W. (2012). *Can purchases make us happier? Perhaps, if we tell others about them.* University of Arizona, Published Doctoral dissertation. Retrieved from https://repository.arizona.edu/handle/10150/297047.

Bauer, M. A., Wilkie, J. E., Kim, J. K., & Bodenhausen, G. V. (2012). Cueing consumerism: Situational materialism undermines personal and social wellbeing. *Psychological Science, 23,* 517–523.

Beatley, T. (2016). *Handbook of biophilic city planning and design.* Washington, D.C: Island Press.

Berman, E. M., West, J. P., & Richter, M. N. (2002). Workplace relations: Friendship patterns and consequences (according to managers). *Public Administration Review, 2,* 217–230.

Bianchi, C., Andrews, L., Wiese, M., & Fazal-E-Hasan, S. (2017). Consumer intentions to engage in s-commerce: A cross-national study. *Journal of Marketing Management, 33*(5–6), 464–494.

Biddle, S. J. H., Mutrie, N., & Gorely, T. (2015). *Psychology of physical activity: Determinants, wellbeing and interventions* (3rd ed.). London, England: Routledge.

Biscaia, R., Correia, A., Rosado, A., Marôco, J., & Ross, S. (2012). The effects of emotions on football spectator's satisfaction and behavioural intentions. *European Sport Management Quarterly, 12,* 227–242.

Boehm, J. K., & Lyubomirsky, S. (2008). Does happiness lead to career success? *Journal of Career Assessment, 16,* 101–116.

Botella, C., Riva, G., Gaggioli, A., Wiederhold, B. K., Alcaniz, M., & Baños, R. M. (2012). The present and future of positive technologies. *Cyberpsychology, Behavior, and Social Networking, 15*(2), 78–84.

Boubekri, M., Cheung, I. N., Reid, K. J., Wang, C.-H., & Zee, P. C. (2014). Impact of windows and daylight exposure on overall health and sleep quality of office workers: A case-control pilot study. *Journal of Clinical Sleep Medicine, 10*(6), 603–611.

Brengman, M., Willems, K., & Joye, Y. (2012). The impact of in-store greenery on customers. *Psychology and Marketing, 29*(11), 807–821.

Brough, A. R., Wilkie, J. E. B., Ma, J., Isaac, M. S., & Gal, D. (2016). Is eco-friendly unmanly? The green-feminine stereotype and its effect on sustainable consumption. *Journal of Consumer Research, 43*(4), 567–582.

Brown, H. S., & Vergragt, P. J. (2016). From consumerism to wellbeing: Toward a cultural transition? *Journal of Cleaner Production, 132,* 308–317.

Brown, D. K., Barton, J. L., & Gladwell, V. F. (2013). Viewing nature scenes positively affects recovery of autonomic function following acute-mental stress. *Environmental Science and Technology, 47,* 5562–5569.

Brown, K. W., Kasser, T., Ryan, R. M., & Konow, J. (2016). Materialism, spending, and affect: An event-sampling study of marketplace behavior and its affective costs. *Journal of Happiness Studies, 17*(6), 2277–2292.

Browning, W. D., Ryan, C. O., & Clancy, J. O. (2014). *14 patterns of biophilic design*. New York, NY: Terrapin Bright Green, LLC. Retrieved from https://www.terrapinbrightgreen.com/wp-content/uploads/2014/09/14-Patterns-of-Biophilic-Design-Terrapin-2014p.pdf.

Bruni, L. (2010). The happiness of sociality. Economics and eudaimonia: A necessary encounter. *Rationality and Society, 22(4), 383–406.*

Burroughs, J. E., & Rindfleish, A. (2011). What welfare? On the definition and domain of transformative consumer research and the foundational role of materialism. In D. G. Mick, S. Pettigrew, C. Pechmann, & J. L. Ozanne (Eds.), *Transformative consumer research for personal and collective wellbeing* (pp. 245–262). New York, NY: Taylor & Francis.

Calvo, R. A., & Peters, D. (2014). *Positive computing: Technology for wellbeing and human potential*. Cambridge, UK: MIT Press.

Cantor, D. E., Morrow, P. C., & Montabon, F. (2012). Engagement in environmental behaviours among supply chain management employees: An organizational support theoretical perspective. *The Journal of Supply Chain Management, 48*(3), 33–51.

Capaldi, C. A., Passmore, H.-A., Nisbet, E. K., Zelenski, J. M., & Dopko, R. L. (2015). Flourishing in nature: A review of the benefits of connecting with nature and its application as a wellbeing intervention. *International Journal of Wellbeing, 5*(4), 1–16.

Caprariello, P. A., & Reis, H. T. (2013). To do, to have, or to share? Valuing experiences over material possessions depends on the involvement of others. *Journal of Personality and Social Psychology, 104*(2), 199–215.

Carnevale, P. J. (2008). Positive effect and decision frame in negotiation. *Group Decision and Negotiation, 17,* 51–63.

Carter, T. J., & Gilovich, T. (2010). The relative relativity of material and experiential purchases. *Journal of Personality and Social Psychology, 98,* 146–159.

Carter, T. J., & Gilovich, T. (2012). I am what I do, not what I have: The differential centrality of experiential and material purchases to the self. *Journal of Personality and Social Psychology, 102,* 1304–1317.

Casais, M., Mugge, R., & Desmet, P. M. A. (2015). Extending product life by introducing symbolic meaning: An exploration of design strategies to support subjective wellbeing. In T. Cooper, N. Braithwaite, M. Moreno & G. Salvia (Eds.), *Product lifetimes and the environment (PLATE) Conference Proceedings,* Nottingham Trent University, CADBE (pp. 44–51).

Casey, D., & Sieber, S. (2016). Employees, sustainability and motivation: Increasing employee engagement by addressing sustainability and corporate social responsibility. *Research in Hospitality Management, 6*(1), 69–76.

Castro Solano, A., & Cosentino, A. C. (2016). The relationships between character strengths and life fulfillment in the view of lay-people in Argentina. *Interdisciplinaria [online], 33*(1), 65–80.

Ceja, L., & Navarro, J. (2011). Dynamic patterns of flow in the workplace: Characterizing within-individual variability using a complexity science approach. *Journal of Organizational Behavior, 32*, 627–651.

Chan, C., & Mogilner, C. (2017). Experiential gifts are more socially connecting than material gifts. *Journal of Consumer Research, 43*(6), 913–931.

Chancellor, J., Layous, K., Margolis, S., & Lyubomirsky, S. (2017). Clustering by wellbeing in workplace social networks: Homophily and social contagion. *Emotion, 17*(8), 1166–1180.

Chancellor, J., Margolis, S. M., & Lyubomirsky, S. (2018). The propagation of everyday prosociality in the workplace. *The Journal of Positive Psychology, 13*, 271–283.

Chi, N., Chung, Y., & Tsai, T. (2011). How do happy leaders enhance team success? The mediating roles of transformational leadership, group affective tone, and team processes. *Journal of Applied Social Psychology, 41*, 1421–1454.

Chiaburu, D. S., & Harrison, D. A. (2008). Do peers make the place? Conceptual synthesis and meta-analysis of coworker effects on perceptions, attitudes, OCBs, and performance. *Journal of Applied Psychology, 93*, 1082–1103.

Chitturi, R. (2009). Emotions by design: A consumer perspective. *International Journal of Design, 3*(2), 7–17.

Chuang, S. C. (2007). Sadder but wiser or happier and smarter? A demonstration of judgment and decision-making. *Journal of Psychology, 141*, 63–76.

Cohn, M. A., Fredrickson, B. L., Brown, S. L., Mikels, J. A., & Conway, A. M. (2009). Happiness unpacked: Positive emotions increase life satisfaction by building resilience. *Emotion, 9*(3), 361–368.

Crede, M., Chernyshenko, O. S., Stark, S., Dalal, R. S., & Bashshur, M. (2007). Job satisfaction as mediator: An assessment of job satisfaction's position within the nomological network. *Journal of Occupational and Organizational Psychology, 80*, 515–538.

Csikszentmihalyi, M. (2006). Introduction. In M. Csikszentmihalyi & I. S. Csikszentmihalyi (Eds.), *A life worth living: Contributions to positive psychology* (pp. 3–14). New York, NY: Oxford University Press.

Dalal, R. S., Baysinger, M., Brummel, B. J., & Lebreton, J. M. (2012). The relative importance of employee engagement, other job attitudes, and trait affect as predictors of job performance. *Journal of Applied Social Psychology, 42*, E295–E325.

De Neve, J.-E., Diener, E., Tay, L., & Xuereb, C. (2013). The objective benefits of subjective wellbeing. In J. Helliwell, R. Layard, & J. Sachs (Eds.), *World Happiness Report* 2013. New York, NY: UN Sustainable Development Solutions Network.

Delmas, M. A., & Pekovic, S. (2013). Environmental standards and labor productivity: Understanding the mechanisms that sustain sustainability. *Journal of Organizational Behavior, 4*, 230–252.

Delmas, M. A., & Pekovic, S. (2018). Organizational configurations for sustainability and employee productivity: A qualitative comparative analysis approach. *Business and Society, 57*(1), 216–251.

Desmet, P. M. A. (2012). Faces of product pleasure: 25 positive emotions in human–product interactions. *International Journal of Design, 6*(2), 1–29.

Desmet, P. M. A., & Hassenzahl, M. (2012). Towards happiness: Possibility-driven design. In M. Zacarias, & J. V. de Oliveira (Eds.), *Human-computer interaction: The agency perspective. Studies in Computational Intelligence* (Vol. 396). Berlin, Gemany: Springer.

Desmet, P. M. A., & Pohlmeyer, A. E. (2013). Positive design: An introduction to design for subjective wellbeing. *International Journal of Design, 7*(3), 5–19.

Dickson-Swift, V., Fox, C., Marshall, K., Welch, N., & Willis, J. (2014). What really improves employee health and wellbeing: Findings from regional Australian workplaces. *International Journal of Workplace Health Management, 7*(3), 138–155.

Diego-Rosell, P., Tortora, R., & Bird, J. J. (2018). International determinants of subjective wellbeing: Living in a subjectively material world. *Journal of Happiness Studies, 19*(1), 123–143.

Diffley, S., Kearns, J., Bennett, W., & Kawalek, P. (2011). Consumer behavior in social networking sites: Implications for marketers. *Irish Journal of Management, 30*(2), 47–65.

Dillard, A. J., Schiavone, A., & Brown, S. L. (2008). Helping behavior and positive emotions: Implications for health and well-being. In S. J. Lopez (Ed.), Positive psychology: Exploring the best in people, Vol. 2. Capitalizing on emotional experiences (pp. 101–114). Westport, CT, US: Praeger Publishers/Greenwood Publishing Group.

Disabato, D. J., Goodman, F. R., Kashdan, T. B., Short, J. L., & Jarden, A. (2016). Different types of wellbeing? A cross-cultural examination of hedonic and eudaimonic wellbeing. *Psychological Assessment, 28*(5), 471–482.

Dittmar, H., Bond, R., Hurst, M., & Kasser, T. (2014). The relationship between materialism and personal wellbeing: A meta-analysis. *Journal of Personality and Social Psychology, 107*(5), 879–924.

Donnelly, G., Iyer, R., & Howell, R. T. (2012). The big five personality traits, material values, and financial wellbeing of self-described money managers. *Journal of Economic Psychology, 33*(6), 1129–1142.

Duckworth, A. L., Kirby, T., Tsukayama, E., Berstein, H., & Ericsson, K. (2010). Deliberate practice spells success: Why grittier competitors triumph at the National Spelling Bee. *Social Psychological and Personality Science, 2,* 174–181.

Edelman. (2017). *Earned brand study, 2017.* Retrieved from https://www.edelman.com/earned-brand.

Eisenberger, R., Jones, J. R., Stinglhamber, F., Shanock, L., & Randall, A. T. (2005). Flow experiences at work: For high need achievers alone? *Journal of Organizational Behavior, 26,* 755–775.

Ekici, A., Sirgy, M. J., Lee, D.-J., Yu, G. B., & Bosnjak, M. (2018). The effects of shopping wellbeing and shopping ill-being on consumer life satisfaction. *Applied Research in Quality of Life, 12*(3), 533–553.

Ekkekakis, P. (2015). Honey, I shrunk the pooled SMD! Guide to critical appraisal of systematic reviews and meta-analyses using the Cochrane review on exercise for depression as example. *Mental Health and Physical Activity, 8,* 21–36.

Ekpu, V. U., & Brown, A. K. (2015). The economic impact of smoking and of reducing smoking prevalence: Review of evidence. *Tobacco Use Insights, 8,* 1–35.

Elci, M., & Alpkan, L. (2009). The impact of perceived organizational ethical climate on work satisfaction. *Journal of Business Ethics, 84,* 297–311.

Felsten, G. (2009). Where to take a study break on the college campus: An attention restoration theory perspective. *Journal of Environmental Psychology, 29*(1), 160–167.

Fliaster, A., & Schloderer, F. (2010). Dyadic ties among employees: Empirical analysis of creative performance and efficiency. *Human Relations, 63,* 1513–1540.

Fokkinga, S., & Desmet, P. M. A. (2012). Darker shades of joy: The role of negative emotion in rich product experiences. *Design Issues, 28*(4), 42–56.

Fredrickson, B. L. (2006). The broaden and build theory of positive emotions. In M. Csikszentmihalyi & I. S. Csikszentmihalyi (Eds.), *A life worth living: Contributions to positive psychology* (pp. 85–103). New York: Oxford University Press.

Fredrickson, B. L., Mancuso, R. A., Branigan, C., & Tugade, M. M. (2000). The undoing effect of positive emotions. *Motivation and Emotion, 24,* 237–258.

Fritz, M. M., & Lyubomirsky, S. (2018). Whither happiness? When, how, and why might positive activities undermine wellbeing. In J. P. Forgas & R. F. Baumeister (Eds.), *The social psychology of living well* (pp. 101–115). New York, NY: Psychology Press.

Fullagar, C. J., & Kelloway, E. K. (2009). Flow at work: An experience sampling approach. *Journal of Occupational and Organizational Psychology, 82,* 595–615.

Gaggioli, A., Riva, G., Peters, D., & Calvo, R. A. (2017). Positive technology, computing, and design: Shaping a future in which technology promotes psychological wellbeing. In M. Jeon (Ed.), *Emotions and affect in human factors and human–computer interaction* (pp. 477–502). London, UK: Academic Press.

Gallup. (2012). *State of the American workplace.* Retrieved from http://www.gallup.com/services/178514/state-american-workplace.aspx.

Ganglmair-Wooliscroft, A., & Wooliscroft, B. (2017). Wellbeing and everyday ethical consumption. *Journal of Happiness Studies*. https://doi.org/10.1007/s10902-017-9944-0.

Gebel, K., Pont, S., Ding, D., Bauman, A. E., Chau, J. Y., Berger, C., … for the CaMos Research Group. (2017). Patterns and predictors of sitting time over ten years in a large population-based Canadian sample: Findings from the Canadian Multicentre Osteoporosis Study (CaMos). *Preventive Medicine Reports, 5,* 289–294.

Geenen, N. Y. R., Hoheluchter, M., Langholf, V., & Walther, E. (2014). The beneficial effects of prosocial spending on happiness: Work hard, make money, and spend it on others? *The Journal of Positive Psychology, 9*(3), 204–208.

Gillet, N., Colombat, P., Michinov, E., Pronost, A., & Fouquereau, E. (2013). Procedural justice, supervisor autonomy support, work satisfaction, organizational identification and job performance: The mediating role of need satisfaction and perceived organizational support. *Journal of Advanced Nursing, 69*(11), 2560–2571.

Goth, U., & Småland, E. (2014). Civic engagement and social capital in ship-preservation work in Norway: The scope, impact, and demographics of formal volunteering and publicly funded engagements. *Nordic Journal of Social Research, 4.* https://doi.org/10.7577/njsr.2071

Grawitch, M., Munz, D., Elliott, E., & Mathis, A. (2003). Promoting creativity in temporary problem-solving groups: The effects of positive mood and autonomy in problem definition on idea-generating performance. *Group Dynamics, 7,* 200 213.

Greening, D. W., & Turban, D. B. (2000). Corporate social performance as a competitive advantage in attracting a quality workforce. *Business and Society, 39,* 254–280.

Guéguen, N., & Stefan, J. (2016). "Green altruism": Short immersion in natural green environments and helping behavior. *Environment and Behavior, 48*(2), 324–342.

Guéguen, N., Meineri, S., & Stefan, J. (2012). "Say it with flowers" … to female drivers: Hitchhikers holding flowers and driver behavior. *North American Journal of Psychology, 14,* 623.

Gwozdz, W., Steensen Nielsen, K., & Müller, T. (2017). An environmental perspective on clothing consumption: Consumer segments and their behavioral patterns. *Sustainability, 9,* 762–789.

Hajli, N. (2015). Social commerce constructs and consumer's intention to buy. *International Journal of Information Management, 35*(2), 183–191.

Harter, J. (2017, December 20). *Dismal employee engagement is a sign of global mismanagement.* Gallup. Retrieved from http://news.gallup.com/opinion/gallup/224012/dismal-employee-engagement-sign-global-mismanagement.aspx.

Headey, B., Muffels, R., & Wooden, M. (2008). Money does not buy happiness: Or does it? A reassessment based on the combined effects of wealth, income and consumption. *Social Indicators Research, 87,* 65–82.

Hefferon, K. M., & Ollis, S. (2006). "Just Clicks": An interpretive phenomenological analysis of professional dancers' experience of flow. *Research in Dance Education, 7*(2), 141–159.

Helliwell, J. F., & Wang, S. (2012). The state of world happiness. In J. F. Helliwell, R. Layard, & J. Sachs (Eds.), *World Happiness Report*. New York, NY: The Earth Institute, Columbia University.

Helliwell, J. F., Layard, R., & Sachs, J. D. (2012). *World Happiness Report.* Retrieved from http://unsdsn.org/wp-content/uploads/2014/02/WorldHappinessReport2013_online.pdf.

Helliwell, J. F., Huang, H., & Wang, S. (2014). Social capital and wellbeing in time of crisis. *Journal of Happiness Studies, 15,* 145–162.

Herrbach, O. (2006). A matter of feeling? The affective tone of organizational commitment and identification. *Journal of Organizational Behavior, 27*(5), 629–643.

Heschong Mahone Group. (2003). *Windows and offices: A study of office worker performance and the indoor environment.* Fair Oaks, CA: CEC, California Energy Commission. Retrieved from http://h-m-g.com/projects/daylighting/summaries%20on%20daylighting.htm.

Higgins, E. (2006). Value from hedonic experience and engagement. *Psychological Review, 113,* 439–460.

Highhouse, S., Hoffman, J. R., Greve, E. M., & Collins, A. E. (2002). Persuasive impact of organziational value statements in a recruitment context. *Journal of Applied Social Psychology, 32,* 1737–1755.

Holt-Lunstad, J., Robles, T. F., & Sbarra, D. A. (2017). Advancing social connection as a public health priority in the United States. *American Psychologist, 72*(6), 517–530.

Hone, L. C., Jarden, A., Duncan, S., & Schofield, G. (2015). Flourishing in New Zealand workers: Associations with lifestyle behaviours, physical health, psychosocial, and work-related indicators. *Journal of Occupational and Environmental Medicine, 57*(9), 973–983.

Howell, R. T., Pchelin, P., & Iyer, R. (2012). The preference for experiences over possessions: Measurement and construct validation of the experiential buying tendency scale. *Journal of Positive Psychology, 7,* 57–71.

Hurst, M., Dittmar, H., Bond, R., & Kasser, T. (2013). The relationship between materialistic values and environmental attitudes and behaviors: A meta-analysis. *Journal of Environmental Psychology, 36,* 257–269.

Huta, V., & Ryan, R. M. (2010). Pursuing pleasure or virtue: The differential and overlapping wellbeing benefits of hedonic and eudaimonic motives. *Journal of Happiness Studies, 11,* 735–762.

Ilies, R., Scott, B. A., & Judge, T. A. (2006). The interactive effects of personal traits and experienced states on intraindividual patterns of citizenship behavior. *Academy of Management Journal, 49,* 561–575.

Ilies, R., Wagner, D., Wilson, K., Ceja, L., Johnson, M., DeRue, S., & Ilgen, D. (2017). Flow at work and basic psychological needs: Effects on well-being. *Applied Psychology, 66*(1), 3–24.

Ivanova, D., Stadler, K., Steen-Olsen, K., Wood, R., Vita, G., Tukker, A., & Hertwich, E. G. (2016). Environmental impact assessment of household consumption. *Journal of Industrial Ecology, 20*(3), 526–536.

Jahncke, H., Hygge, S., Halin, N., Green, A. M., & Dimberg, K. (2011). Open-plan office noise: Cognitive performance and restoration. *Journal of Environmental Psychology, 31*(4), 373–382.

Jimenez, S., Pohlmeyer, A. E., Desmet, P. M. A., & Huzen, G. (2014). Learning from the positive: A structured approach to possibility-driven design. In J. Salamanca, P. Desmet, A. Burbano, G. Ludden, & J. Maya (Eds.), *Proceedings of Colors of Care: The 9th International Conference on Design & Emotion* (pp. 607–615).

Jimenez, S., Pohlmeyer, A. E., & Desmet, P. M. A. (2015). *Positive design reference guide*. Delft: Delft University of Technology.

Jin, B., & Sternquist, B. (2004). Shopping is truly a joy. *The Service Industries Journal, 24*(6), 1–18.

Johnson, K. J., Waugh, C. E., & Fredrickson, B. L. (2010). Smile to see the forest: Facially expressed positive emotions broaden cognition. *Cognition and Emotion, 24,* 299–321.

Jones, D. A., Willness, C. R., & Heller, K. W. (2016). Illuminating the signals job seekers receive from an employer's community involvement and environmental sustainability practices: Insights into why most job seekers are attracted, others are indifferent, and a few are repelled. *Frontiers in Psychology, 7,* 1–16.

Jordan, P. W. (2000). *Designing pleasurable products*. London, UK: Taylor & Francis.

Joye, Y., & Bolderdijk, J.-W. (2014). An exploratory study into the effects of extraordinary nature on emotions, mood, and prosociality. *Frontiers in Psychology, 5,* 1577.

Joye, Y., Willems, K., Brengmen, M., & Wolf, K. (2010). The effects of urban retail greenery on consumer experience. *Urban Forestry & Urban Gardening, 9,* 57–64.

Kahneman, D., & Deaton, A. (2010). High income improves evaluation of life but not emotional wellbeing. *Proceedings of the National Academy of Sciences, 107*(38), 16489–16493.

Kaplan, S. (1995). The restorative benefits of nature: Toward an integrative framework. *Journal of Environmental Psychology, 15*(3), 169–182.

Kasser, T. (2018). Materialism and living well. In E. Diener, S. Oishi, & L. Tay (Eds.), *Handbook of wellbeing*. Salt Lake City, UT: DEF Publishers.

Kasser, T., & Sheldon, K. M. (2002). What makes for a merry Christmas? *Journal of Happiness Studies, 3,* 313–329.

Kasser, T., Rosenblum, K. L., Sameroff, A. J., Deci, E. L., Niemiec, C. P., Ryan, R. M., ... Hawks, S. (2014). Changes in materialism, changes in psychological wellbeing: Evidence from three longitudinal studies and an intervention experiment. *Motivation and Emotion, 38*(1), 1–22.

Keinan, A., & Kivetz, R. (2011). Productivity orientation and the consumption of collectable experiences. *Journal of Consumer Research, 37,* 935–950.

Kellert, S. R. & Calabrese, E. F. (2015). *The practice of biophilic design.* Retrieved from http://www.biophilic-design.com/.

Kellert, S. R., & Wilson, E. O. (1993). *The biophilia hypothesis*. Washington, DC: Island Press.

Kim, S., & Rucker, D. D. (2012). Bracing for the psychological storm: Proactive versus reactive compensatory consumption. *Journal of Consumption Research, 39,* 815–830.

Kim, Y. K., Kang, J., & Kim, M. (2005). The relationships among family and social interaction, loneliness, mall shopping motivation, and mall spending of older consumers. *Psychology & Marketing, 22,* 995–1015.

Kim, J., Kim, Y., & Kim, D. (2017). Improving wellbeing through hedonic, eudaimonic, and social needs fulfillment in sport media consumption. *Sport Management Review, 20*(3), 309–321.

Klarner, P., By, R. T., & Diefenbach, T. (2011). Employee emotions during organizational change—Towards a new research agenda. *Scandinavian Journal of Management, 27*(3), 332–340.

Knight, A. P., & Eisenkraft, N. (2015). Positive is usually good, negative is not always bad: The effects of group affect on social integration and task performance. *Journal of Applied Psychology, 100*(4), 1214–1227.

Knobloch, U., Robertson, K., & Aitken, R. (2017). Experience, emotion, and eudaimonia: A consideration of tourist experiences and wellbeing. *Journal of Travel Research, 56*(5), 651–662.

Koo, Y. (2016). The role of designers in integrating societal value in the product and service development processes. *International Journal of Design, 10*(2), 49–65.

Krekel, C., Ward, G., & De Neve, J.-E. (2019). Employee well-being, productivity, and firm performance: Evidence and case studies. In *Global Happiness and Wellbeing Policy Report 2019* (Chapter 5, pp. 73-94). Dubai, UAE: Global Council for Happiness and Wellbeing. Retrieved from https://s3.amazonaws.com/ghwbpr-2019/UAE/GHWPR19.pdf

Kumar, A., & Gilovich, T. (2015). Some "thing" to talk about? Differential story utility from experiential and material purchases. *Personality and Social Psychology Bulletin, 41,* 1320–1331.

Kumar, A., Mann, T. C., & Gilovich, T. (2014). Questioning the "I" in experience: Experiential purchases foster social connection. *NA—Advances in Consumer Research, 42,* 101–105.

Lambert, L., D'Cruz, A., Schlatter, M., & Barron, F. (2016). Using physical activity to tackle depression: The neglected positive psychology intervention. *Middle East Journal of Positive Psychology, 2*(1), 42–60.

LaTour, K. A., & LaTour, M. S. (2010). Bridging aficionados' perceptual and conceptual knowledge to enhance how they learn from experience. *Journal of Consumer Research, 37,* 688–697.

Lee, L., Frederick, S., & Ariely, D. (2006). Try it, you'll like it: The influence of expectation, consumption, and revelation on preferences for beer. *Psychological Science, 17,* 1054–1058.

Leenders, M. A., Smidts, A., & El Haji, A. (2016). Ambient scent as a mood inducer in supermarkets: The role of scent intensity and time-pressure of shoppers. *Journal of Retailing and Consumer Services*. https://doi.org/10.1016/j.jretconser.2016.05.007.

Lerman, D., & Kachersky, L. (2012). *V-Positive report*. New York, NY: The Center for Positive Marketing at Fordham University.

Lerman, D., & Shefrin, H. (2015). Positive marketing: Introduction to the special section. *Journal of Business Research, 68*(12), 2443–2445.

Lindqvist, E., & Vestman, R. (2011). The labor market returns to cognitive and noncognitive ability: Evidence from the Swedish enlistment. *American Economic Journal: Applied Economics, 3*(1), 101–128.

Lorentzon, B. (2015). *Pactaguideline. 6 månader med 6 timmar. Följeforskning om försök med reducerad arbetstid [Six months with six hours. Ongoing evaluation of reduced work hours].* Gothenburg: Pacta Guideline.

Lount, J. R. B. (2010). The impact of positive mood on trust in interpersonal and intergroup interactions. *Journal of Personality and Social Psychology, 98,* 420–433.

Lyubomirsky, S. (2011). Hedonic adaptation to positive and negative experiences. In S. Folkman (Ed.), *Oxford handbook of stress, health, and coping* (pp. 200–224). New York, NY: Oxford University Press.

McMahan, E. A. (2018). Happiness comes naturally: Engagement with nature as a route to positive subjective wellbeing. In E. Diener, S. Oishi, & L. Tay (Eds.), *Handbook of wellbeing*. Salt Lake City, UT: DEF Publishers.

McMahan, E. A., & Estes, D. (2015). The effect of contact with natural environments on positive and negative affect: A meta-analysis. *The Journal of Positive Psychology, 10*(6), 507–519.

Mick, D. G. (2006). Presidential address: Meaning and mattering through transformative consumer research. *NA—Advances in Consumer Research, 33,* 1–4.

Mick, D. G., Pettigrew, S., Pechmann, C., & Ozanne, J. L. (2011). Origins, qualities, and envisionments of transformative consumer research. In D. G. Mick, S. Pettigrew, C. Pechmann, & J. L. Ozanne (Eds.), *Transformative consumer research for personal and collective wellbeing* (pp. 1–23). New York, NY: Taylor & Francis.

Mignonac, K., & Herrbach, O. (2004). Linking work events, affective states, and attitudes: An empirical study of managers' emotions. *Journal of Business and Psychology, 19*(2), 221–240.

Money, K., Hillenbrand, C., & Camara, N. D. (2009). Putting positive psychology to work in organizations. *Journal of General Management, 34*(3), 21–36.

Morandin, G., Bagozzi, R. P., & Bergami, M. (2013). Brand community membership and the construction of meaning. *Scandinavian Journal of Management, 29,* 173–183.

Morrison, P. S., & Beer, B. (2017). Consumption and environmental awareness. Demographics of the European experience. In H. Shibusawa, K. Sakurai, R. Mizunoya, & S. Ushida (Eds.), *Socioeconomic environmental policies and evaluations in regional science: Essays in Honor of Yoshhiro Higano* (pp. 81–102). Singapore: Springer Monograph Series.

Morrison, M., Gan, S., Dubelaar, C., & Oppewal, H. (2011). In-store music and aroma influences on shopper behavior and satisfaction. *Journal of Business Research, 64*(6), 558–564.

Mower, J. M., Kim, M., & Childs, M. L. (2012). Exterior atmospherics and consumer behavior: Influence of landscaping and window display. *Journal of Fashion Marketing and Management, 16*(4), 442–453.

Mugge, R., Schoormans, J. P. L., & Schifferstein, H. N. J. (2005). Design strategies to postpone consumer' product replacement: The value of a strong person-product relationship. *The Design Journal, 8*(2), 38–48.

Nasr, L., Burton, J., Gruber, T., & Kitshoff, J. (2014). Exploring the impact of customer feedback on the wellbeing of service entities—A TSR perspective. *Journal of Service Management, 25*(4), 531–555.

Nepomuceno, M. V., & Laroche, M. (2015). The impact of materialism and anti-consumption lifestyles on personal debt and account balances. *Journal of Business Research, 68,* 654–664.

Newman, G. E., Diesendruck, G., & Bloom, P. (2011). Celebrity contagion and the value of objects. *Journal of Consumer Research, 38,* 215–228.

Nicolao, L., Irwin, J. R., & Goodman, J. K. (2009). Happiness for sale: Do experiential purchases make consumers happier than material purchases? *Journal of Consumer Research, 36,* 188–198.

Niemiec, R. M. (2013). VIA character strengths: Research and practice (the first 10 years). In H. H. Knoop & A. Delle Fave (Eds.), *Cross-cultural advancements in positive psychology: Vol. 3. Wellbeing and cultures: Perspectives from positive psychology* (pp. 11–29). New York, NY: Springer Science+Business Media.

Norman, D. A. (2004). *Emotional design*. New York, NY: Perseus.

Ong, M. K., & Glantz, S. A. (2004). Cardiovascular health and economic effects of smoke-free workplaces. *The American Journal of Medicine, 117*(1), 32–38.

Owen, N., Healy, G. N., Matthews, C. E., & Dunstan, D. W. (2010). Too much sitting: The population-health science of sedentary behavior. *Exercise and Sport Sciences Reviews, 38*(3), 105–113.

Pancer, E., & Handelman, J. (2012). The evolution of consumer wellbeing. *Journal of Historical Research in Marketing, 4*(1), 177–189.

Parboteeah, D. V., Valacich, J. S., & Wells, J. D. (2009). The influence of website characteristics on a consumer's urge to buy impulsively. *Information Systems Research, 20*(1), 60–78.

Pavliscak, P. (2015, March 12). *A positive design manifesto.* Retrieved from https://soundingbox.com/a-positive-design-manifesto.

Pedragosa, V., Biscaia, R., & Correia, A. (2015). The role of emotions on consumers' satisfaction within the fitness context. *Motriz: Revista de Educação Física, 21*(2), 116–124.

Pencavel, J. (2014). *The productivity of working hours*. IZA Discussion Paper No. 8129. Bonn, Germany: IZA (Institute for the Study of Labor). Retrieved from ftp.iza.org/dp8129.pdf.

Penz, E., Hofmann, E., & Hartl, B. (2017). Fostering sustainable travel behavior: Role of sustainability labels and goal-directed behavior regarding touristic services. *Sustainability, 9*(6), 1056–1073.

Percival Carter, E., & Williams, L. (2014). Prolonging the search for meaning: How hedonic versus eudaemonic consumption experiences shape preference for variety. *NA—Advances in Consumer Research, 42,* 70–75.

Petermans, A., Janssens, W., & Van Cleempoel, K. (2013). A holistic framework for conceptualizing customer experiences in retail environments. *International Journal of Design, 7*(2), 1–18.

Peterson, C., & Seligman, M. E. P. (2004). *Character strengths and virtues: A handbook and classification*. Oxford, UK: Oxford University Press.

Peterson, C., Stephens, J. P., Park, N., Lee, F., & Seligman, M. E. P. (2010). Strengths of character and work. In P. A. Linley, S. Harrington, & N. Garcea (Eds.), *Oxford handbook of positive psychology at work* (pp. 221–231). New York, NY: Oxford University Press.

Pierceall, E. A., & Keim, M. C. (2007). Stress and coping strategies among community college students. *Community College Journal of Research and Practice, 31,* 703–712.

Pinto Pereira, S. M., Geoffroy, M., & Power, C. (2014). Depressive symptoms and physical activity during 3 decades in adult life: Bidirectional associations in a prospective cohort study. *JAMA Psychiatry, 71*(12), 1373–1380.

Pohlmeyer, A. E. (2012). Design for happiness. *Interfaces, 92,* 8–11.

Powdthavee, N. (2008). Putting a price tag on friends, relatives, and neighbours: Using surveys of life satisfaction to value social relationships. *The Journal of Socio-Economics, 37*(4), 1459–1480.

Pratt, M. G., Pradies, C., & Lepisto, D. A. (2013). Doing well, doing good, and doing with: Organizational practices for effectively cultivating meaningful work. In B. J. Dik, Z. S. Byrne, & M. F. Steger (Eds.), *Purpose and meaning in the workplace* (pp. 173–196). Washington, DC: American Psychological Association.

Pressman, S. D., & Cohen, S. (2012). Positive emotion word use and longevity in famous deceased psychologists. *Health Psychology, 31,* 297–305.

Pressman, S. D., Kraft, T. L., & Cross, M. P. (2015). It's good to do good and receive good: The impact of a 'pay it forward' style kindness intervention on giver and receiver wellbeing. *The Journal of Positive Psychology, 10*(4), 293–302.

Rassega, V., Troisi, O., Torre, C., Cucino, V., Santoro, A., & Prudente, N. (2015). Social networks and the buying behavior of the consumer. *Journal of Global Economics, 3*(4), 163–169.

Richins, M. L. (2013). When wanting is better than having: Materialism, transformation expectations, and product evoked emotions in the purchase process. *Journal of Consumer Research, 40,* 1–18.

Romero, E., & Pescosolido, A. (2008). Humor and group effectiveness. *Human Relations, 61*(3), 395–418.

Rosenbaum, M. S., & Massiah, C. (2011). An expanded servicescape perspective. *Journal of Service Management, 22*(4), 471–490.

Rosenbaum, M. S., Otalora, M. L., & Ramirez, G. C. (2016). The restorative potential of shopping malls. *Journal of Retail and Consumer Services, 31,* 157–165.

Rosenbaum, M. S., Ramírez, G. C., & Camino, J. R. (2018). A dose of nature and shopping: The restorative potential of biophilic lifestyle center designs. *Journal of Retailing and Consumer Services, 40,* 66–73.

Rosso, B. D., Dekas, K. H., & Wrzesniewski, A. (2010). On the meaning of work: A theoretical integration and review. *Research in Organizational Behavior, 30,* 91–127.

Ryan, R. M., & Deci, E. L. (2000). Self-determination theory and the facilitation of intrinsic motivation, social development, and wellbeing. *American Psychologist, 55*(1), 68–78.

Ryan, R. M., Huta, V., & Deci, E. L. (2008). Living well: A self-determination theory perspective on eudaimonia. *Journal of Happiness Studies, 9*(1), 139–170.

Sääksjärvi, M., & Hellén, K. (2013). How designers and marketers can work together to support consumers' happiness. *International Journal of Design, 7*(3), 33–44.

Sachs, J. D. (2019). Introduction to the 2019 global happiness and wellbeing policy report. In *Global Happiness and Wellbeing Policy Report 2019* (Chapter 1, pp. 3–8). Dubai, UAE: Global Council for Happiness and Wellbeing. Retrieved from https://s3.amazonaws.com/ghwbpr-2019/UAE/GHWPR19.pdf

Schmitz, T. W., De Rosa, E., & Anderson, A. K. (2009). Opposing influences of affective state valence on visual cortical encoding. *Journal of Neuroscience, 29*(22), 7199–7207.

Schreier, H. M. C., Schonert-Reichl, K. A., & Chen, E. (2013). Effect of volunteering on risk factors for cardiovascular disease in adolescents. *JAMA Pediatrics, 167*(4), 327.

Seligman, M. E. P., & Csikszentmihalyi, M. (2000). Positive psychology: An introduction. *American Psychologist, 55*(1), 5–14.

Seligman, M. E. P., Parks, A., & Steen, T. (2005). A balanced psychology and a full life. In F. Huppert, B. Keverne, & N. Baylis (Eds.), *The science of wellbeing* (pp. 275–283). Oxford, UK: Oxford University Press.

Shin, J., Choi, H. W., Suh, E. M., & Koo, J. (2013). Do happy teenagers become good citizens? Positive affect builds prosocial perspectives and behavior. *Korean Journal of Social and Personality Psychology, 27*, 1–21.

Simões, F. D. (2016). Consumer behavior and sustainable development in China: The role of behavioral sciences in environmental policymaking. *Sustainability, 8*(9), 897–915.

Singhapakdi, A., Lee, D.-J., Sirgy, M. J., & Senasu, K. (2015). The impact of incongruity between an organization's CSR orientation and its employees' CSR orientation on employees' quality of work life. *Journal of Business Research, 68*(1), 60–66.

Sirgy, M. J., & Lee, D. J. (2008). Wellbeing marketing: An ethical business philosophy for consumer goods firms. *Journal of Business Ethics, 77*(4), 377–403.

Sirgy, M. J., Lee, D. J., & Rahtz, D. (2007). Research on consumer wellbeing (CWB): Overview of the field and introduction to the special issue. *Journal of Macromarketing, 27*(4), 341–349.

Sirgy, M. J., Lee, D. J., Yu, G. B., Gurel-Atay, E., Tidwell, J., & Ekici, A. (2016). Self-expressiveness in shopping. *Journal of Retailing and Consumer Services, 30*(3), 292–299.

Sirgy, M. J., Gurel-Atay, E., Webb, D., Cicic, M., Husic-Mehmedovic, M., Ekici, A., ... Johar, J. (2013). Is materialism all that bad? Effects on satisfaction with material life, life satisfaction, and economic motivation. *Social Indicators Research, 110*(1), 349–366.

Söderlund, J., & Newman, P. (2015). Biophilic architecture: A review of the rationale and outcomes. *AIMS Environmental Science, 2*(4), 950–969.

Sohn, M., & Nam, T.-J. (2015). Understanding the attributes of product intervention for the promotion of pro-environmental behavior: A framework and its effect on immediate user reactions. *International Journal of Design, 9*(2), 55–77.

SproutSocial. (2018). *Championing change in the age of social media*. Retrieved from https://sproutsocial.com/insights/data/championing-change-in-the-age-of-social-media/#Key-Findings.

Steger, M. F., & Dik, B. J. (2010). Work as meaning: Individual and organizational benefits of engaging in meaningful work. In P. A. Linley, S. Harrington, & N. Garcea (Eds.), *Oxford handbook of positive psychology and work* (pp. 131–142). New York, NY, US: Oxford University Press.

Steger, M., Kashdan, T., & Oishi, S. (2008). Being good by doing good: Daily eudaimonic activity and wellbeing. *Journal of Research in Personality, 42*, 22–42.

Stephens, J. P., Heaphy, E., & Dutton, J. (2011). High quality connections. In K. Cameron & G. Spreitzer (Eds.), *The Oxford handbook of positive organizational scholarship* (pp. 385–399). New York: Oxford University Press.

St-Pierre, I., & Holmes, D. (2010). The relationship between organizational justice and workplace aggression. *Journal of Advanced Nursing, 66*, 1169–1182.

Suh, A., & Cheung, C. M. K. (2017). Beyond hedonic enjoyment: Conceptualizing eudaimonic motivation for personal informatics technology usage. In A. Marcus & W. Wang (Eds.), *Design, user experience, and usability: Designing pleasurable experiences, DUXU 2017. Lecture notes in computer science* (Vol. 10289). Champaign, IL: Springer.

Suwa, K., Flores, N. M., Yoshikawa, R., Goto, R., Vietri, J., & Igarashi, A. (2017). Examining the association of smoking with work productivity and associated costs in Japan. *Journal of Medical Economics, 20*(9), 938–944.

Teimourpour, B., & Hanzaee, K. (2011). The impact of culture on luxury consumption behaviour among Iranian consumers. *Journal of Islamic Marketing, 2*(3), 309–328.

Thomas, C., & Sharp, V. (2013). Understanding the normalisation of recycling behavior and its implications for other pro-environmental behaviours: A review of social norms and recycling. *Resources, Conservation and Recycling, 79*, 11–20.

Tifferet, S., & Vilnai-Yavetz, I. (2017). Phytophilia and service atmospherics: The effect of indoor plants on consumers. *Environment & Behavior, 49*(7), 814–844.
Todorova, G., Bear, J. B., & Weingart, L. R. (2014). Can conflict be energizing? A study of task conflict, positive emotions, and job satisfaction. *Journal of Applied Psychology, 99*(3), 451–467.
Tsaur, S., Yen, C., & Hsiao, S. (2013). Transcendent experience, flow and happiness for mountain climbers. *International Journal of Tourism Research, 15*(4), 360–374.
Turban, D. B., & Yan, W. (2016). Relationship of eudaimonia and hedonia with work outcomes. *Journal of Managerial Psychology, 31*(6), 1006–1020.
Van Boven, L., & Gilovich, T. (2003). To do or to have? That is the question. *Journal of Personality and Social Psychology, 85,* 1193–1202.
van Dijk, N., Spencer, L., & Ramirez, V. (2014). *Happy country, happy government: How useful are international happiness rankings?* Retrieved from United Nations Research Institute for Development http://www.unrisd.org/happiness.
Velarde, M. D., Fry, G., & Tveit, M. (2007). Health effects of viewing landscapes: Landscape types in environmental psychology. *Urban Forestry and Urban Greening, 6,* 199–212.
Veloutsou, C., & Moutinho, L. (2009). Brand relationships through brand reputation and brand tribalism. *Journal of Business Research, 62*(3), 314–322.
Venhoeven, L. A., Bolderdijk, J. W., & Steg, L. (2013). Explaining the paradox: How pro-environmental behaviour can both thwart and foster wellbeing. *Sustainability, 5,* 1372 1386.
von Thiele, S. U., & Hasson, H. (2011). Employee self-rated productivity and objective organizational production levels: Effects of worksite health interventions involving reduced work hours and physical exercise. *Journal of Occupational and Environmental Medicine, 53*(8), 838–844.
Vringer, K., Heijden, E., Soest, D., Vollebergh, H., & Dietz, F. (2017). Sustainable consumption dilemmas. *Sustainability, 9,* 942–963.
Walker, J., Kumar, A., & Gilovich, T. (2016). Cultivating gratitude and giving through experiential consumption. *Emotion, 16*(8), 1126–1136.
Wang, J., Novemsky, N., & Dhar, R. (2009). Anticipating adaptation to products. *Journal of Consumer Research, 36,* 149–159.
Wang, X., Yu, C., & Wei, Y. (2012). Social media peer communication and impacts on purchase intentions: A consumer socialization framework. *Journal of Interactive Marketing, 26*(4), 198–208.
Waterman, A. S., Schwartz, S. J., & Conti, R. (2008). The implications of two conceptions of happiness (hedonic enjoyment and eudaimonia) for the understanding of intrinsic motivation. *Journal of Happiness Studies, 9,* 41–79.
Wegner, M., Helmich, I., Machado, S., Nardi, A., Arias-Carrion, O., & Budde, H. (2014). Effects of exercise on anxiety and depression disorders: Review of meta-analyses and neurobiological mechanisms. *CNS & Neurological Disorders: Drug Targets, 13*(6), 1002.
Weinstein, N., Przybylski, A. K., & Ryan, R. M. (2009). Can nature make us more caring? Effects of immersion in nature on intrinsic aspirations and generosity. *Personality and Social Psychology Bulletin, 35,* 1315–1329.
Whitmee, S., Haines, A., Beyrer, C., Boltz, F., Capon, A. G., de Souza Dias, B. F., …Yach, D. (2015). Safeguarding human health in the Anthropocene epoch: Report of The Rockefeller Foundation–Lancet Commission on planetary health. *The Lancet, 386*(10007), 1973–2028.
Wiest, M., Schüz, B., Webster, N., & Wurm, S. (2011). Subjective wellbeing and mortality revisited: Differential effects of cognitive and emotional facets of wellbeing on mortality. *Health Psychology, 30*(6), 728–735.
Wolf, K. L. (2005). Trees in the small city retail business district: Comparing resident and visitor perceptions. *Journal of Forestry, 103,* 390–395.
Wrzesniewski, A., LoBuglio, N., Dutton, J. E., & Berg, J. M. (2013). Job crafting and cultivating positive meaning and identity in work. In A. B. Bakker (Ed.), *Advances in Positive Organizational Psychology* (Vol. 1, pp. 281–302). London, UK: Emerald.
Xiao, J. J., & Li, H. (2011). Sustainable consumption and life satisfaction. *Social Indicators Research, 104,* 323–329.

Viswanath, K., Randolph Steele, W., & Finnegan, J. R. (2006). Social capital and health: Civic engagement, community size, and recall of health messages. *American Journal of Public Health, 96*(8), 1456–1461.

Walkiewicz, M., Tartas, M., Majkowicz, M., & Budzinski, W. (2012). Academic achievement, depression and anxiety during medical education predict the styles of success in a medical career: A 10-year longitudinal study. *Medical Teacher, 34*(9), e611–e619.

Yadav, M. S., de Valck, K., Hennig-Thurau, T., Hoffman, D. L., & Spann, M. (2013). Social commerce: A contingency framework for assessing marketing potential. *Journal of Interactive Marketing, 27,* 311–323.

Yan, N., & Eckman, M. (2009). Are lifestyle centres unique? Consumers' perceptions across locations. *International Journal of Retail Distribution and Management, 37*(1), 24–42.

Yoon, J., Pohlmeyer, A. E., & Desmet, P. M. A. (2016). When 'feeling good' is not good enough: Seven key opportunities for emotional granularity in product development. *International Journal of Design, 10*(3), 1–15.

Yuan, L. I., & Dennis, A. R. (2014). *The happiness premium: The impact of emotion on individuals' willingness to pay in online auctions.* Paper presented at the 2014 47th Hawaii International Conference on System Science. Retrieved from https://ieeexplore.ieee.org/stamp/stamp.jsp?arnumber=6758989.

Yeung, J., Zhang, Z., & Kim, T. Y. (2018). Volunteering and health benefits in general adults: Cumulative effects and forms. *BMC Public Health, 18*(1), 8.

Zauberman, G., Ratner, R. K., & Kim, B. K. (2008). Memories as assets: Strategic memory protection in choice over time. *Journal of Consumer Research, 35,* 715–728.

Zelenski, J. M., Dopko, R. L., & Capaldi, C. A. (2015). Cooperation is in our nature: Nature exposure may promote cooperative and environmentally sustainable behavior. *Journal of Environmental Psychology, 42,* 24–31.

Zhong, J. Y., & Mitchell, V.-W. (2012). Does consumer wellbeing affect hedonic consumption? *Psychology and Marketing, 29*(8), 583–594.

Viswanath, K., Randolph Steele, W., & Finnegan, J. R. (2006). Social capital and health: Civic engagement, community size, and recall of health messages. *American Journal of Public Health, 96*(8), 1456-1461.

Chapter 4
Happiness and the Built Environment

Aubrilyn Reeder, Louise Lambert and Nausheen Pasha-Zaidi

Abstract There is growing interest in the physical and natural settings that support physical, social and psychological wellbeing and happiness. In fact, the World Happiness Report has become especially relevant in emerging markets, keen to balance economic growth with social development and environmental sustainability. Matched with population growth in cities and demand for new urban development, this presents an opportunity for public and private sector actors to consider how the built environment, and its associated polices and services, might be harnessed to enable improved happiness. This chapter will briefly describe the key factors which impact the subjective wellbeing measure used to rank countries in the World Happiness Report and explore relationships which exist between some of these factors and the built environment. Further, this chapter includes interviews highlighting the work of private sector companies which have embraced the United Arab Emirate's aspiration for happiness and which have set wellbeing objectives for their built spaces.

4.1 Introduction to the World Happiness Report Ranking

Published by the United Nations Sustainable Development Network (UNSDN), the *World Happiness Report* (WHR) is edited each year by economics and psychology experts Jeffery Sachs, Richard Layard, and John Helliwell. It ranks countries by their average national "happiness score" gathered through the Gallup World Poll.

With contributions from Karim El-Jisr, Vafa Valapour, and Amol Kadam

---

A. Reeder (✉)
United World Infrastructure, Dubai, UAE
e-mail: aubrilyn@gmail.com

L. Lambert
United Arab Emirates University, Al Ain, UAE
e-mail: ltlamber@yahoo.com

N. Pasha-Zaidi
Houston Community College, University of Houston-Downtown, Houston, TX, USA
e-mail: nausheenpasha@outlook.com

L. Lambert and N. Pasha-Zaidi (eds.), *Positive Psychology in the Middle East/North Africa*, https://doi.org/10.1007/978-3-030-13921-6_4

> *Please imagine a ladder with steps numbered from zero at the bottom to ten at the top. The top of the ladder represents the best possible life for you and the bottom of the ladder represents the worst possible life for you. On which step of the ladder would you say you personally feel you stand at this time?*

Fig. 4.1 Cantril's ladder of life

This happiness score is derived from the responses to one single question known as the *Cantril's Ladder of Life*, a measurement developed by Dr. Hadley Cantril in 1965 (Fig. 4.1). A higher score on the ladder corresponds to a higher "happiness score."

The WHR aggregates the individual responses to this question across a span of about three years prior to the report, and calculates a national average to establish a happiness score which is used to determine a nation's rank. The UNSDN was mobilized by the United Nations General Secretariat in 2012 to help inform the Sustainable Development Goals (SDGs) for the 2015–2030 world development agenda—a follow-up to the Millennium Development Goals which drove the agenda from 2000 to 2015. In two separate world happiness reports prior to the adoption of the highly influential SDGs, the director of the UNSDN, Jeffrey Sachs, makes the case, unsuccessfully, for the inclusion of measures of subjective wellbeing within the SDGs (Helliwell, Layard, & Sachs, 2015).

4.1.1 Happiness in the Region

The population weighted mean average happiness score for the Middle East/North Africa (MENA) region is 5.02 (from 2015 to 2017), compared to a mean average of 5.44 for the 153 countries for which there was data available. Within the Gulf Cooperation Council (GCC) nations—Saudi Arabia, Bahrain, Kuwait, Qatar, United Arab Emirates (UAE) and Oman—the mean happiness score is higher at 6.46. The UAE, with an average national happiness score of 6.77, ranks highest among the GCC nations. The mean national happiness average for the countries ranked in the top five for happiness in the 2018 World Happiness Report is 7.56 with the lowest in that group being Switzerland at 7.49 (Helliwell, Layard, & Sachs, 2018).

4.2 Potential Impact of the Built Environment on Happiness

While the WHR ranks nations only according to a single self-reported measure of subjective wellbeing, it has identified six factors—GDP per capita, healthy life expectancy, social support, freedom to make life's choices, perception of corruption,

Table 4.1 Factors influencing how people respond to the Cantril's Ladder as described in the World Happiness Report

GDP per capita	Social support	Healthy life	Generosity	Freedom	Perception of corruption
GDP per capita, purchase power parity defined by World Bank	Social Support defined by Gallup World Poll: "If you were in trouble, do you have relatives or friends you can count on to help you whenever you need them?"	Healthy life expectancy defined by World Health Organization, World Development Indicators	Generosity defined by Gallup World Poll: "Have you donated money in the last month?" Regressed national average of answer on GDP per capita	Freedom to make life's choices defined by Gallup World Poll: "Are you satisfied or dissatisfied with your freedom to choose what you do with your life?" Satisfied 1, Dissatisfied 0	Perception of corruption defined by Gallup World Poll: "Is corruption widespread throughout the government or not?" And: "Is corruption widespread through businesses or not?"

and generosity—which have a strong association with how people evaluate themselves according to the Cantril's Ladder and which help to explain the differences in average scores between countries. The responses to these factors are not used in the happiness ranking score itself, but are believed to be the most influential in how people respond to the Cantril's Ladder prompt. These six factors are described in Table 4.1.

Identifying urban design features which can impact happiness and wellbeing, as defined by the Cantril Ladder of Life score, can be facilitated by considering these six factors. There is especially strong evidence of a dual causal link between social support and happiness, as well as health and happiness (De Neve, Diener, Tay, & Xuereb, 2013; Diener & Chan, 2011). As there are also causal links between social support and health, finding ways in which the built environment can enable enhanced health and social support has the potential for a meaningful impact on both social and individual happiness (Reblin & Uchino, 2008).

4.3 The Built Environment and Health Outcomes

Urban design has particular implications for physical and psychological health. In fact, the WHO (2017) suggests obesity and physical inactivity are, in part, the result of urbanization and passive forms of transportation. Studies estimate that for every additional kilometer walked in the day, there is a corresponding 4.8% reduction in the likelihood of obesity, while each extra hour spent in a car is associated with a 6% greater likelihood of being overweight (Bell, Ge, & Popkin, 2002; Frank, Andresen, & Schmid, 2004; Wen & Rissel, 2008). High urban density, residential density, retail and service density, street-intersection density and land-use diversity, are all associated with better physical, mental and social health. Proximity to and availability of amenities such as restaurants, shops, healthcare facilities, parks, and places of employment have been linked to residential satisfaction, quality of life, and decisions regarding the use of automobiles (Glaeser, Kolko, & Saiz, 2001; Lloyd & Auld, 2003; Southworth, 2005). They also lead to shorter commute times and less urban sprawl, helping the environment as well. As such, these factors deserve careful consideration in urban planning for cities at different scales. Communities in Atlanta, Georgia (USA) for example, with high urban density, greater street connectivity, and increased land-use mix—residential, retail, office, community—were associated with increased walking habits and decreased probabilities for obesity (Frank et al., 2004).

Although it is often considered something decorative or "nice to have" (Lindland, Fond, Haydon, & Kendall-Taylor, 2015), the integration of natural spaces is a vital component of good urban design which supports human and community health. Restoring nature to degraded urban settings has been found to support human wellbeing in several ways (Taylor, Hahs, & Hochuli, 2018). Natural spaces have a positive impact on physical and mental health, sociability, and creativity with reductions in mortality and crime. A Dutch study of the medical records of 340,000 inhabitants showed that a higher percentage of natural space within a one kilometer radius of residential areas correlated with lower incidences of an investigated set of diseases, lower than in areas with less nature (Maas et al., 2009). Depression followed the same inverse relationship whereby a per unit increase in trees per kilometer of street decreased antidepressant medication prescriptions by 1.18 per thousand (Taylor, Wheeler, White, Economou, & Osborne, 2015).

Feeling connected to nature, valuing its presence, and spending time in or near it was also shown to increase psychological wellbeing (Capaldi, Dopko, & Zelenski, 2014; Cervinka, Röderer, & Hefler, 2012), boost longevity (Villeneuve et al., 2012), sleep (Astell-Burt, Feng, & Kolt, 2013), birth outcomes (Donovan, Michael, Butry, Sullivan, & Chase, 2011), and physical activity engagement (Mytton, Townsend, Rutter, & Foster, 2012). A study following over 100,000 women showed that residing in the top quintile of cumulative mean greenness in a 250 m area around one's home was associated with a 12% reduction in all-cause non-accidental mortality, with the strongest association for cancer mortality (James, Hart, Banay, & Laden, 2016). Children especially benefit by spending time in nature, resulting in reductions in stress, anger, and symptoms of ADHD (Faber Taylor & Kuo, 2011; Roe & Aspinall, 2011). Even living in a neighborhood with parks within a 500 m range was shown to reduce children's body mass index (BMI) by age 18 (Wolch et al., 2011).

Topic Box: Healthy Life Expectancy in the MENA Region

The mean healthy life expectancy for the region is 64.62 years (from 2015 to 2017), compared to 63.17 for the 153 countries for which there was data available. Within the GCC countries, the mean healthy life expectancy is somewhat higher at 66.22. The UAE, with a healthy life expectancy of 68.42 years, ranks the highest within the GCC nations and second to Lebanon in the region. The mean healthy life expectancy for the countries ranked in the top five for happiness in the 2018 World Happiness Report is 71.97 years, with the lowest healthy life expectancy of the group being Norway at 71.09 years, requiring an additional 2.67 additional years added to the average for the UAE (Helliwell et al., 2018).

4.4 The Built Environment and Social Support Outcomes

According to the WHR, perceived social support helps explain about 75% of the differences in average national happiness scores between different countries (Helliwell, Huang, & Wang, 2017). To analyze the relationship between social support and Cantril's Ladder scores, the WHR uses data gathered through the Gallup World Poll question: "If you were in trouble, do you have relatives or friends you can count on to help you whenever you need them?" The question addresses different elements of social support (i.e., emotional and instrumental). The beneficial effects of social support on health outcomes and wellbeing have been widely documented. For example, social support is linked to positive affect and life satisfaction among university students (Ammar, Nauffal, & Sbeity, 2013; Matsuda, Tsuda, Kim, & Deng, 2014). In a smaller study, Gülaçto (2010) found that perceived social support, particularly from family members, predicted subjective wellbeing among university students in Turkey. Older people experience similar outcomes when they have someone to count on in times of need. Golden, Conroy, and Lawlor (2009) found that social engagement is linked to lower reports of depression and better quality of life among adults living in a geriatric community. Melchiore and colleagues (2013) note that older adults living in large households with either a spouse, partner or other individuals were more likely to experience high levels of social support; this in turn had an inverse relationship with psychological distress and elder abuse. Regionally, in a review of 22 studies analyzing social support in older people in the Middle East, perceived social support showed a strong association with mental health (Tajvar, Fletcher, Grundy, & Arab, 2013). Perceived social support, in fact, seems to be able to predict life satisfaction without any relevant differences between age groups (Siedlecki, Salthouse, Oishi, & Jeswani, 2014).

4.4.1 Built Environment Factors Impacting Social Support

Urbanization takes a toll on social lives as individuals increasingly prefer to spend their recreational time on electronic media and television rather than outdoors. This is especially the case if the built environment is not supportive of physical activity or mobility (Al Zaabi et al., 2016; Dustin, Bricker, & Schwab, 2010; Gehl, 2006). Less public space, reliance and/or need for transport to access spaces, single person households, and greater social media use are thought to contribute to loneliness as well. Recently identified as a major growing public health issue, loneliness is as harmful to physical health as smoking and sedentary behavior and has been linked to a greater risk of dementia (Cacioppo, Hawkely, & Berntson, 2003; Holt-Lunstad, Smith, Baker, Harris, & Stephenson, 2015; Holwerda et al., 2012). Conversely, having a greater number and quality of social connections, which can be facilitated by having safe welcoming public spaces in which to interact, has been associated with a greatly reduced risk of early death and a host of other positive health outcomes (Holt-Lunstad, Smith, & Layton, 2010; Umberson & Montez, 2010).

Social support and social participation are also affected by the curse of all urban centers: commuting. Psychologically, commuting is rated as the worst part of one's day (Kahneman & Krueger, 2006); yet, effects are moderated if the commute is made with other people. Studies also show that longer commutes are correlated with greater worry, lower likelihood of enjoyment on the previous day, a decrease in feeling rested, as well as neck and back pain, obesity, and high cholesterol, all of which have higher costs and implications for workplaces (Bodea, Garrow, Meyer, & Ross, 2009; Olsson, Gärling, Ettema, Friman, & Fujii, 2013). Many individuals incorrectly assume that a longer commute will pay off. It does not; for every extra hour of weekly commuting time, a 40% increase in salary would be needed to make commuting worthwhile (Stutzer & Frey, 2008). A longitudinal Swedish study (Sandow, 2014) reviewing data between 1995 and 2005 showed that a 45 min commute or more (the figure most accepted beyond which the negative results of commuting compound) further increased the odds of marital separation by 40%, especially if the commuter was the male partner. The effects were worse for women who, as a result of their partner's longer commute, are often left with greater childcare and household responsibilities and more likely to take a lower quality job in exchange.

Long commutes, not surprisingly, have been identified as a precursor to work-family conflict accounting for lower wellbeing scores and greater physical and mental health issues (Hämmig, Gutzwiller, & Bauer, 2009; Jansen, Kant, Kristensen, & Nijhuis, 2003). In US studies, commuting has also been associated with less social participation, lowering social capital (Besser, Marcus, & Frumkin, 2008) which is related to worse health outcomes (Lindström, 2004). Longer commutes also pose a problem for workplaces as the rate of absences and/or sick leave increases the longer one commutes (Hansson, Mattisson, Björk, Östergren, & Jakobsson, 2011). In sum, designers of urban spaces should pay attention to how people get to and from those areas, as well as how they move between them. The spaces should also provide for beauty, nature, walkability, sociability, safety, mobility types (i.e., walkers, strollers, wheelchairs, bicycles, etc.), as well as opportunities for play and discovery for adults and children alike. These features of good design facilitate social connection, physical activity, creativity, good use of time, and a sense of neighborliness (Proyer, 2013).

4.4.2 Social Support in the MENA Region

The mean social support within the region is 0.76 (from 2015 to 2017). This means that an average of 76% of respondents has a person to count on in times of need, compared to 81% for all 154 countries for which there is data available. Neither Oman nor Qatar have data included on this factor. Within the GCC countries (excluding Oman and Qatar), the mean social support value is significantly higher than in the MENA region altogether and somewhat higher than the global average, with 85% of the population saying that they have a person to count on in times of need. The UAE is among the GCC countries faring better at 83%.

4.4.3 Rise of the Happiness Agenda in the Region

The WHR has become especially influential in the UAE. Sheikh Mohammed bin Rashid Al Maktoum, Vice-President and Prime Minister of the UAE and Ruler of the Emirate of Dubai, set out in the UAE Vision 2021 that the country should rank among the five happiest in the world by 2021. The Dubai 2021 Strategy included in 2014 the goal of making Dubai a "City of Happy, Creative, & Empowered People". In 2016, the UAE Minister of State for Happiness was appointed. A year later, Dubai hosted the first Global Dialogue on Happiness, a precursor to the 2017 World Government Summit, and created the Global Happiness Council which published its first policy report in 2018. Like other initiatives in the emerging global city, happiness has become a popular policy topic and inspires innovation in the public and private sector to apply relevant expertise. Attention to happiness and wellbeing has necessarily caught on in areas associated with built environments, including in the UAE. The following case studies demonstrate some of the ways in which private companies concerned with the built environment have integrated happiness and wellbeing into their objectives for built spaces.

4.5 Case Study 1: The Sustainable City in Dubai

The Sustainable City by Diamond Developers is a residential and mixed-use development located in Dubai, UAE. Covering 46 hectares, the development applies sustainability principles to achieve social, economic and environmental outcomes. Completed in 2016, Phase 1 of the development has become an international case study for sustainable living, work, and wellness, with aims to become the first operational Net Zero Energy development in the region. It was voted the "Happiest

Community in the Gulf" by Gulf Real Estate for two years running. Phase 2 of The Sustainable City will comprise Fairgreen International School, a wellness and rehabilitation center, and an Innovation Center for advancing knowledge in urban sustainability.

According to Karim El-Jisr, Executive Director of the SEE Institute, equal importance is given to social, environmental, and economic sustainability. During the planning and design phase (2012–2013), the focus was on how to create an urban space that enhances community building and is conducive to happiness. A number of design elements such as car-free clusters, narrow streets (known as *sikkas* in the region) and an extensive public domain featuring an urban farm were integrated to achieve this. Additionally, given that the climate of the UAE is characterized by high temperatures and sunshine year round, the outdoor environment was designed to maximize shade and encourage people to spend time outdoors. Energy-efficient homes were built by using passive design and integrating solar rooftop photovoltaic systems to generate electricity. The city also offers many sports facilities including bike tracks, rubberized tracks, outdoor fitness stations, an indoor gym, and an exercise pool.

The local culture and heritage of the UAE play an important role in the community as well. With its unique blend of nationalities, Dubai provides opportunities for interfaith and intercultural exchange. The Sustainable City encourages this by facilitating the iftar "blind date" experience during the holy month of Ramadan. Fasting and non-fasting families are matched randomly for the daily iftar, thereby allowing non-Muslim expatriates to experience a private iftar with a neighbor. The Prophet said: "Whoever believes in Allah and the Last Day, should not hurt his neighbor and whoever believes in Allah and the Last Day, should serve his guest generously and whoever believes in Allah and the Last Day, should talk what is good or keep quiet". The community iftar, thus, showcases the hospitality of the region and promotes understanding and socialization among neighbors in the Sustainable City development (Figs. 4.2 and 4.3).

In order to measure wellbeing in the community, proxy indicators of happiness have been utilized: the availability of play and recreation areas, the average number of neighbors every household knows, the frequency of gym/pool usage by residents, and participation in public community events. These include lectures on technologies used by The Sustainable City, lifestyle training courses, and a series called "Let's Talk: TOPIC" that addresses topics of interest to residents such as utility bills, air conditioning, gardening, and pet care. Participation in public celebrations of holidays, town hall gatherings, and dedicated days for children and parents also serve as measures of happiness. El-Jisr notes that investors and landlords have enjoyed a high occupancy rate (almost 90% just two years after completion), while community management has received favorable responses in resolving the concerns of residents.

Being a happy community achieves other benefits as well, such as becoming a visitor attraction, which helps generate footfall to commercial outlets. As studies have shown a positive correlation between happiness and sustainability (Corral-Verdugo, Mireles-Acosta, Tapia-Fonllem, & Fraijo-Sing, 2011; Zidanšek, 2007), planning for happiness through the lens of social, environmental, and economic sustainability

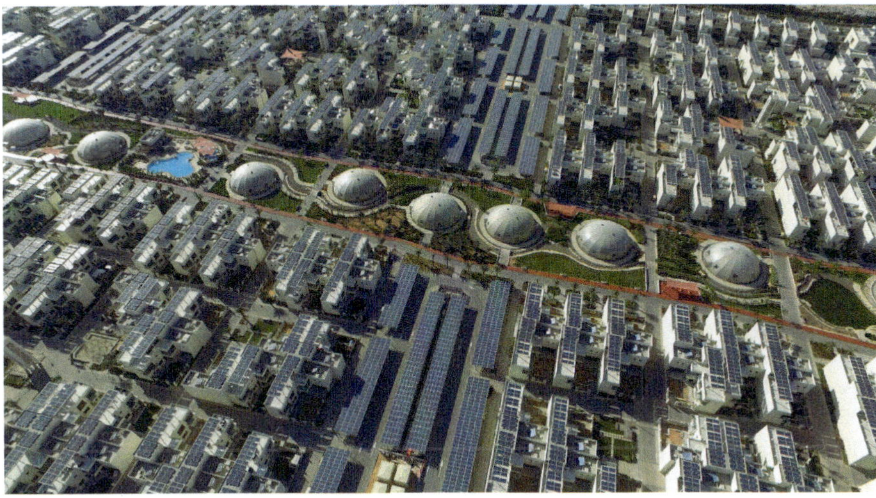

Fig. 4.2 Aerial view of The Sustainable City showing solar rooftops and solar car parks, which help reduce utility bills

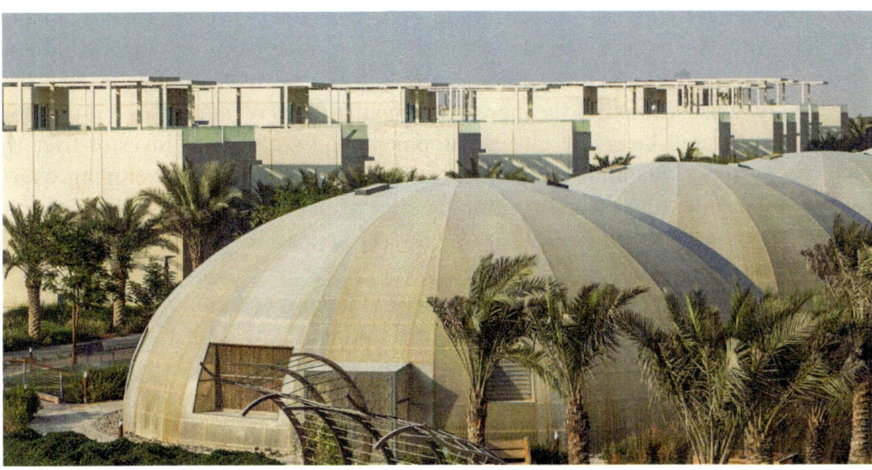

Fig. 4.3 Temperature-controlled bio domes keep the heat outside and provide a unique space for urban farming and community-building

can be feasible economically and result in a community that provides a desirable lifestyle with reduced harm to the environment. Creating a neighborhood, rather than just a place to live, promotes social cohesion, stability, satisfaction with one's home, and pride in and attachment to the community (Bramley, Dempsey, Power, Brown, & Watkins, 2009). Providing a unified and coherent support function is thus an important contribution to creating a shared identity and experience for residents of urban communities. *The Sustainable City* is one such development.

4.6 Case Study 2: The Happier Cities Initiative

United World Infrastructure (UWI) is an infrastructure investment and development company based in Dubai (UAE) and Washington, DC (USA) with 15 years of experience collaborating with public stakeholders in emerging markets to establish national built environment assets to meet growing urban population demands. By witnessing the success of the Dubai city-making model to accommodate population growth, attract investment, and build new industries in an emerging market and the growing urban population demands of the global south, UWI was formed. Most recently, UWI has launched advisory services to advance happier cities through measurement and targeted policy, infrastructure, and service recommendations.

A global trend towards urbanization has been documented (Galea & Vlahov, 2005). Fifty percent of the world's population already resides in urban areas and by 2050 this is expected to reach 70% (UN Department of Economic and Social Affairs, 2018; Zipperer & Pickett, 2012), making the need for better urban design vital. Urban populations are expected to increase by 2.4 billion people in the next 30 years, with Asia and Africa experiencing the most dramatic increases. To accommodate this growth, governments will need to spend 57 trillion USD on infrastructure development over the next 15 years. According to Vafa Valapour, Co-Founder/Principal of UWI, mere investment is not enough; attention to wellbeing through this investment is necessary. Retrofitting existing cities and building new extensions to cities will also be necessary to accommodate the increasing population. UWI addresses this demand with four integrated layers of city development: the creation of investor-friendly policy frameworks, planning people-centric built environments, developing ongoing investment strategies through public-private partnerships, and providing reliable city management services. This all-encompassing approach to development attracts strategic real-estate catalysts such as theme parks, hospitals, and schools to underutilized land and supports emerging markets in meeting economic, environmental, and social objectives for the development. In addition to providing quality municipal services and real estate to meet personal and professional needs, these developments spur new job creation, attract globally mobile talent, and nurture local innovation and skill development, all with the eventual objective of improving GDP per capita, which is considered a key variable to greater subjective wellbeing (McCulla & Smith, 2007). Understanding the power of infrastructure and real estate to transform national outcomes beyond GDP per capita, UWI set its future objectives on improving wellbeing for the residents, workers, and visitors across all of its cities.

Guided by UWI's proprietary Happiness & Wellbeing Index and Framework, the organization launched its *Happier Cities* initiative in 2017. UWI's Happier Cities initiative both informs its current development investments and provides advisory services to governments and government-linked entities to advance the development of happier cities through the built environment and its associated policies, as well as city management services. Based on indices such as The World Happiness Report (UNSDSN), Global Wellbeing (Gallup-Sharecare), the Better Life Index (OECD), Gross National Happiness of Bhutan, and Guidelines for Measuring Subjective

Wellbeing (OECD), UWI's index guides the development of individual and household surveys at the beginning of a project to assess baseline measures of wellbeing and monitor changes over time. The framework helps identify the inputs to the built environment, as well as the associated policies and services which impact wellbeing outcomes. The measures are organized around nine domains: civil, ecological, communal, social, cultural, physical & mental, spiritual, intellectual, and financial. Both subjective measures (known as "happiness measures" to connote an individualized and personal quality) and objective measures (referred to as "wellbeing measures" to connote more observable qualities that may be generalized across groups of people) are utilized. The following provides an overview of the measures in the index:

- **Central Happiness Measures**: The core objective for Happier Cities is to create an environment in which people can improve their overall evaluation of life, their sense of fulfillment, and daily positive emotional experiences. These self-reported measures of happiness—life evaluation, fulfillment, and positive emotions—remain separate from other data gathered and are placed at the center of the model.
- **Happiness Measures in Nine Domains**: The next happiness layer is organized into nine domains around the center. These measures are subjective and specify an area of life to evaluate. This information is gathered from individuals through survey questions which ask them to evaluate satisfaction or happiness in these different domains.
- **Personal Wellbeing Measures in Nine Domains**: Surrounding the core and first layer of happiness measures are the personal wellbeing measures within the nine domains, evaluated at the individual level. These measures consider factors associated with quality of life and improved life evaluation.
- **Collective Wellbeing Measures in Nine Domains**: The outermost layer of the model involves measures of wellbeing collected at the regional or national level. They help connect recommendations to larger national agendas and objectives. Existing public data is reviewed to gather this information. They include the six key factors which the WHR identifies as explaining the majority of the differences between country life evaluation scores; that is, GDP per capita, healthy life expectancy, perceived social support, freedom to make life's choices, perception of corruption, and generosity (Helliwell et al., 2018).

Once data from the UWI Happiness & Wellbeing Index data are gathered and baseline information has been set, the measures are used to identify and drive recommendations for urban inputs needed to improve happiness and wellbeing. Urban inputs are organized into three distinct areas: the built environment, associated policies and, city management services. For each, there is a portfolio of relevant urban inputs which are adapted to the happiness and wellbeing objectives of specific communities (Table 4.2).

UWI's largest development to date, Medini, which is located in Malaysia, demonstrates UWI's approach to developing cities in emerging markets and the influence that city-making in the UAE is having in other parts of the world. Medini is a 2230-acre integrated urban township development located in Iskandar Puteri,

Table 4.2 Happiness and wellbeing recommendations framework

Policy frameworks	Built environments	City services	Effect	Impact
One-stop shop facilitating processes relevant to the domain including: permits for developers, documentation for residents, and start-up requirements for new businesses. Fiscal and non-fiscal incentives for developers and businesses relevant to the domain.	Infrastructure and real-estate outlay and networks relevant to the domain. Smart infrastructure plans relevant to the domain.	Structured partnerships with smart infrastructure developers and operators for services relevant to this domain. Incubation services relevant to this domain.	Collective wellbeing measures; Personal wellbeing measures	Happiness measures

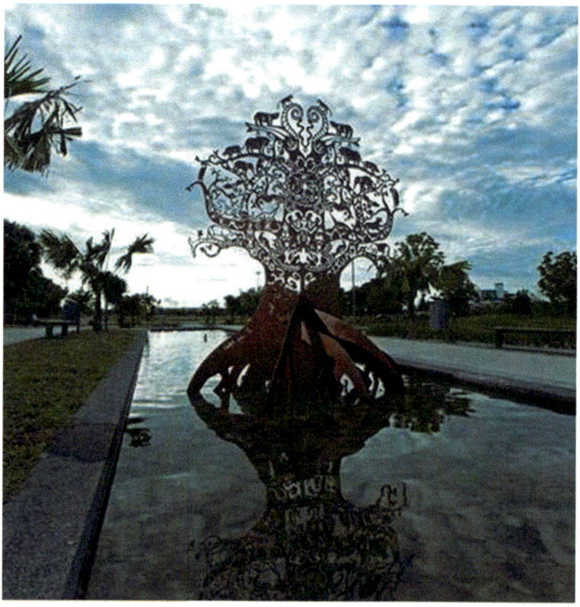

Fig. 4.4 Tree of Life, by Low Khay Hooi. In 2016, Khazanah Nasional launched PublikArt with art works by local artists featured throughout the city to commemorate 10 years of the larger development vision

Iskandar Malaysia, 244 miles from Kuala Lumpur and a 30 min drive from Singapore's Central Business District. Development of the city began in 2007 with full infrastructure in place by 2012. The city is divided into specialized zones focusing on health, finance, leisure and logistics systems to nurture new industries. The complete development process is expected to take between 15 and 20 years (Fig. 4.4).

The city was planned, designed and developed through Medini Iskandar Malaysia (MIM), a public-private partnership incorporated in 2007 by UWI and Iskandar

Investment Berhad (IIB). IIB is owned by state and federal investment agencies with Khazanah Nasional Berhad, the sovereign wealth fund of Malaysia, holding majority ownership. In 2013, the partnership was joined by Mitsui & Co. Ltd. MIM established a special economic zone for the city which allowed an investor-friendly policy framework with fiscal and non-fiscal incentives to attract targeted industries and a one-stop shop to streamline government processes for new businesses, building development, and work visas. Catalyst developments including the first Legoland in Asia with 2 million visitors a year, Gleneagles Hospital, and Pinewood Studios, helped further drive investment and development as well as nurture new economic industries for the region. The city is part of a much larger development vision in the southern corridor of Johor, Malaysia, led by IIB through joint venture partnerships with private sector investors and developers. In 2008, KNB and UWI further established public-private partnerships with additional Middle Eastern partners to facilitate the development of Medini: Global Capital and Development Sdn Bhd. with Mubadala Investment Company from Abu Dhabi (UAE) and Medini Central Sdn Bhd with Kuwait Finance House.

UWI designed the concept masterplan with mixed-use developments (areas where work-, life- and leisure options are co-located for maximum convenience, increased walkability, and decreased commuting times) and 45% of the land reserved for infrastructure and green spaces. Over 20,000 jobs were created through the development projects. According to Valapour, the city has attracted over 2.5 billion USD in foreign direct investments as of 2017. Medini has green and blue spaces which cover approximately 20% of the raw land area with 300 acres designated as open space, including a 22 km walking and bicycle path and 46 public parks operated by Medini Green Parks. These parks include Edible Park, a center and garden which promotes sustainable farming with fruit, vegetable and medicinal trees and Heritage Forest which features flora unique to the Johor. Weekly educational events and demonstrations help residents and visitors learn more about the sustainable food movement and local cooking traditions (Fig. 4.5).

The commitment towards livability has not gone unnoticed. Medini has won the acclaimed "Green Champion Awards" in two categories, "Emerging Green City" and "Smart and Green Infrastructure" from the Institute of Parks and Recreation Singapore (IPRS) and World Urban Parks for its commitment to sustainability, smart infrastructure, and livability. In addition, it has won the "Smart Healthy City and Communities Township" in Iskandar Puteri by the Iskandar Regional Development Authority.

While the methodology for measuring happiness and wellbeing has grown more robust over the past years, the understanding of the impact on these measures by the surrounding environment is growing. Both fields of study continue to evolve and gain greater influence in decision-making. As such, UWI's *Happier Cities* initiative will embrace experimentation in these fields with more researched urban design findings to help move this conversation forward for future built environments.

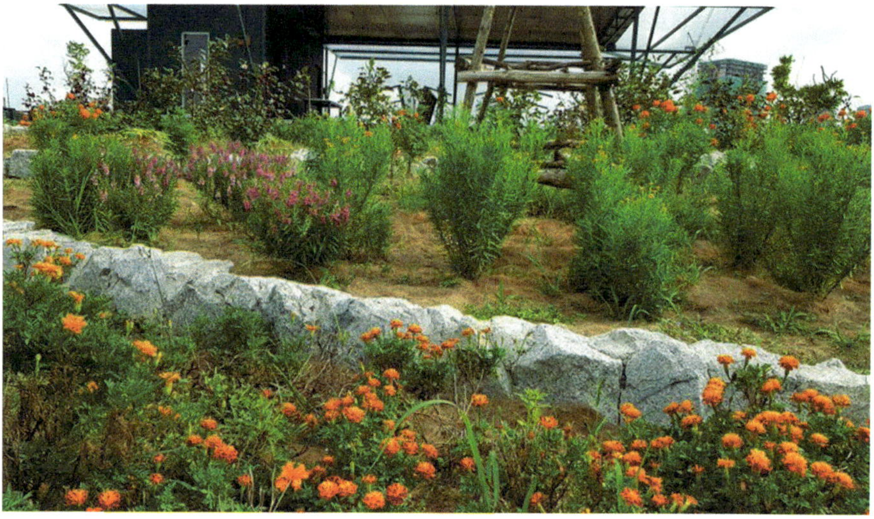

Fig. 4.5 Edible Park opened in February 2018. It is connected to Medini's 22 km bike path and provides 5-acres of edible vegetation and daily events to promote locally grown, sustainable food choices

4.7 Case Study 3: Finding Happiness Across Virtual and Retail Spaces

Greater access to digital environments over the last 30 years has increased the demand for expertise in user experience (UX) design to provide a user-friendly interface between the highly complex foundations of digital environments and their everyday users. However, digital experiences are only one set of channels that impact UX; UX describes the complete experience that end-users, or customers, might have through their interactions with a product or service. This is not a new line of enquiry. In fact, entrepreneurs such as Leonardo Da Vinci, Walt Disney, and industrial designer Henry Dreyfuss have been adjusting systems and operations for hundreds of years to optimize the returns of user experience on productivity and profit (Tariq, 2015). The interaction of human beings and machines has been widely studied and continues to impact industries today. Many of the forerunners of the modern UX field, such as human factors engineering, ergonomics, and human-centered design, focused on maximizing the design of a workplace for greater efficiency or products for better safety. Pioneers in the movement such as Bell Labs helped industries to develop less frustrating experiences for the end-user, hiring a psychologist in the 1940s to inform more usable telephone systems (Nielsen, 2017). Anecdotally, the expression "User Experience" appears to have come from Don Norman, a cognitive psychologist and electrical engineer who created the User Experience Architect's Office at Apple Computers in 1995. In an interview, he described how this came about:

> "I was at Apple and we said, 'The experience of using these computers is weak.' The experience when you first discover it, when you see it in the store, when you buy it…'Oh it can't fit it in the car because it is in this great big box.' And when you finally do get it home, opening the box up and, 'Oh it looks scary, I don't know if I dare put this computer together.' All of that is user experience. It's everything that touches on your experience with the product. That is what we meant when we devised the term user experience and set up the User Experience Architect's office at Apple to try to enhance things" (Norman, 2016).

RBBi, the MENA region's first specialized user experience design and usability consultancy, was founded in 2011 by Amol Kadam and Devesh Mistry in Dubai. Since then, RBBi has helped many top brands and government agencies define and design user experience strategies. Today, RBBi has a multi-disciplinary team of 50 consultants working with clients all over the Middle East and other parts of the world. While RBBi's early projects focused on digital environments and websites for clients, Kadam notes that the rise of "happiness" in the UAE has diversified interest in UX capabilities and services. This has been hastened by the aspirations of Sheikh Mohammed bin Rashid Al Maktoum, the Vice-President and Prime Minister of the UAE and Ruler of Dubai, to make the UAE one of the happiest nations in the world. As such, the government in the UAE has taken up the mantle of setting happiness as part of all customer service objectives for its municipal offices. It further encourages private businesses to do the same. Residents in Dubai are accustomed to ending digital experiences on governmental portals, and in some cases at government service centers, with a set of measures—Smiley Face, Straight Face, or Sad Face—to describe their experience with the delivery of services. These real-time evaluations contribute to a dashboard for UAE ministries to better gauge happiness of customer experiences across the nation. These types of evaluations have helped the market more fully consider UX in both the physical and digital environments.

The concept of "happy users" is well known in the world of UX. In virtual and physical environments alike, there is a requirement that most brands try to include a measure of happiness in their UX framework. When a user completes a task or a service online or offline, each is asked for an emotional response about that service through one simple parameter—Bad, Neutral or Good. UX design in the Middle East, specifically the large urban centers, presents unique challenges as these areas are a melting pot of nationalities, cultures, and languages. There is no generic user. Every brand and every service has the challenge of identifying primary and secondary user segments and then devising a single user experience or, if feasible, multiple user experiences that would appeal to the majority.

In a retail environment like a bank branch, for example, getting a task done easily contributes to a positive emotional experience for an end-user. UX works to facilitate that process and enhance it. In physical environments, UX often considers well-placed signage, queuing terminals, or pleasant customer service executives as well as features which can complement the experience positively such as color, smells and fragrances, and both functional and aesthetic interior design principles. As one of its first projects which required enhancing the physical environment with UX design, RBBi collaborated with the interior design team and the IT team of a local Islamic bank to design an ideal branch pilot. The final design considered every user task from entering the branch to exiting, as well as the full mind-map and set of emotional experiences possible throughout the journey. Analyzing user experiences revealed an overload of digital channels and product cross-sell which could be draining on customers. RBBi limited these experiences to ensure that the user remained in a positive emotional state during the banking experience. Digital tools for employees were added to provide contextual information about the user, including account details and financial tools available on tablets in the waiting area. This provided a win-win situation for both the bank and its customers. Receiving personalized attention and information about relevant products created buy-in from users, while promoting opportunities for the bank employees to sell the products that each customer was interested in.

Airports are another example. The rising interest in happiness in the region has engendered greater interest in expanding the application of UX design to new areas. Like seaports of the last millennium, airports are becoming opportunities for branding the nations in which they are located and enabling new trade hubs. Airport usability as well as a positive user experience is important for inclusion in greater trade networks and passenger transfers. In 2017, RBBi helped craft an overarching UX strategy and set of guidelines for a regional airport. In this project, again the overall user journey was considered. This included passenger arrival at the airport, the navigation of the airport itself, and finally, the destinations served by the facility. Thus, the motivations and expectations of different user groups as well as the stages of the overarching journey were an inherent aspect of the user experience design. Although digital platforms played an important supporting role, the experience in the physical environment took center stage for this project. Thus, way-finding signage, placement and layout of duty-free shops, baggage collection, lounges and accessibility of every touch-point were enhanced to improve the overall emotional experience.

Although most UX and usability projects in the Middle East remain focused on digital experiences, there is a growing interest for organizations, brands, and service providers to realize the full potential of UX within physical environments. By focusing on both physical and digital elements of user experience, RBBi is leading the way for industries in the region to better understand how to implement UX as part of their strategies for sustainability and growth.

4.8 Conclusion

In this chapter, we have explored the impact of built environments, both positive and negative, on happiness and factors strongly correlated with happiness, such as those identified in the WHR—perceived social support and healthy life expectancy. While there is no shortage of subjective wellbeing measures to consider for built environments, we have focused on the life evaluation measure used to rank countries in the WHR for two reasons: its current high relevance in the region noted by its inclusion in the national agenda of the UAE, the UAE Vision 2021, and the identification within the report of several, more concrete measures of wellbeing associated with happiness which help explain the differences in rankings between countries. As private enterprise and investment, as well as government approval are required for large city development projects, there is a potential for proposals with happiness objectives to have a competitive advantage when bidding for projects in the near future. The associated happiness influencers—including social support and healthy life expectancy—provide more concrete intermediary objectives.

Considering rising urbanization, we focused specifically on design relevant to urban areas. As urban environments are linked to a host of related of physical and social issues—lack of physical activity, obesity, depression, stress, and loneliness—we described environments which supported walkability, social interaction, and experiences in nature. Higher density communities, with greater street connectivity and diverse land-uses in a compact area, engender greater walkability through proximity. Ideally, they also decrease the number of cars on the road for short trips because people can walk to retail areas and workplaces, thus decreasing traffic and long commuting times, a harbinger of relationship problems. Public spaces further contribute to greater physical activity, social interactions, and improved health. Additional discussion on ways to improve walking networks with respect to safety, aesthetics, and greater accessibility to needed services and spaces—and in a way which is inclusive and considers the unique needs of women and vulnerable populations—will drive the conversation to a design for happier cities in future. While not discussed in this chapter, greater integration and collaboration between those in the field of user-experience and those in the field of urban planning and building development seems wise in developing the path towards happier cities.

For the Middle East and North Africa, which lags the world mean in happiness and the factors which influence it, improvement to social support and health outcomes can contribute to gains in individuals' overall evaluation of life. With rising urbanization in these nations and the need for new urban development to accommodate it sustainably, now is the time to consider how the built environment can enable improvement to happiness and its influencers. The built environment, often taken for granted as it is simply "there", can be a powerful means of facilitating happiness and wellbeing worldwide. However, understanding how to get "there" will become increasingly important, especially in regions where the environment is still waiting to be built.

References

Al Zaabi, M. A., Shah, S. M., Sheek-Hussein, M., Abdulle, A., Junaibi, A. A., & Loney, T. (2016). Results from the United Arab Emirates' 2016 report card on physical activity for children and youth. *Journal of Physical Activity and Health, 13*(11, Suppl 2), S299–S306.

Ammar, D., Nauffal, D., & Sbeity, R. (2013). The role of perceived social support in predicting subjective wellbeing in Lebanese college students. *The Journal of Happiness & Wellbeing, 1*(2), 121–134.

Astell-Burt, T., Feng, X., & Kolt, G. S. (2013). Does access to neighbourhood green space promote a healthy duration of sleep? Novel findings from a cross-sectional study of 259 319 Australians. *British Medical Journal Open, 3,* e003094.

Bell, A. C., Ge, K., & Popkin, B. M. (2002). The road to obesity or the path to prevention: Motorized transportation and obesity in China. *Obesity Research, 10,* 277–283.

Besser, L. M., Marcus, M., & Frumkin, H. (2008). Commute time and social capital in the US. *American Journal of Preventive Medicine, 34*(3), 207–211.

Bodea, T. D., Garrow, L. A., Meyer, M. D., & Ross, C. L. (2009). Socio-demographic and built environment influences on the odds of being overweight or obese: The Atlanta experience. *Transportation Research Part A: Policy and Practice, 43*(4), 430–444.

Bramley, G., Dempsey, N., Power, S., Brown, C., & Watkins, D. (2009). Social sustainability and urban form: Evidence from five British cities. *Environment and Planning A, 41*(9), 2125–2142.

Cacioppo, J. T., Hawkley, L. C., & Berntson, G. G. (2003). The anatomy of loneliness. *Current Directions in Psychological Science, 12,* 71–74.

Capaldi, C. A., Dopko, R. L., & Zelenski, J. M. (2014). The relationship between nature connectedness and happiness: A meta-analysis. *Frontiers in Psychology, 5,* 976.

Cervinka, R., Röderer, K., & Hefler, E. (2012). Are nature lovers happy? On various indicators of wellbeing and connectedness with nature. *Journal of Health Psychology, 17,* 379–388.

Corral-Verdugo, V., Mireles-Acosta, J. F., Tapia-Fonllem, C., & Fraijo-Sing, B. (2011). Happiness as correlate of sustainable behavior: A study of pro-ecological, frugal, equitable and altruistic actions that promote subjective wellbeing. *Human Ecology Review*, 95–104.

De Neve, J.-E., Diener, E., Tay, L., & Xuereb, C. (2013). The objective benefits of subjective wellbeing. In J. Helliwell, R. Layard, & J. Sachs (Eds.), *World Happiness Report 2013.* UN Sustainable Development Solutions Network: New York, NY.

Diener, E., & Chan, M. (2011). Happy people live longer: Subjective wellbeing contributes to health and longevity. *Applied Psychology: Health and Wellbeing, 3*(1), 1–43.

Donovan, G. H., Michael, Y. L., Butry, D. T., Sullivan, A. D., & Chase, J. M. (2011). Urban trees and the risk of poor birth outcomes. *Health Place, 17,* 390–393.

Dustin, D., Bricker, K., & Schwab, K. (2010). People and nature: Toward an ecological model of health promotion. *Leisure Sciences, 32*(1), 3–14.

Faber Taylor, A., & Kuo, F. E. M. (2011). Could exposure to everyday green spaces help treat ADHD? Evidence from children's play settings. *Applied Psychology: Health and Wellbeing, 3*(3), 281–303.

Frank, L. D., Andresen, M. A., & Schmid, T. L. (2004). Obesity relationships with community design, physical activity, and time spent in cars. *American Journal of Preventive Medicine, 27*(2), 87–96.

Galea, S., & Vlahov, D. (2005). Urban health: Evidence, challenges, and directions. *Annual Review of Public Health, 26,* 341–365.

Gehl, J. (2006). Public spaces for a changing public life. In C. Ward Thompson, & P. Travlou (Eds.), *Open space—People space.* London, UK/New York, NY: Routledge.

Glaeser, E. L., Kolko, J., & Saiz, A. (2001). Consumer city. *Journal of Economic Geography, 1*(1), 27–50.

Golden, J., Conroy, R. M., & Lawlor, B. A. (2009). Social support network structure in older people: Underlying dimensions and association with psychological and physical health. *Psychology, Health & Medicine, 14*(3), 280–290.

Gülaçto, F. (2010). The effect of perceived social support on subjective wellbeing. *Procedia Social and Behavioral Sciences, 2,* 3844–3849.

Hämmig, O., Gutzwiller, F., & Bauer, G. (2009). Work-life conflict and associations with work and nonwork-related factors and with physical and mental health outcomes: A national representative cross-sectional study in Switzerland. *BMC Public Health, 9,* 435.

Hansson, E., Mattisson, K., Björk, J., Östergren, P.-O., & Jakobsson, K. (2011). Relationship between commuting and health outcomes in a cross-sectional population survey in southern Sweden. *BMC Public Health, 11,* 834.

Helliwell, J. F., Layard, R., & Sachs, J. (Eds.). (2015). *World Happiness Report 2015*. New York, NY: Sustainable Development Solutions Network.

Helliwell, J., Huang, H., & Wang, S. (2017). Social foundations of world happiness. In J. Helliwell, R. Layard, and J. Sachs (Eds.), *World Happiness Report 2017*. Retrieved from: https://s3.amazonaws.com/happiness-report/2017/HR17.pdf.

Helliwell, J., Layard, R., & Sachs, J. (Eds.). (2018). *World Happiness Report 2018*. New York, NY: Sustainable Development Solutions Network.

Holt-Lunstad, J., Smith, T. B., & Layton, J. B. (2010). Social relationships and mortality risk: A meta-analytic review. *PLoS Medicine, 7*(7), e1000316.

Holt-Lunstad, J., Smith, T. B., Baker, M., Harris, T., & Stephenson, D. (2015). Loneliness and social isolation as risk factors for mortality: A meta-analytic review. *Perspectives on Psychological Science, 10*(2), 227–237.

Holwerda, T. J., Beekman, A. T., Deeg, D. J., Stek, M. L., van Tilburg, T. G., Visser, P. J., … Schoevers, R. A. (2012). Increased risk of mortality associated with social isolation in older men: Only when feeling lonely? Results from the Amsterdam Study of the Elderly (AMSTEL). *Psychological Medicine, 42,* 843–853.

James, P., Hart, J. E., Banay, R. F., & Laden, F. (2016). Exposure to greenness and mortality in a nationwide prospective cohort study of women. *Environmental Health Perspectives, 124*(9), 1344–1352.

Jansen, N. W. H., Kant, I. J., Kristensen, T. S., & Nijhuis, F. J. N. (2003). Antecedents and consequences of work-family conflict: A prospective cohort study. *Journal of Occupational and Environmental Medicine, 45*(5), 479–491.

Kahneman, D., & Krueger, A. B. (2006). Developments in the measurement of subjective wellbeing. *Journal of Economic Perspectives, 20*(1), 3–24.

Lindland, E., Fond, M., Haydon, A., & Kendall-Taylor, N. (2015). *Nature doesn't pay my bills: Mapping the gaps between expert and public understandings of urban nature and health.* Retrieved from the Frameworks Institute http://frameworksinstitute.org/assets/files/Employment/TKF_mtg_fullreport_final_2015.pdf.

Lindström, M. (2004). Social capital, the miniaturisation of community and self-reported global and psychological health. *Social Science and Medicine, 59*(30), 595–607.

Lloyd, K., & Auld, C. (2003). Leisure, public space and quality of life in the urban environment. *Urban Policy and Research, 21*(4), 339–356.

Maas, J., Verheij, R. A., de Vries, S., Spreeuwenberg, P., Groenewegen, P. P., & Schellevis, G. S. (2009). Morbidity is related to a green living environment. *Journal of Epidemiology and Community Health, 63*(12), 967–973.

Matsuda, T., Tsuda, A., Kim, E., & Deng, K. (2014). Association between perceived social support and subjective wellbeing among Japanese, Chinese, and Korean college students. *Psychology, 5*(6), 491–499.

McCulla, S. H., & Smith, S. (2007). *Measuring the economy: A primer on GDP and the national income and product accounts*. Bureau of Economic Analysis, US Department of Commerce. Retrieved from https://www.bea.gov/sites/default/files/methodologies/nipa_primer.pdf.

Melchiorre, M. G., Chiatti, C., Lamura, G., Torres-Gonzales, F., Stankunas, M., Lindert, J., … Soares, J. F. (2013). Social support, socio-economic status, health and abuse among older people in seven European countries. *PloS One*, *8*(1), e54856.

Mytton, O. T., Townsend, N., Rutter, H., & Foster, C. (2012). Green space and physical activity: An observational study using Health Survey for England data. *Health Place, 18*(5), 1034–1041.

Nielsen, J. (2017). *A 100-year view of user experience.* Nielsen Norman Group. Retrieved from https://www.nngroup.com/articles/100-years-ux/.

Norman, D. (2016). *Don Norman on the term "UX"*. Nielsen Norman Group. Retrieved from https://www.nngroup.com/articles/definition-user-experience/.

Olsson, L. E., Gärling, T., Ettema, D., Friman, M., & Fujii, S. (2013). Happiness and satisfaction with work commute. *Social Indicators Research, 111*(1), 255–263.

Proyer, R. T. (2013). The wellbeing of playful adults: Adult playfulness, subjective wellbeing, physical wellbeing, and the pursuit of enjoyable activities. *European Journal of Humour Research, 1*(1), 84–98.

Reblin, M., & Uchino, B. (2008). Social and emotional support and its implication for health. *Current Opinion in Psychiatry, 21*(2), 201–205.

Roe, J., & Aspinall, P. (2011). The restorative outcomes of forest school and conventional school in young people with good and poor behaviour. *Urban Forestry and Urban Greening, 10*(3), 205–212.

Sandow, E. (2014). Til work do us part: The social fallacy of long-distance commuting. *Urban Studies, 51*(3), 526–543.

Siedlecki, K., Salthouse, T., Oishi, S., & Jeswani, S. (2014). The relationship between social support and subjective wellbeing across age. *Social Indicators Research, 117*(2), 561–576.

Southworth, M. (2005). Designing the walkable city. *Journal of Urban Planning and Development, 131*(4), 246–257.

Stutzer, A., & Frey, B. S. (2008). Stress that doesn't pay: The commuting paradox. *Scandinavian Journal of Economics, 110*(2), 339–366.

Tajvar, M., Fletcher, A., Grundy, E., & Arab, M. (2013). Social support and health of older people in Middle Eastern countries: A systematic review. *Australasian Journal on Ageing, 32,* 71–78.

Tariq, A. (2015). *A brief history of user experience design.* Fast Company. Retrieved from https://www.fastcompany.com/3043024/a-brief-history-of-user-experience-design.

Taylor, L., Hahs, A. K., & Hochuli, D. F. (2018). Wellbeing and urban living: Nurtured by nature. *Urban Ecosystems, 21*(1), 197–220.

Taylor, M. S., Wheeler, B. W., White, M. P., Economou, T., & Osborne, N. J. (2015). Research note: Urban street tree density and antidepressant prescription rates—A cross-sectional study in London, UK. *Landscape and Urban Planning, 136,* 174–179.

Umberson, D., & Montez, J. K. (2010). Social relationships and health: A flashpoint for health policy. *Journal of Health and Social Behavior, 51*(Suppl), S54–S66.

UN Department of Economic and Social Affairs. (2018). *2018 revision of World urbanization prospects*. Retrieved from https://www.un.org/development/desa/publications/2018-revision-of-world-urbanization-prospects.html.

Villeneuve, P. J., Jerrett, M., Su, J. G., Burnett, R. T., Chen, H., Wheeler, A. J., & Goldberg, M. S. (2012). A cohort study relating urban green space with mortality in Ontario, Canada. *Environmental Research, 115*, 51–58.

Wen, L. M., & Rissel, C. (2008). Inverse associations between cycling to work, public transport, and overweight and obesity: Findings from a population based study in Australia. *Preventive Medicine, 46*(1), 29–32.

Wolch, J., Jerrett, M., Reynolds, K., McConnell, R., Chang, R., Dahmann, N., … Berhane, K. (2011). Childhood obesity and proximity to urban parks and recreational resources: A longitudinal cohort study. *Health & Place, 17*(1), 207–214.

World Health Organization (WHO). (2017). *Obesity and overweight.* Retrieved from http://www.who.int/mediacentre/factsheets/fs311/en/.

Zidanšek, A. (2007). Sustainable development and happiness in nations. *Energy, 32*(6), 891–897.

Zipperer, W. C., & Pickett, S. T. A. (2012). Urban ecology: Patterns of population growth and ecological effects. In *eLS*. Chichester: Wiley.

Part II
Education and the Workplace

Chapter 5
Coming Full Circle: Taking Positive Psychology to GCC Universities

Louise Lambert, Rehman Abdulrehman and Cameron Mirza

Abstract The sum of skills that lead to national prosperity has formed the bulk of a new system of inquiry called positive education, the best practises found in teaching along with the principles of positive psychology that focus on the development of student wellbeing versus the remediation of their problems. The positive philosophy differs from mainstream orientations to education by recognizing that even in the absence of problems, attending to student wellbeing and character are essential for good functioning and excellence. Accordingly, in this chapter, we challenge educational institutions to reimagine, redesign and reorganize themselves into "Positive Universities" by harnessing important organizational cultural changes not only for the benefit of students, but for faculty, management, staff, as well as parents and the greater community. We propose to implement character strengths programming to do so. We offer a view of the GCC university landscape and discuss the challenges and opportunities in transforming such learning environments to more positive ones, all the while offering programming ideas and guidance in restructuring these environments accordingly.

5.1 Introduction

As the GCC nations (United Arab Emirates (UAE), Saudi Arabia, Bahrain, Qatar, Kuwait, and Oman) strive to become competitive, knowledge-based post-oil societies, they will require the full participation of their young population as moral, productive, innovative, healthy, and happy agents to join them (Schwalje, 2013).

L. Lambert (✉)
United Arab Emirates University, Al Ain, UAE
e-mail: ltlamber@yahoo.com

R. Abdulrehman
Consulting and Clinical Psychologist, Winnipeg, Canada
e-mail: dr.abdulrehman@clinicpsychology.com

C. Mirza
University of Bahrain, Sakheer, Bahrain
e-mail: cameronmirza10@gmail.com

L. Lambert and N. Pasha-Zaidi (eds.), *Positive Psychology in the Middle East/North Africa*, https://doi.org/10.1007/978-3-030-13921-6_5

Yet, a crucial question remains: are youth ready? But, a more important question is whether universities are fully prepared. While young adults in the GCC are graduating in huge numbers, the quality of their education is debatable, as are their workplace readiness skills and personal character (Kronfol, 2013; Lowden, Hall, Elliot, & Lewin, 2011; Ridge, Shami, Kippels, & Farah, 2014). For instance, many regional schools have relied on substandard quality teaching marked by traditional and rigid methods of rote learning instead of focusing on critical thinking, communication, and problem-solving skills (Pavan, 2014). Further, most universities have programs in place to teach students remedial skills to cope with academic stress, depression and anxiety, but few offer students the skills to learn about themselves or their strengths (Buck, Carr, & Robertson, 2008; Oades, Robinson, Green, & Spence, 2011). In fact, universities generally do not consider their remit to include wellbeing or character development as it is considered a distraction from learning by students, their parents, faculty and administrations alike (White, 2016). Not surprisingly, employers hold universities responsible for failing to equip graduates with the skills that matter (Al Mutairi, Naser, & Saeid, 2014; Kronfol, 2013; Lowden et al., 2011; Sander, 2017) and waste resources compensating for institutional shortfalls, opting to recruit expatriate employees perceived to have a higher level of skill and the personal attributes that contribute to workplace success, like modesty, initiative, and independent thinking instead (Bhayani, 2014; Rutter & Dedoussis, 2016).

Topic Box: Matching Student Skills and Interests to Employment Prospects

A report from Ernst and Young (2015) revealed that only 19% of GCC employers reported feeling that the education system prepared students with the right attitude and behavior for the workplace. Only 16% felt that the education system equipped students with core industry skills and that curricula were in line with the needs of the private sector. Yet, in all GCC nations, when students themselves were asked the same question, 54% in Saudi Arabia and up to 72% in Kuwait felt they possessed such skills. The mismatch between private sector needs and student overconfidence becomes a major barrier in their workforce participation, and more specifically, that of national students. As a result, schemes to increase employment of local nationals across the region are struggling as the number of jobs created in the public sector has been stagnating or is on permanent hold. At the same time, the private sector, where jobs are abundant and expected to rise, continues to fill jobs with expatriates because the required skills among local national applicants are in short supply (Abdalla & Al-Homoud, 2012). It also means there are likely high numbers of graduates who are frustrated and disappointed in their institutions and governments who have failed to fulfill their promise of a good job, one that is well matched to the student's skills and interests, or any job, in exchange for their years of effort toward a post-secondary education. Situations like this are common in the

MENA region. It is cause for concern as many consider this skill-expectation mismatch one of the factors behind rising youth unemployment and events like the Arab Spring (UNDP, 2016).

The skills required for national prosperity form the bulk of what is called positive education (Green, Oades, & Robinson, 2011; Norrish, Williams, O'Connor, & Robinson, 2013; White, 2016), the best practises found in teaching along with the principles of positive psychology (Gillham & Seligman, 1999; Seligman & Csikszentmihalyi, 2000) that focus on the development of student wellbeing and character versus the remediation of problems. The positive philosophy differs from mainstream orientations in education by recognizing that, even in the absence of problems, attending to character is essential (Huppert & So, 2013; Keyes, 2006; Suldo, Thalji, & Ferron, 2011). This approach further coincides with research in positive psychology showing that knowledge, IQ and classroom skills are not enough to succeed. Character, effort, critical thinking and emotional self-regulation count for far more when it comes to success in life (Butler, Pentoney, & Bong, 2017; Duckworth, Kirby, Tsukayama, Berstein, & Ericsson, 2010; Ericsson, Nandagopal, & Roring, 2009; Kautz, Heckman, Diris, ter Weel, & Borghans, 2014). Accordingly, in this chapter, we challenge educational institutions in the GCC region to reimagine, redesign and reorganize themselves into so called Positive Universities and deploy a character strengths approach to do so.

5.2 What is a Positive University?

Education and knowledge are critically important in Islam and great Arab thinkers held the notion of Positive Universities long before the term became fashionable. According to Islamic history, the Prophet Mohammed (peace be upon him) was illiterate, and yet the first word revealed to him from God was "Iqra" or "Read" as a command (Armstrong, 2007). Some would argue that the Quran itself has many scientific principles embedded in the texts, which resulted in Muslims contributing to modern science and culture as a result (e.g., algebra, astronomy, philosophy, and medical ethics) (Al-Hassani, 2012). Mosques were not only places of worship but places for education and other aspects of community life, such as trade (Al-Hassani, 2012). As a result, Muslim civilizations were pivotal in the development of universities, including such monumental ones as Al-Azhar in Egypt (Al-Hassani, 2012). The philosophy of integrating education into community and spiritual life is a concept often considered by Islamic scholars, including the eminent and well respected Imam Al-Ghazali. Learning spaces were not designed solely for trade in mind nor for students to become mere repeaters of knowledge they did not understand; rather, learning spaces focused on developing "whole" individuals, deep thinkers and effective doers capable of reflecting on their contributions to family, the spiritual domain, as well as the civic realm. The original mandate of "whole" universities is a tenet of a positive university as well, and in that sense is not new. Accordingly, to foster such insight, as well as higher order thinking and ability, positive universities focus on the delivery of skills for greater wellbeing and the development of character strengths. This brings questions of curriculum content to the forefront as well as how these skills and strengths are taught (Oades et al., 2011).

Positive universities differ from traditional universities in many ways. The major difference is that their interest is the wellbeing of everyone and not only of students. For example, focusing on improving student learning outcomes alone is a moot point when faculty are overworked and under-stimulated, when academic and administrative staff feel they blindly produce reports no one will read, or when management is frustrated and desperate to find short-term public relation wins at the expense of long-term structural and organizational cultural changes. As a whole, positive universities practise what they preach with positive changes permeating across all levels of the organization, even those that do not immediately affect students on a daily basis and which would not ordinarily be targeted in such efforts. Leadership and distributed leadership matter immensely, and top management plays an important role in adopting these practises by considering issues like integrity, respect and fairness as much as their constituents. They are not caught up in self-congratulatory promotional acts, but quietly strengthen old-fashioned values and virtues and provide evidence for that success. While this does not preclude advertising good work, the primary goal of such positive activities does not begin with public relation concerns in mind.

Positive universities are preventive in nature as well as proactive, predicting what students, faculty, management, employers, and community stakeholders will require rather than taking a spontaneous reactive approach to issues as they arise. They look ahead at regularly programmed intervals to anticipate evolving psychosocial needs, industry and market changes, as well as periodically evaluate their programming and curricula to see if these produce the desired social impact. They also take an exit approach, considering what students need to be successful upon departure rather than solely upon arrival (Francis & Auter, 2017). Their goal is not only to graduate students, but to hand them over ready for the workforce. These universities are also aware that alumni, industry partners, mentors, adult learners, other partner universities and community organizations can act as resources and harness them appropriately. These stakeholders are not only useful for signing Memorandums of Understanding, but also to offer and share regular expertise, guidance, professional exchanges, and opportunities with one another. Parents are considered partners in positive universities and can become effective ambassadors. Opening campuses to the community and offering access to facilities and training opportunities such as continuing professional development or executive education programs are also hallmarks as they impact not only students but the wider society.

5.3 What are Character Strengths?

Character strengths are not the skills one learns in school like architectural drawing or math, but the stable and innate traits used in actions, thoughts, and feelings that lead to individuals being able to draw or do math, such as persistence, courage, honesty, and self-regulation, which lead to excellence over time (see Table 5.1) (Wood, Linley, Maltby, Kashdan, & Hurling, 2011). They can be thought of as positive personality traits (Harzer & Ruch, 2015) or psychological identities by which individuals are best known (Littman-Ovadia, Lazar-Butbul, & Benjamin, 2014; McGrath, 2015a). For example, His Highness Sheikh Mohammed bin Rashid Al Maktoum, Vice-President and Prime Minister of the UAE and Ruler of Dubai, is best known for his drive, leadership and vision, while someone like Bill Gates is known for his creativity and innovation, as well as philanthropy. Peterson and Seligman (2004) consider strengths to be morally valued and universally good by most cultures. Strengths are not meant to facilitate negative functioning or be used towards instrumental or maleficent ends. For example, one does not use the strength of forgiveness to tolerate abuse, humour to insult, or hope to disregard reality. Strengths are also demonstrated across social practices and rituals, as well as by individuals who act as moral exemplars, living a strong life narrative of kindness, love, or integrity as examples. Moral exemplars are socially useful in modeling what strengths are, when to use them, and what their challenges and rewards are. In fact, an entire literature is devoted to identifying such exemplars in cinema for example (Niemiec & Wedding, 2014), where Star Wars characters Finn, Rey and Han Solo offer a means for young adults to learn about moral traits in action (see Sansom, Bretherton, & Niemiec, 2016 for examples).

While natural, strengths are nurtured within families, religions, communities, institutions, and through formal activities like sports, volunteering, competition, travel, work, military service, and recreational clubs like science, photography, or public speaking. Many of these activities are found in universities and the broader community and are all the more important considering the absence of internships, summer and part-time job opportunities, and volunteer positions that place young people in the GCC at a disadvantage compared to their international peers (Al-Waqfi & Forstenlechner, 2012; Singh, Jones, & Hall, 2012).

5.3.1 Of What Use are Character Strengths?

Using one's character strengths appropriately, with the right dose, timing, and in the right context, can trigger opportunities and positive outcomes. For example, identifying and using one's strengths in a new way (i.e., in a different setting, with different people or in a different manner) consistently showed increases in happiness and decreases in depression six months later (Gander, Proyer, Ruch, & Wyss, 2013; Mongrain & Anselmo-Matthews, 2012; Seligman, Steen, Park, & Peterson, 2005), less stress (Park & Peterson, 2006; Peterson & Peterson, 2008), as well as greater

Table 5.1 Character strengths and virtues (Peterson & Seligman, 2004)

Virtue category	Strength
Wisdom & Knowledge: Cognitive strengths that involve learning and using knowledge	1. **Creativity** [originality, ingenuity]: Thinking of novel and productive ways to conceptualize and do things
	2. **Curiosity** [interest, novelty-seeking, openness to experience]: Taking interest in ongoing experience for its own sake; exploring, discovering
	3. **Open-mindedness** [judgment, critical thinking]: Thinking things through and examining them from all sides; weighing evidence fairly
	4. **Love of learning**: Mastering new skills, topics, and bodies of knowledge, whether on one's own or formally
	5. **Perspective** [wisdom]: Providing wise counsel to others; having ways of looking at the world that make sense to oneself and others
Courage: Emotional strengths that involve the will to accomplish goals in the face of difficulties	6. **Bravery** [valor]: Not shrinking from threat, challenge, difficulty, or pain; acting on convictions even if unpopular
	7. **Persistence** [perseverance, industriousness]: Finishing what one starts; persisting in a course of action in spite of obstacles
	8. **Integrity** [authenticity, honesty]: Presenting oneself in a genuine way; taking responsibility for one's feeling and actions
	9. **Vitality** [zest, enthusiasm, vigor, energy]: Approaching life with excitement and energy; feeling alive and activated
Humanity: Relational strengths that involve tending/befriending others	10. **Love**: Valuing close relations with others, in particular those in which sharing and caring are reciprocated
	11. **Kindness** [generosity, nurturance, care, compassion, altruistic love, "niceness"]: Doing favors and good deeds for others
	12. **Social intelligence** [emotional intelligence, personal intelligence]: Being aware of the motives and feelings of other people and oneself
Justice: Civic strengths that underlie a healthy community life	13. **Citizenship** [social responsibility, loyalty, teamwork]: Working well as a member of a group or team; being loyal to the group
	14. **Fairness**: Treating all people the same; being fair and just; not letting personal feelings bias decisions about others
	15. **Leadership**: Encouraging a group of which one is a member to get things done and maintain good relations within the group

(continued)

Table 5.1 (continued)

Virtue category	Strength
Temperance: Self-regulation strengths that protect against excess	16. **Forgiveness and mercy**: Forgiving those who have done wrong; accepting others faults; giving second chances; not being vengeful
	17. **Humility/Modesty**: Letting successes speak for themselves; not regarding oneself as more special than one is or others
	18. **Prudence**: Being careful about one's choices; not taking undue risks; not saying or doing things that might later be regretted
	19. **Self-regulation** [self-control]: Regulating what one feels and does; being disciplined; controlling one's appetites and emotions
Transcendence: These strengths allow for connections to the universe and offer meaning	20. **Appreciation of beauty/excellence** [awe, wonder, elevation]: Appreciating beauty, excellence, performance in many domains of life
	21. **Gratitude**: Being aware of and thankful of the good things that happen; taking time to express thanks
	22. **Hope** [optimism, future-mindedness, future orientation]: Expecting the best in the future and working to achieve it
	23. **Humor** [playfulness]: Liking to laugh and tease; bringing smiles to people
	24. **Spirituality** [religiousness, faith, purpose]: Having coherent beliefs about a higher purpose, the meaning of life

positive affect, self-esteem and a sense of vitality (Wood et al., 2011). The benefits of greater use of character strengths were also evident in the context of leading an active way of life, the pursuit of pleasurable activity, healthy eating, and greater physical fitness (Proyer, Gander, Wellenzohn, & Ruch, 2013).

Of interest to young adults is the usefulness of character strengths in the employment counselling context, where one study showed that young adults who received strengths-based career counselling were significantly more likely to be employed three months post-intervention than those who received traditional services (Littman-Ovadia et al., 2014). Other studies have indicated that the development of character strengths increased the chances of employment and boosted earning power (Lindqvist & Vestman, 2011; Mohanty, 2010). When individuals use their strengths in the workplace, job satisfaction also tended to increase as did the ability to deal with workplace stress (Harzer & Ruch, 2015; Littman-Ovadia & Steger, 2010). However, the most prominent finding was that individuals who identified their strengths in a workplace context increased their likelihood of flourishing compared to employees who had not, while employees who knew and used their strengths showed an 18-times greater likelihood (Hone, Jarden, Duncan, &

Schofield, 2015). Related studies have also shown that when strengths are identified and used, greater ethical and honest decisions are made (James & Chymis, 2004) and moral behaviors observed (Ruch, Bruntsch, & Wagner, 2017). Boosting individual strengths is also of value. Grit (Duckworth, Peterson, Matthews, & Kelly, 2007), the resolve and passion for long-term goals along with sustained effort and interest, has been known to lead to a number of positive outcomes. For example, high-grit individuals attained higher education levels and made fewer career changes over time (Duckworth et al., 2007), and were also more likely to engage with learning experiences of a more challenging nature (Duckworth et al., 2010). The strength of optimism also had positive outcomes, predicting job success and confidence in one's career-related decisions (Creed, Patton, & Bartrum, 2002; Neault, 2002).

Positive effects are not limited to young adults. Studies on primary school students also showed that the use of strengths in new ways led to increases in hope and engagement (Madden, Green, & Grant, 2011), greater student wellbeing (Oppenheimer, Fialkov, Ecker, & Portnoy, 2014), as well as better school achievement and social functioning (Shoshani & Slone, 2013). School-wide character strengths development programs are also well established in other parts of the globe. For example, Proctor et al. (2011) implemented a Strengths Gym program in a UK middle school. Students received instruction in the 24 strengths through class work, self-reflection, group discussion, and homework activities, and relative to a control group, showed increases in life satisfaction and positive affect. Gillham et al.'s (2011) high school program also predicted fewer symptoms of depression, while the popular and often cited Geelong school program in Victoria, Australia (Seligman, Ernst, Gillham, Reivich, & Linkins, 2009) also generated greater student engagement and stronger academic results.

5.4 Which Strengths Make the Biggest Difference?

While strengths are unique to individuals (Mayerson, 2015; Williams, 2016), some combinations lead to greater positive affect and life satisfaction. Curiosity, hope, love, gratitude, and zest show the most consistent and strongest relationships, while modesty, prudence, fairness, spirituality, and forgiveness showed the weakest relationships (see Martínez-Martí & Ruch, 2014; Niemiec, 2013; Proyer et al., 2013). This does not mean that the latter are insignificant, because each of the 24 strengths contributes to overall wellbeing. The ranking relates to the relative impact on wellbeing overall of each individual strength. Strengths have also been categorized by the "heart" (i.e., love, gratitude) and "head" (i.e., open-mindedness, judgement). Research has shown that strengths of the heart were more strongly correlated with wellbeing (Park & Peterson, 2008; Park, Peterson, & Seligman, 2004). Finally, higher scores across all of the strengths correlated positively with life satisfaction, suggesting that good character is related to living a good and happy life (Ruch, Huber, Beermann, & Proyer, 2007). Overall, the findings indicate that the development and a balance of all 24 strengths are necessary for wellbeing and life satisfaction.

Topic Box: Are Character Strengths Universal?

The Values in Action (VIA) classification system (Peterson & Seligman, 2004) was developed by identifying the strengths promoted within various cultures around the world, including the Islamic culture and religion as well as Buddhist, Confucian, Hindu, Athenian, and Judeo-Christian traditions. It also included literary and philosophical sources across historical periods, including the Boy Scouts and Charlemagne's code of conduct for knights (Dahlsgaard, Peterson, & Seligman, 2005)! The work of identifying, assembling, and validating the strengths culminated in six categories of virtues (wisdom, courage, humanity, justice, temperance, and transcendence) under which a total of 24 character strengths are found. Individuals can take the VIA Inventory of Strengths test (VIA-IS; Park & Peterson 2006), available in over 20 languages, on the www.viacharacter.org website. The VIA-IS is considered to have good internal consistency and test-retest reliability (see Niemiec, 2013), including for the Arabic version; see www.viacharacter.org/www/VIA-IS-Arabic-Translation-Psychometrics.

Individuals in 54 nations completed the online VIA-IS (Park, Peterson, & Seligman, 2006) and results showed a high convergence with the 50 US states' endorsement of strengths with Pearson's correlations between 0.73 and 0.99. McGrath (2015b) extended this study to include 75 nations with a total of 1 million VIA participants from 2002 to 2012. Corrected for small national sample sizes, of which the UAE was one, each nation had at least 150 respondents. McGrath showed that the endorsement mean correlation was 0.85 (with a range of 0.49–0.99) and that 55 of the 74 nations exceeded correlations of 0.80. These correlations related to five strengths in particular, indicating that the most endorsed strengths shared between nations showed very high concurrence and included fairness, judgement, honesty, curiosity and kindness. Conversely, spirituality, modesty and prudence were the least endorsed by all nations, except by Indonesia, Pakistan and Kenya who alone endorsed these as part of their top five. These results show that there is a good deal of consistency between what individuals around the world consider to be good character. It also suggests that the construct of character strengths may be one of the most universal to date, serving to allay fears about Western cultural dominance (Baer, 2015).

5.5 Three Approaches to University Level Character Development

Character strengths development programming can take a whole-university approach. Oades et al. (2011) recommend that such efforts target faculty, administration, parents, the university campus residential setting, and work environment,

Opening Session

Students are introduced to the program structure, expectations (i.e., workbook activities, discussion, and participation), and the role you will play. Points to cover:

- Each week, a new strength is covered; homework and workbook activities are expected.
- Students can expect to feel and do better, their grades may improve!
- Students are expected to participate, ask questions, and do their work.
- You, the facilitator, will introduce the strengths, set the activity challenges, ask questions, encourage them to take on new behavior, and cheer on their progress.
- Develop group interaction rules together. For example, treat others as you'd like to be treated, no interruptions or side-conversations, ask curious questions, and encourage one another as needed.

The Lesson

This program is about character strengths, but, what does that mean anyways? Think about 3 people you admire, these could be actors, singers, athletes, or even family members. It's not only what they do; think about what *kind* of person they are. What are their personalities like?

(few minutes: Ask for ideas; write down the strengths or personality characteristics mentioned. Remember, a character strength is not necessarily an action, like "someone sings well", but is the reason for why they sing well, like, "they practice a lot and are committed to being the best". If students give an action, ask what allows or enables the person to do that action.)

Now, let's do that again, but this time thinking about people we do not like. You can select from popular figures. This might be Justin Bieber, or a famous soccer player!

(After a few minutes: Why; what is it about that person's character that makes us not like them?)

Okay, you're starting to understand what we mean by character strengths, the qualities displayed in our thoughts, actions, and feelings that allow us to be who we are. Strengths come out in what we do and how we think and usually lead to good behavior with good outcomes.

Fig. 5.1 Excerpt from opening session (Lambert, 2017)

in addition to students, who represent the main group. Strengths instruction can take a stand-alone format (see Figs. 5.1 and 5.2 for lesson plan examples from Lambert, 2017), the content of which is developed to suit young adults and their concerns, such as stress, job opportunities, relationships, business ventures, decision-making, as well as the concerns of their professors (i.e., workplace stressors and ethical dilemmas, relationship and parenting concerns, or career innovation as examples). Efforts to nurture and develop a university's human resources both professionally and personally are also included in this approach with the recognition that for students to be at their best, faculty, its management and the learning environment must strive for the same.

A second approach uses the same material and content across various activities where the focus is on nurturing strengths in students alone. This approach may entail a more exclusive value proposition targeted at the development of special centres or institutes for character excellence within a university. It may be the case that only selected students or those from certain programs go through such intensive

Integrity: Showing Congruency between What One Does, Feels and Says

Instructor explanation: *Peterson and Seligman (2004) defined integrity as practicing what you preach although it can also be understood as honesty, sincerity, trustworthiness, or honoring commitments, promises, agreements as well as values. We can always count on people with integrity to do what is fair, just and acceptable, and to tell the truth. From parenting to the workplace and in positions of leadership, friendship and intimate relationships, integrity builds trust. Integrity or a lack thereof, is responsible for problems like corruption and social inequality; indeed, most of today's issues are not due to a lack of resources, but ethics and the willingness to act and abide by a code of values, be it professional or personal. It may be that a focus on self-importance, getting social media "likes", and quick monetary returns has negatively impacted the importance of integrity, a topic that only seems to be discussed in the aftermath of business scandals, school cheating, or cases of government corruption.*

Integrity is not only beneficial in limiting potential unethical acts, but for workplace satisfaction and performance as well. For example, the degree to which employees trust their supervisor was positively correlated with one's performance on the job, the level of personal effort given beyond that normally expected, as well as employee's long-term job satisfaction (Dirks & Ferrin, 2002). Further, in high-level executives, integrity played the biggest role in explaining performance differences (Sosik, Gentry, & Chun, 2012). Trusting others to do the right thing has a ripple effect on not only what we do, but how, such that when individuals cannot trust others to do the right thing, they are more likely to engage in unethical behavior themselves. For instance, when students see others cheat, they are more likely to cheat too (Rettinger & Kramer, 2009). Yet, those with strong integrity can overcome negative influences to a greater degree and decide for themselves.
Homework and In-Class Reflection

1. When you make a promise or agree to do something, write it down so that you don't forget. Integrity means doing what you say you'll do, so the list will remind you of what you've said (or at least what not to say if you have no intention of doing it). Be accountable. If you realize you've said yes to something and cannot follow through, let the person know immediately so they can find someone else and move on with their plans. In fact, write a list of all the things you've committed to in the next week and plan your decisions accordingly.
2. At the end of each day, notice the times when you were trying to impress others, like showing off clothes, cars, watches, bags, or when you used the names of others to make yourself appear more important. Reflect on why you felt this was important and consider how it made you look and whether it was helpful in reaching your goals. Try to make this list shorter each day.
3. Have you ever defended your values when it was unpopular? Did you pay a price for it? What was the consequence? How did you feel afterwards? What did you learn from the experience? Would you do it again? Describe what happened in your workbook.

Fig. 5.2 Excerpt from a sample lesson for "Integrity" (taken from Lambert, 2017)

programming accompanied by focused experiential activities included as a form of university internship and/or community service. The benefit of this approach is that it does not come across as a punitive form of additional work but a privileged position into which one is nominated. Graduates from these centres may be expected to take on the status of moral exemplars and act as role models thereafter, adding this training to their CVs with benefits to future employers who gain from this type of quality assurance.

Still, a third more integrated approach involves embedding instruction into existing curriculum whereby strengths can show their expression in almost any course where human behavior is concerned such as English literature, political science, Islamic philosophy, sociology, or business ethics. Selected strengths can be infused into class discussions (i.e., what strength or lack thereof is being demonstrated in a novel's fictional character, business decision, or foreign policy objective?). In this way, all humanities include an examination of human character, a critical aspect of moral analysis that is frequently absent in the classroom and yet, very relevant to real life workplace, parenting or relational concerns. Assessment tasks, personal reflections, interviews, learning and teaching activities can be structured around these strengths so that students become familiar with the notion of character, gain insight and learn to be critical of their own moral choices and hold themselves to a higher standard as a result. This requires significantly more effort on the part of instructors but helps to activate the strengths in as many contexts as possible.

Alongside the VIA, the *Character Strengths and Virtues: A Handbook and Classification* (CSV) diagnostic manual (Peterson & Seligman, 2004) describes the strengths much like the American Psychiatric Association's (2013) *Diagnostic and Statistical Manual of Mental Disorders* (DSM) describes dysfunction. The CSV is used to diagnose individual strengths and is replete with research as well as lists of recommended movies, songs, and novels that are deemed to characterize them. It is used by positive psychologists and strengths coaches to complement the DSM or as a stand-alone diagnostic tool in clinical settings as well as educational and workplace contexts. Yet, despite the growth of the strengths industry in schools and businesses in particular (Niemiec, 2013), the goal of such work is not to increase all strengths indiscriminately or use them across all contexts. Achieving a balance is key (Allan, 2015) as some strengths can complement or undermine one another when used too much, too little, or in certain combinations. For instance, low judgment may undermine the effects of high kindness and leave individuals with unintended outcomes. In fact, a recent study measured the effects of the over and underuse of strengths, showing that both increased depression and social anxiety (Freidlin, Littman-Ovadia, & Niemiec, 2017), although the underuse of strengths contributed to more negative outcomes.

Finally, beyond character and wellbeing, there is real life. Extracurricular activities are where most young people learn the skills for becoming independent adults. Yet, across the GCC nations, high salaries translate into a corresponding plethora of cheap household help (i.e., maids, drivers, cooks, and nannies), who paradoxically undermine such learning. A recent example in one of the author's teaching illustrates this. While undertaking a classroom volunteer project which involved handling and packaging dry foods (i.e., rice) to donate to a labor camp, over half the class did not know how to fold the bottom of a cardboard box for greater support, one had never used scissors before, and another reported not knowing rice was a dry grain. It is little wonder so many students cannot manage many real life challenges themselves; they are never given real life opportunities to learn.

Accordingly, positive universities may want to include a mandatory first year life skills program to not only ensure students know about and can use digital capabilities, but everyday life skills. This could include financial literacy, i.e. how to live within a budget, save money, avoid debt, and distinguish between needs and wants. Resiliency skills would also go a long way as many students find it difficult to tolerate any critical feedback and accept responsibility for failings. Such behaviors are not exactly the qualities of brilliant leaders, industry disruptors, or for that matter, partners and parents! While meaning well, many adults unknowingly contribute to the lack of skill and character development by trying to shield and protect young adults from failure. Yet, the chance to fail in order to learn is exactly what is needed.

All character strengths programming has the goal of helping students *identify* their strengths to achieve a better fit between themselves and the worlds of work, recreation, and relationships, and to *develop* their strengths through activities, self-reflection, and discussion. The "development" approach is broader than the standard "identify and use" approach more commonly used in strengths work. Development avoids limiting individuals to their existing strengths and instead prepares them for real life which requires all of the strengths to be used (Biswas-Diener, Kashdan, & Minhas, 2011). Yet, strengths programming should neither take a compliance nor rewards-based approach (Nesfield, 2016) as the goal is not to tell students what to do, but to facilitate their deliberate contemplation about choices and consequences. Thus, much like children behaving only when their parents are in the room, doing the right thing out of fear or desire for social approval, is not the aim. Instead, it is about understanding the value of doing the right thing when no one is watching. Consequently, such programming focuses on developing insight as to which strengths should be used, under what circumstance and why, so that the range of behavioral and cognitive options becomes broader, the variety of appropriate settings expands, and performance and wellbeing increase as a result.

5.6 Avenues for Future Study

Character strengths are one area in positive psychology where there is much available data. However, regional studies are few and limited to two in the UAE (Lambert, Budhraja, Mullan, & Gupta, 2018; Petkari & Ortiz-Tallo, 2018). Nonetheless, researchers, educators and practitioners can visit the www.viacharacter.org website for a comprehensive listing of studies with which to determine future steps of their own. It is worth reminding that character strength development is not only essential for young people in education, but for all adults in the workplace and everyday life as well.

Examples of future research might involve answering the following questions: Does the use of character strengths (and which ones) change over the duration of time students spend at university and to what aspects of the university environment can these changes be attributed? For instance, does the strength of integrity grow during years spent at university or weaken? If so, what does this say about the university setting? Are these changes due to classroom instruction, the social atmosphere, extracurricular activities like sports, or maturation and development? What are the implications of such findings for university settings and their development as positive institutions? Researchers can rely on longitudinal studies for such answers and experiment with controlled interventions designed to develop such strengths to help effectively prepare students for the workplace.

5.7 Conclusion

As universities look for ways to stand out and recruit top talent, the offer of a character strengths program or positive university can be an attractive proposition for faculty, students and parents alike. Not only focused on academics or extracurricular activities, universities can also offer a moral or psychological element geared not exclusively towards problems but to human excellence and wellbeing. The student experience would be greatly enhanced beyond learning skills, thus providing graduates with a competitive edge in the marketplace and the transferable skills most in demand by employers at present (Sander, 2017). Graduate employability outcomes are becoming increasingly important globally with students attracted to universities that provide a better prospect of employment. Universities can also distinguish themselves from competitors by attracting top faculty not only with the lure of practicing academic excellence but personal excellence as well. Becoming an employer of choice for this reason can be attractive, especially in the current GCC landscape where the number of foreign students continues to grow. This offers a unique form of professional growth within a very broad multicultural context. Having a character strengths programming component would not only attract top student and faculty talent, but ideally, retain such talent with higher standards and practises of moral behavior engrained throughout the organizational culture, including classrooms. Universities can strive to become moral exemplars themselves and boost their reputation, rankings, as well as retention figures in the industry, too.

Character strength education is making a comeback, and young adults should not be overlooked for fear that it may add to a taxing workload or divert resources from learning. Identifying, using and further developing one's character strengths has positive outcomes for learning, ethical behavior, positive affect, social functioning, physical health, job satisfaction, the likelihood of employment, and earning power (Gander et al., 2013; Lindqvist & Vestman, 2011; Littman-Ovadia et al., 2014; Mongrain & Anselmo-Matthews, 2012; Oppenheimer et al., 2014; Proyer et al., 2013; Shoshani & Slone, 2013). Consequently, universities can and should play a role in character formation, not only to meet their own commercial interests, but because they are the ideal institutions in which to grow human capital and best prepare students for a great entry into the world. Universities are the last chance for students to receive the time, space, support and opportunities to contemplate and practise becoming better, more responsible and caring citizens before entering real life contexts. It is only in universities that the contributors to a better society and region can be fully developed.

References

Abdalla, I., & Al-Homoud, M. (2012). Foreign faces in Kuwaiti places: The challenges of human capital utilization in Kuwait. *International Journal of Business and Management, 7*(20), Article 18661.

Al-Hassani, S. T. S. (2012). *1001 inventions: The enduring legacy of Muslim civilization* (3rd ed.). Washington, DC: National Geographic.

Al-Mutairi, A., Naser, K., & Saeid, M. (2014). Employability factors of business graduates in Kuwait: Evidence from an emerging country. *International Journal of Business and Management, 9*(10), 49–61.

Al-Waqfi, M., & Forstenlechner, I. (2012). Of private sector fear and prejudice. *Personnel Review, 41*(5), 609–629.

Allan, B. A. (2015). Balance among character strengths and meaning in life. *Journal of Happiness Studies, 16*(5), 1247–1261.

American Psychiatric Association. (2013). *Diagnostic and statistical manual of mental disorders* (5th ed.). Washington, DC: Author.

Armstrong, K. (2007). *Muhammad: A prophet for our time*. New York, NY: Harper Collins.

Baer, R. (2015). Ethics, values, virtues, and character strengths in mindfulness-based interventions: A psychological science perspective. *Mindfulness, 6*(4), 956–969.

Bhayani, A. (2014). The market route to higher education in UAE: Its rationales and implications. *International Review on Public and Nonprofit Marketing, 11*(1), 75–87.

Biswas-Diener, R., Kashdan, T. B., & Minhas, G. (2011). A dynamic approach to psychological strength development and intervention. *The Journal of Positive Psychology, 6*(2), 106–118.

Buck, B., Carr, S. R., & Robertson, J. (2008). Positive psychology and student engagement. *Journal of Cross-Disciplinary Perspectives in Education, 1*(1), 28–35.

Butler, H. A., Pentoney, C., & Bong, M. P. (2017). Predicting real-world outcomes: Critical thinking ability is a better predictor of life decisions than intelligence. *Thinking Skills and Creativity, 25,* 38–46.

Creed, P. A., Patton, W., & Bartrum, D. (2002). Multidimensional properties of the LOT-R: Effects of optimism and pessimism on career and wellbeing related variables in adolescents. *Journal of Career Assessment, 10,* 42–61.

Dahlsgaard, K., Peterson, C., & Seligman, M. E. P. (2005). Shared virtue: The convergence of valued human strengths across culture and history. *Review of General Psychology, 9*(3), 203–213.

Dirks, K. T., & Ferrin, D. L. (2002). Trust in leadership: Meta-analytic findings and implications for research and practice. *Journal of Applied Psychology, 87,* 611–628.

Duckworth, A. L., Kirby, T., Tsukayama, E., Berstein, H., & Ericsson, K. (2010). Deliberate practice spells success: Why grittier competitors triumph at the National Spelling Bee. *Social Psychological and Personality Science, 2,* 174–181.

Duckworth, A. L., Peterson, C., Matthews, M. D., & Kelly, D. R. (2007). Grit: Perseverance and passion for long-term goals. *Journal of Personality and Social Psychology, 92*(6), 1087–1101.

Ericsson, K. A., Nandagopal, K., & Roring, R. W. (2009). Toward a science of exceptional achievement: Attaining superior performance through deliberate practice. *Annals of New York Academy of Science, 1172,* 199–217.

Ernst & Young. (2015, May 18). *How will the GCC close the skills gap?* Retrieved from http://www.ey.com/em/en/industries/government—public-sector/ey-how-will-the-gcc-close-the-skills-gap.

Francis, J., & Auter, Z. (2017, June 20). *Gallup Blog: 3 ways to realign higher education with todays' workforce.* Retrieved from http://news.gallup.com/opinion/gallup/212522/ways-realign-higher-education-today-workforce.aspx.

Freidlin, P., Littman-Ovadia, H., & Niemiec, R. M. (2017). Positive psychopathology: Social anxiety via character strengths underuse and overuse. *Personality and Individual Differences, 108,* 50–54.

Gander, F., Proyer, R. T., Ruch, W., & Wyss, T. (2013). Strength-based positive interventions: Further evidence on their potential for enhancing wellbeing and alleviating depression. *Journal of Happiness Studies, 14,* 1241–1259.

Gillham, J., Adams-Deutsch, Z., Werner, J., Reivich, K., Coulter-Heindl, V., Linkins, M., Winder, B., … Seligman, M. E. P. (2011). Character strengths predict subjective wellbeing during adolescence. *Journal of Positive Psychology, 6*(1), 31–44.

Gillham, J. E., & Seligman, M. E. (1999). Footsteps on the road to a positive psychology. *Behaviour Research and Therapy, 37,* S163–S173.

Green, S., Oades, L., & Robinson, P. (2011, April). *Positive education: Creating flourishing students, staff and schools.* InPsych, Australian Psychological Society. Retrieved from https://www.psychology.org.au/publications/inpsych/2011/april/green/.

Haj, S. (2009). *Reconfiguring Islamic tradition: Reform, rationality, and modernity*. Stanford, CA: Stanford University Press.

Harzer, C., & Ruch, W. (2015). The relationships of character strengths with coping, work-related stress, and job satisfaction. *Frontiers in Psychology, 6,* 165.

Hone, L. C., Jarden, A., Duncan, S., & Schofield, G. M. (2015). Flourishing in New Zealand workers: Associations with lifestyle behaviors, physical health, psychosocial, and work-related indicators. *Journal of Occupational and Environmental Medicine, 57*(9), 973–983.

Huppert, F. A., & So, T. T. C. (2013). Flourishing across Europe: Application of a new conceptual framework for defining wellbeing. *Social Indicators Research, 110*(3), 837–861.

ICEF Monitor. (2017, October 11). *Dubai strengthens its position as a regional education hub.* Retrieved from http://monitor.icef.com/2017/10/dubai-strengthens-position-regional-education-hub/.

James H. S. Jr., & Chymis A. G. (2004). *Are happy people ethical people? Evidence from North America and Europe* (Working Paper No. AEWP 2004–08). Department of Agricultural Economics. Retrieved from http://ageconsearch.umn.edu/bitstream/26034/1/wp040008.pdf.

Kautz, T. D., Heckman, J., Diris, R., ter Weel, B., & Borghans, L. (2014). *Fostering and measuring skills: Improving cognitive and non-cognitive skills to promote lifetime success.* Organisation for Economic Cooperation and Development. Retrieved from http://www.oecd.org/edu/ceri/Fostering-and-Measuring-Skills-Improving-Cognitive-and-Non-Cognitive-Skills-to-Promote-Lifetime-Success.pdf.

Keyes, C. L. M. (2006). Mental health in adolescence: Is America's youth flourishing? *American Journal of Orthopsychiatry, 76,* 395–402.

Kronfol, N. M. (2013). Demographics and the social reckoning in the Arab region/Démographie et reconnaissance sociale dans la Région arabe. *Eastern Mediterranean Health Journal, 19*(4), 382–388.

Lambert, L. (2017). *Character strengths at university (for a GCC audience): The facilitator's manual.* Retrieved from http://a.co/56f8EWl. ISBN-13: 978-1548597931.

Lambert, L., Budhraja, N., Mullan, C. A., & Gupta, G. (2018). Building life skills through positive education: Evidence from Ras Al Khaimah (UAE). In D. B. Jones & S. Sahraoui (Eds)., *The future of the labour market reform in the Gulf region: Towards a multi-disciplinary, evidence-based and practical understanding* (pp. 136-153). Berlin, Germany: Gerlach Press.

Lindqvist, E., & Vestman, R. (2011). The labor market returns to cognitive and noncognitive ability: Evidence from the Swedish enlistment. *American Economic Journal: Applied Economics, 3,* 101–128.

Littman-Ovadia, H., Lazar-Butbul, V., & Benjamin, B. A. (2014). Strengths-based career counseling: Description and evaluation. *Journal of Career Assessment, 22,* 403–419.

Littman-Ovadia, H., & Steger, M. (2010). Character strengths and wellbeing among volunteers and employees: Toward an integrative model. *Journal of Positive Psychology, 5*(6), 419–430.

Lowden, K., Hall, S., Elliot, D., & Lewin, J. (2011). *Employers' perceptions of the employability skills of new graduates*. Edge Foundation, London, UK: Project Report.

Madden, W., Green, S., & Grant, A. M. (2011). A pilot study evaluating strengths-based coaching for primary school students: Enhancing engagement and hope. *International Coaching Psychology Review, 6*(1), 71–83.

Martínez-Martí, M. L., & Ruch, W. (2014). Character strengths and wellbeing across the life span: Data from a representative sample of German-speaking adults living in Switzerland. *Frontiers in Psychology, 5,* 1253.

Mayerson, N. (2015). "Characterizing" the workplace: Using character strengths to create sustained success. *Kognition & Paedagogik, 96,* 14–22.

McGrath, R. E. (2015a). Integrating psychological and cultural perspectives on virtue: The hierarchical structure of character strengths. *The Journal of Positive Psychology, 10*(5), 407–424.

McGrath, R. E. (2015b). Character strengths in 75 nations: An update. *The Journal of Positive Psychology, 10*(1), 41–52.

Mohanty, M. S. (2010). Effects of positive attitude and optimism on employment: Evidence from the US data. *The Journal of Socio-Economics, 39,* 258–270.

Mongrain, M., & Anselmo-Matthews, T. (2012). Do positive psychology exercises work? A replication of Seligman et al. *Journal of Clinical Psychology, 68*(4), 382–389.

Neault, R. A. (2002). Thriving in the new millennium: Career management in the changing world of work. *Canadian Journal of Career Development, 1*(1), 11–21.

Nesfield, V. (2016). *Character education in a pluralistic context: Can and should we teach values*? Hillary Place Papers (3rd ed.), University of Leeds. Retrieved from http://hpp.education.leeds.ac.uk/wp-content/uploads/sites/131/2016/02/HPP2016-3-Nesfield.pdf.

Niemiec, R. M. (2013). VIA character strengths: Research and practice (The first 10 years). In H. H. Knoop & A. Delle Fave (Eds.), *Wellbeing and cultures: Perspectives on positive psychology* (pp. 11–30). New York: Springer.

Niemiec, R. M., & Wedding, D. (2014). *Positive psychology at the movies 2: Using films to build character strengths and wellbeing* (2nd ed.). Cambridge, MA: Hogrefe.

Norrish, J. M., Williams, P., O'Connor, M., & Robinson, J. (2013). An applied framework for positive education. *International Journal of Wellbeing, 3*(2), 147–161.

Oades, L. G., Robinson, P., Green, S., & Spence, G. B. (2011). Towards a positive university. *The Journal of Positive Psychology, 6,* 432–439.

Oppenheimer, M. F., Fialkov, C., Ecker, B., & Portnoy, S. (2014). Teaching to strengths: Character education for urban middle school students. *Journal of Character Education, 10*(2), 91–105.

Park, N., & Peterson, C. (2006). Methodological issues in positive psychology and the assessment of character strengths. In A. D. Ong & M. van Dulmen (Eds.), *Handbook of methods in positive psychology* (pp. 292–305). New York: Oxford University Press.

Park, N., & Peterson, C. (2008). The cultivation of character strengths. In M. Ferrari & G. Poworowski (Eds.), *Teaching for wisdom* (pp. 57–75). Mahwah, NJ: Erlbaum.

Park, N., Peterson, C., & Seligman, M. E. P. (2004). Strengths of character and wellbeing. *Journal of Social and Clinical Psychology, 23,* 603–619.

Park, N., Peterson, C., & Seligman, M. E. P. (2006). Character strengths in fifty-four nations and the fifty US states. *The Journal of Positive Psychology, 1*(3), 118–129.

Pavan, A. (2014). The New Saudi Educational Renaissance: In between the "Capacity to Aspire" and the "Capacity to Remember". *Higher Education Studies, 4*(5), 37–46.

Peterson, C., & Seligman, M. E. P. (2004). *Character strengths and virtues: A handbook and classification.* New York: Oxford University Press/Washington, DC: American Psychological Association.

Peterson, T. D., & Peterson, E. W. (2008). Stemming the tide of law student depression: What law schools need to learn from the science of positive psychology. *Yale Journal of Health Policy, Law, and Ethics, 9*(2).

Petkari, E., & Ortiz-Tallo, M. (2018). Towards youth happiness and mental health in the United Arab Emirates: The path of character strengths in a multicultural population. *Journal of Happiness Studies, 19*(2), 333–350.

Proctor, C., Tsukayama, E., Wood, A. M., Maltby, J., Eades, J. F., & Linley, P. A. (2011). Strengths gym: The impact of a character strengths-based intervention on the life satisfaction and wellbeing of adolescents. *Journal of Positive Psychology, 6,* 377–388.

Proyer, R. T., Gander, F., Wellenzohn, S., & Ruch, W. (2013). What good are character strengths beyond subjective wellbeing? The contribution of the good character on self-reported health-oriented behavior, physical fitness, and the subjective health status. *Journal of Positive Psychology, 8,* 222–232.

Ridge, N., Shami, S., Kippels, S., & Farah, S. (2014). *Expatriate teachers and education quality in the Gulf Cooperation Council* (Policy Paper No. 11). The Sheikh Saud bin Saqr Al Qasimi Foundation for Policy Research. Retrieved from http://www.alqasimifoundation.com/en/publication/21/expatriate-teachers-and-education-quality-in-the-gulf-cooperation-council.

Ruch, W., Bruntsch, R., & Wagner, L. (2017). The role of character traits in economic games. *Personality and Individual Differences, 108,* 186–190.

Ruch, W., Huber, A., Beermann, U., & Proyer, R. T. (2007). Character strengths as predictors of the "good life" in Austria, Germany and Switzerland. In Romanian Academy, George Barit Institute of History, Department of Social Research (Ed.), *Studies and researches in social sciences* (Vol. 16, pp. 123–131). Cluj-Napoca, Romania: Argonaut Press.

Rutter, R., & Dedoussis, E. (2016). Workforce localisation and change management: The view from the Gulf. In A. Goksoy (Ed.), *Organizational change management strategies in modern business* (pp. 301–327). Hershey, PA: Business Science Reference.

Sander, L. (2017, February 28). *Lack of workers with 'soft skills' demands a shift in teaching.* The Conversation. Retrieved from http://theconversation.com/lack-of-workers-with-soft-skills-demands-a-shift-in-teaching-73433.

Sansom, L., Bretherton, R., & Niemiec, R. M. (2016). Doing the right thing: Character, moral goodness and Star Wars. *PsycCRITIQUES, 61*(25), Article 10.

Schwalje, W. (2013). *A conceptual model of national skills formation for knowledge-based economic development in the Arab world.* Al Qasimi Foundation. Retrieved from http://www.alqasimifoundation.com.

Seligman, M. E. P., & Csikszentmihalyi, M. (2000). Positive psychology: An Introduction. *American Psychologist, 55,* 5–14.

Seligman, M. E. P., Ernst, R. M., Gillham, J., Reivich, K., & Linkins, M. (2009). Positive education: Positive psychology and classroom interventions. *Oxford Review of Education, 35*(3), 293–311.

Seligman, M. E. P., Steen, T. A., Park, N., & Peterson, C. (2005). Positive psychology progress: Empirical validation of interventions. *American Psychologist, 60,* 410–421.

Shoshani, A., & Slone, M. (2013). Middle school transition from the strengths perspective: Young adolescents' character strengths, subjective wellbeing, and school adjustment. *Journal of Happiness Studies, 14*(4), 1163–1181.

Singh, A., Jones, D. B., & Hall, N. (2012). Talent management: A research based case study in the GCC region. *International Journal of Business and Management, 7*(24), 94–107.

Suldo, S. M., Thalji, A., & Ferron, J. (2011). Longitudinal academic outcomes predicted by early adolescents' subjective wellbeing, psychopathology, and mental health status yielded from a dual-factor model. *Journal of Positive Psychology, 6*(1), 17–30.

United Nations Development Programme (UNDP). (2016). *Arab human development report: Youth and the prospects for human development in a changing reality.* New York, NY: UNDP. Retrieved from http://hdr.undp.org/sites/default/files/reports/2699/ahdr2016en.pdf.

White, M. A. (2016). Why won't it stick? Positive psychology and positive education. *Psychology of Wellbeing, 6,* 2. Retrieved from https://doi.org/10.1186/s13612-016-0039-1.

Williams, G. (2016). Discovering the professional within: How identifying our character strengths can help build our ideal career and success. *PsychTalk, 85,* 5–9.

Wood, A. M., Linley, P. A., Matlby, J., Kashdan, T. B., & Hurling, R. (2011). Using personal and psychological strengths leads to increases in wellbeing over time: A longitudinal study and the development of the strengths use questionnaire. *Personality and Individual Differences, 50,* 15–19.

Chapter 6
Saudi Arabia's Road to Positivity: Positive Psychology Education and Research

Saddiga Jaber Al-Ghalib, Shaden Abdul-Hakeem Al-Khalifah, Afeefah Y. Salim and Rana Abdulrahman Hafed Dahlawi

Abstract In April 2016, a new vision for the Kingdom of Saudi Arabia was revealed on national TV. The ambitious blueprint outlines a long-term plan for diversifying the country's oil based economy. Set forth by Crown Prince Mohammad bin Salman, the Vision 2030 places Saudi citizens in the center of its quest for a post-oil era by recognizing Saudis as an untapped resource necessary for the country's new economic plan. The vision sets forth a number of goals, one of which is improving the social, physical and psychological wellbeing of Saudis. In this chapter, we provide an overview of a growing positive psychology movement in the Kingdom, as well as the accelerating effects recent economic and social reforms have had on the movement. Additionally, we briefly discuss how the predominant religion of Saudi Arabia, Islam, contributes to positive psychology, the beginning of positive psychology education in the nation and, the prospect of an indigenous positive psychology as a result of establishing the Kingdom's first positive psychology research lab.

6.1 Introduction

Islamic civilization began to flourish in the 8th century due to the contributions of Muslim scholars to science, philosophy, mathematics, medicine, and psychology. Early Muslim scholars wrote extensively about the tenets of human nature although the word "psychology" was not used at the time to describe this particular field of knowledge. The scholars called it "Ilm-al-Nafs" or self-knowledge. Many of their works appear as the basis for many psychological theories, ideas and practices of the modern age. Their works were specifically blended with Islamic philosophy and ideas that are decoded from the holy book of Muslims, the Quran (Haque, 2004). Concurrently, the word "science" comes from a Greek word that means "knowledge" or "to know". The science of the self is considered the basis for all other sciences in Islam: as the Prophet Muhammad (PBUH) said: "He who knows himself knows Allah (God)". Thus, in Islamic tradition, there is no schism between religion and

S. J. Al-Ghalib (✉) · S. A.-H. Al-Khalifah · A. Y. Salim · R. A. H. Dahlawi
Effat University, Jeddah, Saudi Arabia
e-mail: salghalib@effatuniversity.edu.sa

L. Lambert and N. Pasha-Zaidi (eds.), *Positive Psychology in the Middle East/North Africa*, https://doi.org/10.1007/978-3-030-13921-6_6

science, as is the norm in the West, because science and religion are considered complementary and not contradictory. After the demise of the Islamic civilization, the Muslim civilization entered its Dark Ages and lost its excellence in science as its focus was diverted to expand the boundaries of the Islamic empire (Khodayarifard et al., 2016; Rezaeitalarposhti & Rezaeitalarposhti, 2013).

Recently, a trend has been emerging where psychologists are giving importance to spirituality and utilizing religious teachings or practices as psychological interventions. For example, mindfulness, religious coping, Acceptance and Commitment Therapy (ACT), etc., have been adapted from religious origins. Khodayarifard and colleagues (2016) state that Islamic spirituality, in terms of its focus on positive thinking, is a source that has not yet been comprehensively and extensively investigated.

Topic Box: Prevalence of Psychological Disorders in Saudi Arabia

No studies to date have examined the prevalence of psychological disorders, nor provided an accurate depiction of current rates of psychological problems in Saudi Arabia. Despite this, researchers looking into the area of mental health research can find useful information in a few studies. Becker, AlZaid, and AlFaris (2002) examined the prevalence of somatization and depression among outpatients from a primary health care facility in Riyadh. The self-administered Patient Health Questionnaire (PHQ) was given to a sample of 431 patients (45.9% male and 54.1% female). The participant's ages ranged between 18 and 80 with the majority of them under 50 (75%). The results indicated a 19.3% prevalence of somatization (69% females), 13.5% prevalence of generalized anxiety disorder (68.2% females), 20% prevalence of depression (67.4% females), and 10.2%, (79.4% females) prevalence of panic disorder. Al Gelban (2009) examined the prevalence of psychiatric symptoms among high school students aged between 14 and 19. The Symptom Checklist 90 (SCL-90-R) was used in a sample of 545 young people. The all-female participants were recruited from 10 schools in Abha. According to the researchers: 16% of participants reported symptoms of phobic anxiety, 15% reported symptoms of psychoticism, 14% anxiety, 14% somatization, and 14% reported symptoms of depression.

6.2 The Positive Islamic Psychology Movement

In earlier times, psychology focused on the negative side of human psychology; in particular, how to alleviate mental illness. However, at the end of the 20th century, psychologist Martin Seligman challenged the focus of psychology on disease and established a "positive psychology", which aimed instead to develop the positive side of human psychology. He believed that psychology had been missing an important role in society; that is, working for the betterment of society by enhancing wellbeing and flourishing. His 2011 book described "flourishing" as the outcome of specific scientifically-backed practices that help make life worth living and promote wellbeing. Seligman initially selected happiness as the ultimate goal of positive psychology. Soon, he realized this was naïve. He stated in his earlier book "Authentic Happiness" (2002) that happiness is in fact, only one aspect of achieving wellbeing and flourishing. He introduced his theory of wellbeing called PERMA (Seligman, 2011), where positive emotions, engagement, relationships, meaning and accomplishment are essential to human wellbeing. In order to flourish, an individual has to strive towards enhancing these elements. Support through scientific research for his theory was offered as well as detailed examples of how to use positive psychology in different circumstances. Table 6.1 provides a brief explanation of each element of the PERMA model.

The PERMA model and other theories found under the umbrella of positive psychology are familiar to Muslims. A plausible cause for this would be that in Islam, the Holy Quran and the Prophet Muhammad (PBUH) always encouraged Muslims to stay positive even in the face of adversity. The following Hadith (Prophets' saying) advises people to stay positive: "Whoever abstains from asking others, Allah will make him contented, and whoever tries to make himself self-sufficient, Allah will make him self-sufficient. And whoever remains patient, Allah will make him patient. Nobody can be given a blessing better and greater than patience" (Sahih Al-Bukhari). The Quran gives Muslims many solutions to live a fulfilling life and enhance their wellbeing like patience, thinking positively, developing optimism and relying on prayer: "O you who have believed, seek help through patience and prayer. Indeed, Allah is with the patient" (Quran 2:153). This particular chapter also mentions that God does not give a soul a hardship that it cannot endure. Another chapter states that with every difficulty there will be ease (Quran 94:6). Abu Hurayrah, one

Table 6.1 PERMA: a brief review (Seligman, 2011)

Essential elements	Description
Positive emotions	Feeling good and experiencing more positive emotions by contemplating one's past, present and future
Engagement	Acknowledging and using one's personal strengths to be more consciously engaged in work and other activities and enjoying optimal moments in a state of flow as a result
Relationships	Spending time to maintain strong relationships and being authentically connected to other people allows one to feel supported and be able to offer support to others in return
Meaning	Dedicating time to accomplish goals that are greater than one's individual interests, such as community work, charity, political causes, environmental causes, faith, etc., which allow one to live a purposeful existence
Accomplishment	Working on establishing and reaching ones goals that motivate them and give them a sense of accomplishment and success

of the companions of the Prophet Muhammad (PBUH), reported him to have said: "Allah the Most High said, 'I am as My servant thinks (expects) I am. I am with him when he mentions Me. If he mentions Me to himself, I mention him to Myself; and if he mentions Me in an assembly, I mention him in an assembly greater than it. If he draws near to Me a hand's length, I draw near to him an arm's length. And if he comes to Me walking, I go to him at speed" (Sahih Al-Bukhari).

Having faith and anticipating that good things will come is important to living a life filled with meaning and purpose. The principles of Islamic Positive Psychology are derived from the Holy Book and the teachings of Prophet Muhammad (PBUH). Muslim scholars have taken the initiative to use the knowledge that was already given to humans hundreds of years ago and refine it to serve the purposes of modern societies. Muslim and Arab psychologists have recently started the trend of making use of religious or spiritual practices such as prayer, Tasbeeh, etc., as positive psychology interventions as well as clinical interventions (Abdullah, 2014). The following verses from the Holy Quran and Hadiths express how Islam attempts to get its followers to become positive individuals living fruitful lives and gives solutions to help them rid their worries.

- "And your Lord says: Call upon Me, I will answer you; surely those who are too proud to worship Me shall soon enter hell abased" (Quran 40:60).
- "Whoever does a lot of Istighfar (asking for forgiveness), Allah will provide him a way out of each concern he has, and will solve all his troubles, and will provide him with livelihood from sources that were not known to him" (Sahih Al-Bukhari, Muslim).
- "The strong believer is better and more beloved to Allah than the weak believer, although there is good in each. Desire that which will bring you benefit, and seek help from Allah and do not give way to incapacity. If something happens to you, do not say, 'If only I had done such-and-such.' Rather say, 'The decree of Allah. He does what He will.' Otherwise you will open yourself up to the action of Shaitan" (Muslim).

Saudi Arabia is a country that views itself as the heart of the Arab and Islamic nations. It is very proud of its Islamic historical and cultural legacy and the country has recently come to recognize the importance of preserving its heritage and Islamic values to promote national unity. In the recently established Vision 2030, the country acknowledged that the happiness and fulfillment of its citizens and residents is important and has stated that this goal can be achieved only through the promotion of physical, psychological and social wellbeing (Vision 2030, 2016).

6.3 Saudi Arabia's Positive Vision

On September 26, 2017, the Saudi representative at the United Nations, Abdullah bin Yahya Al-Moalimi, took the stand to make an announcement regarding the lifting of the ban on women driving (Alarabia, 2017). Families around the country had gathered to hear a reading of the royal decree made on national TV. Issued by King Salman, the historic decree overturned a decade long ban on women driving. This change came as part of a series of sweeping economic and social reforms modernizing life in Saudi Arabia. A few months prior to giving women the right to drive, another policy was overturned allowing women access to attend sporting events held at football stadiums in three major cities. Girls in public schools were also given the right to play sports and receive physical education, while the guardianship law (a law limiting women's freedom of mobility and autonomy) was also loosened. Today, Saudi women can work and obtain driving licenses without the presence or written permission of a male guardian. Women have grown stronger after years of facing challenges and the government has begun taking the lead in improving the state of women's rights and reducing the gender gap in the Kingdom.

In an effort to revitalize Saudi culture, the government has also overturned a ban on cinemas and music events. The move came as a result of de-regulating the entertainment industry in the Kingdom. This change in policy brought to the surface a growing arts scene, one that was kept underground for many years. Local talent is now encouraged to participate in exhibitions and cultural events by the help of the government as well as organizations like Community Jameel (Community Jameel, n.d.). The government has also revealed plans for developing more cultural venues such as libraries and museums as part of its vision for 2030.

The vision, revealed in 2016 by Crown Prince Muhammad bin Salman, is an ambitious blueprint that outlines a long-term plan for diversifying the country's oil-based economy. Women and Saudi youth are key features of this vision. Young Saudis are recognized as an asset to be harnessed because they make up more than half of the population. Thus, the vision sets forth a goal to close the gap between higher education outputs and the requirements of the job market. Additionally, 50% of university graduates in the Kingdom are women yet, they make up only 22% of the workforce. This number is estimated to grow up to 30% in the upcoming years (Vision 2030, 2016).

> "One of our most significant assets is our lively and vibrant youth. We will guarantee their skills are developed and properly deployed. While many other countries are concerned with aging populations, more than half of the Saudi population is below the age of 25 years. We will take advantage of this demographic by harnessing our youth's energy and by expanding entrepreneurship and enterprise opportunities. Saudi women are yet another great asset. We will continue to develop their talents, invest in their productive capabilities and enable them to strengthen their future and contribute to the development of our society and economy" (Vision 2030, 2016).

The vision designed by Crown Prince Muhammad Bin Salman has generated a great sense of motivation and optimism among Saudis. The current sociopolitical discourse in the country is charged with feelings of excitement and hope for the future. These reforms have driven many Saudis to believe in the 2030 vision; among those most enthusiastic are members of the positive psychology movement. The theme "Vibrant Society: With fulfilling lives" is one component of the vision that has received near universal praise from members of the movement. In it, the Saudi citizen is recognized as a key component, necessary for a post-oil era. Accordingly, the vision describes a plan to promote the physical, social, and psychological wellbeing of Saudis. In fact, two projects described in this chapter, the Positive Psychology and Wellbeing Research Lab and the Positive Psychology Symposium, were inspired by the plans and goals described in this theme.

> "Saudi Arabia has enormous untapped opportunities and a rich blend of natural resources, but our real wealth lies in our people and our society. The happiness and fulfillment of citizens and residents are important to us. At the heart of our vision is a society in which all enjoy a good quality of life, a healthy lifestyle, and an attractive living environment. Our goal is to promote and reinvigorate social development in order to build a strong and productive society" (Vision 2030, 2016).

The prospect of concepts such as happiness and personal wellbeing becoming goals of future public policy is an indication of an underlying shift in the government's approach to increasing citizen's productivity. This shift has resonated with members of the positive psychology movement in the country and has inspired many of their current projects that promote the philosophy and practice of the discipline.

6.4 A Growing Movement of Positive Psychology and Other Practices

Among the rapid economic and social changes taking place in Saudi Arabia, there is a trend of people incorporating positive psychology into their daily lives. Saudi citizens have taken up practices such as healthy eating, growing organic food, exercising, meditation, mindfulness, yoga, journaling, etc. to live meaningful and fulfilling lives. Workplaces are incorporating team building activities and other practices to create a positive and motivating atmosphere. Companies have finally come to the understanding that employees have needs apart from salaries that affect job satisfaction and productivity (Alahmadi, 2002; Alotaibi, Paliadelis, & Valenzuela, 2015; Hamad & Al Kwifi, 2015). For example, job stress levels can negatively affect job satisfaction. Saudi Arabia is reported to have high levels of job stress and workplace violence (54%), especially in the private sector (Alzalabani, 2017).

The Saudi Arabian workforce has just begun focusing on enhancing the newly developed concept of psychological capital, defined as "the extent to which an individual operates in a positive psychological state, and this state is characterized by high self-efficacy, optimism, hope, and resiliency" (Idris & Manganaro, 2017, p. 251). Idris and Manganaro (2017) highlight the importance of measuring such psychological constructs which can allow managers to create training programs and provide adequate support to help promote a better work environment. Enhanced psychological capital has many benefits, some of which are greater organizational commitment, positive organizational citizenship behaviors, lower employee absenteeism, and greater motivation, engagement, achievement, and higher job satisfaction (Datu, King, & Valdez, 2016; Pradhan, Jena, & Bhattacharya, 2016). Studies have shown that having positive attitudes such as hope and optimism have a significant positive relationship with altruism and sportsmanship behaviors (Alessandri et al., 2012; Van Dyne, Vandewalle, Kostova, Latham, & Cummings, 2000). Vision 2030 encourages employers to instill these attitudes in their employees.

Many initiatives are popping up around Saudi Arabia, especially in the larger cities. Government officials such as Prince Khalid Al-Faisal, Advisor to the Custodian of the Two Holy Mosques and Prince of Makkah region, have started initiatives for the betterment of society such as "How to be a Role Model" campaign. This campaign aims to promote community service and teaches young students social responsibility. Many projects such as the Makkah Schools Maintenance Project were started under this campaign. These stem from the notion that Islam urges people to become good role models in all aspects of life (Jabalomar, 2017). 'Community Jameel' is a social enterprise that was started in 2003 and which generated a range of initiatives that aim to promote and contribute to enhancing positive societal change and economic sustainability. It helps individuals by offering various trainings, creating jobs, and supporting businesses that help communities transform themselves. A notable investment by this particular organization is that it supports local artists by showcasing their art (Community Jameel, n.d.).

Saudi Arabia is also taking steps to support the establishment of networking hubs and other organizations that provide a positive and creative space for young entrepreneurs to develop their business ideas and follow their ambitions. These organizations promote empowerment, social responsibility, a positive work environment and provide opportunities for getting social support. Some examples of such organizations are Riyadh Hub, Shababuna Creative Hub, and Vibes. Shababuna Creative Hub is currently in the midst of creating educational toys and stationary items that reflect Islamic values for kids and teens. The United Nations Development Programme in Saudi Arabia is another large initiative designed to maintain and enhance environmental wellbeing in the country. Their goal is to conserve biodiversity and protect wildlife to maintain ecological equilibrium. They also plan to make the country energy efficient in the next 20 years by comprehensively using energy efficiency standards and labels (United Nations Development Programme, n.d.).

An increasing number of events focused on wellbeing are also being initiated. For example, Creative Mornings Jeddah Chapter arranges talks and events where people can share and express their views on chosen topics (Creative Mornings, n.d.). They can connect with one another and get inspired by others' experiences. Many workshops on topics that come under the umbrella of positive psychology are being offered to people within the country, especially in cities like Jeddah and Riyadh. While the public is on the right path, the means they use to reach the goal of a better country do not necessarily have scientific backing. There is a growing need for positive psychology research to be generated. Interventions that are based on the people's needs and Saudi Arabian society and culture are urgently required as most positive psychology practices are adopted from the West. While these practices are not necessarily harmful, they are also not necessarily appropriate for the culture of Saudi Arabia as they were created with western population needs in mind.

Topic Box: Hamza Iskandar

Hamza Iskandar is a prominent figure in the positive psychology movement in Saudi Arabia. In 2012, the young man's journey of positivity started with a cancer diagnosis. The fearless warrior decided within two hours of receiving the news to spend the rest of his life fighting cancer and taboos surrounding it. Through his "I fight cancer with a smile" campaign, the young man fought against misconceptions surrounding the disease. In an interview with the MD Anderson Cancer Center at the University of Texas, Hamza said: "People back home are scared of cancer. They don't ever want to talk about it. I want to teach them that it's not a death sentence. You don't have to be afraid."

Throughout his life, Hamza advocated a positive reframing of cancer related language. In one of his initiatives he collaborated with a local hospital, The International Medical Center (IMC), to change the name of their cancer unit from "IMC Cancer Patient Center" to "IMC Cancer Fighter Center". Hamza spent most of his time giving motivational speeches and visiting cancer fighters in hospitals around the Kingdom and neighboring countries. He was a strong believer in the importance of support and a positive environment for cancer warriors, saying, while describing the purpose of his Cancer Support Center: "I hope I can change people's ideas about cancer patients and spread positive vibes instead of negative ones, because that is what a support system is all about." Despite passing away in 2017 due to bronchitis-related complications, Hamza's message of optimism continues to inspire others inside and outside the positive psychology movement.

6.5 Developments in the Research Culture of Saudi Arabia

Since 2002, the Saudi government has exhorted great efforts to increase research productivity in the country. These efforts have led to the development of a research infrastructure and the emergence of a culture that appreciates scientific pursuits. Yet, despite these advancements, research productivity in the fields of psychology and mental health is still in its infancy. A climate conducive to scientific research in Saudi Arabia began to emerge when the Saudi government developed a long-term vision of science, technology, and innovation (STI). The aim of this vision is to transfer the Saudi economy from oil-based to knowledge-based, placing the Kingdom among the highest-ranking countries in science, technology and innovation by the year 2025 (Al-Swailem, 2014). Following the development of this vision, the government focused its efforts on increasing research productivity in public, medical and academic settings. For instance, new ministry and government research centers were established, increasing the number of research facilities in public settings to 46.

According to a 2013 estimate, these centers produced 2119 studies in the fields of medicine, engineering, agriculture, water desalination, environment and humanities (Alshayea, 2013).

For the promotion of creativity and innovation, the government also established a variety of institutions in different cities around the Kingdom. The "Foundation for Giftedness & Creativity" and the "Riyadh Charitable Foundation for Science" are two institutions playing a key role in raising awareness for the scientific and technical support available to inventors and scientists (Alshayea, 2013). Additionally, a National Medical and Health Research strategy was developed as part of the Kingdom's STI vision for 2025, the goal of which is to promote research in medical and health sciences to further the health and wellbeing of Saudis. A national committee was assembled to develop a list of priority research areas to become the focus of this strategy and after a careful assessment of the current prevalence and incidence of diseases, the committee identified nine priority research areas. Notably, mental health research is emphasized, along with disability and neurodegenerative diseases (Koenig, 2014).

Further, research in academic settings was encouraged through initiatives such as the "Research Excellence Centers". This initiative had two phases during which 14 research centers including three Nanotechnology Institutes were established in different universities around the Kingdom, with the Center of Research Excellence in Renewable Energy and the King Abdullah Institute for Nanotechnology as examples. These efforts have indeed promoted a culture of research in the Kingdom and initiated the development of a research infrastructure. Yet, despite the many strides made, research productivity in the area of psychology and mental health research remains low. In fact, according to a recent study looking at mental health research publications in the Arab world between the years 2006 and 2012, Saudi Arabia had a decline in mental health research. Hence, it moved down from its rank of second highest in terms of research publications between 1996 and 2006 to fifth highest between 2006 and 2012 (Jaalouk, Okasha, Salamoun, & Karam, 2012; Karam & Itani, 2015). No signs of improvement can be found in psychology departments around the country and most research can be described as fragmented, non-accumulative and conducted mostly for short-term purposes such as the obtainment of a degree or work promotion.

Despite the current poor situation of research productivity in the areas of psychology and mental health, there are reasons to expect a future increase in research activity after the introduction of the 2030 Vision. As noted, the recent change in government priorities has placed the overall wellbeing of Saudi citizens at the heart of its future plans. Consequently, this inspired a team of four women, the authors of this chapter, to establish not only the first positive psychology research lab in the Kingdom, but the first of only two across the entire Middle East/North Africa (MENA) region.

Topic Box: An Early Example of a Woman Scholar in Psychology

Today, female scholars are recognized as essential to the development of an inclusive scientific view of the world and human behavior. Yet throughout history, cultural notions of gender and cognitive disparities between men and women have intersected with science and affected the practice of research in academia (Keller, 1995). When examining the history of female scholars who challenged the gender roles of their time, Mary Whiton Calkins comes to mind. The psychologist and philosopher established the first psychology research lab at a liberal arts college in Boston, Massachusetts. In 1891, women in the United States were given limited opportunities to learn and work in higher education. Calkins, who taught at the all girls Wellesley College, was one of the few women in her time to learn and teach experimental psychology. The new, laboratory-based field was a transition from the old, non-empirical psychology called, at the time, "Mental Philosophy". As an instructor of experimental psychology, Calkins received her education at the hands of William James, Josiah Royce, and Hugo Münsterberg. Yet, as a woman, she was denied a degree from Harvard University despite fulfilling all the requirements for a Ph.D. (Furumoto, 1980). She instead received an offer for a Ph.D degree from Radcliffe College (the only institution for girls associated with Harvard), but refused to accept it as an act of activism against the discriminatory system applied by institutions at the time (Furumoto, 1980).

6.6 The Beginning of Positive Psychology Education in Saudi Arabia

In 1999, Queen Effat Al-Thunyan established the University of Effat in southeast Jeddah. The Queen, who was born and raised in Turkey along with her spouse, the late King Fasisal bin Abdulaziz, institutionalized the formal education of girls in Saudi Arabia. Despite strong resistance from the conservative and religious community in the Kingdom, the couple managed to establish multiple schools and colleges for girls (Hamdan, 2005; Kechichian, 2015). Effat University became the first private institution for higher education in Saudi Arabia. This world renowned university is a testament to the Queen's vision. Strengthened by her legacy, the university has pioneered many advancements in women's education. It was the first institution in Saudi Arabia to offer Architecture, Electrical & Computer Engineering, Entrepreneurship, Visual and Digital Production, Operation and Information Management, Energy Engineering, Islamic Finance Management, Urban Design and many more courses exclusively to women. Effat University is also the first educational institution in the MENA region to offer Positive Psychology as a course to its students. It was included in the new program adopted by the psychology department at the university

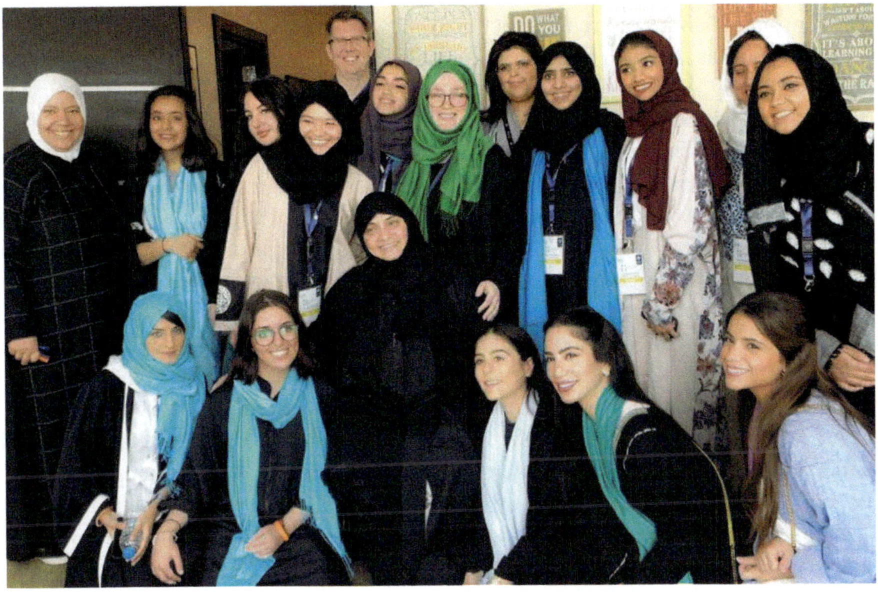

Fig. 6.1 Positive psychology at Effat University with Dr. Saddiga Al-Ghalib

with the aim of exposing its students to newer subfields of psychology such as cyber psychology, sports psychology, and forensic psychology. It was first offered in the fall of 2013 as a technical elective for psychology undergraduates.

The Positive Psychology course offered at Effat University became one of the most popular technical electives offered by the department. Students were skeptical at the start, as they initially believed that positive psychology was solely about happiness. However, their perceptions changed as they realized what positive psychology was really about, exploring topics such as flow, mindfulness, gratitude, forgiveness, hope, love, optimism, wellbeing, etc. The course includes fun activities such as debates, campaigns, guest speakers and offers an opportunity to test some positive psychology interventions. Over the years, students emerge from the course enlightened with new knowledge that will not only help them in their professional lives but also enhance their personal ones (Fig. 6.1).

6.7 The Positive Psychology and Wellbeing Research Lab (PPWRL)

Dr. Saddiga Al-Ghalib, an Assistant Professor of Psychology (and first author of this chapter), became the informal spokesperson for positive psychology at Effat University as she came to know about the subject throughout her own personal struggles. After trying many practices, she stumbled upon a positive psychology intervention which had a great impact on her life. She used a combination of Islamic practices such as Tasbeeh and scientific positive interventions to enhance her personal wellbeing. She then started teaching positive psychology at Effat University. One of her senior students conducted a study that found high levels of depression, anxiety and stress in nearly 860 university students. The results were shocking and intriguing at the same time. This made her ponder whether there was a solution for this issue as there was clear evidence of the presence of high levels of distress in Saudi college students. In 2017, Afeefah Yahya Salim, a psychology senior at Effat University, presented her thesis on the Jeddah Mindful Program (below). The project examined the effectiveness of a newly developed mindfulness intervention. Although the sample was small, the study yielded promising results and Afeefah, along with her supervisor Dr. Al-Ghalib, received positive feedback from the majority of the participants. Consequently, the pair started to further test the program.

A few months later, Dr. Al-Ghalib, Afeefah, Shaden Alkhalifan and Rana Dahlawi gathered to discuss the potential of developing further programs similar to the Mindful Jeddah program. Shortly after, the discussion progressed to address the necessity of having a place where like-minded individuals could come together to examine the factors affecting people's mental health and wellbeing as well as develop culturally-sensitive and evidence-based interventions to promote the social, spiritual, physical and psychological wellbeing of individuals in society. That conversation led the four women to develop the idea of establishing a positive psychology research lab. In the months following, the team developed an official proposal to establish the lab. Each member contributed a different set of skills, experiences, and knowledge to the team, and talked about their goals and motivations that fueled their passion for this project (Fig. 6.2).

Dr. Al-Ghalib and Afeefah's goal is to further develop positive psychology interventions and programs. Shaden is driven to provide the students of Effat

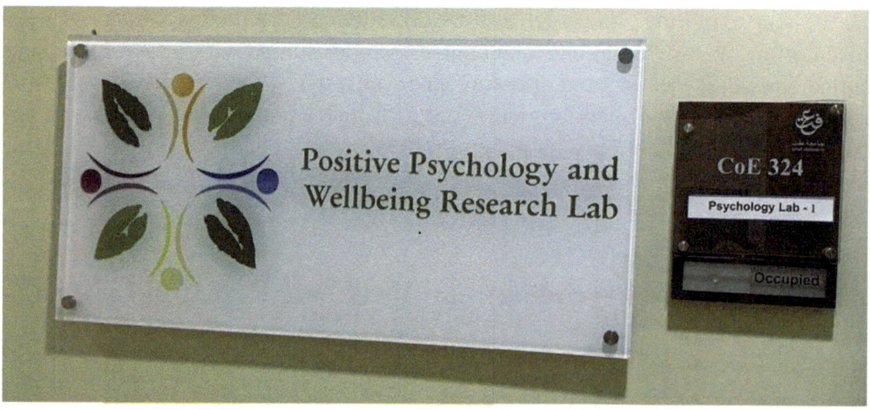

Fig. 6.2 The positive psychology & Wellbeing Research Lab (PPWRL) is located in the Psychology Department at Effat University

University with the same research opportunities she received abroad, while Rana's passion for experimental psychology made her eager to contribute to a growing culture of research in the Kingdom. The team members went on to shape the vision and mission for the lab and on April 29, 2018, the *Positive Psychology & Wellbeing Research Lab* (PPWRL) was established. Located in the psychology department at Effat University, the five-room lab is equipped with a meeting room, reception area, storage and observation room with double mirrors overlooking a testing room. A sound and camera system were set up in the observation room along with a library housing books on a variety of topics such as mindfulness, happiness, leadership, wisdom, and positive psychology.

6.7.1 Mission and Vision of the Lab

As the first of its kind, the PPWRL vision is to lead the positive psychology movement in Saudi Arabia and significantly improve the wellbeing of individuals in our society. The founders of the PPWR Lab define positive psychology as the scientific study of human flourishing and an applied approach to optimal functioning (Positive Psychology Institute). It also includes the study of strengths and virtues that enable individuals, communities and organizations to thrive. Positive psychology as a field is grounded in the belief that people want to lead meaningful and fulfilling lives, to cultivate what is best within them, and to enhance their experiences of love, work, and play (Seligman, 2009). As for psychological wellbeing, the founders define it in accordance with the PERMA Model, stating that wellbeing consists of Positive Emotions, Engagement, Relationships, Meaning, and Accomplishments (Seligman, 2011). Within this theoretical framework, the founders developed the lab's mission to include conducting multidisciplinary research in the fields of positive psychology and wellbeing and to translate the findings of this research into practice by producing evidence-based interventions tailored to serve the Saudi population. In addition, the lab aims to help academics by providing services and opportunities for research, education, training and the dissemination of knowledge and awareness in Saudi society. Thus, the lab has the following four functions that work simultaneously to help the founders achieve their mission: research, assessment development, community services, and professional services.

- **Research**: The lab aims to produce cutting edge research that investigates the practical implications of positive psychology theories in improving the wellbeing of individuals in Saudi society. The research function aims to create programs that have gone through rigorous scientific procedures that target the needs of the population that will adopt these programs into their daily lives.
- **Assessment**: The lab aims to validate and culturally adapt assessments widely used in clinical settings such as psychiatric hospitals, counseling centers and clinics within the Kingdom. Multiple scales have been developed as a result, i.e., the Women Driving Scale (see below).

- **Community Services**: The lab offers workshops and lectures, and arranges for events to educate the public on the theory and practice of positive psychology, as well as raise awareness of the importance of research in clinical practice. It also aims to provide students and academics alike with assistance and guidance to help them develop their research skills.
- **Professional Service**: One of the future plans for the lab is to provide local professionals, who apply a positive psychology approach to their practice, with a virtual and physical space to help them connect with new clients and other professionals in the field.

6.7.2 Research Assistant Program

The PPWR Lab is in a unique position to facilitate the growth of the scientific literature representing an understudied population such as the one in Saudi Arabia. The lab, with its location at an all-girls university, has the potential to play a key role in nurturing the female perspective in scientific research, particularly in the area of mental health research where a history of white male dominance has influenced the treatment and conceptualization of mental health problems among women and minorities. Thus, the lab offers a Research Assistant Program (RA) designed to increase research productivity. The program is an investment in the students of Effat University who the founders believe can be trained to make valuable contributions to the growing body of literature in mental health and wellbeing.

The RA Program offered at the lab is based on a research assistant model that was developed by the founders in 2017. The model aims to develop the research skills of undergraduate students and enable them to undertake an individual or collaborative research project. The model is composed of four levels: Pre-Foundation, Foundation, Intermediate, and Advanced. Each is designed to achieve certain learning outcomes. RAs can gradually develop their research skills as they move from one level to the next. A training program with theoretical and practical components is designed for each level. The program is composed of lectures, workshops and a set of lab duties tailored to meet each level's learning objectives.

Effat students from all majors are welcomed to apply to the lab's RA Program. Applicants are required to complete an online course about the ethics of research on human subjects. The course is followed by an online exam given by the Saudi National Committee of Bioethics (NCBE). The committee is responsible for "developing and monitoring compliance with bio/medical research ethics and standards in Saudi Arabia" (Al-Swailem, 2018). Students taking the NCBE course are expected to learn about the laws governing research in the Kingdom and the legal history behind the evolution and implementation of these laws.

After successful completion of the NCBE course and exam, applicants are invited for an interview with one of the lab founders. Based on the applicant's performance in the exam and during their interview, they are placed into one of the four available levels. Once accepted into the lab, RAs are briefed about lab policies and procedures and assigned tasks, which can vary from administrative in nature, to research specific depending on their level. During their time in the Program, RAs are required to attend lectures and workshops designed to meet the learning objectives of their level. For instance, lectures on the scientific method and an SPSS workshop for beginners are mandatory in the foundational level.

By the end of the program year, RAs interested in advancing to the next level must meet minimum requirements for promotion. Since the goal of the program is to encourage research among undergraduates, RAs advancing to the next level must show an understanding of the different elements involved in the research process. For instance, in order to move from pre-foundation to foundation, RAs must develop a research question, while moving from foundation to intermediate requires the development of a hypothesis. By the time they reach the advanced level, they will have a complete plan for a research project preparing them to undertake an individual or collaborative project. The RA program is in its early stages of development. The first implementation of the program was in January 2018, with six RAs now enrolled. The effectiveness of the RA model will be evaluated in the light of RA's feedback and used to make improvements.

6.8 Planting the Seeds for an Indigenous Positive Psychology

Rao, Donaldson, and Doiron (2015) conducted a study to review the literature on positive psychology in the MENA region. The most popular topic of interest was subjective wellbeing including life satisfaction and happiness. Positive psychology research in the MENA region has been taking a distinctive direction as most of the predictors of wellbeing that are studied are spirituality, religion, family and social support as opposed to the western trend of studying character strengths, resilience, hope, growth and gratitude. Further analysis of the literature revealed that two main approaches are being used to enrich positive psychology research in the region. The first includes developing and studying constructs that help in building positive qualities in individuals and improve their quality of life, while the second involves applying positive constructs with the aim of helping develop coping skills and overcoming adversity. Although the research is in its infancy, the enthusiasm of researchers and the interest being generated in the topic makes up for it. The PPWR lab is in the midst of conducting several studies covering a range of topics under positive psychology and targets its research to the growing psychological needs and issues of the Saudi population. Our current research projects are featured below in Table 6.2.

Table 6.2 Current research projects at the PPWR Lab

Program	Description
The Mindful Jeddah Program in Saudi Academic Society	Jon Kabat-Zinn, founder of the Mindfulness Based Stress Reduction Program, describes mindfulness as the "awareness that arises through paying attention, on purpose, in the present moment, non-judgmentally" (Kabat-Zinn, 2003, 2012, p. 1). Mindfulness is the practice of being self-aware of the here and now, whereas a lack of mindfulness is as if you are putting your brain in autopilot. Mindfulness also involves a non-judging and non-identifying attitude (Hollis-Walker & Colosimo, 2011). The aim of this experimental study was to investigate the effectiveness of a new mindfulness based wellbeing program—Mindful Jeddah Program—on a Saudi academic group. A total of 26 participants completed a 3-week program after being randomly assigned to either the control group or experimental group. A paired sample t-test revealed that the Mindful Jeddah program had a significant effect on life satisfaction. However, no significant effect was seen on variables of wellbeing, stress, anxiety and spirituality (Al-Ghalib & Salim, 2018).
The Mindful Jeddah Program in Saudi Workplaces	Mindfulness can act as an effective tool in buffering the negative effects of stress that have become a reality in many people's working lives. Using mindfulness techniques as a way to improve the way people relate to one another can enhance corporate culture by creating a more caring and friendlier workplace. However, almost all of these programs have been made with the Western and European population in mind and there are almost no comprehensive and culturally-sensitive mindfulness-based wellbeing programs in Arab society. The aim of this study was to test the effectiveness of a newly established mindfulness training program called the 'Mindful Jeddah' Program in a Saudi Arabian workplace.
Benefits of gratitude: interventions applied to a Saudi Arabian Academic Society	Gratitude is a construct that cannot be easily classified, as it is has been considered a moral virtue, emotion, attitude, personality trait, habit and coping response. This study will benefit society by creating awareness about the benefits of gratitude interventions and the importance of Islamic values to Muslims. Practicing gratitude has multiple benefits; better quality of life, greater happiness, wellbeing and sleep quality, lower levels of depression, anxiety, aggression and stress, better relationships, etc. (Bhullar, Surman, & Schutte, 2015; Jacobsen, 2013). Yet, the literature on the relationship between gratitude and spirituality is limited. Most interventions that make use of gratitude exercises were developed in the West. The aim of this study was to look at the benefits of an Islamic based intervention on an Arab population that comprises a majority of Muslims. The literature, although limited, supports the notion that an intervention that is inclusive of the spiritual needs of the Muslim population is more efficient (Al-Seheel & Noor, 2016). The research project is comprised of two studies that use different approaches to examine gratitude, wellbeing, spirituality, life satisfaction, emotions, depression, stress, anxiety and happiness.

(continued)

Table 6.2 (continued)

Program	Description
Validating the School Spirit Scale in a University in Jeddah, Saudi Arabia	School spirit means representing one's school proudly through actions that paint the school and community in a positive light, and which demonstrate student's love for it. However, research suggests that student dissatisfaction ranging from intellectual and social detachment to apathy has risen in the last decades (Terzian, 2004). Universities in Saudi Arabia seem to be facing low levels of school spirit; however, no steps have been taken to measure it. The aim of this research was to determine the level of school spirit in a private university in Jeddah, Saudi Arabia and offer solutions for improvement. It also aims to examine whether there is a relationship between school spirit, happiness, and motivation. This study will be significant for educational institutions in Saudi Arabia and is the first of its kind to be conducted in the nation. As a result of this study, a scale will be developed which can be used as an example for other educational institutions.
Relationship between obesity and psychological wellbeing: a case study in Saudi Arabia	Obesity has become a global epidemic and major risk factor for the development of disability, co-morbidities, and premature death. Medical factors include easily diagnosed issues such as hormonal imbalances; however, regional psychological factors contributing to the development of obesity are often more complicated to determine (Razzak, Qawas, El-Metwally, Harbi, & Al-Shujairi, 2017). The study examines obesity/overweight and its prevalence, risk and protective factors, weight loss interventions and psychological wellbeing. An alarming 75% of people in Saudi Arabia have been categorized as obese or overweight (Alqarni, 2016), while one in four males and one in three females in the adult population of Saudi Arabia have been diagnosed with obesity (Memish et al., 2014).
Public perception of women driving: relationships with personality and effects on wellbeing	Driving for women in Saudi Arabia has been a debate for ages. Finally, the Saudi government has granted its female citizens the right to do so. Consequently, there is a dire need to examine the public's opinion on Saudi women driving in a scientific manner. This research will be divided into three separate studies across three different time frames. The study aims to examine the relationship between an individual's perception of Saudi women driving and their level of openness. Another aim is to discover how the affordance of women driving in Saudi Arabia affects their wellbeing and satisfaction with life. These perception will illustrate the direction of where national social changes may be headed in the future (Al-Ghalib, Salim, Al-Khalifah, & Dahlawi, 2018).

6.9 The Positive Psychology Symposium

Following the establishment of the PPWR Lab, the first Positive Psychology Symposium in the Middle East was held on March 29, 2018. The goal of this symposium was to amplify the voices of scholars in the field of positive psychology and highlight research activity in this region of the world. Effat University, as a leading figure of the Positive Psychology Movement in Saudi Arabia, organized and hosted the symposium. The two-day event showcased recent research developments underpinning best practices and innovations in the field of positive psychology. The annual symposium aims to:

- Promote the scientific understanding and implementation of positive psychology through various evidence-based methodologies.
- Encourage young people to embrace positive psychology in their lives.
- Understand the relationship between Islamic values and psychology.
- Promote positive psychology research in the Kingdom of Saudi Arabia, the countries of the Gulf Cooperation Council (GCC), and the Middle East/North Africa (MENA) region.

The symposium provided a platform for seven scholars from different countries to present their papers on a variety of topics in the field. For instance, Irwan Nuryana Kurniawan, from Universitas Islam Indonesia presented two papers titled "Exploring and Validating the Questionnaire of Takwa to Allah Taala with Indonesian Islamic Boarding School Students" and "Constructing and Validating Psychological Instrument Al-Akhlaq Al-Karimah Quality of Life for Indonesian Muslims". Muhammad Safdar, Gulfam Ali Safdar, Muhammad Abdul Malik and Kamran Masood from the International Islamic University in Islamabad, Pakistan presented their paper on "Positive Psychology and Islamic Spiritualization".

The event had two keynote speakers, Dr. David Creswell, and Dr. Louise Lambert. An associate professor of psychology from Carnegie Mellon University (USA), Dr. Creswell is a researcher in the field of positive psychology and interested in understanding human resilience, stress, and coping. He discussed his most recent research exploring various stress management techniques that can alter coping and stress. More specifically, he is exploring how the use of simple strategies such as self-affirmation, rewarding activities, and cognitive reappraisal can buffer stress and improve problem solving under pressure. Dr. Louise Lambert, Editor of the Middle East Journal of Positive Psychology (and lead editor of this book), discussed her experiences developing evidence-based positive psychology intervention programs. She also discussed research trends in the region and the potential for the development of an indigenous positive psychology.

During the second day of the symposium, a panel discussion titled "Youth Matter" was held for the purpose of engaging young Saudis and including them in the positive psychology discourse generated by the event. The panelists discussed the importance of reaffirming the role of young Saudis in the Kingdom and the ways in which positive psychology philosophy and practice could facilitate that goal. Moderated by Ms. Rozana Al-Banawi (Leadership Development Coach and Consultant), the session was enriched by the different points raised by a diverse group of panelists; Mr. Khalid Sendi (Relationship and Self Development Therapist), Mrs. Nirmeen Alireza (Founding Head of Nün Academy and Kunskapsskolan's Education Director), Dr. Majed Ashi (a psychology consultant), Ms. Afnan Tash (Business Graduate and an owner of the Mihrab المحراب Store). Following the panel discussion, attendees of the symposium were invited to attend several workshops addressing different areas within the field including; a mindfulness workshop given by Dr. Al-Ghalib and Dr. Creswell, a workshop on building relationships delivered by Mr. Sindi, a workshop on positive thinking in the workplace given by Dr. Laila J. Al-Ghalib (Dean of Student Affairs, Al-Rayan Colleges), and a workshop of the use of positive psychology interventions by Dr. Louise Lambert.

6.10 Conclusion

The Kingdom of Saudi Arabia is currently on the brink of one of the biggest transformations in its history. The series of sweeping economic and social reforms redefining life in Saudi is an indication of a greater shift in government priority. As a result, happiness and subjective wellbeing are expected to be part of future public policy. This prospect has inspired many of the projects initiated by members of the positive psychology movement in the Kingdom. The growing movement in Saudi Arabia has manifested itself in a variety of initiatives and projects undertaken by individuals, corporations, government officials and organizations. As Muslims, a majority of Saudis are able to connect Islamic philosophy with the theory and practice of positive psychology, with serious potential for the development of an indigenous positive psychology coming as a result of recent positive psychology education and research activities pioneered by Effat University. The Positive Psychology and Wellbeing Research Lab is only just the beginning.

References

Abdullah, F. (2014). Virtues and character development in Islamic ethics and positive psychology. *International Journal of Education and Social Science, 1*(2), 69–77.

Al Gelban, K. S. (2009). Prevalence of psychological symptoms in Saudi secondary school girls in Abha, Saudi Arabia. *Annals of Saudi Medicine, 29*(4), 275–279.

Alahmadi, H. A. (2002). Job satisfaction of nurses in Ministry of Health hospitals in Riyadh. *Saudi Arabia. Saudi Medical Journal, 23*(6), 645–650.

Alessandri, G., Vecchione, M., Tisak, J., Deiana, G., Caria, S., & Caprara, G. V. (2012). The utility of positive orientation in predicting job performance and organisational citizenship behaviors. *Applied Psychology, 61,* 669–698.

Al-Ghalib, S. J., & Salim, A. Y. (2018). A mindfulness based intervention to enhance university student wellbeing in Saudi Arabia. *Middle East Journal of Positive Psychology, 4*(1), 142–157.

Al-Ghalib, S. J., Salim, A. Y., Al-Khalifah, S., & Dahlawi, R. A. (2018). Perceptions of women's driving in Saudi Arabia: Relationship with openness to experience and happiness. *Middle East Journal of Positive Psychology, 4*(1), 102–125.

Alotaibi, J., Paliadelis, P. S., & Valenzuela, F. (2015). Factors that affect the job satisfaction of Saudi Arabian nurses. *Journal of Nursing Management, 24*(3), 275–282.

Alqarni, S. S. (2016). A review of prevalence of obesity in Saudi Arabia. *Journal of Obesity & Eating Disorders, 2*(2), 25.

Al-Seheel, A. Y., & Noor, N. M. (2016). Effects of an Islamic-based gratitude strategy on Muslim students' level of happiness. *Mental Health, Religion & Culture, 19*(7), 686–703.

Alshayea, A. (2013). Scientific research in the Kingdom of Saudi Arabia: Potential for excellence and indicators of underdevelopment. *Higher Education Studies, 3*(5), 47–51.

Al-Swailem, A. M. (2014). Saudi national science, technology and innovation plan towards knowledge based economy. *BMC Genomics, 15*(Suppl 2), 02.

Al-Swailem, A. M. (2018). *Introduction: National committee of bio ethics.* Retrieved April 29, 2018, from http://bioethics.kacst.edu.sa/About.aspx.

Alzalabani, A. H. (2017). Antecedents of job satisfaction in Saudi Arabia: Impact of industrial sector. *International Journal of Business and Management, 12*(11), 61–72.

Becker, S., AlZaid, K., & AlFaris, E. (2002). Screening for somatization and depression in Saudi Arabia: A validation study of the PHQ in primary care. *International Journal of Psychiatry in Medicine, 32*(3), 271–283.

Bhullar, N., Surman, G., & Schutte, N. S. (2015). Dispositional gratitude mediates the relationship between a past-positive temporal frame and wellbeing. *Personality and Individual Differences, 76,* 52–55.

Community Jameel. (n.d.). *Our initiatives—Together for good.* Retrieved April 29, 2018, from https://www.cjameel.org/en/initiatives.

Creative Mornings. (n.d.). *About|CreativeMornings/Jeddah.* Retrieved April 30, 2018, from https://creativemornings.com/cities/jed/about.

Datu, J. A., King, R. B., & Valdez, J. P. (2016). Psychological capital bolsters motivation, engagement, and achievement: Cross-sectional and longitudinal studies. *The Journal of Positive Psychology, 13*(3), 260–270.

Furumoto, L. (1980). Mary Whiton Calkins (1863–1930). *Psychology of Women Quarterly, 5*(1), 55–67.

Hamad, M. O., & Al Kwifi, O. S. (2015). Factors influencing job productivity: A case study of the Kingdom of Saudi Arabia. *Journal for Global Business Advancement, 8*(3), 326.

Hamdan, A. (2005). Women and education in Saudi Arabia: Challenges and achievements. *International Education Journal, 6*(1), 42–64.

Haque, A. (2004). Psychology from Islamic perspective: Contributions of early Muslim scholars and challenges to contemporary Muslim psychologists. *Journal of Religion and Health, 43*(4), 357–377.

Hollis-Walker, L., & Colosimo, K. (2011). Mindfulness, self-compassion, and happiness in non-meditators: A theoretical and empirical examination. *Personality and Individual Differences, 50*(2), 222–227.

How Saudi Arabia's UN Envoy Announced the Women Driving Decree. (2017, September 27). *Alarabia English.* Retrieved April 29, 2018, from https://english.alarabiya.net/en/News/gulf/2017/09/27/Saudi-envoy-to-UN-breaks-news-of-permission-for-women-to-drive-amid-applause-.html.

Idris, A. M., & Manganaro, M. (2017). Relationships between psychological capital, job satisfaction, and organizational commitment in the Saudi oil and petrochemical industries. *Journal of Human Behavior in the Social Environment, 27*(4), 251–269.

Jaalouk, D., Okasha, A., Salamoun, M. M., & Karam, E. G. (2012, November). Mental Health Research in the Arab world. *Social Psychiatry and Psychiatric Epidemiology, 47,* 1727–1731.

Jabalomar. (2017). *In the framework of Prince Khalid Al-Faisal's Initiative "How to be a role model".* Retrieved from https://jabalomar.com.sa/في-إطار-مبادرة-الامير-خالد-الفيصل-كيف-ن.

Jacobsen, D. (2013). *Bibliography of workplace gratitude.* Retrieved from http://www.globoforce.com/gfblog/2013/the-power-of-workplace-gratitude-a-brief-bibliography/.

Kabat-Zinn, J. (2003). Mindfulness-based stress reduction (MBSR). *Constructivism in the Human Sciences, 8*(2), 73–107.

Kabat-Zinn, J. (2012). *Mindfulness for beginners: Reclaiming the present moment—and your life.* Boulder, CO: Sounds True.

Karam, E., & Itani, L. (2015). Mental health research in the Arab world: An update. *BJPsych International, 12*(S1), S-25–S-28.

Kechichian, J. A. (2015). *Iffat Al Thunayan: An Arabian Queen.* Eastbourne: Sussex Academic Press.

Keller, E. F. (1995). *Reflections on gender and science.* New Haven, CT (USA): Yale University Press.

Khodayarifard, M., Ghobari-Bonab, B., Akbari-Zardkhaneh, S., Zandi, S., Zamanpour, E., & Derakhshan, M. (2016). Positive psychology from Islamic perspective. *International Journal of Behavioral Sciences, 10*(1), 77–83.

Koenig, H. G. (2014). Mental health care in Saudi Arabia: Past, present and future. *Open Journal of Psychiatry, 4,* 113–130.

Memish, Z. A., El Bcheraoui, C., Tuffaha, M., Robinson, M., Daoud, F., Jaber, S., … Al Rabeeah, A. A. (2014). Obesity and associated factors: Kingdom of Saudi Arabia. *Preventing Chronic Disease, 11,* E174.

Pradhan, R. K., Jena, L. K., & Bhattacharya, P. (2016). Impact of psychological capital on organizational citizenship behavior: Moderating role of emotional intelligence. *Cogent Business & Management, 3*(1).

Rao, M. A., Donaldson, S. I., & Doiron, K. M. (2015). Positive psychology research in the Middle East and North Africa. *Middle East Journal of Positive Psychology, 1*(1), 60–76.

Razzak, H., Qawas, A., El-Metwally, A., Harbi, A., & Al-Shujairi, A. (2017). The prevalence and risk factors of obesity in the United Arab Emirates. *Saudi Journal of Obesity, 5*(2), 57.

Rezaeitalarposhti, A., & Rezaeitalarposhti, A. (2013). Psychology from Islamic perspective: Contributions of Quran to contemporary psychologists. *International Research Journal of Applied and Basic Sciences, 6*(11), 1590–1595.

Seligman, M. (2009, September 25). *Positive Psychology Center Report (Rep.).* Retrieved April 30, 2018, from https://www.sas.upenn.edu/psych/seligman/ppcreport2009.pdf.

Seligman, M. E. P. (2002). *Authentic happiness*. New York, NY: Free Press.

Seligman, M. E. P. (2011). *Flourish: A visionary new understanding of happiness and wellbeing*. New York, NY: Free Press.

Shababuna Creative Hub. (n.d.). *A new platform for social innovation.* Retrieved April 30, 2018, from http://lfalsharif.wixsite.com/creativehub.

Terzian, S. G. (2004). The elusive goal of school spirit in the comprehensive high school: A case history, 1916–1941. *The High School Journal, 88*(1), 42–51.

United Nations Development Programme. (n.d.). *Environment and energy.* Retrieved April 30, 2018, from http://www.sa.undp.org/content/saudi_arabia/en/home/ourwork/environmentandenergy/overview.html.

Van Dyne, L., Vandewalle, D., Kostova, T., Latham, M. E., & Cummings, L. L. (2000). Collectivism, propensity to trust and self-esteem as predictors of organizational citizenship in a non-work setting. *Journal of Organizational Behavior, 21,* 3–23.

Vision 2030. (2016, May 8). *Vision 2030.* Retrieved from http://vision2030.gov.sa/en.

Chapter 7
Positivity at Work: It's Not a Contradiction!

Louise Lambert, Elizabeth Topolskaya, Meg A. Warren and Mansoor Anwar Habib

Abstract While the benefits of greater organizational positivity are gaining popularity, the means to increase it are less well known. Too many organizations still take a traditional approach that focuses on reducing problems rather than increasing or leveraging human emotions and potential. With the recent attention to happiness at work in the United Arab Emirates, and increasingly across the region of the Gulf Cooperation Council, we make the case for greater positivity in organizations. We posit that positivity increases productivity, profits, employee engagement, and commitment, and reduces turnover and sick leave. Positivity is not a naïve endeavor that wastes organizational resources and time, but rather an evidence-based pathway for broadening individual perspectives, ideas, and actions with a demonstrable effect on the building of psychological resources useful to employees in the present and future. Insights are offered as to how HR personnel and managers can use the science of positive psychology to increase positivity in the workplace by exploring strategies such as social capitalization, health initiatives, expression of gratitude, acts of kindness, character strengths, and undertaking a Best Self exercise. We conclude with a case study of the telecom company *du* and highlight its practices for increasing organizational wellbeing.

L. Lambert (✉)
United Arab Emirates University, Al Ain, UAE
e-mail: ltlamber@yahoo.com

E. Topolskaya
Pearson Education, Dubai, UAE
e-mail: elizabeth@topolskaya.com

M. A. Warren
Western Washington University, Bellingham, WA, USA
e-mail: meg@megwarren.com

M. A. Habib
du Telecom, Dubai, UAE
e-mail: mansoor.anwar@du.ae

L. Lambert and N. Pasha-Zaidi (eds.), *Positive Psychology in the Middle East/North Africa*, https://doi.org/10.1007/978-3-030-13921-6_7

7.1 Introduction

Despite a wealth of research that shows that fulfillment at work and the happiness of workers is critical to productivity (Warren, Donaldson, & Luthans, 2017), leaders and managers still overlook these aspects (Ulrich, 2013). Much like traditional psychology, the idea of "fixing the broken" unfortunately still prevails in many organizations (Linley, Harrington, & Garcea, 2013), despite lip service otherwise. Leaders often focus on targets and attaining profits because of a false belief that those are the only ways of creating high performing workplaces. Paradoxically, such an approach not only dehumanizes the workplace but also predicts worse outcomes for the sustainability of organizations (Mayerson, 2015; Mills, Fleck, & Kozikowski, 2013).

7.1.1 Positivity: The Humane Thing to Do

In today's world, the expectations of employees have changed. Work is a calling for many professionals who see beyond its financial rewards towards the fulfilment of personal aspirations (Rosso, Dekas, & Wrzesniewski, 2010). It is where they aspire to use their strengths, express themselves in careers that reflect their values and satisfy a desire to work under competent and morally principled leaders. Considering that people work throughout their adult lifetimes, and spend a majority of their waking hours at the workplace, it is inevitable to think of work as a source of meaning and purpose as well as a place where identities are shaped (Rosso et al., 2010; Warr & Clapperton, 2010). Work is more than a paycheck; individuals also want to be happy there. Paying attention to the human side of the workplace and creating an environment that is uplifting and meaningful is an important ethical contribution that businesses can offer society.

While high oil revenues and a large expatriate labor pool have made the notion of human capital investment redundant in much of the Gulf Cooperation Council (GCC) region, prioritizing the development of human capital and its talents has become the new untapped competitive resource (Gallup, 2018a). In fact, the work on positivity has taken visible and tangible strides in the region. A Minister of State for Happiness and Wellbeing in the United Arab Emirates (UAE) has been appointed; several national initiatives promote happiness at work; organizations like *A Great Place to Work*® now have offices in Saudi Arabia and Qatar; Kuwait's AlNowair group is undertaking large-scale program initiatives across their nation's enterprises, universities, and schools. In light of such developments, we feel that a formal introduction to the field of positive psychology is timely and warranted for the HR professional. Consequently, we review a handful of positive psychology interventions that may be of use in the workplace and dispel some misconceptions about implementing a focus on happiness at work. We conclude with a short case study on the work being done at the *du* offices in the UAE.

7.1.2 Positivity: The Smart Thing to Do

Although it is indisputable that attention to employee wellbeing is the humane thing to do, is it also the smart thing to do? In other words, is there a business case to be made for positivity? The evidence suggests that there is. For instance, studies suggest that happier employees are more productive (see review of 36 studies, van de Voorde, Paauwe, & van Veldhoven, 2012). Specifically, greater levels of job satisfaction, long-term wellbeing and short-term positive affect predicted up to a 12% increase in productivity (greater output and without a loss in quality), a 6% value-added measure per hours worked, an increase in future stock market performance across several industries, and greater organizational profits (Bockerman & Ilmakunnas, 2012; Edmans, 2012; Ford, Cerasoli, Higgins, & Decesare, 2011; Judge, Thoreson, Bono, & Patton, 2001; Kaplan, Bradley, Luchman, & Haynes, 2009; Oswald, Proto, & Sgroi, 2015; Ulrich, 2013). Forming an upward spiral, greater productivity in turn, feeds back towards greater psychological wellbeing for employees (Donald et al., 2005). Further, costly rates of absenteeism and turnover are also reduced when employees experience more positive emotions (Pelled & Xin, 1999). A large review (Erdogan, Bauer, Truxillo, & Mansfield, 2012) suggests that employees with higher levels of satisfaction with life have lower turnover intentions and a stronger commitment to their organizations. Higher wellbeing, perhaps through the mediating factor of commitment, is also related to higher income in the present and future (Deneve & Oswald, 2012; Graham, Eggers, & Sandip, 2004; Judge, Piccolo, Podsakoff, Shaw, & Rich, 2010), suggesting that not only do organizations reap the financial benefits of positivity and wellbeing, but employees can too.

Consequently, we call for greater attention to employee happiness and wellbeing, and specifically a major component of it: the experience of positive emotions. In fact, evidence for this business case is easy to make with Berry, Mirabito and Baun (2010) showing that a wellbeing program initiated by Johnson & Johnson had reaped 2.71USD for every 1USD spent. Several studies have shown returns on wellbeing investments although some have shown poor returns due, in part, to ineffective implementation, communication, monitoring, and incentivization, a lack of organizational and managerial support, and/or use of sporadic one-off activities designed to be nothing more than an afternoon's entertainment rather than part of a comprehensive evidence-backed and policy supported wellbeing program. Such investments are not only the smart thing to do for financial returns including the softer dividends of employee loyalty, morale and organizational reputation, but the right thing to do from an ethical and legal perspective as wellbeing is quickly becoming government regulated (Stoewen, 2016). Thus, we echo previous efforts toward this new research agenda (Klarner, By, & Diefenbach, 2011). To support our stance, we outline the Broaden and Build Theory (Fredrickson, 2001, 2006) to understand the importance of positivity and the means by which employers and employees can increase the frequency of positive emotional experiences.

7.2 Positive Work and Organizations

This chapter adopts a positive psychology lens, which has inspired a new sub-field of psychology that focuses on identifying, building, and generating individual and community strengths, positive experiences, and virtues (Seligman & Csikszentmihalyi, 2000). It differs from a traditional psychological approach, which targets distress, ill-functioning or abnormality (Bolier et al., 2013), and whereby practitioners focus on remediating negative states in order to restore functioning to previous levels. Yet, treating only negative states merely leaves individuals at pre-dysfunctional levels, which for many may only have been satisfactory or even mediocre. In fact, researchers argue that only removing negative states leaves individuals vulnerable for future distress as the skills for building a more positive foundation are neither mobilized nor maximized (Fournier et al., 2010; Layous, Chancellor, Lyubomirsky, Wang, & Doraiswamy, 2011; Wood & Joseph, 2010). Positive psychology instead focuses not exclusively on removing the negatives (although there remains a need for this), but also on building and augmenting positive strengths, emotions, and experiences in order for individuals and organizations to exceed what is considered normal and attain greater states of excellence (Seligman & Csikszentmihalyi, 2000; Wood & Tarrier, 2010).

In this manner, the field is focused on what makes life worthwhile by determining how and which experiences and emotional interactions contribute to greater health, meaning, relationships, engagement, and daily satisfaction, while maximizing functioning, productivity, and creativity (Csikszentmihalyi, 2009; Linley, Joseph, Harrington, & Wood, 2006). In the realm of the workplace, positive organizational behavior (Luthans, 2002) and positive organizational scholarship (Cameron, Dutton, & Quinn, 2003) espouse a similar philosophy. Positive organizational behavior is concerned with building positive psychological capacities at the individual and team level, while positive organizational scholarship primarily focuses on creating organizational structures, processes, routines, and conditions that support thriving at work. Collectively, these specific positive foci and other emergent topics in organizational and work-related theory, research, and application have been collectively termed the field of "positive work and organizations" (Warren et al., 2017). Schaufeli and Salanova (2010) call this workplace development a new period of "amplition". The focus of organizations is on the long-term investment in human capital alongside the development of sustainable interventions and focused towards the health and wellbeing of all employees, not just those who typically would have received attention for their problematic behaviors or responses. Examples of research interests examined through a lens of positivity include: positive group dynamics, career callings, positive leadership development, positive workplace ethics and corporate social responsibility (for a review see Mills et al., 2013).

7.3 What Do We Mean by "Positivity"?

Happiness and positivity are sometimes used synonymously as an all-encompassing word which, in the research literature, has been assessed by a variety of approximate measures such as subjective wellbeing, satisfaction with life, psychological wellbeing, or engagement, and is likely to continue in this manner until consensus emerges on its definition (Diener, 1984; Hart & Sasso, 2011; Joseph & Wood, 2010; Kashdan, Biswas-Diener, & King, 2008; Norrish & Vella-Brodrick, 2008). Positivity is also conceptualized as a dispositional trait, mood, and emotion (Barsade & Gibson, 2007). For our purposes, we use the definition of positivity provided by Fredrickson (2001, 2006) as the experience of any positive emotion, no matter how brief or seemingly inconsequential. Examples of positive emotions include passion (Vallerand, 2008), a strong preference for a liked, valued, and chosen activity that defines individuals; pride (Tracy & Robins, 2007), a feeling of self-worth motivated by maintaining a positive self-concept, others' respect, and status; elevation (Algoe & Haidt, 2009), the warm, emotional lift individuals receive when observing others partake in excellence and good deeds that inspire them to do the same; and admiration (Haidt & Seder, 2009), the response to others' talent, or fame and the consequent desire to build relationships with them and learn.

7.4 Positivity and the Broaden and Build Theory

An important theory in positive psychology and the field of wellbeing in general, is Barbara Fredrickson's Broaden and Build Theory (2001, 2006). She argues that positive emotions serve an undeniably important purpose: They transform individuals by bringing about physiological, cognitive, psychological and social changes in the present and with benefits that reach into the future as well.

The *broadening* component of the theory is that positive emotions (i.e., joy, curiosity, love, interest, awe, gratitude, optimism, etc.) expand individual thought-action repertoires (Fredrickson, 2001, 2006), which can lead to a greater number and higher quality of solutions generated for a given problem, as well as higher cognitive flexibility and creativity (Amabile, Barsade, Mueller, & Staw, 2005; George & Zhou, 2007; Labroo & Patrick, 2009). Individuals under the influence of positivity integrate new information more easily, make better decisions, and recognize opportunities more quickly (Nesse & Ellsworth, 2009). They also experience an expanded visual range and benefit from consequent increases in perception, focus, and attention (Schmitz, De Rosa, & Anderson, 2009; Wadlinger & Isaacowitz, 2006). These responses prompt stronger motivation and the willingness to learn and play (Fredrickson & Branigan, 2005; Johnson, Waugh, & Fredrickson, 2010). Positive emotions even reduce other-race bias such that individuals notice race less, bringing people together under more cooperative and altruistic conditions (Johnson & Fredrickson, 2005). Thus, the broadening effects that occur under the influence of positive emotions lead individuals to manage immediate opportunities more successfully and *build* a repository of resources (i.e., health, social, psychological, and cognitive) over time. In contrast, negative emotions hinder cognition, attention, and physiological responses in the face of problems or opportunities (negativity hypothesis, Carver, 2003; Cosmides & Tooby, 2000).

7.4.1 Positivity and Health

Employee health is an important issue for organizations. Considerable research studies show the high costs of organizational sick leave (i.e., absenteeism) when employees experience greater stress and poor health (Azagba & Sharaf, 2011; Pelled & Xin, 1999). In addition, research shows that "presenteeism", where people go to work even when they are sick because of strict policies, also leads to loss of productivity (Miraglia & Johns, 2016). Thus, whether or not the effects of health and stress are immediately visible through absenteeism, or remain obscured due to presenteeism, the adverse impact on productivity is clear. Positivity makes an important contribution to mitigating poor health outcomes and, as such, reducing instances of low productivity. Positive emotions protect against stress by reducing the time spent in fight-or-flight conditions and the unnecessary waste of physiological resources. During stressful events, the sympathetic nervous system stimulates the production of stress hormones. However, positive emotions enable the organism to return to baseline more quickly and achieve physiological recovery more effectively. Thus, positivity has an "undoing effect" of harmful physiological consequences of stress on the body and enables individuals to cope with difficulty and return to their pre-stress levels of functioning more effectively (Fredrickson, Mancuso, Branigan, & Tugade, 2000). Positivity is further linked with individuals taking more health-promoting actions such as avoiding smoking, partaking in exercise and physical activity, and eating more healthily (Blanchflower, Oswald, & Stewart-Brown, 2012; Grant, Wardle, & Steptoe, 2009). Thus, positivity can have immediate and lasting effects on employee health and productivity.

7.4.2 Positivity, Learning and Creativity

In today's fast-paced world, organizations have an interest in leading the market through high levels of creativity and innovation. Just as critical is the need for agility that comes through knowledge development and learning at the individual, team, and organizational levels. Positive emotions facilitate learning by fostering a sense of empowerment, openness and eagerness to absorb new information, resulting in an accumulation of knowledge and broadening of one's intellectual potential (Fredrickson, 2006). As positive emotions broaden the spectrum of thoughts and allow individuals to see the fuller picture, it also leads to enhanced creativity and new ideas that may change and expand an individual's views (Fredrickson, 2004). Learning and creativity can lead to important innovations in organizations. Thus, positivity can support organizations in creating an environment that is conducive for such development and being at the cutting-edge of change.

7.4.3 *Positivity and Social Influence*

The ability to network and develop social skills has become important in a knowledge-based, service-oriented business world. Positive emotions can assist in acquiring social resources through greater openness, which leads to better social connections (Aron, Norman, Aron, McKenna, & Heyman, 2000), cooperation and collaborative actions in negotiations (win-win deals, Carnevale, 2008), as well as trust (Lount, 2010). Moreover, through positivity, individuals can more easily build supportive social networks and create long-lasting bonds that are inspiring during good times, and helpful in difficult ones (Kok, Catalino, & Fredrickson, 2008). Simply having one good friend at work can influence an employee to remain with the organization and not quit when times are stressful, boost employee engagement by a factor of seven compared to employees without friends at work, and give the sense that someone is interested in their personal and professional development (Gallup, 2012, 2018b).

7.4.4 *Positivity, Efficacy and Resilience*

Positive emotions have an effect on psychological resources (Fredrickson, 2001) such as self-efficacy (Bandura, 2008) and resilience (Werner, 1990), both of which facilitate success in the workplace. Efficacy beliefs involve the conviction that individuals can assume courses of action that will help them achieve their goals as they believe they have the ability to influence their own outcomes. These beliefs are known to increase under the influence of positive emotions (Bandura, 2001). As individuals feel more positive and have stronger efficacy beliefs, they are more likely to stick with a given activity (i.e., be resilient and perseverant), excel in it, and as a result feel more positive (Salanova, Llorens, & Schaufeli, 2011). Further, higher resiliency is related to the increased use of task-oriented coping strategies during the process, which predict more adaptive emotional outcomes over time, such as lower depression and greater life satisfaction (Smith, Saklofske, Keefer, & Tremblay, 2016). Similarly, ego-resilience, the ability to bounce back from stress and resume normal activity, is also known to increase with greater positivity (Cohn, Fredrickson, Brown, Mikels, & Conway, 2009; Fredrickson, Cohn, Coffey, Pek, & Finkel, 2008; Ong, Bergeman, Bisconti, & Wallace, 2006). In sum, positive emotions help accrue resources that are useful for employees for the present and future, and also serve as positive workplace assets that are integral to the success of the whole organization.

7.5 Is Positivity Overrated?

The question of whether positivity should be prioritized in organizations has been a frequent subject of debate and we posit that greater attention to emotions overall can be helpful in detecting where attention is needed. Emotions, whether positive or negative, reflect the mood of the organizational culture, effectively signaling its health and climate. Positive emotions can be a sign of harmonious relationships and a safe, trusting environment built on credibility and fairness, while negative emotions can point to stress, conflictual workplace relationships, a lack of fairness, or other problems like discrimination, which deserve attention. Emotions are not good or bad in themselves, but symptoms of current realities that lead to certain outcomes and which may be more conducive in some contexts than others.

For example, opponents of positivity argue that negative emotions are of greater importance in the workplace when there is a degree of risk (i.e., financial or safety) as these can signal the need to act or face an upcoming failure. They would then serve as a warning, misgiving, or miscalculation that requires attention and can offer valuable learning (Klarner et al., 2011). Evidence would also suggest that excessive positivity can lead to risk-taking behavior and a lower ability to appropriately respond to one's reality, although much of this reasoning extends to clinical populations (Gruber, 2011; McNulty, 2010; Tan & Forgas, 2010; Warren, 2011). Positive emotions experienced too intensely and at inopportune times have also been associated with undesirable and unintended consequences (Gruber, Mauss, & Tamir, 2011). Managers would do well to reign in too much positive affect lest unintended negative consequences arise as a result (Lam, Spreitzer, & Fritz, 2014).

It is also well documented that employees who are actively discouraged from showing negative affect suffer from emotional exhaustion, or happiness fatigue, with implications for workplace engagement (Ybema & van Dam, 2014). Other criticisms are centered around the rise of the happiness industry where human resource management is asked to do more with less and capitalize on the psychology of employees as a source of economic profit and competitiveness (Ehrenreich, 2009). This has created a subsequent shift in responsibility for wellbeing on the part of the employer to the employee and offers a rationale for intrusive types of psychological interventions that effectively decontextualize the workplace from its employees (Pykett & Cromby, 2017) and overlook the importance of enabling structures, systems and routines which are inherent to good workplaces.

While these claims have merit, we nonetheless contend that the long-term effects of genuine and unforced positive emotions, i.e., the building of physical, cognitive, social and psychological resources and their immediate adaptive benefits, need far greater attention than organizations currently provide. What we posit instead is a greater degree of organizational flexibility and balance in harnessing the power of the positive alongside the sometimes necessary negative view, and less of the opinion that positivity is merely an add-on, staff perk, or frivolous trend. To understand how to harness the power of positive emotions, we review several strategies.

7.6 Positive Psychology Interventions (PPIs)

PPIs are interventions primarily designed to promote wellbeing (and not merely remove distress) and emphasize the positive versus exploring weaknesses or problems (Parks & Biswas-Diener, 2013). In two large meta-analyses, these empirically derived interventions have shown moderate effectiveness in increasing happiness and decreasing depression and negative emotions over time (Bolier et al., 2013; Sin & Lyubomirsky, 2009). To date, PPIs have primarily been used in clinical and health-care settings (Lambert D'raven, Moliver, & Thompson, 2015; Seligman, Rashid, & Parks, 2006), online (Parks, Della-Porta, Pierce, Zilca, & Lyubomirsky, 2012), and more recently, in organizational settings (for a review in organizational settings see Meyers, Van Woerkom, & Bakker, 2013; for a review of clinical PPIs see Lambert D'raven & Pasha-Zaidi, 2014). The benefits of using these PPIs include the elicitation of positive responses from employees, which reinforces future use of PPIs, boosting the organizations' social climate in terms of social cohesion and prosocial behavior (Salanova, Llorens, Acosta, & Torrente, 2013).

Here, we review selected PPIs that have demonstrated effectiveness, are relevant for the HR professional and of interest to the individual employee for use within and outside the workplace. We include both organizational and individual interventions because the most effective means to transform organizational wellbeing is when both parties take responsibility in creating a more positive and productive workplace (Laine & Rinne, 2015; Spence, 2015). This effectively creates a psychological contract of sorts: The gains expected from one's organization should be proportionate to those of the employee's own contributions (Salanova et al., 2013). Our aim is not to offer an exhaustive list of possible interventions, but rather a starting point for organizations, HR personnel or managers who may be looking for a pathway to greater positivity.

7.6.1 Acts of Kindness

Simple and effective, kind acts can range from small actions like giving a thank-you note, complimenting a colleague's efforts, to implementing larger group-based activities, such as volunteering for charity organizations or making team donations. As long as it involves acting in the service or interest of others, its results have the intended effects and constitute an intervention (Lyubomirsky, Sheldon, & Schkade, 2005; Nelson et al., 2015). Kindness can help employees become less conscious of their problems, integrate themselves into work teams and gain a feeling of control over their tasks (Post, 2005). Kind acts also generate positive responses from others in the form of gratitude or other positive emotions like joy and inspiration, and help recipients see themselves as good people, boosting self-esteem along the way (Boehm & Lyubomirsky, 2009). Spending money on others or donating individually or as an office can also increase happiness (Borgonovi, 2008; Dunn, Aknin, & Norton, 2014).

Employees can collectively perform kind acts to benefit the community and create a sense of meaning and purpose for themselves (Rosso et al., 2010). Secret acts of kindness can improve the emotional state of fellow employees and reduce hedonic adaptation, a process where people become accustomed to their surroundings and lose interest as a result (Armenta, Jacobs Bao, Sheldon, & Lyubomirsky, 2014). With more employees practising kindness, organizations can transform workplace atmospheres and develop more collegial and successful teams. However, these acts must not be forced because inauthenticity is easy to spot and detrimental to relationships.

7.6.2 Gratitude

Gratitude has become a topic of interest in recent years (Fehr, Fulmer, Awtrey, & Miller, 2017). Individuals can experience greater positivity by expressing gratitude, the act of attending to one's surroundings, appreciating its positive attributes and showing recognition via deliberate positive deeds and words (DeWall, Lambert, Pond, Kashdan, & Fincham, 2012). Interventions can include counting one's daily blessings or keeping a diary and reflecting on positive things that happened in the workplace that day (Emmons & McCullough, 2003). Employees can write a heartfelt letter of thanks to a colleague, client, or supervisor who is helpful or supportive (Boehm, Lyubomirsky, & Sheldon, 2011; Lyubomirsky, Dickerhoof, Boehm, & Sheldon, 2011), or recollect and re-experience positive emotions, reinforcing the relationship with the addressee simultaneously. Consistently expressing gratitude over a period of one month has also been associated with decreases in depression and increases in subjective wellbeing for the writer (Seligman, Steen, Park, & Peterson, 2005). The expression of gratitude can generate more moral and prosocial behaviour in others (Grant & Gino, 2010) and inhibit the experience and expression of anger (DeWall et al., 2012). In organizations, gratitude can be incorporated through words of thanks addressed to employees during meetings, through public nominations of individuals who provided exemplary support and service. It can also be documented on employee portals or a gratitude wall that can motivate others to share nominations. Formal employee recognition programs can also be developed where the recognition and praise of the efforts of many (versus identifying one's success at the expense of others) are planned, regular, and a shared endeavor, embedded as part of the organizational culture (Roberts, Dutton, Spreitzer, Heaphy, & Quinn, 2005).

7.6.3 Using Character Strengths

Character strengths are positive trait-like attitudes that are reflected in thoughts, feelings, and behaviors and are considered to be innate capacities through which one can achieve high functionality (Park & Peterson, 2008; Peterson & Seligman, 2004). Examples of strengths include perseverance, courage, honesty, self-regulation, leadership, and humor. Employees can take the VIA Survey of Character Strengths at www.viacharacter.org or discover their strengths by doing a Reflected Best Self activity (Spreitzer, Stephens, & Sweetman, 2009), a 360-degree evaluation that involves asking colleagues, clients, family and friends to identify situations when a person was at their best and what strengths were being used at that moment. Using character strengths at work can result in significant boosts to performance and wellbeing. For instance, Harzer and Ruch (2012) found that regularly using at least four character strengths at work improved one's work experience and made it more likely that employees considered their work a calling versus a mere job. The same researchers (2015) found that using strengths at work also protected individuals against stress, while using strengths that are consistent with those demanded by the workplace was related to high levels of workplace satisfaction and boosted positive emotions, the feeling of engagement, and the meaning one attached to the job (Harzer & Ruch, 2013; Lavy & Littman-Ovadia, 2017).

Mayerson (2015) suggests that identifying character strengths may help in the recruitment and selection of personnel for a better fit between employee capabilities and the soft skills required by many jobs. Similarly, the VIA survey can serve as a diagnostic tool that helps the selection of work team members. For instance, employees who score high on the strengths of creativity, integrity, citizenship, fairness, and social intelligence may be considered a good fit for a high functioning diverse team, but a poor fit for a team in which everyone is high on leadership and where power conflicts might result. Including the VIA as part of employee annual reviews, as many local organizations already do, can help in the identification and development of strengths so that team members can complement each other and offer a broad range of strengths to boost organizational performance. Further, it can be a critical ingredient to support task-related job crafting (Berg, Dutton, & Wrzesniewski, 2013; Wrzesniewski, Berg, & Dutton, 2010). Job crafting is a way of modifying job tasks within a job description for a better "fit" (Williams, 2016) by changing the order of tasks, swapping tasks with others, doing them in a manner that suits strengths better, or taking on adjacent or more difficult tasks as a way to achieve upward or lateral mobility within the organization.

7.6.4 *Best Possible Self*

Layous, Nelson, and Lyubomirsky (2013) propose another reflection-oriented method to increase positive emotions which may be useful at work. This intervention consists of imagining what one's best self would be and describing this in detailed writing over a period of several days. Employees may consider how they would be at their best in their work roles and with colleagues, doing specific tasks in the immediate future, or envisioning how they see their careers develop over time. The next phase of this activity involves specifying the steps one would take to make this future vision of the self possible. The future reflection encourages individuals to be proactive in achieving workplace goals and can fuel both individual and organizational growth. This strategy, like the VIA, can be included as part of one's annual review where employees themselves set their own goals and where managers can also learn about and support employees' visions in ways they could not before.

When individuals repeatedly accomplish their goals, a sense of achievement generates positive emotions and motivation in the immediate term, and individuals can also attain and increase new levels of subjective wellbeing over time (Cummins, Li, Wooden, & Stokes, 2014; Headey, 2010; Latham, 2012). Research on the Best Self activity has shown that even when the associated steps do not come to fruition, individuals obtain a boost in positive affect, greater flow experiences, social relatedness (Layous et al., 2013), and optimism (Peters, Meevissen, & Hanssen, 2013). In a variation, Boehm et al. (2011) asked participants to write about their best overall life (i.e., work, social life, health, hobbies, etc.) and this too resulted in a boost in life satisfaction. Employees working in teams can try this exercise as a group and consider what their "best team" would look like and what they could achieve over time and how.

7.6.5 *Capitalization*

Relationships are prominent contributors to wellbeing (Seligman, 2011) and equally so in the workplace, despite the fact that individuals routinely overlook the pleasure of connecting with others and assume they will be happier in solitude (Epley & Schroeder, 2014). Relationships are so important at work that having a work-friend can boost engagement sevenfold (Gallup, 2001). Workplace relationships also impact health. Studies show the likelihood of early death and illness is predicted by a lack of social networks and this likelihood is greater than the risks of smoking and obesity (Holt-Lunstad, Smith, Baker, Harris, & Stephenson, 2015; Holt-Lunstad, Smith, & Layton, 2010; Pressman et al., 2005). Similarly, a meta-analysis recently showed that a social circle at work significantly contributed to both physiological and psychological health (Steffens, Haslam, Schuh, Jetten, & van Dick, 2017).

There are many ways to boost relationships. One is to give employees a physical space in which to socialize, talk, and mingle, another is to give them time to do so by encouraging outings, lunches, breakfast meet and greets—all ways to establish trust, rapport and safety, and to know who is working on what. Relationships can also be boosted by modelling care, interest and positivity (Sandstrom & Dunn, 2014). Any interaction, professional, familial or otherwise, can benefit from active constructive capitalization (Gable, Gonzaga, & Strachman, 2006; Gable & Reis, 2010), responding to and sharing good news with others in a manner that allows positive emotions to be maximized. By changing how employees respond to one another, i.e., from indifference to interest or enthusiasm, corporate cultures can be changed via the transmission of positive emotions through their networks, three degrees of separation to be exact (Fowler & Christakis, 2008). Employees can also take on others' emotions by mirroring facial expressions, body language and tone of voice (Hess & Fischer, 2014). Contagion can come from leadership or group members (Barsade & Knight, 2015). Thus, it is critical to set the right tone.

7.6.6 Health

Lastly, it is vital to pay attention to the physical health of employees, given that individuals who accumulate physical resources take fewer sick leaves and are more productive. Physical activity is increasingly being recognized as an intervention to boost positive emotions, positive mood, minimize workplace stress and work-related fatigue, as well as enhance workplace performance (de Vries et al., 2016; Hyde, Conroy, Pincus, & Ram, 2011; Josefsson, Lindwall, & Archer, 2014; Loehr & Schwartz, 2001). Organizations can build in more movement across the office and consider holding standing or walking meetings to reduce the effects of a sedentary lifestyle (although further research is needed to examine the effectiveness of such meetings). They can also modify office layouts to ensure more frequent movement (e.g., lunch rooms located at a distance from office areas) (de Vries et al., 2016) to offset "sitting disease", a contributor to all-cause mortality, the incidence of cancer, type 2 diabetes, and cardiovascular disease irrespective of time spent in daily exercise and also more dangerous than the effects of smoking (Biswas et al., 2015; Lee, Artero, Sui, & Blair, 2010). These benefits can be further enhanced if the walking or movement breaks can be done in a nearby park, natural area, or developed green space, as these are also contributors to positivity (Bratman, Daily, Levy, & Gross, 2015). Organizations can facilitate employees' wellbeing and positivity by providing for and investing in health facility access, low-cost or free memberships, technology such as treadmill computer desks, corporate sporting events or other community based sports programs.

Topic Box: At *du*, Happiness Starts with Wellness by Dr. Mansoor Anwar Habib

Experts agree that promoting a healthy lifestyle plays a role in happiness. We, at *du* Corporate Offices, concur. With the Board of Directors' support in 2010, health and wellness were positioned within the company's strategic objectives. The first step was linking 5% of executive employee performance to the achievement of positive gains on glucose, cholesterol, and weight indicators, and rewarding those who achieved their desired health goals. Since, the wellness department has created many health events and competitions. Our biggest annual event, launched in 2011, is the "Biggest Winner", where employees have lost over 3000 kgs in the past five years! Contestants are introduced to exercise classes in the company's fitness club, which promotes happiness, a friendly relationship between staff members, and interrupts the work day. We work hard to impress upon employees that they can use these facilities anytime as it is a common problem in organizations that while employees have access to these spaces, they feel penalized using them as they are perceived to be "playing" versus "working".

As a result, the *du* team has received many awards over the years and was appointed the best UAE sports team in 2016. In the past three years, we have focused on employee participation in fitness competitions like the Desert Challenge, Spartan Race (receiving the largest Corporate Team award for 2016 with 200 + employees), and Sandstorm Challenge. We have also created clubs for football, basketball, swimming, badminton, and tennis, appointing employees to organize inter-departmental competitions. A team was also created to organize women's events, through which female employees and wives of employees have participated in the Dubai Women's Run. A *du* employee even won the race during Sheikha Hind bin Maktoum's Women's Sport Championship in 2016. Last year, we launched "Women's Health Day", a working day held at the Dubai Ladies Club, to promote sporting activities, relaxation and yoga. *du* has also transformed a floor of the company's headquarters into an integrated fitness club led by a group of qualified trainers, to provide monthly fitness and yoga classes and dedicated women's classes. Each floor has a recreational room with pool tables, table tennis and PlayStation. We've created photography and reading clubs to unleash the creative and literary passions of employees and build a sense of purpose. We offer a series of interactive positivity workshops to empower employees with the skills to boost their levels of happiness as well.

du wellness program results show consistent decreases in medical insurance expenses and in sick-day absences from 4 to 2.5 days per year. Our employee engagement scores also increased from 4.4 three years ago, to 4.66 at the end of 2016. With such outcomes, the company is allocating more resources for innovative activities to enhance the health and happiness of employees. We have over 2000 staff from over 60 countries and 50% of our senior management team and customer-facing staff are UAE nationals. We have more than 6.5 million mobile customers (nearly 50% market share), 555,000 fixed line subscribers, 180,000 home services subscribers and over 70,000 businesses choosing our services. Our successes have allowed our annual revenue to now exceed AED 10 billion.

7.7 Last Words

Managers and organizations in the region may be tempted to take the easy way and simply give employees salary raises rather than invest effort and time in undertaking interventions to improve wellbeing. But, studies are clear—money is not a good substitute (assuming wages are fair, equitable, and provide adequately for living and human dignity). Increases in income merely produce short-term spikes in happiness to which employees quickly adapt (Kahneman & Deaton, 2010; Lyubomirsky, 2011) and cannot make a bad workplace feel like a good one. Further, organizations may not be interested in wellbeing for other reasons. The high number of expatriates in the GCC countries of 85% and more in the UAE and Qatar, and more than half in other GCC nations could be one reason (European University Institute, 2016). Private organizations generally are not considered places in which resources or time is spent nurturing wellbeing as expatriate employees, especially the labor classes, are considered highly expendable, in abundant supply from around the globe, and easily made redundant (Dedoussis & Rutter, 2016). Yet, we make a case that reinvesting in new hires (with visa, housing, medical, and travel costs), as well as retraining employees with the associated loss of organizational memory in the transfer of knowledge and skills, is costly in the short and long run and can jeopardize an organization's long-term sustainability.

Further, positivity efforts themselves should not be used to overlook dysfunctional workplace practices. In fact, Laine and Rinne (2015) suggest that organizational efforts often fail and even backfire when the climate in which they are implemented lacks trust, transparency, and honest communication as employees view efforts with suspicion and resistance. Organizations must first take responsibility for their own practices and then proactively develop and take leadership in implementing and modeling positivity interventions as a way to invest in their employees instead of viewing PPIs as a cost, form of remediation, or worse, punishment (Allen & McCarthy, 2016). Overzealous organizations as well as individuals (Held, 2002) should thus be cautious in their messaging around the use of positivity and be careful not to enforce happiness either, especially in the face of popular rankings, competitions and other reporting trends. We have already heard of several local organizations chastising employees for not being "Happiness Compliant". They could alienate employees and increase their propensity to burn out under the additional emotional labor required to demonstrate positivity, teamwork, and contentment (Choi & Kim, 2015; Grandey, Fisk, & Steiner, 2005; Hülsheger, & Schewe, 2011).

To this effect, Spence (2015) suggests posing the obvious question to employees: "What one thing could this organization do to improve your experience on the job?" (p. 117). More pressing needs may be identified such as better parking, more flex-time, a lunch room, or better internal communication. While listening to employee needs seems so basic, it is astonishing that so few organizations take the time to do it. It is also advisable to undertake any such efforts in small, manageable chunks. As a cautionary tale, a large organization (kept anonymous to protect identity), that had several disgruntled employees, asked a similar question for the first time ever on a company-wide platform. Managing the deluge of emotions and feedback became such a massive challenge that the platform had to be shut down within 48 hours. This is not to suggest that one must not ask the question, but rather to deploy such feedback mechanisms in measured and achievable ways. As employees may have different attitudes and levels of receptiveness towards positivity interventions, it is wise to begin by making small, manageable organizational changes that employees themselves feel are needed (Allen & McCarthy, 2016; Terjesen, Jacofsky, Froh, & DiGiuseppe, 2004). Managers should also pay attention to what currently generates positive emotions in the organization (Judge & Ilies, 2004). Is it equitable treatment, the offer of instrumental support, effective and timely praise? Capitalizing on positive experiences that are already present in the office can pave the way for the introduction and development of greater workplace positivity, as it is experienced as being in alignment with the norm.

HR practitioners also need to consider the cultural context, organizational setting, as well as individual worldviews in which these PPIs might be used. This is especially the case in the UAE and other GCC countries where expatriates from almost 190 nations are represented in the workplace and who account for the majority of the country's population. For instance, considering "other"-oriented PPIs (e.g., good deeds) versus "self"-oriented interventions (e.g., goal setting; Lambert D'raven & Pasha-Zaidi, 2014; Lyubomirsky & Layous, 2013) may be more appropriate when working with individuals from more collectivist cultures (Al-Krenawi & Graham, 2000; Lambert, 2008), where members are more likely to value interpersonal relations (i.e., social obligations, interdependence) than personal achievements and independence (Pflug, 2009; Uchida & Ogihara, 2012). Nonetheless, there is evidence that these orientations are becoming more individualistic over time (Whiteoak, Crawford, & Mapstone, 2006) and may differ based on context. For example, Al-Esia and Skok (2014) noted that within the UAE, Emiratis may fluctuate between collectivism and individualism based on who they are speaking with. Collectivism was reflected to a greater degree in interactions with other nationals or those with whom they had strong social bonds, whereas individualistic behaviors were the norm in interactions with foreign co-workers.

Finally, as positive work and organizations research relies upon evidence against which to stake its claims, so should the responsible HR professional seeking to make organizational changes. Determining how positivity programs can be used and to what ends, requires a careful reading of the literature to identify relevant and solid scientific evidence from this still emerging field (Mills et al., 2013). HR professionals must measure the effectiveness of their efforts and not be afraid to replace strategies that do not meet their needs or achieve their goals. Ambitious HR managers may also want to partner with academics and publish their results to further develop the field (Mills et al., 2013) and help the employment landscape achieve greater wellbeing. These strategies will not only help boost the wellbeing of organizations and their employees, but, as Mayerson (2015) suggests, produce great value to stakeholders, customers, and the broader community, as well as solidify, legitimize, and elevate the role and position of HR departments.

References

Al-Esia, Z., & Skok, W. (2014). Arab knowledge sharing in a multicultural workforce: A dual case study in the UAE. *Arabian Journal of Business and Management Review, 4*(4), 1–10.

Al-Krenawi, A., & Graham, J. R. (2000). Culturally sensitive social work practice with Arab clients in mental health settings. *Health and Social Work, 25*(1), 9–22.

Algoe, S., & Haidt, J. (2009). Witnessing excellence in action: The "other praising" emotions of elevation, gratitude, and admiration. *The Journal of Positive Psychology, 4*(2), 105–127.

Allen, M. S., & McCarthy, P. J. (2016). Be happy in your work: The role of positive psychology in working with change and performance. *Journal of Change Management, 16*(1), 55–74.

Amabile, T. M., Barsade, S. G., Mueller, J. S., & Staw, B. (2005). Affect and creativity at work. *Administrative Science Quarterly, 50,* 367–403.

Armenta, C. N., Jacobs Bao, K., Sheldon, K. M., & Lyubomirsky, S. (2014). Is lasting change possible? Lessons from the Hedonic Adaptation Prevention model. In K. M. Sheldon & R. E. Lucas (Eds.), *Can happiness change? Theories and evidence* (pp. 57–74). New York, NY: Elsevier.

Aron, A., Norman, C., Aron, E., McKenna, C., & Heyman, R. (2000). Couples' shared participation in novel and arousing activities and experienced relationship quality. *Journal of Personality and Social Psychology, 78*(2), 273–284.

Azagba, S., & Sharaf, M. F. (2011). Psychosocial working conditions and the utilization of health care services. *BMC Public Health, 11,* 642 (Open Access).

Bandura, A. (2001). Social cognitive theory: An agentic perspective. *Annual Review of Psychology, 52,* 1–26.

Bandura, A. (2008). Reconstrual of "free will" from the agentic perspective of social cognitive theory. In J. Baer, J. C. Kaufman, & R. F. Baumeister (Eds.), *Are we free?: Psychology and free will* (pp. 86–127). Oxford, UK: Oxford University Press.

Barsade, S. G., & Gibson, D. E. (2007). Why does affect matter in organizations? *Academy of Management Perspectives, 21,* 36–59.

Barsade, S. G., & Knight, A. J. (2015). Group affect. *Annual Review of Organizational Psychology and Organizational Behavior, 2*(1), 21–46.

Berg, J. M., Dutton, J. E., & Wrzesniewski, A. (2013). Job crafting and meaningful work. In B. J. Dik, Z. S. Byrne, & M. F. Steger (Eds.), *Purpose and meaning in the workplace* (pp. 81–104). Washington, DC: American Psychological Association.

Berry, L., Mirabito, A. M., & Baun, W. B. (2010). *What's the hard return on employee wellness programs?* Mays Business School Research Paper No. 2012-68. Retrieved from https://ssrn.com/abstract=2064874.

Biswas, A., Oh, P. I., Faulkner, G. E., Bajaj, R. R., Silver, M. A., Mitchell, M. S., et al. (2015). Sedentary time and its association with risk for disease incidence, mortality, and hospitalization in adults: A systematic review and meta-analysis. *Annals of Internal Medicine, 162*(2), 123–132.

Blanchflower, D. G., Oswald, A. J., & Stewart-Brown, S. (2012). Is psychological wellbeing linked to the consumption of fruit and vegetables? *Social Indicators Research, 114*(3), 785–801.

Bockerman, P., & Ilmakunnas, P. (2012). The job-satisfaction-productivity nexus: A study using matched survey and register data. *Industrial and Labor Relations Review, 65,* 244–262.

Boehm, J. K., & Lyubomirsky, S. (2009). The promise of sustainable happiness. In S. J. Lopez (Ed.), *Handbook of positive psychology* (2nd ed., pp. 667–677). Oxford, UK: Oxford University Press.

Boehm, J. K., Lyubomirsky, S., & Sheldon, K. M. (2011). A longitudinal experimental study comparing the effectiveness of happiness-enhancing strategies in Anglo Americans and Asian Americans. *Cognition and Emotion, 25,* 1152–1167.

Bolier, L., Haverman, M., Westerhof, G. J., Riper, H., Smit, F., & Bohlmeijer, E. (2013). Positive psychology interventions: A meta-analysis of randomized controlled studies. *BMC Public Health, 13*(1), 119.

Borgonovi, F. (2008). Doing well by doing good. The relationship between formal volunteering and self-reported health and happiness. *Social Science and Medicine, 66,* 2321–2334.

Bratman, G. N., Daily, G. C., Levy, B. J., & Gross, J. J. (2015). The benefits of nature experience: Improved affect and cognition. *Landscape and Urban Planning, 138,* 41–50.

Cameron, K. S., Dutton, J. E., & Quinn, R. E. (2003). Foundations of positive organizational scholarship. In K. S. Cameron, J. E. Dutton, & R. E. Quinn (Eds.), *Positive organizational scholarship: Foundations of a new discipline* (pp. 3–13). San Francisco, CA: Berrett-Koehler Publishers Inc.

Carnevale, P. J. (2008). Positive effect and decision frame in negotiation. *Group Decision and Negotiation, 17,* 51–63.

Carver, C. S. (2003). Pleasure as a sign you can attend to something else: Placing positive feelings within a general model of affect. *Cognition and Emotion, 17,* 241–261.

Choi, Y. G., & Kim, K. S. (2015). A literature review of emotional labor and non-task behavior. *Universal Journal of Management, 3*(4), 143–147.

Cohn, M., Fredrickson, B., Brown, S., Mikels, J., & Conway, A. (2009). Happiness unpacked: Positive emotions increase life satisfaction by building resilience. *Emotion, 9,* 361–368.

Cosmides, L., & Tooby, J. (2000). Evolutionary psychology and the emotions. In M. Lewis & J. M. H. Jones (Eds.), *Handbook of emotions* (pp. 91–115). New York, NY: Guilford.

Csikszentmihalyi, M. (2009). The promise of positive psychology. *Psychological Topics, 18*(2), 203–211.

Cummins, R., Li, N., Wooden, M., & Stokes, M. (2014). A demonstration of set-points for subjective wellbeing. *Journal of Happiness Studies, 15*(1), 183–206.

de Vries, J. D., Claessens, B. J. C., van Hooff, M. L. M., Geurts, S. A. E., van den Bossche, S. N. J., & Kompier, M. A. J. (2016). Disentangling longitudinal relations between physical activity, work-related fatigue, and task demands. *International Archives of Occupational and Environmental Health, 89*(1), 89–101.

Dedoussis, E.-V., & Rutter, R. N. (2016). Workforce localisation and change management: The view from the Gulf. In A. Goksoy (Ed.), *Organizational change management strategies in modern business* (pp. 301–327). Hershey, PA: Business Science Reference.

DeNeve, J. E., & Oswald, A. J. (2012). Estimating the influence of life satisfaction and positive affect on later income using sibling fixed effects. *PNAS: Proceedings of the National Academy of Sciences, 109*(49), 19953–19958.

DeWall, C. N., Lambert, N. M., Pond, R. S., Jr., Kashdan, T. B., & Fincham, F. D. (2012). A grateful heart is a non-violent heart: Cross-sectional, experience sampling, longitudinal, and experimental evidence. *Social Psychological and Personality Science, 3*(2), 232–240.

Diener, E. (1984). Subjective wellbeing. *Psychological Bulletin, 95,* 542–575.

Donald, I., Taylor, P., Johnson, S., Cooper, C., Cartwright, S., & Robertson, S. (2005). Work environments, stress, and productivity: An examination using ASSET. *International Journal of Stress Management, 12*(4), 409–423.

Dunn, E. W., Aknin, L. B., & Norton, M. I. (2014). Prosocial spending and happiness: Using money to benefit others pays off. *Current Directions in Psychological Science, 13*(2), 347–355.

Edmans, A. (2012). The link between job satisfaction and firm value, with implications for corporate social responsibility. *Academy of Management Perspectives, 26*(4), 1–19.

Ehrenreich, B. (2009). *Bright-sided: How the relentless promotion of positive thinking has undermined America.* New York, USA: Metropolitan Books.

Emmons, R. A., & McCullough, M. E. (2003). Counting blessings versus burdens: An experimental investigation of gratitude and subjective wellbeing in daily life. *Journal of Personality and Social Psychology, 84,* 377–389.

Epley, N., & Schroeder, J. (2014). Mistakenly seeking solitude. *Journal of Experimental Psychology: General, 143*(5), 1980–1999.

Erdogan, B., Bauer, T. N., Truxillo, D. M., & Mansfield, L. R. (2012). Whistle while you work: A review of the life satisfaction literature. *Journal of Management, 38,* 1038–1083.

European University Institute. (2016). *GCC total population and percentage of nationals and foreign nationals in GCC countries (national statistics, 2010–2016) (with num-*

bers). Retrieved from http://gulfmigration.eu/gcc-total-population-percentage-nationals-foreign-nationals-gcc-countries-national-statistics-2010-2016-numbers/.

Fehr, R., Fulmer, A., Awtrey, E., & Miller, J. (2017). The grateful workplace: A multilevel model of gratitude in organizations. *Academy of Management Review, 40,* 182–209.

Ford, M. T., Cerasoli, C. P., Higgins, J. A., & Decesare, A. L. (2011). Relationships between psychological, physical, and behavioural health and work performance: A review and meta-analysis. *Work and Stress: An International Journal of Work, Health and Organisations, 25*(3), 185–204.

Fournier, J. C., DeRubeis, R. J., Hollon, S. D., Dimidjian, S., Amsterdam, J. D., Shelton, R. C., et al. (2010). Antidepressant drug effects and depression severity: A patient-level meta-analysis. *Journal of the American Medical Association, 303*(1), 47–53.

Fowler, J. H., & Christakis, N. A. (2008). The dynamic spread of happiness in a large social network. *BMJ: British Medical Journal, 337*, a2338.

Fredrickson, B. L. (2001). The role of positive emotions in positive psychology: The broaden-and-build theory of positive emotions. *American Psychologist, 56,* 218–226.

Fredrickson, B. L. (2004). Gratitude, like other positive emotions, broadens and builds. In R. A. Emmons & M. E. McCullough (Eds.), *The psychology of gratitude* (pp. 145–166). New York, NY: Oxford University Press.

Fredrickson, B. L. (2006). The broaden-and-build theory of positive emotions. In M. Csikszentmihalyi & I. S. Csikszentmihalyi (Eds.), *A life worth living: Contributions to positive psychology* (pp. 85–103). New York, NY: Oxford University Press.

Fredrickson, B. L. (2009, June). *Positive interventions: Theory, research, and practice.* Paper presented at the meeting of the First World Congress on Positive Psychology, Philadelphia, PA.

Fredrickson, B. L., & Branigan, C. (2005). Positive emotions broaden thought-action repertoires: Evidence for the broaden-and-build model. *Cognition and Emotion, 19*(3), 313–332.

Fredrickson, B. L., Cohn, M. A., Coffey, K. A., Pek, J., & Finkel, S. M. (2008). Open hearts build lives: Positive emotions, induced through loving-kindness meditation, build consequential personal resources. *Journal of Personality and Social Psychology, 95,* 1045–1062.

Fredrickson, B. L., Mancuso, R. A., Branigan, C., & Tugade, M. M. (2000). The undoing effect of positive emotions. *Motivation and Emotion, 24*(4), 237–258.

Gable, S. L., Gonzaga, G. C., & Strachman, A. (2006). Will you be there for me when things go right? Social support for positive events. *Journal of Personality and Social Psychology, 91,* 904–917.

Gable, S. L., & Reis, H. (2010). Good news! Capitalizing on positive events in an interpersonal context. *Advances in Experimental Social Psychology, 42,* 195–257.

Gallup. (2001, September 15). *The collective advantage.* Retrieved from http://www.gallup.com/businessjournal/787/collective-advantage.aspx.

Gallup. (2012). *State of the American Workplace*. Retrieved from http://www.gallup.com/services/178514/state-american-workplace.aspx.

Gallup. (2018a, January 22). *Untapped human capital is the next great global resource.* Retrived from http://news.gallup.com/opinion/gallup/225725/untapped-human-capital-next-great-global-resource.aspx.

Gallup. (2018b, February 26). *Why a best friend at school matters for students and teachers.* Retrieved from http://news.gallup.com/opinion/gallup/228125/why-best-friend-school-matters-students-teachers.aspx.

George, J. M., & Zhou, J. (2007). Dual tuning in a supportive context: Joint contributions of positive mood, negative mood, and supervisory behaviors to employee creativity. *Management Journal, 50,* 605–622.

Graham, C., Eggers, A., & Sandip, S. (2004). Does happiness pay? An exploration based on panel data from Russia. *Journal of Economic Behavior & Organization, 55,* 319–342.

Grandey, A. A., Fisk, G. M., & Steiner, D. D. (2005). Must "service with a smile" be stressful? The moderate role of personal control for American and French employees. *Journal of Applied Psychology, 90*(5), 893–904.

Grant, A., & Gino, F. (2010). A little thanks goes a long way: Explaining why gratitude expressions motivate prosocial behavior. *Journal of Personality and Social Psychology, 98*(6), 946–955.

Grant, N., Wardle, J., & Steptoe, A. (2009). The relationship between life satisfaction and health behaviour: A cross-cultural analysis of young adults. *International Journal of Behavioral Medicine, 16,* 259–268.

Gruber, J. (2011). When feeling good can be bad: Positive emotion persistence (PEP) in bipolar disorder. *Current Directions in Psychological Science, 20,* 217–221.

Gruber, J., Mauss, I. B., & Tamir, M. (2011). A dark side of happiness? How, when, and why happiness is not always good. *Perspectives on Psychological Science, 6,* 222–233.

Haidt, J., & Seder, P. (2009). Admiration and awe. *Oxford Companion to Affective Science* (pp. 4–5). New York, NY: Oxford University Press.

Hart, K. E., & Sasso, T. (2011). Mapping the contours of contemporary positive psychology. *Canadian Psychology, 52,* 82–92.

Harzer, C., & Ruch, W. (2012). When the job is a calling: The role of applying one's signature strengths at work. *Journal of Positive Psychology, 7,* 362–371.

Harzer, C., & Ruch, W. (2013). The application of signature character strengths and positive experiences at work. *Journal of Happiness Studies, 14*(3), 965–983.

Harzer, C., & Ruch, W. (2015). The relationships of character strengths with coping, work-related stress, and job satisfaction. Frontiers in Psychology, 6, 165.

Headey, B. (2010). The set point theory of wellbeing has serious flaws: On the eve of a scientific revolution. *Social Indicators Research, 97,* 7–21.

Held, B. S. (2002). The tyranny of the positive attitude in America: Observation and speculation. *Journal of Clinical Psychology, 58*(9), 965–991.

Hess, U., & Fischer, A. (2014). Emotional mimicry: Why and when we mimic emotions. *Social and Personality Psychology Compass, 8,* 45–57.

Holt-Lunstad, J., Smith, T. B., & Layton, J. B. (2010). Social relationships and mortality risk: A meta-analytic review. *PLoS Medicine, 7*(7), e1000316.

Holt-Lunstad, J., Smith, T. B., Baker, M., Harris, T., & Stephenson, D. (2015). Loneliness and social isolation as risk factors for mortality: A meta-analytic review. *Perspectives on Psychological Science, 10*(2), 227–237.

Hülsheger, U. R., & Schewe, A. F. (2011). On the costs and benefits of emotional labor: A meta-analysis of three decades of research. *Journal of Occupational Health Psychology, 16,* 361–389.

Hyde, A. L., Conroy, D. E., Pincus, A. L., & Ram, N. (2011). Unpacking the feel-good effect of free-time physical activity: Between- and within-person associations with pleasant-activated feeling states. *Journal of Sport & Exercise Psychology, 33*(6), 884–902.

Johnson, K. J., & Fredrickson, B. L. (2005). "We all look the same to me": Positive emotions eliminate the own-race bias in face recognition. *Psychological Science, 16,* 875–881.

Johnson, K. J., Waugh, C. E., & Fredrickson, L. (2010). Smile to see the forest: Facially expressed positive emotions broaden cognition. *Cognitive & Emotion, 24*(2), 299–321.

Joseph, S., & Wood, A. (2010). Assessment of positive functioning in clinical psychology: Theoretical and practical issues. *Clinical Psychology Review, 30,* 830–838.

Josefsson, T., Lindwall, M., & Archer, T. (2014). Physical exercise intervention in depressive disorders: Meta-analysis and systematic review. *Scandinavian Journal of Medicine and Science in Sports, 24*(2), 259–272.

Judge, T. A., Piccolo, R. F., Podsakoff, N. P., Shaw, J. C., & Rich, B. L. (2010). The relationship between pay and job satisfaction: A meta-analysis of the literature. *Journal of Vocational Behavior, 77,* 157–167.

Judge, T. A., & Ilies, R. (2004). Is positiveness in organizations always desirable? *Academy of Management Executive, 18*(4), 151–155.

Judge, T. A., Thoreson, C. J., Bono, J. E., & Patton, G. K. (2001). The job satisfaction-job performance relationship: A qualitative and quantitative review. *Psychological Bulletin, 127,* 376–407.

Kahneman, D., & Deaton, A. (2010). High income improves evaluation of life but not emotional wellbeing. *Proceedings of the National Academy of Sciences, 107*(38), 16489–16493.

Kaplan, S. A., Bradley, J. C., Luchman, J., & Haynes, D. (2009). The role of positive and negative affectivity in job performance: A meta-analysis. *Journal of Applied Psychology, 94,* 162–176.

Kashdan, T., Biswas-Diener, R., & King, L. (2008). Reconsidering happiness: The costs of distinguishing between hedonics and eudaimonia. *Journal of Positive Psychology, 3*(4), 219–233.

Klarner, P., By, R. T., & Diefenbach, T. (2011). Employee emotions during organizational change: Towards a new research agenda. *Scandinavian Journal of Management, 27,* 332–340.

Kok, B. E., Catalino, L. I., & Fredrickson, B. L. (2008). The broadening, building, buffering effects of positive emotions. In S. J. Lopez (Ed.), *Positive psychology: Exploring the best of people: Vol. 3 capitalizing on emotional experiences* (pp. 1–19). Westport, CT: Greenwood Publishing Company.

Labroo, A., & Patrick, V. (2009). Providing a moment of respite: Why a positive mood helps seeing the big picture. *Journal of Consumer Research, 35*(5), 800–809.

Laine, P., & Rinne, R. (2015). Developing wellbeing at work: Emerging dilemmas. *International Journal of Wellbeing, 5*(2), 91–108.

Lam, C. F., Spreitzer, G., & Fritz, C. (2014). Too much of a good thing: Curvilinear effect of positive affect on proactive behaviors. *Journal of Organizational Behavior, 35,* 530–546.

Lambert, L. (2008). A counselling model for young women in the United Arab Emirates: Cultural considerations. *Canadian Journal of Counselling, 42*(2), 16–33.

Lambert D'raven, L., Moliver, N., & Thompson, D. (2015). Happiness intervention decreases pain and depression and boosts happiness among primary care patients. *Primary Health Care Research & Development, 16*(2), 114–126.

Lambert D'raven, L., & Pasha-Zaidi, N. (2014). Positive psychology interventions: A review for counselling practitioners. *Canadian Journal of Counselling and Psychotherapy/ Revue Canadienne de Counseling et de Psychothérapie, 48*(4), 383–408.

Latham, G. P. (2012). Motivate employee performance through goal setting. In E. A. Locke (Ed.), *Handbook of principles of organizational behavior: Indispensable knowledge for evidence-based management* (2nd ed., pp. 161–178). Hoboken, NJ, USA: John Wiley & Sons Inc.

Lavy, S., & Littman-Ovadia, H. (2017). My better self: Using strengths at work and work productivity, organizational citizenship behavior and satisfaction. *Journal of Career Development, 44*(2), 95–109.

Layous, K., Chancellor, J., Lyubomirsky, S., Wang, L., & Doraiswamy, P. (2011). Delivering happiness: Translating positive psychology intervention research for treating major and minor depressive disorders. *Journal of Alternative and Complementary Medicine, 17*(8), 675–683.

Layous, K., Nelson, S. K., & Lyubomirsky, S. (2013). What is the optimal way to deliver a positive activity intervention? The case of writing about one's best possible selves. *Journal of Happiness Studies, 14,* 635–654.

Lee, D., Artero, E. G., Sui, X., & Blair, S. N. (2010). Mortality trends in the general population: The importance of cardiorespiratory fitness. *Journal of Psychopharmacology (Oxford, England), 24*(4_supplement), 27–35.

Linley, P. A., Harrington, S., & Garcea, N. (2013). Finding the positive in the work of work. In P. A. Linley, S. Harrington, & N. Garcea (Eds.), *The Oxford handbook of positive psychology and work* (pp. 3–9). New York, NY: Oxford University Press.

Linley, P., Joseph, S., Harrington, S., & Wood, A. (2006). Positive psychology: Past, present, and (possible) future. *Journal of Positive Psychology, 1*(1), 3–16.

Loehr, J., & Schwartz, T. (2001). The making of a corporate athlete. *Harvard Business Review, 79*(1), 120–128.

Lount, J. R. B. (2010). The impact of positive mood on trust in interpersonal and intergroup interactions. *Journal of Personality and Social Psychology, 98,* 420–433.

Luthans, F. (2002). The need for and meaning of positive organizational behavior. *Journal of Organizational Behavior, 23,* 695–706.

Lyubomirsky, S. (2011). Hedonic adaptation to positive and negative experiences. In S. Folkman (Ed.), *Oxford handbook of stress, health, and coping* (pp. 200–224). New York: Oxford University Press.

Lyubomirsky, S., Dickerhoof, R., Boehm, J. K., & Sheldon, K. M. (2011). Becoming happier takes both a will and a proper way: An experimental longitudinal intervention to boost wellbeing. *Emotion, 11,* 391–402.

Lyubomirsky, S., Sheldon, K. M., & Schkade, D. (2005). Pursuing happiness: The architecture of sustainable change. *Review of General Psychology, 9,* 111–131.

Lyubomirsky, S., & Layous, K. (2013). How do simple positive activities increase wellbeing? *Current Directions in Psychological Science, 22,* 57–62.

Mayerson, N. (2015). "Characterizing" the workplace: Using character strengths to create sustained success. *Kognition & Paedagogik, 96,* 14–27.

McNulty, J. K. (2010). When positive processes hurt relationships. *Current Directions in Psychological Science, 19,* 167–171.

Meyers, M. C., van Woerkom, M., & Bakker, A. B. (2013). The added value of the positive: A literature review of positive psychology interventions in organizations. *European Journal of Work and Organizational Psychology, 22*(5), 618–632.

Mills, M. J., Fleck, C. R., & Kozikowski, A. (2013). Positive psychology at work: A conceptual review, state-of-practice assessment, and a look ahead. *The Journal of Positive Psychology, 8*(2), 153–164.

Miraglia, M., & Johns, G. (2016). Going to work ill: A meta-analysis of the correlates of presenteeism and a dual-path model. *Journal of Occupational Health Psychology, 21*(3), 261–283.

Nelson, S. K., Della Porta, M. D., Jacobs Bao, K., Lee, H. C., Choi, I., & Lyubomirsky, S. (2015). "It's up to you": Experimentally manipulated autonomy support for prosocial behavior improves wellbeing in two cultures. *The Journal of Positive Psychology, 10,* 463–476.

Nesse, R. M., & Ellsworth, P. C. (2009). Evolution, emotions, and emotional disorders. *American Psychologist, 64*(2), 129–139.

Norrish, J., & Vella-Brodrick, D. (2008). Is the study of happiness a worth scientific pursuit? *Social Indicators Research, 87*(3), 393–407.

Ong, A. D., Bergeman, C. S., Bisconti, T. L., & Wallace, K. A. (2006). Psychological resilience, positive emotions, and successful adaptation to stress in later life. *Journal of Personality and Social Psychology, 91,* 730–749.

Oswald, A. J., Proto, E., & Sgroi, D. (2015). Happiness and productivity. *Journal of Labor Economics, 334,* 789–822.

Park, N., & Peterson, C. (2008). Positive psychology and character strengths: Application to strengths-based school counseling. *Professional School Counseling, 12,* 85–92.

Parks, A. C., & Biswas-Diener, R. (2013). Positive interventions: Past, present and future. In T. Kashdan & J. Ciarrochi (Eds.), *Bridging acceptance and commitment therapy and positive psychology: A practitioner's guide to a unifying framework* (pp. 140–165). Oakland, CA: New Harbinger.

Parks, A., Della Porta, M., Pierce, R. S., Zilca, R., & Lyubomirsky, S. (2012). Pursuing happiness in everyday life: The characteristics and behaviors of online happiness seekers. *Emotion, 12,* 1222–1234.

Pelled, L. H., & Xin, K. R. (1999). Down and out: An investigation of the relationship between mood and employee withdrawal behavior. *Journal of Management, 25,* 875–895.

Peters, M. L., Meevissen, Y. M. C., & Hanssen, M. M. (2013). Specificity of the best possible self intervention for increasing optimism: Comparison with a gratitude intervention. *Terapia Psicologica, 31*(1), 93–100.

Peterson, C., & Seligman, M. E. P. (2004). *Character strengths and virtues: A handbook and classification.* Oxford, UK: Oxford University Press.

Pflug, J. (2009). Folk theories of happiness: A cross-cultural comparison of conceptions of happiness in Germany and South Africa. *Social Research Indicators, 92*(3), 551–563.

Post, S. G. (2005). Altruism, happiness and health: It's good to be good. *International Journal of Behavioral Medicine, 12*(2), 66–77.

Pressman, S., Cohen, S., Miller, G. E., Barkin, A., Rabin, B. S., & Treanor, J. J. (2005). Loneliness, social network size, and immune response to influenza vaccination in college freshmen. *Health Psychology, 24,* 297–306.

Pykett, J., & Cromby, J. (2017). Mapping happiness, managing urban emotions. In V. Higgins & W. Larner (Eds.), *Assembling neoliberalism: Expertise, practices, subjects* (pp. 195–216). USA: Palgrave MacMillan.

Roberts, L. M., Dutton, J. E., Spreitzer, G. M., Heaphy, E. D., & Quinn, R. E. (2005). Composing the reflected best-self portrait: Building pathways for becoming extraordinary in work organizations. *Academy of Management Review, 30,* 712–736.

Rosso, B. D., Dekas, K. H., & Wrzesniewski, A. (2010). On the meaning of work: A theoretical integration and review. *Research in Organizational Behavior, 30,* 91–127.

Salanova, M., Llorens, S., Acosta, H. C., & Torrente, P. (2013). Positive interventions in positive organizations. *Terapia Psicológica, 31,* 101–113.

Salanova, M., Llorens, S., & Schaufeli, W. B. (2011). "Yes, I can, I feel good, and I just do it!" On gain cycles and spirals of efficacy beliefs, affect, and engagement. *Applied Psychology, 60*(2), 255–285.

Sandstrom, G. M., & Dunn, E. W. (2014). Is efficiency overrated? Minimal social interactions lead to belonging and positive affect. *Social Psychological and Personality Science, 5*(4), 437–442.

Schaufeli, W. B., & Salanova, M. (2010). How to improve work engagement? In S. L. Albrecht (Ed.), *Handbook of employee engagement. Perspectives, issues, research and practice* (pp. 399–415). Northampton, MA: Edward Elgar.

Schmitz, T. W., De Rosa, E., & Anderson, A. K. (2009). Opposing influences of affective state valence on visual cortical encoding. *Journal of Neuroscience, 29*(22), 7199–7207.

Seligman, M. E. P. (2011). *Flourish: A visionary new understanding of happiness and wellbeing.* New York, NY: Free Press.

Seligman, M. E. P., & Csikszentmihalyi, M. (2000). Positive psychology: An introduction. *American Psychologist, 55*(1), 5–14.

Seligman, M. E. P., Rashid, T., & Parks, A. C. (2006). Positive psychotherapy. *American Psychologist, 61,* 774–788.

Seligman, M. E. P., Steen, T., Park, N., & Peterson, C. (2005). Positive psychology progress: Empirical validation of interventions. *American Psychologist, 60*(5), 410–421.

Sin, N. L., & Lyubomirsky, S. (2009). Enhancing wellbeing and alleviating depressive symptoms with positive psychology interventions: A practice-friendly meta-analysis. *Journal of Clinical Psychology, 65,* 467–487.

Smith, M. M., Saklofske, D. H., Keefer, K. V., & Tremblay, P. F. (2016). Coping strategies and psychological outcomes: The moderating effects of personal resiliency. *The Journal of Psychology: Interdisciplinary and Applied, 150*(3), 318–332.

Spence, G. B. (2015). Workplace wellbeing programs: If you build it they may NOT come…because it's not what they really need! *International Journal of Wellbeing, 5*(2), 109–124.

Spreitzer, G., Stephens, J. P., & Sweetman, D. (2009). The Reflected Best Self field experiment with adolescent leaders: Exploring the psychological resources associated with feedback source and valence. *The Journal of Positive Psychology, 4*(5), 331–348.

Steffens, N. K., Haslam, S. A., Schuh, S. C., Jetten, J., & van Dick, R. (2017). A meta-analytic review of social identification and health in organizational contexts. *Personality and Social Psychology Review, 21*(4), 303–335.

Stoewen, D. L. (2016). Wellness at work: Building healthy workplaces. *The Canadian Veterinary Journal, 57*(11), 1188–1190.

Tan, H. B., & Forgas, J. P. (2010). When happiness makes us selfish, but sadness makes us fair: Affective influences on interpersonal strategies in the dictator game. *Journal of Experimental Social Psychology, 46,* 571–576.

Terjesen, M. D., Jacofsky, M., Froh, J., & DiGiuseppe, R. (2004). Integrating positive psychology into schools: Implications for practice. *Psychology in the Schools, 41*(1), 163–172.

Tracy, J., & Robins, R. (2007). The psychological structure of pride: A tale of two facets. *Journal of Personality and Social Psychology, 92*(3), 506–525.

Uchida, Y., & Ogihara, Y. (2012). Personal or interpersonal construal of happiness: A cultural psychological perspective. *International Journal of Wellbeing, 2*(4), 354–369.

Ulrich, D. (2013). Forward: The abundant organization. In P. A. Linley, S. Harrington, & N. Garcea (Eds.), *The Oxford handbook of positive psychology and work* (pp. xvii–xxii). New York, NY: Oxford University Press.

Vallerand, R. (2008). On the psychology of passion: In search of what makes people's lives most worth living. *Canadian Psychological Association, 49*(1), 1–13.

van de Voorde, F. C., Paauwe, J., & van Veldhoven, M. J. P. M. (2012). Employee wellbeing and the HRM-organizational performance relationship: A review of quantitative studies. *International Journal of Management Reviews, 14*(4), 391–407.

Wadlinger, H. A., & Isaacowitz, D. M. (2006). Positive mood broadens visual attention to positive stimuli. *Motivation and Emotion, 30,* 89–101.

Warr, P., & Clapperton, G. (2010). *The joy of work?* London, UK: Routledge.

Warren, M. A., Donaldson, S. I., & Luthans, F. (2017). Taking positive psychology to the workplace: Positive organizational psychology, positive organizational behavior, and positive organizational scholarship. In M. A. Warren & S. I. Donaldson (Eds.), *Scientific advances in positive psychology* (pp. 195–227). Santa Barbara, CA: Praeger.

Warren, S. (2011). What's wrong with being positive? In P. Linley, S. Harrington, & N. Garcea (Eds.), *Oxford handbook of positive psychology and work* (pp. 313–322). New York, NY: Oxford University Press.

Werner, E. E. (1990). Protective factors and individual resilience. In R. Meisells, & J. Shonkoff (eds.), *Handbook of early intervention* (pp. 97–116). Cambridge, UK: Cambridge.

Whiteoak, J. W., Crawford, N. G., & Mapstone, R. H. (2006). Impact of gender and generational differences in work values in an Arab culture. *Thunderbird International Business Review, 48*(1), 77–91.

Williams, G. (2016). Discovering the professional within: How identifying our character strengths can help build our ideal career and success. *PsychTalk, 85,* 5–9.

Wood, A. M., & Joseph, S. (2010). The absence of positive psychological (eudemonic) wellbeing as a risk factor for depression: A ten year cohort study. *Journal of Affective Disorders, 122,* 213–217.

Wood, A. M., & Tarrier, N. (2010). Positive clinical psychology: A new vision and strategy for integrated research and practice. *Clinical Psychology Review, 30*(7), 819–829.

Wrzesniewski, A., Berg, J. M., & Dutton, J. E. (2010). Turn the job you have into the job you want. *Harvard Business Review, 88,* 114–117.

Ybema, J. F., & van Dam, K. (2014). The importance of emotional display rules for employee wellbeing: A multigroup comparison. *The Journal of Positive Psychology, 4*(9), 366–376.

Part III
Measurement: Research Trends and Challenges

Chapter 8
Big Data and Wellbeing in the Arab World

Aamna Al-Shehhi, Ian Grey and Justin Thomas

Abstract The rapid and widespread usage of social media platforms, such as Twitter, Facebook and Instagram has given rise to unprecedented amounts of user-generated data. This data contains expressions reflecting users thoughts, opinions and affective states. Systematic explorations of this type of data have begun to yield valuable information about a variety of psychological and cultural variables. To date however, very little of this research has been undertaken in the Arab world. It is important to extend this type of macro-level big data analysis across cultures and languages as each situation is likely to present different methodological challenges and to reveal findings particular to the sociocultural context. This chapter examines research—much of it our own—exploring subjective wellbeing in the United Arab Emirates (UAE) using data from Twitter and explores the findings from cross-linguistic analysis of happiness (positive–negative affective patterns of language use) and other variables associated with subjective wellbeing in the region. Additionally, we explore temporal patterns of happiness observed in relation to Ramadan and other events of sociopolitical and religio–cultural significance. The UAE focus is discussed with reference to broader trends in data science, sentiment analysis and hedonometry.

8.1 Introduction

The 21st century has been witness to many technological changes and foremost amongst these has been the accelerated digitisation of people's social lives. The thoughts and feelings of millions of people around the globe are expressed daily on

A. Al-Shehhi
Khalifa University of Science and Technology, Abu Dhabi, UAE
e-mail: aamena.shehhi@gmail.com

I. Grey (✉)
School of Social Sciences, Lebanese American University, Beirut, Lebanon
e-mail: Ian.grey@zu.ac.ae

J. Thomas
Zayed University, Abu Dhabi, UAE
e-mail: justin.thomas@zu.ac.ae

L. Lambert and N. Pasha-Zaidi (eds.), *Positive Psychology in the Middle East/North Africa*, https://doi.org/10.1007/978-3-030-13921-6_8

various online platforms and the enormous growth of social media usage witnessed on Facebook, Twitter and Google has led to the accumulation of huge amounts of data (referred to as "Big Data"). These vast datasets have attracted the attention of social scientists as a potential means to provide a greater understanding of various aspects of human behaviour, and a rapidly expanding body of research is now testifying to the power of Big Data to provide insight into a range of psychological questions. However, not only does the use of Big Data facilitate addressing questions but the answers resulting from its use may be as robust, or even more so, than what is currently associated with existing traditional methodologies. For instance, Schwartz et al. (2013a) analysed the language used in tweets from 1300 different US counties and reported that Twitter content was as predictive of the subjective wellbeing of people living in those counties as that measured by representative surveys, over and above established demographic and socio-economic controls like age, gender, ethnicity, income, and education. Other research suggests that social media platforms like Twitter can capture more information about issues such as county-level atherosclerotic heart disease than robust epidemiological models that include socio-economic status, key demographics and health variables like smoking, diabetes and hypertension (Eichstaedt et al., 2015). Finally, other research suggests that Facebook-language-based predictions of personality seem to be about as good as a friend's rating (Park et al., 2014) and that Twitter language can reflect psychological differences with respect to differing political orientations (Sylwester & Purver, 2015).

The present chapter contributes to this new research agenda by showing how Big Data can improve not only our understanding of subjective wellbeing but how it also provides new means to investigate aspects of wellbeing on a scale not possible until now. We first provide a brief overview of why subjective wellbeing has become an important topic in psychological research and how it is conceptualized, and follow by identifying common methods of analysis used in social media and their respective advantages and disadvantages. Finally, we report several of our key studies based on social media data for the United Arab Emirates (UAE), noting the insights and challenges associated with such research in Arab-speaking countries. We argue that the convergence of the rise in interest in aspects of psychological wellbeing and the availability of large cross-linguistic datascapes offers the potential to both present and address important psychological questions for the Arab World.

8.2 The Beginnings and Proof of Concept

A key question from the outset regarding the relevancy of social media to answer psychological questions is; are there sufficient similarities between online digital behaviour and behaviour in the real world? In answering this, many authors point to a seminal study conducted by Google in 2009 (Google, 2009; Olson, Konty, Paladini, Viboud, & Simonsen, 2013), demonstrating that simply by measuring the frequency of online search queries related to the common flu, in addition to topics such as flu symptoms and medications, the spread of flu through the United States could be accurately tracked (Cook, Conrad, Fowlkes, & Mohebbi, 2011). What was particularly important about the study was not only that the use of search terms correlated with the occurrence of flu on the ground but that Google's estimates of future occurrences of the illness were about two weeks ahead of those made by leading medical authorities in the US, and with a very high degree of accuracy between the estimates provided by Google and the data reported by the Centers for Disease Control. This study served as an initial proof of concept suggesting that both the Internet and its data could be used to measure a variety of variables about people that concerned them at a social level. This research was pivotal in demonstrating that when people search for information online, the data revealed by these search patterns can be reflective of the relative importance of their concerns.

8.3 Psychology and Big Data

While the above study points to a possible convergence between online behaviour and aspects of behaviour in the real world, the question that arises is whether wellbeing can be studied as effectively by accessing or monitoring the behaviour of individuals on digital platforms? A traditional limitation of most psychology studies in this domain is that the number of people involved is small, often no more than 50–150 people. While even the largest studies number a few thousand, the ability of these small numbers to generalize to larger populations remains a major criticism of the field. Researchers ask whether the use of Big Data and techniques similar to those employed in the Google flu study can be used to garner insights into the wellbeing of individuals as the potential to access millions of people in contrast to traditional psychological studies relying on self-report is immense. For instance, Facebook alone has approximately one billion users. Thus, rather than rely on generalizations from small samples to entire populations, which have only a limited degree of success, it is possible to get estimates about entire populations or large proportions of given populations owing to their participation in bigger data sets. Moreover, with so many people, a closer and more nuanced look at different subgroups is possible; for example, understanding how women differ from men, young from old, and so forth. However, there is one key additional advantage; social media users tend to behave in more naturalistic ways than is the case with traditional methodologies like surveys, improving ecological validity. The behaviour of people online appears highly similar to natural settings where they talk about things they care about with their friends in what they consider to be private environments. As such, we analyse the language people use on social media, addressed later.

8.4 Subjective Wellbeing

Over the last two decades, there has been a growing body of work that evaluates human wellbeing based on self-reporting by individuals and groups. Generally referred to as measures of subjective wellbeing (SWB), these studies attempt to measure "satisfaction" with their quality of life (Diener, Suh, Lucas, & Smith, 1999). SWB has been defined as the sum of a person's affective and cognitive needs and though SWB is often assumed to be restricted to happiness, the term in fact covers a wider range of concepts, comprising at least three components: life evaluation (i.e., satisfaction with one's life or with specific domains), affect (i.e., the balance between positive and negative emotions) and eudemonia (i.e., the extent to which a person has realised their potential and has a meaningful life) (Diener et al., 1999).

The basis of using SWB as a metric is to measure the extent to which human needs are being met and how individuals perceive their quality of life. Because these measures have been typically based on the judgments of survey respondents rather than on more easily quantifiable inputs of money and material goods, there have always been concerns that these "subjective" measures are not factually based and therefore less valid than "objective" measures like GDP. Yet, as noted by several authors, objective measures such as life expectancy, rates of disease, and GDP are only proxies for wellbeing that have been identified through the subjective judgment of decision-makers; "hence the distinction between objective and subjective indicators is somewhat illusory" (Costanza et al., 2007, p. 268). There is also a concern that there are cultural differences that make it difficult to compare the results across different ethnic, gender, age, religion, and other cultural boundaries (Morrison, Jebb, Tay, & Diener, 2018). However, comparisons of reported wellbeing and per capita GDP have shown that beyond a certain income level, happiness does not increase significantly with additional income and economic gains beyond the threshold no longer correlate with increases in wellbeing (Inglehart, 1997). As a result, ways to help identify as accurately as possible how SWB can be meaningfully assessed, in addition to how these metrics can determine the impact of policies on the lives of individuals are being sought. Measuring subjective wellbeing is not without its challenges; most notably, SWB is not always revealed by people's behaviour or choices and accessing meaningful data typically requires large representative surveys which are time-consuming and financially costly, as well as limited in coverage, time and space. This eliminates the possibility of measuring SWB with the appropriate time-cycle frequency and to posess local relevance for policymakers that is necessary for decision-making.

8.5 Happiness as Policy Agenda

Happiness has become largely interchangeable with subjective wellbeing, which is to say, an experiential state that contains a globally positive affective tone. To date, social scientists have conceptualised and measured happiness in at least two different ways. One of these is what is termed "affect balance", which examines the relative balance between pleasant and unpleasant emotional states, and is thus primarily the sum of how one feels at different moments. The second, life satisfaction, goes beyond momentary feelings to elicit an evaluative assessment of one's life as a whole (Linley, Maltby, Wood, Osborne, & Hurling, 2009).

Spreading across many countries, the "happiness agenda" is not without detractors. Research has shown that having purpose and meaning in life is associated with a number of positive outcomes such as increases in overall wellbeing and life satisfaction, better mental and physical health, increased resiliency, enhanced self-esteem, and reduced likelihood of depression. In contrast, happiness as an affective state is paradoxical in that the more importance people place on being happy, the more they appear to become unhappy and prone to being depressed (Mauss, Tamir, Anderson, & Savino, 2011). For example, individuals who put most emphasis on being happy report less frequent positive emotions, less satisfaction with life, and substantially more depressive symptoms than people who do not have happiness as a priority. Further, individuals that value happiness the most also seem to report less psychological wellbeing. It seems that the very pursuit of happiness seems to thwart its attainment (Mauss et al., 2011).

Another study asked nearly 400 Americans aged between 18 and 78 whether they thought their lives were meaningful and/or happy (Baumeister, Vohs, Aaker, & Garbinsky, 2013). Examining their self-reported attitudes toward meaning in life, happiness, and their interactions with a number of other variables such as stress levels, spending patterns, and having children, the researchers found that while a meaningful life and happy life overlap, they are different. The researchers report that leading a happy life appears linked with what they conceptualise as being a "taker" while leading a meaningful life corresponded with being a "giver". Those people identified as happy obtained joy from receiving benefits from others while people leading meaningful lives obtained joy from giving to others. Happiness without meaning appeared to characterize a relatively shallow, self-absorbed or even selfish life in which things went well, where needs and desires were easily satisfied, and difficult situations were avoided. They concluded that meaning transcends the self while happiness is about giving the self what it wants.

Collectively, these results fit the overall view that having one's needs satisfied, being able to obtain what one wants and needs, and feeling good more often than bad are central to happiness but have relatively little to do with a meaningful life. People are happy when they get what they want. Meaning, on the other hand, is to be found elsewhere. In sum, happiness is important but it is not all there is to wellbeing, nor is it the only thing that ought to be valued. The above suggests that there are critical nuances in the measurement of subjective wellbeing, which are important considerations when approaching data obtained from social media platforms.

8.6 The Language of Social Media

Every day millions of people share their thoughts and feelings through simple text messages written on various social media platforms such as Facebook and Twitter, with such platforms in general creating an unprecedented amount of written language, significant amounts of which are publicly available. Twitter users alone write approximately 500 million messages every day (Krikorian, 2013). An immediate implication of the corpus of written language accumulating on such platforms is that it represents a massive source of rich psychological data with substantial scientific potential. The task confronting researchers is to develop methods that can meaningfully and effectively access this data. Whereas in the past researchers relied on either historical language samples such as literature or prompted participants to write new text, social media provides researchers with the natural language of millions of people with relative ease.

Several characteristics of social media language render it useful for research. First, social media language is typically written in natural social settings such as homes and schools and captures communication among friends, family members and acquaintances. Second, time-consuming prospective studies, whereby researchers track pre-identified variables over a period of time, are less necessary as data can be retroactively accessed for research purposes. Third, social media users disclose information about themselves at high rates; for many users, a frequent topic of discussion is themselves (Naaman, Boase, & Lai, 2010) and as such, social media users typically present their true selves and not mere idealized versions (Mitja et al., 2010). Social media language is a rich source of data; Twitter is particularly popular because it allows researchers to access massive amounts of data quickly, cost-effectively, and without having to obtain any informed consent from users.

Thus, the fundamental unit of analysis of data from social media is the language people use and the underlying premise is that this written language represents a quantifiable signal that can be used to assess a variety of psychological issues as diverse as personality traits (Bogg, 2017; Sap et al., 2014; Schwartz et al., 2013a) to depression (Coppersmith, Dredze, & Harman, 2014). Social media provides unprecedented access to unforced natural language that affords substantial increases in ecological validity (i.e., the extent to which findings can be generalized to real life settings) compared to that provided by traditional survey methodologies.

8.7 Methods to Investigate Language

Language patterns on social media platforms are generally studied using one of two formats: closed vocabulary or open-vocabulary approaches. With relatively few exceptions, psychological studies have used a closed vocabulary or word-counting approach to analysing such language. This method starts with lists of words that are combined into categories (e.g., pronouns) based on theory, followed by a count of the relative frequency of these words within a body of text. As this approach begins with predefined categories of words, it has been described as closed vocabulary. The closed-vocabulary approach scans the text for keywords that are retrieved from a predefined dictionary. Sometimes, these dictionaries contain only a few dozen highly specific words. Most however, comprise thousands. For example, the LabMT dictionary that is used in several studies contains 10,000 words that were rated by Amazon Mechanical Turk on a scale from sad to happy.

The most popular dictionary in SWB research, however, is the Linguistic Inquiry and Word Count (LIWC; Pennebaker, Chung, Ireland, Gonzales, & Booth, 2007), which comprises more than 6000 words assigned to one or more dimensions. The LIWC was developed to capture multiple psychological dimensions (Pennebaker & King, 1999). Words were first compiled from dictionaries, thesauri, existing questionnaires, and other sources, and then independently rated by three or more judges for inclusion in each category (Pennebaker & Francis, 1996; Pennebaker & King, 1999). The 2001 version includes 64 categories within nine main types (affective, social, sensory, biological, and cognitive processes; verbs; relativity, function and miscellaneous words) and has been translated into 12 languages. An updated version (LIWC2015) appeared in April 2016 (www.liwc.net), automatically counting word frequencies for 64 psychologically relevant categories, such as "function words" (e.g., articles, pronouns, conjunctions), "affective processes" (e.g., happy, cried, nervous), and "social processes" (e.g., pal, friend, talk). The dimensions most frequently used by SWB researchers are positive and negative emotion words and dimensions related to specific emotions such as sadness or anger. Though a simple interface, LIWC nonetheless allows text to be turned into numeric values. The program passes text through a "processor" (i.e., tokenizer and word counter) and provides the frequency that a user mentions each category. Frequencies can be adjusted by the total number of words as users differ in the number of words they write, which is also the probability that any random word in a document belongs to a given category. The relative frequencies can then be summarized descriptively, correlated with other variables, or used as predictors in regression analyses. LIWC is easy to use and widely accepted as a validated method to study language patterns; yet, it comprises a limited number of words and does not work well for colloquial language, leading some to question its validity for the analysis of social media language (Luhmann, 2017).

On the other hand, open-vocabulary approaches are not based on an a priori defined list of words but instead use statistical and probabilistic techniques to identify relevant language patterns or topics (i.e., clusters of words frequently used together) in order to find potentially meaningful clusters of words in large samples of natural language (e.g., Grimmer & Stewart, 2013; O'Connor, Bamman, & Smith, 2011; Schwartz et al., 2013b; Yarkoni, 2010). Open-vocabulary methods do not rely on a priori word or category judgments; rather, they extract a comprehensive collection of language features from the text being analysed. In contrast to closed-vocabulary methods, open-vocabulary methods characterize a language sample by the relative use of (a) single, uncategorized words; (b) non-word symbols (e.g., emoticons, punctuation); (c) multiword phrases; and (d) clusters of semantically related words identified through unsupervised methods, or topics. Because these language features are not identified a priori, these methods can accommodate neologisms and unconventional language use. As such, open-vocabulary methods extract more and richer features of language samples.

As an example, Schwartz et al. (2013a) applied an open-vocabulary approach called differential language analysis (DLA) to a large collection of social media messages and identified 2,000 clusters of words or topics. For example, one topic included the words "love", "sister", "friend", "world", "beautiful", "precious", and "sisters", and a second topic included "government" "freedom", "rights", "country", "political", and "democracy". These topics are generated in a data-driven, "bottom-up" manner, as opposed to the theory-driven, "top-down" methods used in closed-vocabulary approaches. Evidence suggests that open-ended approaches outperform closed vocabulary approaches when developing prediction models of language use associated with gender (Schwartz et al., 2013a). In addition, open-vocabulary methods appear to outperform closed-vocabulary methods when predicting the personality of online users in several studies (e.g., Gill, Nowson, & Oberlander, 2009). Open-vocabulary based predictions of SWB also tend to exhibit greater predictive validity than closed-vocabulary-based predictions. In one study, life satisfaction was less strongly correlated with words identified using a closed-vocabulary approach than with topics identified using an open-vocabulary approach (Luhmann, 2017). However, the downside is that open-vocabulary approaches require more sophisticated statistical skills and computational abilities although they are less labour intensive than closed vocabulary approaches in that they do not require the construction of a priori categories.

Despite the relative advantage of open-vocabulary approaches, closed-vocabulary methods remain popular in analyses of social media language (Golbeck, Robles, & Turner, 2011; Holtgraves, 2011; Sumner, Byers, Boochever, & Park, 2012). Within computer science and related fields, researchers have used closed-vocabulary analyses to study how well social media language can predict a user's personality (Mitja et al., 2010). For example, Golbeck et al. (2011) used a closed vocabulary approach to analyse the language written in the personal profiles and messages of Facebook users, who also completed personality measures. Relative uses of LIWC word categories (e.g., positive emotions, social processes) were then used as predictors in statistical models where the outcomes were self-reports of personality. When applied to a new sample of users, these models predicted users' personality traits better than chance, with the authors concluding that "users' Big Five personality traits can be predicted from the public information they share on Facebook" (Golbeck et al., 2011, p. 260).

8.8 Accessing Social Media Data

The social media analytics process involves four distinct steps which are data discovery, collection, preparation and analysis. Accessing social media data begins with raw data which can include comments, shares, likes, mentions, impressions, messages, profiles and hashtag use. Once a particular dataset is selected (e.g., Twitter, or Facebook), the data are typically accessed through an application programming interface (API), which is a format that enables computer programs to communicate with one another. More importantly, an API is also an interface for researchers to collect data from a given social media service. Through small program scripts, researchers can access the API to retrieve, store, and manipulate digital traces left by the users of a service for subsequent empirical analysis. Part of the attraction of API-based research is that the collection, organization, cleaning, preservation and analysis of data can be automated making APIs highly efficient research tools (Lomborg & Bechmann, 2014). Some social media companies such as Twitter provide publically available API's. However, they typically do not provide full and unlimited access to the entire social media dataset and is restricted to the data provided by the company. As such, API research can suffer from a lack of transparency regarding the data output and quality (i.e., the data that the company selects to make available for use with an API). Comparisons between social media platforms are also made difficult by the fact that there are differences between companies in terms of what they give access to.

To date, most API research has been conducted with Twitter as it has been traditionally quite open in terms of access to its database. Facebook API researchers are required to request permission to collect non-public data from participants through a Facebook app, while Twitter makes a random sample of all public tweets available in real time, which can be accessed through the Twitter API (https://dev.twitter.com/streaming/public) and only requires a Twitter account to access. Upon registering, an API key, API secret, access token, and access secret are received by the user. Following this, a blank Twitter application is created, from which data can be selected and retrieved. This can include tweets, user information, entities (metadata and contextual information), and places. As part of the code, a destination for the data is specified, such as a CSV file or database. Twitter places limits on how much information can be requested each hour as a free user (1% random feed per day; alternatively, data based on a specific criterion, such as geographic location can also be requested). Often, meta-data about each social media post is needed, such as the time it was posted, location, and by whom it was posted. Some information (e.g., time of posting) is easy to extract through the API; other information can be inferred from user profiles.

The data accessed through the API form a database with language data (social media posts and their metadata) and associated outcome variables either at the individual, group, or region level. The language data in its raw form is not suited for quantitative analysis as at this stage it remains only a sequence of characters. The next step, tokenization, refers to the process of breaking up posts or sentences into meaningful tokens or words, which may be known dictionary words, misspellings, punctuation, netspeak (e.g., lol, brb), emoticons (e.g., "<3" is a heart, ":)" is a smiling face), and other variations. Sequences of letters are automatically identified with adjustments made to separate punctuation from words. Related to this is that as the API selected for usage with a dataset influences the kinds of research questions that can be meaningfully asked, it is important that researchers have sufficient computational skills or work alongside others who do in order to use social media APIs.

8.8.1 Social Media and Wellbeing

Analysis of social media data can provide a macro-level perspective on various aspects of human behaviour and related psychological variables. As noted, closed-vocabulary approaches, of which there are several examples, are widely used in social media analysis. In psychological research, closed-vocabulary approaches have most commonly been implemented through the LIWC program (Pennebaker et al., 2007). For example, by applying a priori created lexica across thousands of Facebook users and blogs and millions of word instances, extraversion was positively corelated to using more positive emotion words, whereas neuroticism related to using more negative emotion and swear words (Gill et al., 2009; Sumner, Byers, & Shearing, 2011). In over 140 million words from nearly 20,000 blogs, older and male bloggers tended to use more words related to religion, politics, business, and the Internet. Conversely, younger and female bloggers used more personal pronouns, conjunctions, fun, romance, and swear words (Argamon, Koppel, Pennebaker, & Schler, 2007). Across 16,000 Twitter users and two million tweets, Christians used more religious, positive emotion, and social process words, whereas atheists used more negative emotion and insight words (Ritter, Preston, & Hernandez, 2014). In millions of Facebook posts, positive and negative emotion expressions even appear to be related to local weather reports (Coviello et al., 2014).

As mentioned previously, happiness and life satisfaction are correlated but conceptually and functionally distinct (Diener, Diener, Choi, & Oishi, 2018; Diener, Ng, Harter, & Arora, 2010; Diener, Oishi, & Tay, 2018; Lucas, Diener, & Suh, 1996). To date, most approaches using social media have tapped into emotional aspects of wellbeing (i.e., happiness) and these appear to yield valid indicators of emotional wellbeing, as indicated by studies showing that the use of closed vocabulary approaches fluctuate in weekly and diurnal patterns in a manner similar to self-reported emotional wellbeing, and also by studies reporting moderate correlations of these measures with self-reported emotional wellbeing (Luhmann, 2017). For life satisfaction, however, the correlations between self-reported scores and alternative indicators are typically weaker suggesting that individual-level life satisfaction cannot yet be fully predicted reliably from people's digital traces.

Social media research on happiness has been mostly limited to studying positive and negative affect, also called sentiment analysis. Watson, Clark and Tellegen (1988) present a two-dimensional model of human emotion, where one dimension represents the valence of affective states—positive and negative—and a second dimension reflects the level of physiological arousal—high and low. These states are highly dynamic and influenced by internal and external stimuli, such as the weather, social interactions and our subjective interpretations of such external events. These affective states can be expressed in written or spoken language, reflected in English by words such as "happy", "sad", "excited", or "bored". Increasingly, people use social media platforms such as Twitter to express their current status, including direct or indirect references to their affective states. This phenomenon provides researchers with an opportunity to explore affective states as a function of time and place and concerning a specified attitude object (e.g., religion, politics, or smoking).

Sentiment analysis aims to extract and quantify subjective opinions or feelings from the words people use on social media platforms and can be valuable to those interested in monitoring and promoting community or even national wellbeing. Its techniques have been successfully applied across a range of topics including the exploration of public sentiment across time and in response to major events or political occurrences (Diaz, Gamon, Hofman, Kıcıman, & Rothschild, 2016). This interest has led to the development and refinement of sentiment analytic techniques. For instance, a technique known as the Hedonometer and Valence Shift Word Graphs were used to study the affective linguistic trends of song lyrics and blogs posts over time (Dodds & Danforth, 2010); the authors concluded that the happiness (greater expressed positive affect, relative to negative affect) of song lyrics declined from the 1960 to 1990s and then remained stable after 1995. Other studies have attempted to explore temporal patterns in affective states over varying durations (Dodds, Harris, Kloumann, Bliss, & Danforth, 2011). For instance, one study examined affective rhythms across 84 countries using LIWC and developed a lexicon for measuring positive and negative affect from Twitter data (Tausczik & Pennebaker, 2010). They found largely universal diurnal patterns across countries, such that the early part of the day was associated with heightened positive affect, which reached a peak around 6:00 am and then decreased over the duration of the day. This study also found that the weekday morning positivity pattern shifts by two hours during the weekend. Other Twitter studies exploring the temporal dynamics of happiness using the Hedonometer have also observed pronounced weekly patterns; weekends tend to be more positive than early weekdays.

In a business context, Twitter data and sentiment analytics have been employed to measure customer satisfaction within the hospitality industry. One study conducted with hotels in Las Vegas found that the Twitter-derived sentiment correlated well with hotel rankings provided by guests. Exploring the meteorological relationship to mood, another Twitter study used OpinionFinder sentiment lexicon and Profile of Mood States (POMS) to extract sentiment. This data was correlated with data from U.S. meteorological agencies such as temperature, rainfall, snow depth, and wind. High temperatures were associated with fatigue, anger and reduced depression, while snow was associated with increased depression, and precipitation with decreased tiredness (Li, Wang, & Hovy, 2014).

In summary, the sentiment analytic Twitter studies have produced findings that are consistent with intuition and highly convergent with findings obtained via other research methods and data sources. Yet, the majority of this work has focused on the English language. There is a need to extend such inquiry further and explore the validity and reliability of sentiment analytic techniques across sociocultural and linguistic contexts.

8.8.2 Beyond Sentiment Analysis

Beyond transient affective states such as happiness, relatively few studies have focused on self-referential tweets using a template driven retrieval strategy to explore life satisfaction, a more trait-like component of subjective wellbeing. Twitter-derived estimates of life satisfaction appear relatively stable across time (i.e., no temporal patterning) and uninfluenced by seasonal transition, celebrity deaths or political crises (Yang & Srinivasan, 2016). Additionally, Twitter users categorized as "satisfied" as opposed to "dissatisfied" showed patterns in their tweets consistent with previous findings in the subjective wellbeing literature. For example, the "satisfied" group expressed significantly more positive and less negative affective words. They also used less profanity and were significantly more positive about religion than their "dissatisfied" counterparts. The research of Schwartz et al. (2013b) is particularly important when moving beyond sentiment analysis. They analysed tweets originating in 1293 US counties for which results from life satisfaction surveys were independently available. Using lexicon features (LIWC and PERMA, a special lexicon founded on Seligman's (2011) wellbeing research) and LDA derived topic features, they built models to predict life satisfaction at the county level. Consistent with general life satisfaction research in psychology, terms and topics about physical activity and social engagement were positively related to subjective wellbeing, while disengagement words (sleepy, tired) related negatively to wellbeing.

A recent study by Yang and Srinivasan (2016) offers a good example of a top-down or theory-driven approach to examining life satisfaction using a large Twitter two-year dataset. Using the Satisfaction with Life Scale (SWLS) (Diener, Emmons, Larsen, & Griffin, 1985) they derived a set of template-driven, retrieval strategies to obtain tweets conveying self-ratings of life satisfaction. Life satisfaction has received relatively little attention in social media research, largely due to difficulties in operationalizing the term. The SWLS scale (Diener et al., 1985) provided the basis for lexicon retrieval and analysis, and has been cited more than 9800 times and used in many areas, including positive psychology. Starting with a SWLS survey statement (Step 1), the authors first obtained an initial set of equivalent statements through crowdsourcing with MTurk (Step 2). For example, the sentence "my life is peachy" is synonymous with the SWLS statement 3 (I am satisfied with my life). Next, they manually generalized the statements into templates (Step 3) which identified equivalent expressions. Identified words in a template could be substituted by a variety of synonyms from a lexicon or a dictionary (e.g., happy, delighted, content are synonymous in this context). Two sets of templates to retrieve tweets expressing life satisfaction versus life dissatisfaction were developed. Dissatisfaction templates had their own synonym sets, e.g., "sad, depressing, miserable". Then, they built 16 retrieval strategies (search queries) from each template (Step 4). The strategies differed along two dimensions: (1) the number of intervening words allowed in a template (P) and (2) the number of words allowed before or after a text segment that satisfies the template asking questions ("Is my life good?") were filtered out (Yang & Srinivasan, 2016). Using this methodology, the authors were able to extract expressions of satisfaction and dissatisfaction with life. Consistent with their definitions, trends in life satisfaction posts appear resilient to external events (political, seasonal, etc.) unlike affect trends reported by previous researchers (Dodds et al., 2011). Comparing users, they found differences between satisfied and dissatisfied users in several linguistic, psychosocial and other features. For example, the latter post more tweets expressing anger, anxiety, depression, sadness and on death.

Twitter is by no means the only source of big data to help identify relationships between wellbeing and other variables as it also appears that people's use of search terms on Google reveals much about wellbeing. In a key study, Algan and colleagues (2016) built a wellbeing indicator from a combination of search keyword groups derived from Google Trends. Search terms were grouped into twelve domains that reflected three aspects of wellbeing: material conditions (job search, job market, financial security and home finance), social aspects (family stress, family time, civic engagement and personal security), and finally, health and wellness (healthy habits, health conditions, summer activities and education, and ideals). A key methodological strength of the study however was the use of factor analysis to create meaningfully composite terms. For instance, the category family stress contained the following component keywords (domesticabuse, marriagehelp, marriageprob, marriagecounseling, familysupport, custody and womensshelter). The researchers report that a number of search categories were consistently associated with lower subjective wellbeing such as job search, financial security, and family stress. Conversely, search terms related to civic engagement and healthy habits were positively related to wellbeing. Overall, this research suggests that the online use of key search terms can be used to build an index of subjective wellbeing.

8.9 Big Data, Wellbeing and the Gulf Countries

To date, few studies have investigated aspects of wellbeing using data from social media platforms in the Gulf countries. However, given the widespread use of social media in these countries, considerable potential exists to investigate various aspects of wellbeing (Sulaiman & Aquil, 2015). A handful of studies have been conducted suggesting that the use of this data may render meaningful insights. We describe these studies in detail and examine their implications for the future of wellbeing research in the region.

8.9.1 Hedonometer: Using Both Arabic and English

Al-Shehhi et al. (in press) examined the affective component of subjective wellbeing (happiness) in the UAE using a large 2015 dataset extracted from Twitter. More than 8 million Twitter messages (tweets) written in Arabic and English were analysed. Numerous cross-linguistic differences were observed, including significant differ-

The technique is based on using 10222 English words to calculate the overall emotional content of a given text or dataset. The 10222 words had previously been rated for happiness from 1 (least happy) to 9 (most happy). The equation below explains how the total happiness of a given text or tweet is computed.

$$h_{avg}(T) = \frac{\sum_{i=1}^{N} h_{avg}(w_i) f_i}{\sum_{i=1}^{N} f_i} = \sum_{i=1}^{N} h_{avg}(w_i) p_i \quad \ldots\ldots\ldots (1)$$

Where:

T *is a given text*

N *is unique words in* T

w_i *is a given word in the text*

f_i *is the frequency of the ith word* w_i

Δh_{avg} *is the range of words to exclude;* $5 - \Delta h_{avg} < h_{avg} < 5 + \Delta h_{avg}$

$h_{avg}(w_i)$ *average happiness of word* w_i,

it is a natural tuning parameter; by default, we can choose $\Delta h_{avg}=1$ *to, balance the sensitivity* versus robustness.

$p_i = \frac{f_i}{\sum_{i=1}^{N} f_i}$ is the normalized frequency

Fig. 8.1 The Hedonometer Algorithm based on Dodds et al. (2011)

ences in the number of tweets, followers and friends associated with users of English and Arabic. The main purpose of this study was to explore "happiness", that is, social media sentiment (the use of positive and negative words on social media). More specifically, the study aimed to explore whether the use of such terms would correspond with times when people report feeling more or less positively. This study, the first in the Arabian Gulf region, used the hedonometer 2.0 algorithm detailed in Fig. 8.1.

Using the above-mentioned lexicon-based sentiment analytic tool (Hedonometer) and applying it to English and Arabic, we were able to explore temporal patterns in happiness (sentiment). The findings were rich and corresponded closely to intuitive hypotheses. For example, in Arabic and in English, Friday was the "happiest day" (see Fig. 8.2). In the UAE, Friday is the start of the weekend when schools, colleges and many businesses take a break.

Interestingly, the low point of the week in Arabic was Sunday (the start of the working week in the UAE); in English however (see Fig. 8.2), Monday was the low sentiment point. This relates to the large number of expatriates working in the UAE,

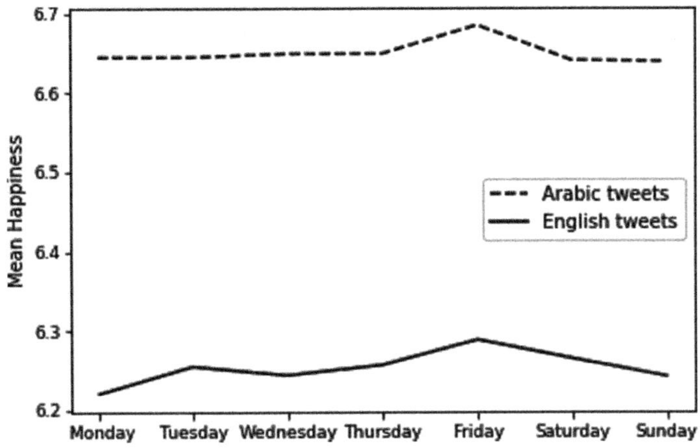

Fig. 8.2 UAE Twitter sentiment (happiness) by days of the week

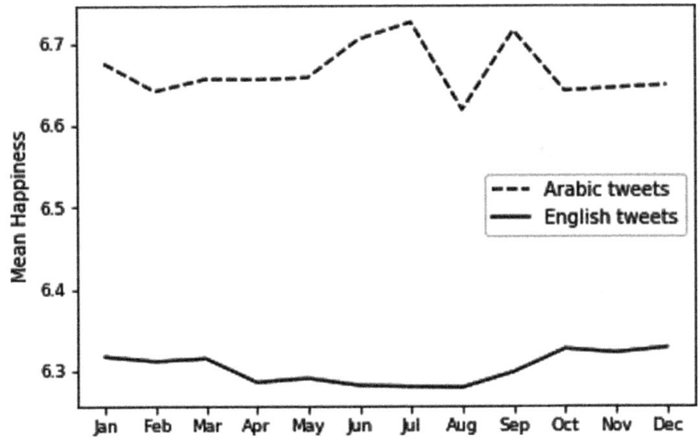

Fig. 8.3 UAE Twitter sentiment (happiness) by months

who come from nations where Monday might be the start of the week given their work with international offices. One interpretation of this finding is that among expatriates (English users), something like an emotional body clock has not yet recalibrated to the new working environment, where the workweek starts on Sunday and not Monday as it did back home. Other findings indicated that 7:00 am was the happiest hour, but may relate to the fact that individuals are tweeting more prior to starting their work day and less as the day progresses. The happiest months differ based on language, and notable patterns are also observed in relation to Ramadan and other events of socio-political and religio-cultural significance in the nation (Fig. 8.3).

The UAE becomes unbearably hot in the summer; people are mostly restricted to indoor activities and this may account for the low points in the English language tweets observed in June through August. It is also when many expatriates leave for their summer and school breaks. In Arabic however, there is a spike in June and July and again in September, with August becoming a low point. This pattern is explained in terms of the Holy month of Ramadan and its corresponding two Eid holidays. In 2015, Ramadan took place during June with Eid al Fitr (a celebration marking the end of Ramadan) in July. In September, there was another big holiday, marking the end of the Hajj pilgrimage (Eid al Adha). These patterns overlap with religio-cultural events being associated with elevated happiness as expressed through social media. The happiest day of the year in the English tweets was New Year's Eve; in Arabic, it was Eid al-Fitr. It is worth noting that religion is still widely practised among the indigenous communities of the Arabian Gulf and is also an important source of national identity, social identity and wellbeing (Thomas, 2014).

8.9.2 Religiosity

Religion often provides people meaning in their lives and is widely viewed as contributing to wellbeing for many individuals (Smith, McCullough, & Poll, 2003). In a study of UAE Twitter data, Thomas, Al-Shehhi and Grey (2018) explored religiosity and the use of profanity among the UAE's Twitter users. Religiosity, similar to happiness, was operationalised as a lexicon, comprising words that unambiguously associated with Islamic religious practice (e.g., Masjid, Mosque, Salah, and Wudu). In this lexicon-driven, cross-linguistic (Arabic/English) analysis of 152 million tweets, the team first looked at differences in language use among users. They found that Arabic users sent a lot more tweets than English users (see Table 8.1).

Although Arabic users represent only 16% of the sample, they account for more than 50% of the tweets. This pattern might be related to the demography of the UAE, where the Arabic speaking citizens are a minority, but also a relatively young minority. UAE citizens comprise around 12% of the population, with a younger median age than the expatriate population (National Bureau of Statistics (NBS), 2009). The discrepancy in tweet frequency by language might also reflect cultural differences (individualism/collectivism) in internet usage (see Würtz, 2005), or

Table 8.1 Tweets by language and unique users

	Tweets	Tweets (%)	Unique users	Users (%)
Arabic	82,065,108	53.69	88,280	16.61
English	42,235,907	27.63	404,689	76.15
Other[a]	28,534,712	18.67	38,444	7.23

[a]There were 64 languages recorded. After Arabic and English, Urdu, Tagalog and Hindi were most frequently used

cultural differences in communication style, high versus low context communication (Hall, 2000), with culture manifesting itself in the online world; however, we are only just beginning to investigate this phenomenon and its implications for wellbeing.

Beyond the linguistic differences in tweet frequency, this study also found patterns of religiosity that support intuitive hypotheses and others that challenge conventional wisdom. Regarding religiosity, Friday (Islam's holy day) was associated with an increase in the overall proportion of religiosity related vocabulary used in Arabic. Similarly, Ramadan (Islam's holiest Month) was associated with a substantial increase in religious sentiment (English and Arabic) and a month-long decrease in the frequency of Arabic obscenity (see Fig. 8.4).

As highlighted in Fig. 8.4, religiosity peaks during the first week of Ramadan then quickly returns to pre-Ramadan levels for much of the month, before again rising during the last week. This pattern seems analogous to the idea of the "hedonic treadmill", where an event (e.g., receipt of a gift) gives rise to elevated positive affect, before a rapid return to a set point (Diener, Lucas, & Scollon, 2006). The dawning of the event, in this case, Ramadan, gives rise to heightened religiosity, which quickly returns to baseline levels (religiosity set-point). The second rise in religiosity during the last week of Ramadan might reflect the religious significance of Laylat Al-Qadr (The Night of Power). The Night of Power is said to be the night when the first verses of the Quran were revealed to the Prophet Muhammad and Muslims are encouraged to perform a special night vigil prayer (Qiam ul Lail) at this time, an activity associated with an abundance of blessings. According to the Quran, "The night of Qadr is better than a thousand months" (97:3). Nobody knows when Laylat Al-Qadr is, however, it is agreed that it falls on one of the last ten nights of Ramadan. The seeking of Laylat Al-Qadr explains the resurgence of religiosity in the UAE Twitter data corresponding with the last week of Ramadan.

This study also explored gender differences, based on a relatively small subset of the data (confirmed males and females), finding some expected and unexpected

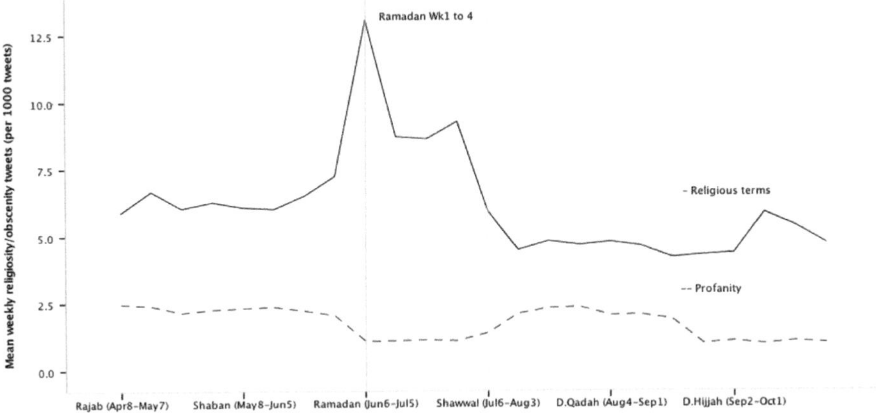

Fig. 8.4 UAE Twitter sentiment (Arabic religiosity) by months

gender differences. Gender was assumed by Twitter display names, i.e., Fatima/Mariam versus Mohammed. Proportionally, females (Fatima's and Mariam's) tweeted in English more than males (Mohammed's). This might be explained in terms of females outperforming males in tertiary education in the UAE. Almost all colleges and universities in the UAE use English as the language of tuition and previous research has documented greater female participation in tertiary education, as well as higher academic performance (Thomas, Al-Marzooqi, & Raynor, 2012). It might be that female Twitter users in the UAE have greater English language proficiency and feel more comfortable tweeting in English. However, this linguistic gender difference could equally be framed as males being more proficient in Arabic and perhaps less Western acculturated. At least one previous study in the UAE has suggested that Western acculturation is greater among UAE females (Ghubash, Daradkeh, Al-Muzafari, El-Manssori, & Abou-Saleh, 2001).

In addition to tweeting more in Arabic, males also expressed more religiosity, both in English and Arabic. This greater public expressivity of religiosity may reflect traditional gender roles in Islam, where males are encouraged to pray in the mosque and women encouraged to pray at home. Similarly, Islamic public service roles, such as Imam (prayer leader), have typically been restricted to men. That said, past research typically reports elevated religiosity among women (Miller & Stark, 2002; Schnabel, 2015). Although previous research has focused on Christian denominations, some studies show a similar, although less pronounced, pattern among Muslims (Stark, 2002). The present atypical findings (females expressing less religiosity than males) are interpretable within the socialisation hypothesis of female religiosity, which suggests that social expectations contribute to females reporting greater religiosity than males (Schnabel, 2015). Social media, however, affords people a degree of anonymity and this might lessen the pressure to conform to social expectations. There are alternative interpretations. For example, among Muslims, female social media users might be highly atypical of the general Muslim female population of the UAE, while their male counterparts are more representative. Such a situation might arise due to pervasive gender-role expectations concerning social interaction. For example, within some households, it might be argued that a "good Muslim woman" does not speak to, or share information with strangers on the Internet.

This same study also examined the use of profanity (obscenities). Although often used casually, profanity can be associated with the expression of negative affect (anger). Looking at the Twitter data in Arabic, revealed patterns are consistent with previous research exploring English curse-words (Wang, Chen, Thirunarayan, & Sheth, 2014), where males used more obscenities than females. This pattern, however, was reversed in English, where females proportionally used more obscenity than males. In cases where English was a second language, using English obscenity might be less emotive. Previous research among bilingual (Turkish/English) speakers has found that using obscenity (e.g., whore) in the second language evoked significantly less autonomic reactivity (emotion) than it did in the first language (Harris, Aycicegi, & Gleason, 2003). This affective attenuation (dampening of emotion) associated with second language use might also explain the far higher rate of English obscenity across the whole dataset. The UAE is a bilingual nation with English widely spoken in education and at the workplace, while Arabic remains widely spoken at home by UAE citizens and Arab expatriates (Mourtada-Sabbah, Al-Mutawa, Fox, & Walters, 2008). This study is important in highlighting some of the variables that need to be considered when exploring wellbeing in the context of a Gulf nation.

8.9.3 I Versus We: Exploring Self-concept on Twitter Using Arabic and English

Past research has indicated that a strong sense of belonging and the expectation of social support act as a buffer to self-esteem and wellbeing (Haslam, Jetten, Postmes, & Haslam, 2009). Viewing oneself (self-concept) as belonging to valuable social groups is another important variable potentially impacting wellbeing. The cultural influence hypothesis suggests that people from individualistic societies tend to emphasise more personal attributes (tall, athletic, geeky) when articulating their self-concepts, while individuals from collectivist societies place greater emphasis on social attributes (Emirati, Muslim, Father). A study by our team (Thomas et al., in prep) explored this hypothesis based on an extract of Twitter data for the UAE. In the first study, the team randomly extracted a thousand user biographies. A user biography (bio) is a short narrative statement, typically written by the user, about the user, which can be viewed as a snapshot of the individual's self-concept. Bios were explored using structured content analysis and the differences in self-concept between English and Arabic users were quantified. In a second study, using an expanded dataset, the team used the LIWC software to explore differences between individuals with biographies uniquely characterised by either group (we, our, us) or self (I, mine, me) referential linguistic constructs ($N = 62{,}038$). In line with the study's predictions, Arabic users mentioned more social attributes than their English speaking counterparts. Conversely, English speakers mentioned more personal attributes. Study Two found that self-referentiality was associated with the more frequent mention of personal attributes, while group-referentiality (us, our, we) was associated with social attributes. Participants who were more social in their orientation (bios mentioning we, us, our) also had tweets that expressed more positive and less negative affect than their self-referential counterparts. In sum, the Big Data extracted from social media platforms such as Twitter, offers a potentially useful means of exploring wellbeing relevant constructs across cultures.

8.10 Challenges to Big Data Analysis in Arab Countries

While the use of Big Data to formulate and answer psychological questions, particularly around aspects of wellbeing in Arabic speaking countries is in its infancy, there are two challenges confronting researchers in the Arab world. Firstly, there is an absence of dictionaries similar to the LIWC for the easy analysis of Arabic. At present, researchers must develop dictionaries for closed language analytic methods by hand. The second challenge is that many of the words used are simultaneously commonly used forenames (polysemy). For instance, Sa'eed is the Arabic word for happy yet is also a common male forename. As a result, using words such as happy in sentiment analysis is made highly problematic resulting in many false positives. Psycholinguists and data scientists will need to collaborate on developing more sophisticated search and quantification strategies for the Arabic language for progress to be made.

8.11 Conclusion

Big Data has great potential in the study of wellbeing. Traditional survey methodologies for the assessment of wellbeing are beset by a range of problems relating to response biases and heuristics such as acquiescence, extreme responding, random responding, digit preferences, primacy and recency effects, demand characteristics, consistency bias and priming effects (Miller, 2017). Though not without its methodological considerations, Big Data at its core relies on natural language and is not particularly prone to these considerations. Social media analysis, such as those reported here, might help further explore the rate and direction of social change in rapidly developing Arabian Gulf states such as the UAE. These surveillance methods offer obvious advantages over self-report survey methodologies in that the data are less influenced by socially desirable responding and other forms of reactivity (Ritter et al., 2014). Social media use frequently involves individuals conversing with one another on wide-ranging topics, freely expressing attitudes, fears and aspirations. In addition to this relative ecological validity, the sample sizes that can be obtained through social media are unparalleled in direct survey work. It is this sample size that silences many potential criticisms, such as the fact that some tweets are posted by news agencies, or commercial entities. Similarly, some tweets are not a reflection of a person's thoughts or emotional state as they might simply be a quoting a celebrity or the lyrics of a song, etc. Big Data however, will typically ensure that such noise is overwhelmingly drowned out by the mass of data that is reflective of people's genuine concerns and sentiment (Dodds et al., 2011). When it comes to helping social scientists learn more about happiness and wellbeing in the MENA/GCC region, the future of Big Data is bright indeed.

References

Algan, Y., Beasley, E., Guyot, F., Higa, K., Murtin, F., & Senik, C. (2016, May 10). *Big data measures of wellbeing: Evidence from a Google wellbeing index in the United States*. OECD Statistics Working Papers, 2016/03. Paris, France: OECD Publishing.

Al Shehhi, A., Thomas, J., Welsch, R., Grey, I. M., Woon, W. L., & Aung, A. (in press). Arabia Felix 2.0: A cross-linguistic twitter analysis of the temporal patterns of happiness in the United Arab Emirates. *EPJ Data Science Journal*.

Argamon, S., Koppel, M., Pennebaker, J., & Schler, J. (2007, September). Mining the blogosphere: Age, gender and the varieties of self-expression. *First Monday*, *12*(9).

Baumeister, R., Vohs, K., Aaker, J., & Garbinsky, E. (2013). Some key differences between a happy life and a meaningful life. *The Journal of Positive Psychology, 8*(6), 505–516.

Bogg, T. (2017). Social media membership, browsing, and profile updating in a representative U.S. sample: Independent and interdependent effects of big five traits and aging and social factors. *Frontiers in Psychology*, *8*, 1122.

Cook, S., Conrad, C., Fowlkes, A., & Mohebbi, M. (2011). Assessing Google flu trends performance in the United States during the 2009 influenza virus A (H1N1) pandemic. *PLoS ONE, 6*(8), e23610.

Coppersmith, G., Dredze, M., & Harman, C. (2014). Quantifying mental health signals in Twitter. In *Proceedings of the Workshop on Computational Linguistics and Clinical Psychology: From Linguistic Signal to Clinical Reality* (pp. 51–60).

Costanza, R., Fisher, B., Ali, S., Beer, C., Bond, L., Boumans, R., … Snapp, R. (2007). Quality of life: An approach integrating opportunities, human needs, and subjective wellbeing. *Ecological Economics*, *61*(2–3), 267–276.

Coviello, L., Sohn, Y., Kramer, A., Marlow, C., Franceschetti, M., & Christakis, N. (2014). Detecting emotional contagion in massive social networks. *PLoS ONE, 9*(3), e90315.

Diaz, F., Gamon, M., Hofman, J., Kıcıman, E., & Rothschild, D. (2016). Online and social media: Data as an imperfect continuous panel survey. *PLoS ONE, 11*(1), e0145406.

Diener, E., Suh, E. M., Lucas, R. E., & Smith, H. L. (1999). Subjective wellbeing: 3 decades of progress. *Psychological Bulletin, 125*, 276–302.

Diener, E., Diener, C., Choi, H., & Oishi, S. (2018a). Revisiting "Most People Are Happy"—And discovering when they are not. *Perspectives on Psychological Science, 13*(2), 166–170.

Diener, E., Emmons, R. A., Larsen, R. J., & Griffin, S. (1985). The satisfaction with life scale. *Journal of Personality Assessment, 49*, 71–75.

Diener, E., Oishi, S., & Tay, L. (2018b). Advances in subjective wellbeing research. *Nature Human Behavior, 2*(4), 253–260.

Diener, E., Lucas, R. E., & Scollon, C. N. (2006). Beyond the hedonic treadmill: Revising the adaptation theory of wellbeing. *American Psychologist, 61*(4), 305–314.

Diener, E., Ng, W., Harter, J., & Arora, R. (2010). Wealth and happiness across the world: Material prosperity predicts life evaluation, whereas psychosocial prosperity predicts positive feeling. *Journal of Personality and Social Psychology, 99*(1), 52–61.

Dodds, P., & Danforth, C. (2010). Measuring the happiness of large-scale written expression: Songs, blogs, and presidents. *Journal of Happiness Studies, 11*(4), 441–456.

Dodds, P. S., Harris, K. D., Kloumann, I. M., Bliss, C. A., & Danforth, C. M. (2011). Temporal patterns of happiness and information in a global social network: Hedonometrics and Twitter. *PLoS ONE, 6*(12), e26752, 1–26.

Eichstaedt, J. C., Schwartz, H. A., Kern, M. L., Dziurzynski, L., Lucas, R. E., Agrawal, M., … Ungar, L. H. (2013). Characterizing geographic variation in wellbeing using tweets. In *Proceedings of the 7th International AAAI Conference on Weblogs and Social Media (ICWSM), July 8–1, 2013*, Boston, MA.

Eichstaedt, J. C., Schwartz, H. A., Kern, M. L., Park, G., Labarthe, D. R., Merchant, R. M., … Seligman, M. E. P. (2015). Psychological language on Twitter predicts county-level heart disease mortality. *Psychological Science*, *26*(2), 159–169.

Gill, A. J., Nowson, S., & Oberlander, J. (2009). What are they blogging about? Personality, topic and motivation in blogs. In E. Adar, M. Hurst, T. Finin, N. S. Glance, N. Nicolov, & B. L. Tseng (Eds.), *Proceedings of the 3rd International ICWSM Conference* (pp. 18–25). The AAAI Press.

Golbeck, J., Robles, C., & Turner, K. (2011). Predicting personality with social media. In *Proceedings of the 2011 Annual Conference on Human Factors in Computing Systems* (CHI EA 2011; May 7–12, 2011) (pp. 253–262). Vancouver, BC, Canada.

Google. (2009). *Google flu trends*. Retrieved from www.google.org/flutrends.

Grimmer, J., & Stewart, B. (2013). Text as data: The promise and pitfalls of automatic content analysis methods for political texts. *Political Analysis, 21*(3), 267–297.

Ghubash, R., Daradkeh, T. K., Al-Muzafari, S. M. A., El-Manssori, M. E., & Abou-Saleh, M. T. (2001). Al Ain community psychiatric survey IV: Socio-cultural changes (traditionality-liberalism) and prevalence of psychiatric disorders. *Social Psychiatry and Psychiatric Epidemiology, 36,* 565–570.

Hall, E. T. (2000). Context and meaning. In L. Samovar & R. E. Porter (Eds.), *Intercultural communication: A reader* (pp. 34–43). Belmont, CA: Wadsworth Publishing Co.

Harris, C. L., Aycicegi, A., & Gleason, J. B. (2003). Taboo words and reprimands elicit greater autonomic reactivity in a first language than in a second language. *Applied Psycholinguistics, 24,* 561–579.

Haslam, S. A., Jetten, J., Postmes, T., & Haslam, C. (2009). Social identity, health and wellbeing: An emerging agenda for applied psychology. *Applied Psychology: An International Review, 58*(1), 1–23.

Holtgraves, T. (2011). Text messaging, personality, and the social context. *Journal of Research in Personality, 45*(1), 92–99.

Inglehart, R. (1997). *Modernization and postmodernisation: Cultural, economic and political change*. Boston, MA: Princeton University Press.

Krikorian, R. (2013, August 16). *New Tweets per second record, and how!* (Web Log Post). Retrieved May 14, 2018, from https://blog.twitter.com/engineering/en_us/a/2013/new-tweets-per-second-record-and-how.html

Li, J., Wang, X., & Hovy, E. (2014). What a nasty day: Exploring mood-weather relationship from Twitter. In *Proceedings of the 23rd ACM International Conference on Conference on Information and Knowledge Management, CIKM 2014* (pp. 1309–1318). New York, USA: ACM.

Linley, P., Maltby, J., Wood, A., Osborne, G., & Hurling, R. (2009). Measuring happiness: The higher order factor structure of subjective and psychological wellbeing measures. *Personality and Individual Differences, 47*(8), 878–884.

Lomborg, S., & Bechmann, A. (2014). Using APIs for data collection on social media. *The Information Society, 30*(4), 256–265.

Lucas, R. E., Diener, E., & Suh, E. (1996). Discriminant validity of wellbeing measures. *Journal of Personality and Social Psychology, 71*(3), 616–628.

Luhmann, M. (2017). Using Big Data to study subjective wellbeing. *Current Opinion in Behavioral Sciences, 18,* 28–33.

Mauss, I. B., Tamir, M., Anderson, C. L., & Savino, N. S. (2011). Can seeking happiness make people happy? *Paradoxical effects of valuing happiness. Emotion, 11*(4), 807–815.

Miller, A., & Stark, R. (2002). Gender and religiousness: Can socialization explanations be saved? *American Journal of Sociology, 107*(6), 1399–1423.

Miller, P. (2017). Is there a future for surveys? *Public Opinion Quarterly, 81,* 205–212.

Mitja, D., Back, J., Vazire, S., Gaddis, S., Schmukle, S., Egloff, B., et al. (2010). Facebook profiles reflect actual personality, not self-idealization. *Psychological Science, 21*(3), 372–374.

Morrison, M., Jebb, A., Tay, L., & Diener, E. (2018). Subjective wellbeing across the lifespan worldwide: The role of culture and changing priorities. Under review with *Psychology and Aging.*

Mourtada-Sabbah, N., Al-Mutawa, M., Fox, J. W., & Walters, T. (2008). Media as social matrix in the United Arab Emirates. In A. Alsharekh & R. Sprinborg (Eds.), *Popular culture and political identity in the Arab Gulf States*. London, UK: SAQI in association with The London Middle East Institute at SOAS.

Naaman, M., Boase, J., & Lai, C. (2010). Is it really about me? Message content in social awareness streams. *Proceedings of the ACM Conference on Computer Supported Cooperative Work, CSCW* (pp. 189–192).
NBS. (2009). *Population estimates (2006–2009)* (p. 10). United Arab Emirates: UAE National Bureau of Statistics.
O'Connor, B., Bamman, D., & Smith, N. A. (2011). Computational text analysis for social science: Model assumptions and complexity. In *2nd Workshop on Computational Social Science and Wisdom of the Crowds (NIPS, 2011)*. Retrieved from http://repository.cmu.edu/cgi/viewcontent.cgi?article=1201&context=lti.
Olson, D. R., Konty, K. J., Paladini, M., Viboud, C., & Simonsen, L. (2013). Reassessing Google flu trends data for detection of seasonal and pandemic influenza: A comparative epidemiological study at three geographic scales. *PLoS Computational Biology, 9*(10), e1003256.
Park, G., Schwartz, H. A., Eichstaedt, J. C., Kern, M. L., Kosinski, M., Stillwell, D. J., ... Seligman, M. E. P. (2014). Automatic personality assessment through social media language. *Journal of Personality and Social Psychology, 108*(6), 934–952.
Pennebaker, J., Chung, C., Ireland, M., Gonzales, A., & Booth, R. (2007). *The development and psychometric properties of LIWC 2007* (www.LIWC.net, Austin, TX).
Pennebaker, J., & Francis, M. E. (1996). Cognitive, emotional, and language processes in disclosure. *Cognition and Emotion, 10*(6), 601–626.
Pennebaker, J., & King, L. A. (1999). Linguistic styles: Language use as an individual difference. *Journal of Personality and Social Psychology, 7*(6), 1296–1312.
Ritter, R. S., Preston, J. L., & Hernandez, I. (2014). Happy tweets: Christians are happier, more socially connected, and less analytical than atheists on Twitter. *Social Psychological and Personality Science, 5*(2), 243–249.
Sap, M., Park, G., Eichstaedt, J., Kern, M., Ungar, L., & Schwartz, H. A. (2014). Developing age and gender predictive lexica over social media. In *Proceedings of the 2014 Conference on Empirical Methods in Natural Language Processing, EMNLP*, 2014.
Schnabel, L. (2015). Review of why are women more religious than men. *Secularism and Nonreligion, 4*(1), Article 7.
Schwartz, H. A., Eichstaedt, J. C., Kern, M. L., Dziurzynski, L., Lucas, R. E., Agrawal, M., ... Ungar, L. H. (2013a). Characterizing geographic variation in wellbeing using Tweets. In *Proceedings of the 7th International AAAI Conference on Weblogs and Social Media (ICWSM)*. Boston, MA.
Schwartz, H. A., Eichstaedt, J. C., Kern, M. L., Dziurzynski, L., Ramones, S. M., Agrawal, M., ... Ungar, L. H. (2013b). Personality, gender, and age in the language of social media: The open-vocabulary approach. *PLoS ONE, 8*(9), e73791.
Seligman, M. E. P. (2011). *Flourish: A visionary new understanding of happiness and wellbeing*. New York, NY: Free Press.
Smith, T. B., McCullough, M. E., & Poll, J. (2003). Religiousness and depression: Evidence for a main effect and the moderating influence of stressful life events. *Psychological Bulletin, 129*(4), 614–636.
Stark, R. (2002). Physiology and faith: Addressing the "universal" gender difference in religious commitment. *Journal for the Scientific Study of Religion, 41*(3), 495–507.
Sulaiman, R., & Aquil, A. (2015). Growth patterns of social media in Arab gulf states: An analytic study. *Social Networking, 4*, 23–32.
Sumner, C., Byers, A., Boochever, R., & Park, G. (2012). Predicting dark triad personality traits from Twitter usage and a linguistic analysis of Tweets. In *Proceedings of the 11th International Conference on Machine Learning and Applications, ICMLA*.
Sylwester, K., & Purver, M. (2015). Twitter language use reflects psychological differences between democrats and republicans. *PLoS ONE, 10*(9), e0137422.
Sumner, C., Byers, A., & Shearing, M. (2011). Determining personality traits and privacy concerns from Facebook activity. *Black Hat Briefings* (pp. 197–221).
Tausczik, Y., & Pennebaker, J. (2010). The psychological meaning of words: LIWC and computerized text analysis methods. *Journal of Language and Social Psychology, 29*(1), 24–54.

Thomas, J. (2014). *Psychological wellbeing in the Gulf states: The new Arabia Felix*. London, UK: Palgrave Macmillan.

Thomas, J., Al-Marzooqi, A., & Raynor, M. (2012). Marital status and gender as predictors of undergraduate academic performance: A United Arab Emirates context. *Learning and Teaching in the Gulf, 9*(2), 1–9.

Thomas, J., Al-Shehhi, A., & Grey, I. (2018, Accepted). The sacred and the profane: Social media and temporal patterns of religiosity in the United Arab Emirates. *Journal of Contemporary Religion*.

Wang, W., Chen, L., Thirunarayan, K., & Sheth, A. P. (2014, February 15–19). *Cursing in English on Twitter.* Paper presented at the 17th ACM conference on Computer supported cooperative work & social computing, Baltimore, Maryland, USA.

Watson, D., Clark, L. A., & Tellegen, A. (1988). Development and validation of brief measures of positive and negative affect: The PANAS scales. *Journal of Personality and Social Psychology, 54,* 1063–1070.

Würtz, E. (2005). A cross-cultural analysis of websites from high-context cultures and low-context cultures. *Journal of Computer-Mediated Communication, 11*(1), Article 13.

Yang, C., & Srinivasan, P. (2016). Life satisfaction and the pursuit of happiness on Twitter. *PLoS ONE, 11*(3), e0150881.

Yarkoni, T. (2010). Personality in 100,000 Words: A large-scale analysis of personality and word use among bloggers. *Journal of Research in Personality, 44*(3), 363–373.

Chapter 9
Because a Citation and a Contribution are Not the Same: A Path for (Positive) Psychology Research

Louise Lambert, Nausheen Pasha-Zaidi and Annie E. Crookes

Abstract Psychology research normally focuses on investigating questions specific to psychological interest, like distress or wellbeing, along with the methodologies used to generate such findings. However, the availability of research in published form is subject to a variety of criteria. So, what gets published, and more precisely, by whom and why? As psychology and the dissemination of psychological research become increasingly globalized, it is worth asking whether there are inherent biases and systems of privilege that may influence the answers to these questions and what the effects of such biases are. The concept of privilege is especially apt as academic publishing has historically been and continues to be a Caucasian enterprise of Western nations. This is not in dispute. Rather, this chapter examines how privilege permeates the publishing system. It explores how such systems affect the study of psychology in general as well as the emerging regional field of positive psychology, along with the implications of academic privilege for non-Western researchers.

9.1 Introduction

Publishing or more aptly, worrying about publishing, is one thing all academics share. Typical questions are: "Will I get published this year and in which journal?" Or: "Do I take my chances (and waste time between teaching, grading, meetings, parenting, exercising, eating, and sleeping) and risk rejection (again!) in another top-tiered journal that, as a matter of course, rejects 85% to 90% of all submissions?" Demoralized and frustrated, they wonder whether they are good enough, if they will

L. Lambert (✉)
United Arab Emirates University, Al Ain, UAE
e-mail: ltlamber@yahoo.com

N. Pasha-Zaidi
Houston Community College, University of Houston-Downtown, Houston, TX, USA
e-mail: nausheenpasha@outlook.com

A. E. Crookes
Heriot Watt University, Dubai, UAE
e-mail: crookesannie@gmail.com

L. Lambert and N. Pasha-Zaidi (eds.), *Positive Psychology in the Middle East/North Africa*, https://doi.org/10.1007/978-3-030-13921-6_9

ever be part of the blessed 10%, or whether the system is rigged after all. It is not only early-career researchers who have such doubts. In time, most academics begin to question whether claims that the system is biased may be warranted and whether Western researchers, audiences and topics of relevance are prioritized. They might consider whether the journal impact factor is faulty (Archambault & Larivière, 2009) or even manipulated (Falagas & Alexiou, 2008). They may even wonder whether, as a group of academics, they have become complacent in their tacit acceptance of and participation in such a system by sticking to topics that meet the needs of high ranking journals and institutions.

These questions are not new and as psychology and the dissemination of psychological research become increasingly globalized, they become even more salient. In this chapter, publication bias, Western bias, topic bias, and all things related are explored with respect to psychology and the newly emerging field of positive psychology. We explore the conundrum in which researchers find themselves regarding the expected accumulation of citations that often results in meaningless publications with little scientific value instead of clear social contribution. We conclude by offering what we hope are viable solutions for their work.

9.2 How Did We Get Here?

Considered the currency of researchers (Paulus, Rademacher, Schäfer, Müller-Pinzler, & Krach, 2015) and the vehicle through which a science of psychology professes to understand human behavior (Arnett, 2009), academic journals are part of a global system of publishing through which millions of scholars, publishers and institutions of higher education contribute and communicate knowledge. Journal publications are a benchmark of professional quality and often the only major factor in the evaluation and promotion of academic faculty in higher education (Lehmann, Jackson, & Lautrup, 2006; Ravenscroft, Liakata, Clare, & Duma, 2017). Yet, this scholarly enterprise may carry with it an implicit bias grounded in pre-existing privilege that serves to perpetuate the global sociopolitical status quo and may not be conducive to the growth of psychology itself.

9.2.1 Money and Place Matter

The number of peer-reviewed journals is immense with over 57,000 titles identified as of 2011 (Cope & Philips, 2014), and at least 624 journals in psychology alone as of 2008 (García-Martínez, Guerrero-Bote, & de Moya-Anegón, 2012). Additionally, there are 10,000 open-access journals (Directory of Open Access Journals, n.d.), and if non-English journals are included, those that contain non-English abstracts, or those that are not yet indexed or do not always appear in directories, there are countless more. Yet, despite these numbers, publications tend to be concentrated in a few countries due to the financial backing of governments and private sector organizations.

For example, using the Scimago Institutions Rankings resource, an evaluation tool designed by Scopus to assess the research output of universities and research institutions, García-Martínez et al. (2012) made several finds. Of the 159 countries publishing in psychology from 2003 to 2008, the 40 most productive (with over 200 cited papers) published 98% of all documents, with the rest produced by the remaining 119 nations. The US was in first place, accounting for 48% of the world's psychology documents. The UK came second with a gap of 75% to the US output, followed by Canada with another gap of nearly 50%. Different methodologies produce the same results. Using a spatial distribution tool to determine the cities from which the most highly cited psychology papers emerged, researchers (Bornmann, Leydesdorff, & Krampen, 2012) discovered that select US and UK cities, followed by locations in the Netherlands, Israel, and Australia, were the top psychology output producers, creating what they considered to be an "Anglo-American agglomeration effect" (pp. 541), reflecting the Caucasian research enterprise of Western nations (Hartmann et al., 2013; National Center for Education Statistics, 2015; Rao & Donaldson, 2015).

In contrast, a 2010 study (Osman & Afifi, 2010) showed that psychology publications in the Gulf Cooperation Council (GCC) nations (Bahrain, Oman, Qatar, Saudi Arabia, Kuwait, and United Arab Emirates (UAE)) numbered just under 200 studies collectively between 1989 and 2008, thus representing a mere 1% of biomedical research. Among countries within the broader Middle East/North African (MENA) region, Israel produces over 80% of psychology research with the next most productive country being Iran at 5% (Biglu, Chakhmachi, & Biglu, 2014). A review of English-language positive psychology MENA publications (Rao, Donaldson, & Doiron, 2015) showed increases in recent years, with a total of 53 English articles identified between 1998 and 2013. Israel was again responsible for much of this growth. Science-Metrix (2010) similarly recorded global trends in research output using Thomson Reuters Web of Science data across the past 30 years and showed that the publication growth rate from the MENA region quadrupled, with Iran and Turkey leading the way.

These top-producing countries have research funding in common. Money allows researchers from top-funded countries to undertake research activity, participate in conferences, disseminate and avail themselves of information, and most importantly, access for-profit journals to remain professionally current. Research funding allows a climate of knowledge to be produced and nurtured within and between top universities, government agencies, and foundations, which in turn, support and contribute to research. Yet, the flow of money also creates a cyclical pattern of privilege where studies from these areas are better received as they fit with, reflect and create what is considered accepted, mainstream knowledge cited the world over. In contrast, researchers in countries with fewer resources and access to funding find themselves on the periphery as they have more difficulty getting funds, grants, and attention for work that is often distant from the mainstream, and consequently, unpublished (Arnett, 2008; Gone, 2011; Rozin, 2007). Yet, this may be exactly the type of research that is needed in that region.

9.2.2 Those Impact Factors!

As journals are a forum for the dissemination of knowledge and serve a key position in the evaluation of research, criteria exist to help determine their quality. The "Journal Impact Factor" (JIF) was created in the 1960s by the Institute for Scientific Information (ISI) as a way to determine which journals were most important in their respective disciplines. The JIF is the ratio of the number of citations received by an article published in a particular journal in one year to the number of articles published by that journal in the preceding two years. Thus, the JIF determines whether a particular journal is included in its respective index. It contributes to the higher status of larger journals and increases with the number of journals published in a particular discipline and the number of articles published in a specific journal (Cameron, 2005).

As it is recalculated annually, articles that are highly cited can raise the JIF of a journal in any given year. The result is that journals may pressure authors to cite other papers published in their repository, or authors may self-cite excessively, contributing to an inflated JIF for the journal in which their article appears (Bartneck & Kokklemans, 2011). Chorus and Waltman (2016) suggest that journals often request that authors frame their submissions in relation to recently published papers from that journal, or accept manuscripts upon condition that authors cite them. Authors themselves often pre-emptively and gratuitously include published papers from that journal to increase their chances of publication. Not surprisingly, they found that since 2000 there has been a significant increase in journal self-citation malpractice. Thomson Reuters, the agency that publishes the Journal Citation Reports and where the calculation metrics for thousands of JIFs can be found, acknowledges the danger of inflated self-citations and has taken to naming and shaming such journals on an annual list and suppressing them altogether until they improve their practices.

Although the JIF plays a role in determining the quality of published research, its growing use in academia for decisions related to hiring, tenure, contractual decisions and salaries also contributes to a recurring pattern of privilege (Lehmann et al., 2006; Ravenscroft et al., 2017). As any journal can propose its inclusion in an ISI index, selection criteria such as availability of citation data, timeliness and frequency of publication, and abstracts written in English often limit the diversity of indexed journals. To evaluate new journals, the ISI investigates the publishing record of authors and members of the journal's editorial board, who are often hand-picked and invited from within a circle of prominent and already established researchers with an emphasis on their citation record as well as other journals where their articles have been published (Testa, 2003).

9.2.3 English Please

The criteria upon which to base a journal's worthiness for inclusion in the ISI index is also questionable. The Thomson Reuters website notes the importance of including high quality international and regional journals in ISI indexes. Yet critics identify the tendency of ISI indexes to be biased towards English language publications as well as those originating in the US (Crespi & Geuna, 2008). The English language greatly impacts the citation and download data used to measure the quality of papers and journals (Guerrero-Bote & de Moya-Anegón, 2014), and the privilege enjoyed by English-medium journals appears to be substantiated. Testa (2009), Senior Director at the ISI, states that, as English is the universal language of science, Thomson Reuters focuses on journals that publish full text in English, or at least English bibliographic information, and going forward "it is clear the most important texts for the international research community, and particularly in the natural sciences, will have to have their full text published in English" (p. 70).

English is considered the default language and standard for excellence in scientific communication and dissemination of academic research (Bornmann et al., 2012; Hicks, Wouters, Waltman, de Rijcke, & Rafols, 2015), and more than 90% of indexed social science journals use all or some English (Bornmann et al., 2012). There are practical reasons for English as the lingua franca. Gordin (2015) explains that a monolingual research world reduces the unnecessary duplication of effort in the discovery of knowledge. Agreement on, or at least the accepted use of, English also decreases territorial disputes over who discovered and developed particular concepts, theories or findings first, and allows science to progress more smoothly as the focus can remain on knowledge. Yet, despite the efficiencies of a unilingual system, English is not the language of the majority of researchers around the world, and this necessarily presents a problem in the successful publication of one's work (Lages, Pfajfar, & Shosham, 2015). The privileged position of Western academia and English as the lingua franca of research means that non-English research is ignored, dismissed and/or downgraded (Arnett, 2008). However, it also means that English research is potentially misunderstood, unused or inapplicable to non-English scholars. Yet, the burden of learning English in terms of effort and time (which may be better devoted to doing actual research), falls to the non-English majority world with seemingly few options available, thus confirming that Western, English-medium scholarship indeed holds a higher status in academia.

9.2.4 Is Your Sample WEIRD?

The term "WEIRD" was coined to represent Western, Educated, Industrialized, Rich, and Democratic research populations—the easily accessible undergraduate psychology student samples that set the standard for what is considered normal regarding the generalizability of findings (Henrich, Heine, & Norenzayan, 2010). These WEIRD samples are pervasive in the psychology literature as more than 90% of the published research emerges from the US despite the fact that it only accounts for 5% of the world's population (Arnett, 2008, 2009; Bermant, Talwar, & Rozin, 2011). Theoretical constructs developed on WEIRD samples and applied outside a WEIRD sociocultural context are additionally disseminated in textbooks and by default, have come to be used as proxies for not only Americans, but for the rest of the world as well (Bennis & Medin, 2010; Christopher, Wendt, Marecek, & Goodman, 2014). The norm has become so prevalent that any study using non-WEIRD samples is often considered ungeneralizable and is likely to be rejected by many high impact journals.

While positive psychology appears to have done better than mainstream psychology with fewer college and more community samples, it too reflects an overrepresentation of Caucasian participants. Still, Rao and Donaldson (2015) note that while there are more Caucasian female than male participants in the extant literature, there is also an underrepresentation of females as first authors with less than half of positive psychology articles having a female first author. In terms of addressing race and ethnicity, they add that positive psychology mirrors the trend in other areas of psychology, with little emphasis being placed on diversity of participants, samples, and research topics. Efforts to increase cultural representation in research have done little to improve the situation (Arnett, 2008; Hartmann et al., 2013; Rao et al., 2015), nor have they resulted in greater awareness on the part of researchers about the cultural origins of a US-centric psychology (Christopher et al., 2014).

In the US itself, research has shown that despite an increased awareness of the need to attend to ethnic minorities and cross-cultural issues, little has changed. Hartmann et al. (2013) found that across APA/APS journals, the highest percentage of articles devoted to cross-cultural issues was 6% while among non-APA/APS first-tier journals, the figure ranged between 2% and 14%. Representation of minorities and cross-cultural research was higher in journals that were not top-tier, had no impact factor and limited readership, and which were devoted to cross-cultural issues as their mandate. However, researchers working in these areas may be at a disadvantage as their research draws on smaller bodies of evidence and smaller sample sizes. Given the limited availability of grant funding, theoretical advancements that are applicable to the diversity of the world's population may progress more slowly as fewer people investigate lesser-studied topics. This predictably results in lower productivity and less value being placed on such issues (Gone, 2011). Thus, even when cross-cultural research is undertaken, it tends to be focused within a Western context, or edited to be marketable to a Western journal audience.

9.2.5 Are Reviewers WEIRD Too?

This lack of diversity extends to editorial boards (Hartmann et al., 2013), where authors and reviewers alike may submit their work or offer their services to journals with a cultural representation more like their own or those of their research participants. Whether by preference for more culturally-aligned journals or by choice of opting out of journals that may be considered more representative of (white) "Americans only" (Arnett, 2008), these practices serve to perpetuate the lack of cultural representations in top-tier journals and relegate diversity to low JIF journals with poor readership.

Not limited to psychology, Lages et al. (2015) interviewed 42 marketing researchers from the MENA region who had been rejected by Western and/or international journals. Among many issues, they stated that editors and reviewers had little interest in the region and challenged authors about why and how their findings were of interest to Western audiences, even though the journals were purported to be international or focused on issues of culture and development. In other cases, limited knowledge of the region was obvious in the reviewer comments. For example, the region was neither identified nor adequately discussed beyond the fact that authors used a "different context". Others reported the fact that top journals did not publish single non-US country studies, greatly limiting the ability to get one's work published. These findings support the premise that the task of showing relevance falls on non-Western researchers, rather than obliging Western researchers to demonstrate their relevance for non-Western audiences. The difficulty of becoming a member of the "Western research establishment", the entry price for which was to pursue topics of Western concern over local issues with a stifling of local knowledge as a result, was also noted as a barrier to getting one's work published.

That bias occurs is not surprising, and its impact can be extrapolated to the review and grant process as well. In a US study, Inbar and Lammers (2012) found that one in six social psychologists reported being somewhat or more inclined to discriminate against conservative researchers by refusing to invite them for a conference or reviewing their work. A further one in four stated they would vote against them in grant application reviews. Most telling was that respondents, all social psychologists, did not think this bias existed. While conducted in the US, it is not a stretch to consider how in-group favoritism and out-group exclusion would affect researchers with non-Western topics and worldviews.

9.3 It's Not Your Imagination

Akin to an all-boys club, Coyne (2012) addressed the privileged access that is afforded to certain researchers by journals. The free pass occurs when editors invite experts or renowned researchers to submit an article. As it is solicited, the review process, designed to identify the limitations of a manuscript and address errors, is bypassed or cursory at best. This limits the objectivity of the findings or commentary provided. Further, who qualifies as an expert is often determined by popularity, leadership in a professional organization, committee membership, informal cliques, friendships, or whether a financial, professional, or publicity gain is possible. This privilege boosts a researchers' scientific credibility disproportionately compared to their contribution and amplifies a journal's prestige unfairly.

The process is not without detractors. Wong and Roy (2017) charge the field of positive psychology in particular with elitism, an "invitation-only" academic system operated by "mutual admiration" and the citing and publishing of colleagues' work, which they contend has led to a breakdown of critical thinking and unflinching acceptance of anything published by self-appointed leaders. It is easy to identify these leaders who continue to enjoy academic prestige through world class travel, summit attendance and the reward of having one's name on a report without a corresponding substantial contribution. These namesake figures are not always esteemed for what they continue to do, but for what they have done in the past. When homages like these are included in journals, the work of more critical and relevant researchers with less brand value may be overlooked, impoverishing science as a result.

This practice has also led to the exclusion or denigration of prior work in an effort to position and legitimize a newly demarcated field like positive psychology (Lomas, 2015), the exclusion or downgrading of new and upcoming researchers, or of experts in other domains who may shed further light on findings or discredit them with alternative explanations. In the face of the privileged position afforded to such researchers and their claims, readers assume that controversies are settled or that evidence exists where it does not, or worse, that no competing viewpoints exist. These assumptions are fueled by virtue of privileged research being featured in a top-tier journal while critiques are not included in these special issues or relegated to lower-tier publications not referenced in top-tier publications. What is more disturbing about the practice is the effect on inexperienced researchers who are exposed to limited views, as well as on consumers and organizations who, in the case of positive psychology, spend important financial resources in a domain that is being "over-used for commercial interests" (Wong & Roy, 2017) and becoming more of an industry on some days than a science.

9.3.1 Hot or Not?

Experts appear to have a monopoly when it comes to deciding what is worthwhile to study. As a result of such expert opinions, many research questions with value for society or science are overlooked. The obvious risk is that such judgements are influenced by personal interests of the experts or their chances for future funding and subsequent publicity and fame. In response, scores of voluntary, eager researchers embark to study such declared hot topics and help in documenting growing interest. Yet, as a result of research piling up in some areas, holes are created in others (Rozin, 2007). While cold topics attract less funding, there are still good reasons to study them. The benefits include having one's work stand out more easily, generating a bigger impact as the first few studies in an area generally yield the greatest findings, facing less competition, putting one's name to something new, and having less literature to read.

Further, researchers, by virtue of searching online, tend to obtain search query results that deliver the most popular citations. The fact that most journals still block free access to their articles with paywalls also means that researchers increasingly reference fewer, but first appearing articles in searches, and they reference from fewer journals, too (Evans, 2008). Hot topics generally flow from where power is already consolidated with the effect that non-Western topics rarely reach a level of importance. Yet, from a scientific perspective, findings from the periphery significantly add to a deeper understanding of social issues and expand the boundaries of psychological science everywhere. However, it is often the case that cold-topic researchers are penalized for going against the mainstream, often by necessity due to their locality and participant base (Rozin, 2007). In this respect, not only has mainstream psychological research failed the local diversity of those it claims to represent (Arnett, 2008, 2009; Hartmann et al., 2013), it has made psychological science less productive at a global level as well (Kirschener, 2013).

9.3.2 When Nothing Happens

Publication bias is a growing issue in psychology, especially in the wake of claims about its lack of replicability for a number of key findings. The Open Science Collaboration (2015) produced a damning report about their attempts to replicate 100 well-established findings in psychology, noting that while 97% of the original studies had statistically significant results, only 36% of the replications did. Gilbert, King, Pettigrew, and Wilson (2016) were among the most critical of that report, citing flaws in the methodology and stating that psychology had no greater replication failures than other sciences (although low replication rates elsewhere are not an excuse for our own) and that other studies did find support (see Klein et al., 2014).

Beyond the replication issue is also the fact that the majority of null findings are never published as researchers have learned that it is pointless to submit them, with the effect of local knowledge production suppressed in favor of pleasing the gatekeepers of high JIF publications (Hicks et al., 2015). This has implications for non-mainstream countries when it comes to psychology research as findings are indeed very likely not to coincide with mainstream findings, and thus, remain invisible to science and the local environments for which they would have particular relevance. Even undergraduate students show concern that their dissertations, theses or research will be poorly assessed if the analysis does not reach significance, despite it being a finding in itself. But an emphasis on p-values is not enough: If the sample size is very large, even a small difference between groups can show statistical significance, which is why effect size should also be reported in articles (Sullivan & Feinn, 2012).

Perhaps all findings, whether positive, negative or null, should be openly published and freely accessible so that researchers can decide what is important and meaningful for themselves (van Assen, van Aert, Nuijten, & Wicherts, 2014). Yet, given the time required to read thousands of papers and the difficulty with which to determine the scientific worth of a paper, the indispensability of peer reviewers remains. Another option is to mandate the pre-registry of experimental analyses (see OFSPreprints https://osf.io/preprints/ and Nosek, Ebersole, DeHaven, & Mellor, 2017) so that the shame of null findings is dispelled and researchers can be exposed more often to studies not going as predicted.

Facilitating the publication of non-significant findings alongside the wider literature would go far. The Journal for Negative Results in Bio Medecine (JNRBM) (https://jnrbm.biomedcentral.com) and in psychology, the Journal of Articles in

Support of the Null Hypothesis (http://www.jasnh.com) are examples. PLOS ONE also published a collection of null, negative and inconclusive results underlining the importance of such studies. Yet, these initiatives are not well known, with the JNRBM removed from the BiomedCentral listing in 2017. Despite the need for null findings towards the advancement of research, it remains difficult for journals to attract readers and submissions within the current publishing system given that, much like tabloids, consumers prefer to read about extraordinary results. The null finding, while scientifically important, is little more than a "nothing happened" report and of decreasing interest, especially as more journals enter the market and with greater competition among them.

9.3.3 The Purse or Its Logo: Branded Findings

It would be nice to think that "other" people created such a biased system, but in all truthfulness, researchers are part of the problem. Moriarty (2016) asked academics to reflect upon moments where they were called upon to evaluate grant proposals, promotions or prospective colleagues and where they used JIF's as the sole criteria from which to do so, without even reading the publications themselves. Outsourcing judgments of quality to for-profit journals may be common in positive psychology too. Yet, by doing do, it is not the content of the articles that is critically assessed, but the journal's brand name.

Such judgements are not conducive to developing psychology, or positive psychology for that matter. However, it is admittedly difficult for researchers to become aware of the assumptions their work and practices carry (Christopher & Hickinbottom, 2008), as issues of culture, in-group favoritism or implicit, albeit often unintended biases, are bigger than any one of us. Each individual is a product of their culture and society (Christopher et al., 2014) and often inattentive to their cultural worldviews, which seem natural and moral over time (Fessler, 2010; Gone, 2011). Yet, as privileged groups set the standard for acceptable social norms, group members remain blind to the benefits they derive as a result (Johnson, 2006; Kendall, 2006). Consequently, it is perhaps neither science nor psychology that is the problem, but the structures and practices inherent in these systems that facilitate and reinforce a reliance on dominant ideologies and norms to the exclusion of certain groups and in ways that affect their professional livelihoods. Yet, the fear of doing otherwise and going against the grain carries the threat of potential career suicide. Even journals and their editors play it safe and go with what reviewers suggest, accepting mainstream findings and preferring study replications over novel unorthodox findings (Lynch, Alba, Krishna, Morwitz, & Gurhan-Canli, 2012).

9.4 Recommendations

The following recommendations are offered for the development of a better publishing system by which researcher's work can be fairly judged, equally shared, and have a greater social impact.

9.4.1 Look Closer to Home

One solution is to shift the dominant focus of research production to smaller and more numerous focal points around the world through more varied angles of research. Decentralization is already taking place due to the internet's democratizing effects in terms of who holds the right to produce and disseminate information. Consequently, the number of open-access journals is increasing (Laakso et al., 2011), especially in positive psychology with the *Middle East Journal of Positive Psychology* (UAE), *Journal of Happiness and Wellbeing* (Turkey), *Iranian Journal of Positive Psychology* (Iran), and the *Indian Journal of Positive Psychology* (India) appearing in the last years. Many were started as a response to local work being judged as unrepresentative and irrelevant to the Western mainstream. These journals offer researchers the chance to investigate concepts from within their culture and/or nation with the intent that the information produced will be relevant to the respective region (Bornmann et al., 2012). While not top-tier, researchers have an interest in supporting such journals as they often represent the only platforms for the publication of local work. By submitting to them, they can help to develop the regional scientific field of psychology.

9.4.2 Translate, Min Fadlik

Online journals have the added benefit of providing open access and being freely available. Yet, for these journals to be accessed and to meet the aims of information dissemination on a global scale, they must nonetheless meet academic research standards (Paton, Househ, & Malik, 2013) and provide, at a minimum, secondary abstracts in English. At the same time, existing journals must also strive to offer abstracts and/or articles in languages other than English, regardless of the journals origins, audience, or nation-specific content (Bornmann et al., 2012). To this effect, built-in automated translation services could be an asset, while a global crowd-sourced mass translation of psychology research articles could accomplish great things. To further facilitate broader linguistic access and interest, more frequent special issues of international or regional interest could be prioritized by mainstream journals in order to raise the profile of other regions and concepts to which mainstream Western audiences are not normally exposed (Lages et al., 2015).

9.4.3 TripAdvisor for Psychology

An additional advantage of Open Access journals is their ability to garner immediate feedback. Much like a TripAdvisor or Amazon online product review, academics and researchers of various disciplines as well as students can comment, critique, or extend a study's discussion directly with the author(s). Traditional review processes make researchers vulnerable to few, anonymous and potentially biased reviewers (Harris, 2018) who determine whether the work of thousands of dollars and many years is "acceptable" and worthy of being read by others. As it is impossible for all reviewers to be familiar with specific methods, adequately trained to evaluate statistics, or knowledgeable enough about all aspects of a topic, an open review process, in effect, removes the judgment of quality from their hands and opens the door for more dialogue about topics, participants, methods, and the generalizability of findings.

Opening commentary and debate may help the field arrive at consensus more quickly than is the case with for-profit journals that have a turnaround time of nine months to two years. Open commentary can also push the boundaries of science more effectively as consumers are exposed to views not otherwise available, given that journals do not, as a rule, invite feedback from readers. This can also make journals and reviewers more accountable for the science that is disseminated. A post-publication review can further provide a space for readers to ask or comment upon cultural, regional, or religious relevance or obtain information that was not indicated due to word count limitations.

9.4.4 Decolonizing Research Methods

Participatory research methods have been espoused by indigenous groups who have become increasingly vocal in their response to traditional research methods. "Past researchers have disempowered communities, imposed stereotypes that reinforced internalized racism, and conducted research that benefited the careers of individual researchers, or even science at large, but brought no tangible benefit to the communities struggling with significant health disparities. Many tribal nations have provided accounts of researchers who have exploited tribes by coming in, taking information from tribal members, and providing nothing in return" (Simonds & Christopher, 2013, p. 2186). As social constructs are value-laden, researchers studying cultures that are not their own may overlook nuances that are obvious to local community members. Decolonizing research practices allows those who are most affected by the research to have a say in developing appropriate questions, reviewing current literature, exploring the findings, and playing an integral role in the research process. An extension of this would be to publish one's research intentions and garner feedback before the study begins to help shape the ways in which studies can best address gaps in knowledge. Researchers may already be doing this with their colleagues or within their departments, depending on the relationships they have and the composition of their research team. Extending pre-study reviews to members of the academic community as well as concerned stakeholders can ensure science is both relevant and accountable.

9.4.5 Demand Transparency

All journals, especially dominant English-speaking ones, should by default require authors to explicitly state who constituted their research sample and how this selection impacted the relevance of their findings for global (and local) audiences. While protocols like these are considered standard science (Hicks et al., 2015), the inconsistent enforcement of such practices is common, and often the biggest culprits are Western researchers engaging in the false consensus bias as they assume, for example, everyone knows where Nebraska is (Mills, Wu, Gagnier, Heels-Ansdell, & Montori, 2005; Yousefi-Nooraie, Shakiba, & Mortaz-Hejri, 2006). In fact, it is rare to see such declarations in Western studies, yet non-mainstream researchers are routinely asked to state their case. Making this mandatory for all researchers will force attention to such issues and make the assumptions of the work explicit. While the burden of understanding how bias and privilege operate rests on everyone, non-English or non-Western authors are tasked with holding journals accountable for diversity by asking where reviewers and board members are from, how diversity is represented, or why little representation exists. Offering to become a reviewer or board member may be a helpful nudge for journals to address these issues.

Topic Box: Got "Likes"?

Altmetrics is the count of how many times an article is mentioned on Facebook, Twitter, blogs, other social media outlets, the nightly news, or print media and has come to symbolize academic worth. And while we scoff at using "Likes" as an indicator of quality, Altmetrics nonetheless tell us what is important to people. Presumably if an article gets downloaded, posted, re-tweeted, or commented on, it has generated interest. Although this does not mean an article was read or understood, it does hold value for people in some way. Sleep, relationships, self-esteem, high blood pressure, parenting and yoga might not be the stuff of stellar academia, but frequently accessed literature like this might suggest that for the average person, such issues are not resolved and require better laymen's communication. Where Altmetrics scores become harmful is when, like JIFs, they are the sole measure of whether work is of high quality, and whether peers pass a performance review or obtain grants. These metrics, literally a researcher's version of Facebook "Likes", may transform science into sensationalist PR. Given that recent research shows that false news travels faster along Twitter than verifiable news (Vosoughi, Roy, & Aral, 2018), it is important to consider that humans are the ones making judgments about what is considered worthy of transmitting and as social scientists, we should be aware of our own biases.

9.4.6 Make Friends

Research is inherently a social process and having personal contact with other researchers is not only effective but predicts the likelihood of a successful paper as well. For example, being in the same building (versus different buildings on the same or different university campuses) produced papers that were of higher quality, published in better quality journals, and 45% more likely to be cited, as collaboration is facilitated by proximity, ease of communication, impromptu meetings, and lower costs to the exchange of ideas (Lee, Brownstein, Mills, & Kohane, 2010). The clustering effect (Sohn, 2016) is vital to facilitate such research networks. Professional travel—whether in the form of a semester abroad, teaching exchanges, completing a PhD overseas, or networking at international conferences—is of great benefit (Rodrigues, Nimrichter, & Cordero, 2016). More than that, cultural exchanges stimulate intellectual and creative enterprises, making relevant the many issues under study that are common to humanity versus those uniquely found in one's home country. Yet, much like the privilege and systemic bias that pervades publishing, limitations exist as many academics are limited in their travel by their passports, access to funds, as well as gender and childcare issues (Rodrigues et al., 2016).

Institutions can take the lead in developing partnerships with other research units, universities or organizations around the globe to facilitate their work and eventual publication in international journals. Researchers from higher-tiered institutions can also act as reviewers in lower-tier journals and provide much needed feedback on submitted work. They can also submit their articles to lower-tier journals in an effort to help raise journal profiles and the work of authors who publish in them. While these forms of partnership do not necessarily help researchers from high-impact countries, they do help those from low-impact countries (Guerrero Bote, Olmeda-Gómez, & de Moya-Anegón, 2013). It is important, however, to note that such collaborations can be mutually beneficial and should not be interpreted as charity, but as a way to decentralize influence.

9.4.7 Forget Metrics, Show Impact

The move away from academic impact towards a demonstration of how one's work has social impact is a growing phenomenon (Bornmann, 2012; Donovan, 2008;

Park, 2009; Taylor, 2009). The Leiden Manifesto (see Hicks et al., 2015) and the San Francisco Declaration on Research Assessment (DORA) are two examples. Increasingly frustrated by an obsession with metrics, the Manifesto puts forward ten principles, one of which includes measuring the performance of the researcher against the mission of the institution or group. Rather than focus on academic impact, the merits of the researcher's work are considered against the tasks or goals set forth for social development, policy, or industry needs. So far, the UK and Australia have made concrete moves for research to help advance social goals (Hicks et al., 2015). Similarly, the DORA declaration (www.ascb.org/dora/), to which a number of high profile US organizations and individuals have signed up, calls on researchers to categorically reject JIF as a criterion for the evaluation of academic success in favor of actual scientific content. This move may allow the identification of quality research on a diverse range of topics otherwise overlooked due to its non-inclusion in high-impact journals. This, in turn, can deepen, broaden, and boost the relevance of psychology, positive psychology, as well as other disciplines worldwide (Schmid, 2013).

Academic institutions can adopt a policy requiring researchers to produce a single annual paper derived from real social need. Every spring, institutions, industry, business, government, non-profits and stakeholders (i.e., members of the affected community) meet to set forth their challenges. Researchers choose to address those topics the coming academic year with the intention of addressing local needs while soliciting ongoing open-review feedback from stakeholders to evaluate project effectiveness. This would reduce the burden on researchers to choose a topic that may not be considered valuable by others in the scientific community and decrease the influence of superstar academics setting research agendas three continents away. It can also have a positive effect on the competitive climate that reigns in universities as a result of the "publish or perish" culture. The collaborative nature of such work can strengthen ties with communities and allow researchers to learn from others they normally would not team up with, and who, through their taxes, tuition or donations, in fact, subsidize and/or benefit from the work. This would help to counter the current practice of researchers undertaking topics of little interest or value to community stakeholders, yet using that same research to increase their personal or institutional status instead (Chalmers, Essali, Rezk, & Crowe, 2012).

While the effect of a social needs focus is hard to measure, Ravenscroft et al. (2017) suggest a comprehensive influence beyond academia that shows broad effects on health, policy, economic, social or environmental issues. Donovan (2008) proposes that research with a social impact would, for example, add to a nation's social capital or inform public policy debates, and by default, necessitate inquiry into local issues. By taking a step beyond academic impact, researchers are more accountable to the contexts in which they publish rather than to the discipline or the for-profit journals they serve, using what are often public funds (Moriarty, 2016). More must be done to advance proactive research into social, health, and education needs. It will help governments, businesses and philanthropic organizations as well as ordinary people recognize the value of research and how it can benefit policy decisions, industry practices, as well as personal choices. Only when researchers and their publication systems become more accountable to the public and less to one another will research become less biased and more relevant to society.

9.4.8 Ask Better Questions

Researchers can have greater social impact by simply asking better research questions (Rozin, 2009). Replicating endless Western findings or creating more measurement scales among the thousands already in existence does little to advance the field, or one's career for that matter. This singular focus on novelty before the proper validation of existing tools for example, is often short-sighted and reflects the obsession of publishing for publishing's sake. In fact, an older, yet still relevant study of research practices across the Arabic-speaking world (Zebian, Alamuddin, Maalouf, & Chatila, 2007) highlighted that a large majority of researchers "adopted theories, concepts, and measures wholesale, without critique or adaptation" (p. 106), which resulted in nothing more than repetitive and imitative research producing little utility or value for society (Yang, 2012).

Although positive psychology is new, we already see such practices in the MENA/GCC region where interventions are promoted without questioning their philosophical or cultural origins, or giving thought to the people or the socio-political contexts for which they were designed. The field of psychology, and positive psychology too, is Western and thus, heavily culture-bound (Bermant et al., 2011; Pandey, 2011; Wong, 2013a), prompting a need to explore, expand, and include non-Western views and understandings of wellbeing. As Wong (2013b) declared, the second wave in positive psychology (Positive Psychology 2.0) is to go global and consider the full richness of wellbeing from diverse cultural and religious views, entailing more research from within single cultures and between them. Only an act of courage will get researchers to orient their studies towards answering those questions with the very good possibility of never getting published as a result.

9.4.9 Not Everyone Is Good at Everything

To expect that all academics be proficient in research and publishing is unrealistic and reminiscent of old-school management styles where roles and rules are applied to all without respect or recognition for the professional and personal strengths of individual employees. Diener (2016) argues that psychology departments review their expectations and consider who is better positioned to take on particular activities. Multiple roles exist such as research, service, teaching, advising, outreach, public speaking, etc., and fitting those roles to employees may be more effective than demanding that all faculty members excel at all of them, or worse, persist doing them moderately or poorly. Some professors are great at teaching and raise the standards for student learning, while others love research and find statistical analysis the idea of a great afternoon. Greater honesty in where strengths exist would go a long way in improving psychology departments. Overlooking individual strengths means many talents are underused for some faculty, while weaker strengths may be overused, producing great frustration, lack of job satisfaction, and dramatic departures to industry instead. Diener further contends that while universities spend much time attracting faculty, once hired, they do little to provide for their continued excellence. While most offer types of continuing education, these are often offered to all faculty in general (thus, interesting no one) and are neither incentivized nor made mandatory. The result is that scholars do not attend them, remaining blissfully unaware of, and overconfident in their declining knowledge. Consequently, maintaining a focus on their narrow areas of specialization—often the topic of their dissertation from yesteryear—prevents them from developing professionally.

9.5 Implications for Positive Psychology in the MENA Region

What are the implications of this system for positive psychology in the MENA region? One major consideration is the applicability of positive psychology research and practices for local communities. Given that wellbeing in the region is related to collectivism, political stability and Islamic worldviews (Lambert D'raven & Pasha-Zaidi, 2014), these areas should be given priority in the development of an indigenous positive psychology and the dissemination and application of positive psychology research. A great deal of interdisciplinary conversations have been occurring regarding the use of the Islamization of Knowledge (IOK) framework for creating paradigms that are relevant to Muslim populations. Al-Attas (1993) and Al-Faruqi (1989) are two scholars who have contributed to the IOK framework, which attempts to revitalize and normalize Islamic scholarship that unfortunately has been in decline since the end of the Golden Age of Islam (circa 750 AD–1250 AD). This would require positive psychology in the MENA region to be inclusive of research methods that take into consideration the metaphysical aspects of human experiences, something that is not done in Western psychology. In doing so, we would need to be mindful of the diversity of the region itself and promote research that reflects Islamic principles of plurality and critical thinking, as these are not products of Western social science, but rather inherent to an Islamic historical legacy.

Thus, the first step for overcoming bias in publishing and research and to decentralize the existing power structures is to revive the notion of critical education in the MENA region. This does not mean that we throw away the scientific method, but rather that we develop paradigms that are reflective of human experiences in this area of the world, instead of only relying on the adaptation of existing measures and theories. Al-Attas (1993) in particular noted the importance of including intuition as a valid tool in the scientific method. Considering that researchers use intuition along with prior research as part of the interpretation of both quantitative and qualitative data, this is neither a stretch, nor something that should be considered unscientific in psychology.

As a second step, developing more graduate programs that focus on regional research would certainly be one approach to increase the training and availability of local researchers who are familiar with the context and prevailing worldviews so that valid perspectives can be added to the extant literature. This does not need to be a lone venture, but as noted, can be done through developing university partnerships, especially with countries that currently hold prominent positions in the field. Many universities in Western industrialized countries already offer programs that provide opportunities for students in the MENA region to work with students and faculty in the West. Such partnerships would provide opportunities for growth and understanding on both sides of the world and are an option that is increasingly utilized by universities.

Yet, one of the challenges to creating more opportunity for diverse perspectives is the fact that decentering existing structures often exposes power dynamics that are resistant to change (Anderson, 2014). Thus, equality for "others" may feel like a loss of privilege for those who reap the benefits of their higher position in academia. Another challenge is the lack of understanding of positive psychology in the region. While introduced in 1998 (by then President of the American Psychological Association, Dr. Martin Seligman), many of our colleagues in the UAE have still not heard of it or, if they have, contend it is pseudoscience, despite it being a heavily promoted UAE national vision since 2016. This suggests that their knowledge is greatly outdated and not in line with the more general scientific advances in psychology overall. Additionally, as the hard sciences like engineering and medicine continue to have higher prestige in the region, "soft" sciences such as psychology may not receive the same attention or value from academics. This further reduces the ability to create a regional psychology, much less an indigenous positive psychology that can produce research to decenter existing knowledge. Finally, there continues to be an appreciation of Western knowledge and institutions that often outweighs local efforts. In academic hiring decisions in the region, for example, advertisements often indicate that they are looking for candidates who have experience with Western-style education. In our own experiences, we have seen how candidates with Western qualifications are more likely to receive interviews and job offers than those who have obtained their degree from a local university. If academics in the MENA region are not confident in their ability to educate young adults and create scientific knowledge, then how can those who are currently leading the field be convinced that equal opportunity for diverse perspectives will actually produce relevant and important information for the wider scientific community?

9.6 Conclusion

There is a growing dissatisfaction with the academic publishing industry. Academics have increasingly noted the biases in what (and who) is funded, sampled, and which authors and topics are given preferential treatment. A key message is that academic merit should shift to a focus on social impact and the public dissemination of knowledge over a mere emphasis on publishing anything in traditional for-profit, academic journals. It is nonsensical that academic success is currently measured on publishing a large number of articles, which are cited and read by a very small number of academics from within one's field (Diener, 2016), rather than publishing a small number of articles which can be read, reviewed and discussed by all. In fact, Remler (2014) argues that any given article is read by a stunning average of three people, while Meho (2007) estimates that about 90% of published research is indeed, never at all cited! While public dissemination holds a risk that only "marketable" topics or headline grabbing findings will be given access, with some planning, this may still be a better solution for ensuring fairer and open access to dissemination than the current system. In sum, we urge a return to a focus on quality research that adds to the knowledge base of the area in which it was conducted and for whom it purports to represent instead of a narrow and ill-conceived focus on prestige and rankings that only lead to a "publish or perish" approach, filled with redundant studies of little value for the majority of the world. We have noted some of the main challenges to this shift. With a concerted effort, we believe the MENA region can be a leader in the creation and dissemination of positive psychology research, on its own and for itself, and in collaboration with other international researchers.

References

Al-Attas, S. M. N. (1993). *Islam and secularism*. Kuala Lumpur: International Institute of Islamic Thought and Civilization (ISTAC).

Al-Faruqi, I. R. (1989). *Islamization of knowledge: General principles and work plan* (2nd ed.) Herndon, VA: International Institute of Islamic Thought.

Anderson, K. (2014). *Modern misogyny*. New York, NY: Oxford University Press.

Archambault, É., & Larivière, V. (2009). History of the journal impact factor: Contingencies and consequences. *Scientometrics, 79*(3), 635–649.

Arnett, J. J. (2008). The neglected 95%: Why American psychology needs to become less American. *American Psychologist, 63*(7), 602–614.

Arnett, J. J. (2009). The neglected 95%, a challenge to psychology's philosophy of science. *American Psychologist, 64*(6), 571–574.

Bartneck, C., & Kokkelmans, S. (2011). Detecting h-index manipulation through self-citation analysis. *Scientometrics, 87*(1), 85–98.

Bennis, W. M., & Medin, D. L. (2010). Weirdness is in the eye of the beholder. *Behavioral and Brain Sciences, 33*(2), 85–86.

Bermant, G., Talwar, C., & Rozin, P. (2011). To celebrate positive psychology and extend its horizons. In K. M. Sheldon, T. B. Kashdan, & M. F. Steger (Eds.), *Designing positive psychology: Taking stock and moving forward* (pp. 430–438). Oxford, UK: Oxford University Press.

Biglu, M. H., Chakhmachi, N., & Biglu, S. (2014). Scientific study of Middle East countries in psychology. *Collnet Journal of Scientometrics and Information Management, 7*(2), 293–296.
Bornmann, L. (2012). Measuring the societal impact of research. *EMBO Reports, 13*(8), 673–676.
Bornmann, L., Leydesdorff, L., & Krampen, G. (2012). Which are the "best" cities for psychology research worldwide? *Europe's Journal of Psychology, 8*(4), 535–546.
Cameron, B. D. (2005). Trends in the usage of ISI bibliometric data: Uses, abuses, and implications. *Portal: Libraries and the Academy, 5*(1), 105–125.
Chalmers, I., Essali, A., Rezk, E., & Crowe, S. (2012). *Is academia meeting the needs of non-academic users of the results of research?* Health in the Occupied Palestinian Territory 2012 (Conference Abstract). Retrieved from http://www.thelancet.com/health-in-the-occupied-palestinian-territory-2012.
Christopher, J. C., & Hickinbottom, S. (2008). Positive psychology, ethnocentrism, and the disguised ideology of individualism. *Theory & Psychology, 18,* 563–589.
Christopher, J. C., Wendt, D. C., Marecek, J., & Goodman, D. M. (2014). Critical cultural awareness: Contributions to a globalizing psychology. *American Psychologist, 69*(7), 645–655.
Chorus, C., & Waltman, L. (2016). A large-scale analysis of impact factor biased journal self-citations. *PLoS ONE, 11*(8), e0161021.
Cope, B., & Phillips, A. (Eds.). (2014). *The future of the academic journal*. Cambridge, UK: Chandos Publishing.
Coyne, J. C. (2012, April 11). Authors, don't call us, we'll call you. *Psychology Today.* Retrieved from https://www.psychologytoday.com/blog/the-skeptical-sleuth/201204/authors-don-t-call-us-we-ll-call-you.
Crespi, G., & Geuna, A. (2008). An empirical study of scientific production: A cross-country analysis, 1981–2002. *Research Policy, 37*(4), 565–579.
Diener, E. (2016). Improving departments of psychology. *Perspectives on Psychological Science, 11*(6), 909–912.
Directory of Open Access Journals. (no date). *About DOAJ.* Retrieved from https://doaj.org/about.
Donovan, C. (2008). The Australian Research Quality Framework: A live experiment in capturing the social, economic, environmental, and cultural returns of publicly funded research. *New Directions for Evaluation, 118,* 47–60.
Evans, J. A. (2008). Electronic publication and the narrowing of science and scholarship. *Science, 321*(5887), 395–399.
Falagas, M. E., & Alexiou, V. G. (2008). The top-ten in journal impact factor manipulation. *Archivum immunologiae et therapiae experimentalis, 56*(4), 223.
Fessler, D. M. T. (2010). Cultural congruence between investigators and participants masks the unknown unknowns: Shame research as an example. *Behavioral and Brain Sciences, 33*(2), 32.
García-Martínez, A. T., Guerrero-Bote, V. P., & de Moya-Anegón, F. (2012). World scientific production in psychology. *Universitas Psychologica, 11*(3), 699–717.
Gilbert, D. T., King, G., Pettigrew, S., & Wilson, T. D. (2016). Comment on "Estimating the reproducibility of psychological science". *Science, 351*(6277), 1037a–1037b.
Gone, J. P. (2011). Is psychological science a-cultural? *Cultural Diversity & Ethnic Minority Psychology, 17*(3), 234–242.
Gordin, M. D. (2015). Absolute English. *Aeon Magazine*. Retrieved from http://aeon.co/magazine/science/how-did-science-come-to-speak-only-english/.
Guerrero-Bote, V. P., & de Moya-Anegón, F. (2014). Relationship between downloads and citations at journal and paper levels, and the influence of language. *Scientometrics, 101*(2), 1043–1065.
Guerrero Bote, V. P., Olmeda-Gómez, C., & de Moya-Anegón, F. (2013). Quantifying the benefits of international scientific collaboration. *Journal of the American Society for Information Science and Technology, 64,* 392–404.
Harris, R. (2018, February 24). *Scientists aim to pull peer review out of the 17th century*. NPR. Retrieved from https://www.npr.org/sections/health-shots/2018/02/24/586184355/scientists-aim-to-pull-peer-review-out-of-the-17th-century.

Hartmann, W. E., Kim, E. S., Kim, J. H. J., Nguyen, T. U., Wendt, D. C., Nagata, D. K., et al. (2013). In search of cultural diversity, revisited: Recent publication trends in cross-cultural and ethnic minority psychology. *Review of General Psychology, 17*(3), 243–254.

Henrich, J., Heine, S. J., & Norenzayan, A. (2010). The weirdest people in the world? *Behavioral and Brain Sciences, 33*(2–3), 61–83.

Hicks, D., Wouters, P., Waltman, L., de Rijcke, S., & Rafols, I. (2015). Bibliometrics: The Leiden Manifesto for research metrics. *Nature, 520*(7548), 429–431.

Inbar, Y., & Lammers, J. (2012). Political diversity in social and personality psychology. *Perspectives on Psychological Science, 7*(5), 496–503.

Johnson, A. G. (2006). *Privilege, power, and difference* (2nd ed.). New York, NY: McGraw-Hill.

Kendall, F. E. (2006). *Understanding white privilege: Creating pathways to authentic relationships across race*. New York, NY: Routledge.

Kirschner, M. (2013, June 14). A perverted view of "impact" [Editorial]. *Science, 340*(6138), 1265.

Klein, R. A., Ratliff, K. A., Vianello, M., Adams, R. B., Bahník, Š., Bernstein, M. J., … Nosek, B. A. (2014). Investigating variation in replicability: A "Many Labs" replication project. *Social Psychology, 45*(3), 142–152.

Laakso, M., Welling, P., Bukvova, H., Nyman, L., Björk, B.-C., & Hedlund, T. (2011). The development of open access journal publishing from 1993 to 2009. *PLoS ONE, 6*(6), e20961.

Lages, C. R., Pfajfar, G., & Shosham, A. (2015). Challenges in conducting and publishing research on the Middle East and Africa in leading journals. *International Marketing Review, 32*(1), 52–77.

Lambert D'raven, L., & Pasha-Zaidi, N. (2014). Happiness strategies among Arab university students in the United Arab Emirates. *The Journal of Happiness & Wellbeing, 2*(1), 1–151.

Lee, K., Brownstein, J. S., Mills, R. G., & Kohane, I. S. (2010). Does collocation inform the impact of collaboration? *PLoS ONE, 5*(12), e14279.

Lehmann, S., Jackson, A. D., & Lautrup, B. E. (2006). Measures for measures. *Nature, 444*, 1003–1004.

Lomas, T. (2015). Positive cross-cultural psychology: Exploring similarity and difference in constructions and experiences of wellbeing. *International Journal of Wellbeing, 5*(4), 60–77.

Lynch, J. G., Alba, J. W., Krishna, A., Morwitz, V. G., & Gurhan-Canli, Z. (2012). Knowledge creation in consumer research: Multiple routes, multiple criteria. *Journal of Consumer Psychology, 22*(4), 473–485.

Meho, L. I. (2007). The rise and rise of citation analysis. *Physics World, 20*(1), 32–36.

Mills, E., Wu, P., Gagnier, J., Heels-Ansdell, D., & Montori, V. M. (2005). An analysis of general medical and specialist journals that endorse CONSORT found that reporting was not enforced consistently. *Journal of Clinical Epidemiology, 58*, 662–667.

Moriarty, P. (2016, March 14). *Addicted to the brand: The hypocrisy of a publishing academic.* Impact of Social Sciences Blog. Retrieved from http://eprints.lse.ac.uk/id/eprint/66673.

National Center for Education Statistics. (2015). *Characteristics of postsecondary faculty.* Retrieved from http://nces.ed.gov/programs/coe/pdf/coe_cuf.pdf.

Nosek, B. A., Ebersole, C. R., DeHaven, A. C., & Mellor, D. T. (2017, August 24). *The preregistration revolution*. Retrieved from osf.io/2dxu5

Open Science Collaboration. (2015). Estimating the reproducibility of psychological science. *Science, 349*(6251), aac4716–aac4716.

Osman, O. T., & Afifi, M. (2010). Troubled minds in the Gulf: Mental health research in the United Arab Emirates (1989-2008). *Asia–Pacific Journal of Public Health, 22*(3), 48S–53S.

Pandey, S. (2011, Nov 22–24). *Positive psychology: Blending strengths of western, eastern and other indigenous psychologies.* Paper presented at 1st International Conference on Emerging Paradigms in Business & Social Sciences (EPBSS-2011), Middlesex University, Dubai, United Arab Emirates.

Park, D. C. (2009). Publishing in the psychological sciences: Enhancing journal impact while decreasing author fatigue. *Perspectives on Psychological Science, 4*, 36–37.

Paton, C., Househ, M., & Malik, M. (2013). The challenges of publishing on health informatics in developing countries. *Applied Clinical Informatics, 4*(3), 428–433.

Paulus, F. M., Rademacher, L., Schäfer, T. A. J., Müller-Pinzler, L., & Krach, S. (2015). Journal impact factor shapes scientists' reward signal in the prospect of publication. *PLoS ONE, 10*(11), e0142537.

Rao, M. A., & Donaldson, S. I. (2015). Expanding opportunities for diversity in positive psychology: An examination of gender, race, and ethnicity. *Canadian Psychology/Psychologie Canadienne, 56*(3), 271–282.

Rao, M. A., Donaldson, S. I., & Doiron, K. M. (2015). Positive psychology research in the Middle East and North Africa. *Middle East Journal of Positive Psychology, 1*(1), 60–76.

Ravenscroft, J., Liakata, M., Clare, A., & Duma, D. (2017). Measuring scientific impact beyond academia: An assessment of existing impact metrics and proposed improvements. *PLoS ONE, 12*(3), e0173152.

Remler, D. (2014, April 23). *Are 90% of academic papers really never cited? Reviewing the literature on academic citations.* London School of Economics and Political Science. Retrieved from http://blogs.lse.ac.uk/impactofsocialsciences/2014/04/23/academic-papers-citation-rates-remler/.

Rodrigues, M. L., Nimrichter, L., & Cordero, R. J. B. (2016). The benefits of scientific mobility and international collaboration. *FEMS Microbiology Letters, 363*(21), fnw247. https://doi.org/10.1093/femsle/fnw247.

Rozin, P. (2007). Exploring the landscape of modern academic psychology: Finding and filling the holes. *American Psychologist, 62,* 754–766.

Rozin, P. (2009). What kind of empirical research should we publish, fund and reward? A different perspective. *Perspectives on Psychological Science, 4,* 435–439.

Schmid, S. L. (2013, September 3). Beyond CVs and impact factors: An employer's manifesto. [Perspective]. *Science,* https://doi.org/10.1126/science.caredit.a1300186. Retrieved from http://sciencecareers.sciencemag.org/career_magazine/previous_issues/articles/2013_09_03/caredit.a1300186.

Science-Metrix. (2010 February). *30 years in science: Secular movements in knowledge creation. Montreal, Canada: Science-Metrix.* Retrieved from http://www.science-metrix.com/30years-Paper.pdf.

Simonds, V. W., & Christopher, S. (2013). Adapting Western research methods to indigenous ways of knowing. *American Journal of Public Health, 103*(12), 2185–2192.

Sohn, E. (2016). Collaboration: The geography of discovery. *Nature, 533,* S40–S42.

Sullivan, G. M., & Feinn, R. (2012). Using effect size—or why the P value is not enough. *Journal of Graduate Medical Education, 4*(3), 279–282.

Taylor, S. E. (2009). Publishing in scientific journals: We're not just talking to ourselves any more. *Perspectives on Psychological Science, 4,* 38–39.

Testa, J. (2003). The Thomson ISI journal selection process. *Serials Review, 29*(3), 210–211.

Testa, J. (2009). The Thomson Reuters journal selection process. *Transnational Corporations Review, 1*(4), 59–66.

van Assen, M. A. L. M., van Aert, R. C. M., Nuijten, M. B., & Wicherts, J. M. (2014). Why publishing everything is more effective than selective publishing of statistically significant results. *PLoS ONE, 9*(1), e84896.

Vosoughi, S., Roy, D., & Aral, S. (2018). The spread of true and false news online. *Science, 359*(6380), 1146–1151.

Wong, P. T. P. (2013a). Cross-cultural positive psychology. In K. Keith (Ed.), *Encyclopedia of Cross-Cultural Psychology.* Oxford, UK: Wiley Blackwell Publishers. Retrieved from http://www.drpaulwong.com/cross-cultural-positive-psychology/.

Wong, P. T. P. (2013b). *Chinese positive psychology: What is the ancient Chinese secret to resilience and happiness?* Retrieved from http://www.meaning.ca/archives/archive/art_Chinese-PP_P_Wong.htm.

Wong, P. T. P., & Roy, S. (2017). Critique of positive psychology and positive interventions. In N. J. L. Brown, T. Lomas, & F. J. Eiroa-Orosa (Eds.), *The Routledge international handbook of critical positive psychology.* London, UK: Routledge. Retrieved from www.drpaulwong.com/critique-of-positive-psychology.

Yang, K.-S. (2012). Indigenous psychology, Westernized psychology, and indigenized psychology: A non-Western psychologist's view. *Chang Gung Journal of Humanities and Social Sciences, 5*(1), 1–32.

Yousefi-Nooraie, R., Shakiba, B., & Mortaz-Hejri, S. (2006). Country development and manuscript selection bias: A review of published studies. *BMC Medical Research Methodology, 6,* 37.

Zebian, S., Alamuddin, R., Maalouf, M., & Chatila, Y. (2007). Developing an appropriate psychology through culturally-sensitive research practices in the Arabic speaking world: A content analysis of psychological research conducted between 1950 and 2004. *Journal of Cross-Cultural Psychology, 38*(2), 91–122.

Chapter 10
Measuring Wellbeing: How and Why?

Louise Lambert, Lauren Hotchkiss and Holli-Anne Passmore

Abstract A focus on wellbeing and happiness in social discourse has necessarily raised questions about how to appropriately measure and manage wellbeing, and about the validity of reported subjective experiences. Historically, objective measures have monopolized the arena of wellbeing, as it was believed that a single measure, like GDP, income, education, or crime rates accurately reflected a state of psychosocial prosperity in nations. More recently, a sole reliance on such indicators is increasingly being discouraged. Governments are urged to consider wellbeing and happiness a public good and not a private individual matter. In this chapter we discuss why it is important to measure the subjective aspects of wellbeing and how a theoretical orientation can help in this regard. We propose tools to develop a dashboard and present a number of best practise recommendations gleaned from the empirical literature. While we target recommendations at government bodies, we encourage corporations, organizations, educational institutions, and health care providers to follow suit and include the collection of wellbeing data in their efforts.

10.1 Introduction

A focus on wellbeing and happiness in government discourse has raised concerns about how the measurement and management of wellbeing can be appropriately handled. Concerns involve the validity of using subjective (or self-report) measures to assess national levels of wellbeing and prosperity. Historically, single objective measures (e.g., GDP, income tax, hospital admission rates) monopolized the arena of national wellbeing assessment as it was believed that such objective measures

L. Lambert (✉)
United Arab Emirates University, Al Ain, UAE
e-mail: ltlamber@yahoo.com

L. Hotchkiss · H.-A. Passmore
University of British Columbia, Vancouver, BC, Canada
e-mail: hotchkissl@alumni.ubc.ca

H.-A. Passmore
e-mail: passmoreh@alumni.ubc.ca

L. Lambert and N. Pasha-Zaidi (eds.), *Positive Psychology in the Middle East/North Africa*, https://doi.org/10.1007/978-3-030-13921-6_10

accurately depicted nations' levels of psychosocial prosperity. Recently however, exclusive use of such measures is felt to be passé (Adler & Seligman, 2016; Forgeard, Jayawickreme, Kern, & Seligman, 2011; Stiglitz, Sen, & Fitoussi, 2009; Weijers & Jarden, 2013), given the recognition that, once governments have provided for basic needs like shelter and security, second-order needs become vital such as a sense of belonging, identity, and self-actualization (Adler & Seligman, 2016; Diener, Oishi, & Lucas, 2015; Diener & Seligman, 2004). As such, governments must consider wellbeing and happiness a public good and not a mere facet of private life (Thin, 2011). In this chapter, we discuss why it is important to measure subjective aspects of individual wellbeing and happiness. We propose several tools to develop what is called a dashboard measure (a multi-dimensional approach where high, moderate, low, or absent wellbeing can be easily illustrated) and offer a number of best practise recommendations gleaned from the empirical literature in an attempt to guide data collection entities.

10.2 Why Measure Wellbeing at All?

There are many reasons to measure and track subjective wellbeing. Such data are imperative for benchmarking purposes to determine whether changes in wellbeing have resulted from government policies, actions, and institutional arrangements and to which extent. For instance, measurement can determine whether the introduction of maternity leave, national childcare, labor reforms, or a minimum wage have had any effect on wellbeing and if so, in what direction (Frey & Stutzer, 2017). Wellbeing data provide vital information for the development and refinement of public policy and enable agencies to determine which sectors (e.g., labor, health, education, etc.) may be most implicated (Canaviri, 2016). Tracking wellbeing data can also indicate where incongruities exist between government services or amenities meant to address wellbeing needs and the wellbeing outcomes actually achieved. Such data can then inform decisions to redirect resources towards those services and amenities wherein the enhancement of wellbeing can be most effectively actualized. For instance, if neither pleasure, nor satisfaction and health are generated through the use of outdoor gyms, why invest in them if sporting activities by the beach are shown to be better utilized and to generate more value?

Live emotional data (that is, how people feel "on the spot") can be useful in assessing the immediate effects of daily patterns in, for example, traffic flow or queuing for services, as well as the immediate wellbeing effects of major social and political events. Live data acts as a type of Twitter-feed for emotional expression, and allows for possible immediate intervention by government agencies. Events or regulations regarding activities eliciting positive emotions (e.g., outdoor public markets, concerts, closing hours of parks or physical activity facilities) could be extended; announcements evoking confusion could be promptly clarified, or events inducing panic, fear, or aggression could trigger the additional presence of security forces. Retrospective use of live emotional data can also be useful when planning for future events (indicating which to further develop or repeat) and when considering longer-term changes to policy. If data show, for example, that stress levels caused by work commutes or waiting for government services are particularly high at certain times of the day or week, legislation, programs, or policies could be introduced to reduce this stress by staggering work and school opening hours. Equally, if data show that parenting or social isolation are commonly noted in conjunction with emotions indicating reduced wellbeing, then parenting, family support, and community-engagement programs could be bolstered, and awareness campaigns launched to ensure that people are fully informed of these enhanced resources. Additionally, participatory decision-making processes, such as those often used in urban planning, can be informed by live emotional data (Zeile, Resch, Exner, & Sagl, 2015).

Utilization of broad and wide-ranging wellbeing measures of various kinds also allows for an evaluation of how wellbeing in one domain may affect another, like undermining or synergistically enhancing effects elsewhere (Helliwell, Layard, & Sachs, 2012). For example, strong scores in positive physical health behaviors may, when considered in isolation, indicate good overall public health. However, given that the effects of loneliness are as detrimental to physical health as are smoking and sedentary behavior, corresponding weak scores in social wellbeing may weaken that same state of physical health (Cacioppo, Hawkely, & Berntson, 2003; Holt-Lunstad, Smith, Baker, Harris, & Stephenson, 2015).

Measurement of wellbeing also facilitates a longitudinal understanding of the distribution of wellbeing. For instance, age and gender reversals in wellbeing levels are common. Globally, women prior to the age of 50 report greater degrees of happiness, laughter, enjoyment, and feeling rested, but thereafter, experience a drop and are surpassed by men in all four categories (Fortin, Helliwell, & Wang, 2015). Thus, greater granularity in the data regarding patterns and levels of wellbeing across ages, as well as national regions, cities, or rural spaces can permit refined adjustments in ways that are relevant and exacted to specific needs. This same granularity can help limit financial waste across high-wellbeing areas where the effects of interventions will be negligible in comparison to low-scoring areas. An example of the spatial distribution of wellbeing (Canaviri, 2016; Helliwell et al., 2012; O'Donnell, 2013; Pykett & Cromby, 2017) was illustrated in a US study of physical and mental health where inequalities in longevity of up to 25 years were found between neighborhoods a mere 10 miles apart (Evans, Zimmerman, Woolf, & Hayley, 2012). This suggests that despite equal provision of government services, differential access to and use of provisions and services reflects the status of certain groups as well as differences in lifestyle and attitudes towards care, all of which impact wellbeing outcomes (Chartier et al., 2014). The juncture between wellbeing and environmental contexts, perceptions, sociopolitical dynamics and culture can emerge through detailed longitudinal tracking and provides a foundation upon which governments can build targeted interventions to create changes in the wellbeing of specific groups.

A final reason for the tracking of wellbeing data is to facilitate the international comparability of data (Bronsteen, Buccafusco, & Masur, 2014; OECD, 2013). Between-nation analyses help determine how factors like progressive taxation (a higher tax rate for the rich that leads to greater social equality and subjective wellbeing; Oishi, Schimmack, & Diener, 2012), green spaces (Alcock, White, Wheeler, Fleming, & Depledge, 2014; Mensah, Andres, Perera, & Roji, 2016), or levels of economic freedom (the degree to which one is free to enter and compete in markets, as well as the protection of persons and property; Gropper, Lawson, & Thorne, 2011) impact wellbeing. Additional factors known to contribute to wellbeing include low levels of corruption (Tay, Herian, & Diener, 2014) and quality systems of governance such as rule of law, political stability, government accountability, and regulatory quality (Ott, 2011). While there are commonalties across nations, the impact of culture, as well as historical, political, and social events, also influence the wellbeing of nations.

Measurement tools reflect quality of life dimensions, such as personal mastery and self-actualization. Thus, measuring wellbeing reveals what is important and valued. Yet, it is not only governments that benefit from knowing such information. Benefits also emerge at the individual level. Merely being asked about what matters allows individuals to pay greater attention to their own wellbeing and prompts them to make decisions to optimize their happiness (Bakker, Burger, van Haaren, Oerlemans, & Veenhoven, 2015). For example, Bakker et al. (2015) asked about one's happiness by indicating in what activities one participated and what effect these had. Compared to simply rating one's level of overall happiness, the more detailed measure reported a 2% increase in aggregate happiness equivalent to the effect of a 600€ annual rise in salary. While small, this study suggests that attending to the specifics of one's happiness can serve a mutually beneficial purpose of providing data to policymakers and enhancing greater individual wellbeing. The potential to expand what is asked of constituents is a further avenue of development.

In sum, measurements help prioritize wellbeing. As the adage says, attention goes to what is measured and what is measured becomes valued (Diener et al., 2015). In short, when indices of wellbeing exist and are utilized, it is difficult for authorities to ignore the data generated by them. Moreover, governments can be held accountable for progress towards national wellbeing fulfillment and become more responsive by doing what is necessary to achieve socially desired goals and outcomes, resulting in greater service efficiencies in the process (Diener et al., 2015; Weijers, 2014).

10.3 A Theoretical Orientation for Measurement

Theoretical frameworks are influential structures designed to support inquiry and can be likened to lenses which influence both what is observed and how it is interpreted (Schram, 2006). Consequently, a good theory, upon which to base the selection of indicators to be measured, is one aspect. It helps make sense of that data based on the theory's presuppositions about wellbeing. Another aspect is to know when and where to intervene to make a difference. A good theoretical model will effectively guide these increasingly difficult decisions, while a haphazardly constructed model (or none at all) will cause much confusion when the amount of collected data grows. Unfortunately, the use of a theoretical model or framework is often overlooked in the measurement of wellbeing. Yet, it is essential in appropriately guiding the selection of measured indicators. Moreover, a theoretical framework offers avenues through which to improve wellbeing itself (Canaviri, 2016; Gander, Proyer, & Ruch, 2016; Linton, Dieppe, & Medina-Lara, 2016).

While there are many wellbeing theoretical frameworks, we highlight five models for which an accumulated body of empirical evidence exists. These models consider human functioning across many domains (what people do), in addition to considering personal aspirations, experiences, and life evaluations (how people feel as a result of what they do). Thus, these models best approximate how individuals live their lives (Kern, Waters, Adler, & White, 2015; Keyes, 2005; Waterman et al., 2010). The models highlighted below also capture aspects of both hedonic (feeling good) and eudaimonic (functioning well) wellbeing. They stand in contrast to hedonic-focused models like Subjective Wellbeing (SWB; Diener, 1984) which mainly capture the experience of positive and negative emotions plus a cognitive component of life satisfaction, and therefore offer a limited picture of wellbeing. The distinction between hedonia and eudaimonia is vital, and it is incumbent upon data collection agencies to target a complete picture of wellbeing. Indeed, hedonia (a focus on immediate, short-lived, pleasant emotions and experiences) and eudaimonia (a focus on human potential, growth, and striving according to one's values) constitute two aspects of wellbeing across which the majority of theories exist (Carlisle, Henderson, & Hanlon, 2009; Lambert, Passmore, & Holder, 2015). It is important to note that the term "wellbeing" is widely preferred to "happiness" as wellbeing encompasses a broader array of constructs and nuanced facets (Hart & Sasso, 2011; Joseph & Wood, 2010; Linton et al., 2016). This broader approach can help governments to achieve what Pawelski (2016) referred to as "fractal flourishing … an ideal that holds out for the wellbeing of individuals *and* groups, that values happiness in the short-term *and* long-term, and that seeks approaches that work locally *and* globally" (p. 363).

10.3.1 Psychological Wellbeing (PWB)

The PWB model (Ryff, 1989) comprises six dimensions, reflecting health, wellness, and full functioning. This model puts forth that the highest human goal is activity in line with character virtues that are embedded within an array of individual needs, ultimately striving for the pursuit of excellence in domains of health, employment, relationships, and security. PWB focuses on functioning and personal growth and includes the following dimensions: (1) Self-Acceptance: liking, knowing, and accepting the self; (2) Relationships with Others: positive social relationships reflecting an ability to empathize and show affection; (3) Personal Growth: the development of potential and the capitalization of new challenges; (4) Purpose: creating direction, defining goals, and deciphering meaning; (5) Environmental Mastery: the ability to choose and create fitting environments which involves the ability to control one's internal and external world; and (6) Autonomy: a sense of independence emerging from taking responsibility and acting for one's self. Ryff (1989) operationalized PWB and provided a measure for its assessment (see Table 10.2).

10.3.2 Self-determination Theory (SDT)

SDT (Ryan & Deci, 2000) proposes that individuals have three basic psychological needs—autonomy, competence, and relatedness—which need to be satisfied to achieve wellbeing. Autonomy refers to the desire to organize one's experiences by exerting control over one's chosen goals. Competence relates to feelings of effectiveness in the completion of tasks. Relatedness refers to the feeling of belonging one has with others and is based on the need to care for and love others, as well as the need to be cared for and loved by them. As individuals meet these basic psychological needs through goal pursuits, wellbeing increases such that persistence, psychological health, and better performance emerge. Years of research supports SDT's validity and efficacy across a wide variety of domains like the workplace (Gagné & Deci, 2005) and academia (Black & Deci, 2000).

10.3.3 PERMA

Seligman's (2002) precursor to the PERMA model was termed the authentic happiness framework and includes the pathways of pleasure, engagement, and meaning. The Pleasant Life, considered the first pathway, is geared towards the maximization and generation of positive emotions and experiences. Engagement, the second path, is characterized by the connection individuals feel to their activities, which rely on and develop their character strengths, and which facilitate growth. The third, Meaning, is strongly associated with a eudaimonic view and includes using one's strengths in the service of positive institutions like volunteering or religion. In 2011, Seligman revised this model and proposed the PERMA model, whereby the original pathways, pleasure (P), engagement (E), and meaning (M), were combined with positive relationships (R) and accomplishments (A). The model is nonetheless strongly contested given its intuitive development in the absence of theoretical evidence (see Goodman, Disabato, Kashdan & Kauffman, 2018). However, research that has directly tested it, seems to supports its validity (Coffey, Wray-Lake, Mashek, & Branand, 2014).

10.3.4 Flourishing

Keyes (2002, 2005) first proposed the term "flourishing" to refer to a complete state of mental health. Keyes' model encompasses three different mental health statuses: flourishing, languishing, and moderate mental health. Flourishing is a state of strong subjective wellbeing and optimal psychological and social functioning. It is indicated not only by evidence of healthy functioning, such as feeling good and functioning well, but also by a concurrent absence of psychopathology (mental illness). Flourishing contrasts with languishing, defined as a state of stagnation and emptiness characterized by low subjective wellbeing and low psychological and social wellbeing. Mentally healthy individuals who are neither languishing nor flourishing are considered to experience moderate mental health. Keyes' (1998) measure incorporates psychological wellbeing, subjective wellbeing, and social wellbeing, dimensions felt to reflect an ideal state of mental health as the criteria involve assessments of emotion, personal criteria for self-evaluation, and public criteria to evaluate social functioning.

10.3.5 Eudaimonic Wellbeing (EWB)

EWB (Waterman et al., 2010) is positioned as the feeling arising from living a eudaimonic lifestyle, in which the individual enacts qualities they determine congruent with how it is right to live. This lifestyle reflects a high quality of life derived from the development of potential and fulfillment of goals and is based on both subjectively determined aspects as well as on activity. It is not simply a measure of how one feels. EWB is composed of six categories: (1) Effort, (2) Self-discovery, (3) Enjoyment, (4) Purpose and meaning, (5) Development of one's potentials, and (6) Involvement. Although EWB correlates positively with Ryff's (1989) PWB as well as with Diener's (1984) SWB, these three models are distinguishable and each contributes differentially to wellbeing (Waterman et al., 2010).

10.4 What to Measure?

The measurement of wellbeing is admittedly complex, and choosing a wellbeing assessment tool can be difficult. There is an overwhelming multitude of over 160 indices wellbeing measures currently in use (OECD, 2008). An average of eight new tools has been designed every five years since the 1980s, with the majority having been developed in the last decade (Linton et al., 2016). Given that no formal agreement exists about which domains of wellbeing or which wellbeing indicators should be included in government assessments (Canaviri, 2016; Cooke, Melchert, & Connor, 2016; Linton et al., 2016), measures are often chosen arbitrarily. Choices range from material living standards (i.e., income, consumption), physical health and health status, education, political voice and governance, and the number and quality of social connections (Stiglitz et al., 2009), to crime, employment, and recreation indices (Epley & Mohan, 2008), and subjective indicators such as attitudes to life, cultural values, and perceptions (White, 2009). The development of positive psychology in recent years has sparked a new trend, that of focusing on the presence of positive emotions (exemplified by Gallup's 2017 Global Emotions Report) and spirituality (Linton et al., 2016) in order to account for a full view of wellbeing. Adding to the difficulty for governments to achieve consistency in measuring wellbeing, is the fact that the variety of measures also points to the involvement of several disciplines, like medicine and sociology (Cooke et al., 2016; Linton et al., 2016). Despite this, the freedom to experiment within sociocultural contexts is nonetheless a bonus for researchers. Choosing measures with the greatest empirical weight allows for consistency with other data collection bodies and provides confidence in the validity and reliability of emergent data.

Policymakers' healthy skepticism of subjective data adds further concern to the assessment of wellbeing, given psychology's reliance on self-report measures (Diener et al., 2015; Nikolova, 2016), which admittedly can suffer from response bias, demand characteristics, the effects of priming, and lack of insight and accurate memory, as well as variability in the personal and cultural interpretation of questions (Cromby, 2011). Rebuttals to these criticisms of self-report measures stress that it is paternalistic and undemocratic to disallow individuals to be the final judge of their own experience and evaluators of how they feel about their lives (Binder, 2014). Indeed within the science of positive psychology, subjective experiences are the focal point of all investigation. Given that happiness and wellbeing stem from individual perceptions and experiences, self-report measures (considered suitable for negative emotions and experiences) are considered a valid representation of one's feelings. While some amount of bias is recognized, it is not considered unduly large by itself or in comparison to natural biases that also exist in objective measures (Baumeister, Vohs, & Funder, 2007; Diener & Ryan, 2009; Kurtz & Lyubomirsky, 2008). Overall, self-report measures of wellbeing are well established by experts in the field as reliable and valid instruments that can be used to make comparisons between nations, communities, and individuals (Cooke et al., 2016; Helliwell & Barrington-Leigh, 2010).

Data collection agencies have three options in determining which measurement route to pursue (Musikanski, Polley, Cloutier, Berejnoi, & Colbert, 2017). Firstly, established measures can be used, the benefits of which include existing and rigorous standards of validity and reliability. Second, agencies can establish measures of their own, although validity, reliability, and other tests of statistical power may be of concern and must be achieved (especially across multiple languages). The third preferred choice for most institutions and governments is to adapt existing measures to their specific contexts.

Regardless of the option chosen, we recommend that data collection entities take an open-source data dashboard approach—that is, the use of multiple measures at once (Wallace & Schmueker, 2012)—which show the performance of individual indicators and illustrate where high, moderate, or low wellbeing exists by geographical location, age, gender, socio-economic status, nationality, etc., and that is updated frequently and instantly. This approach allows for transparency across ministries as well as across stakeholders (e.g., university research units) from which to generate analyses. Transparency facilitates better decision-making and reduces potential conflict between entities who might contest investing in one area or sector over another; it also means the rationale for investments is clear to all. Finally, a visual dashboard is advantageous as most people prefer to see data rather than read it (see Fig. 10.1 for a dashboard measure example).

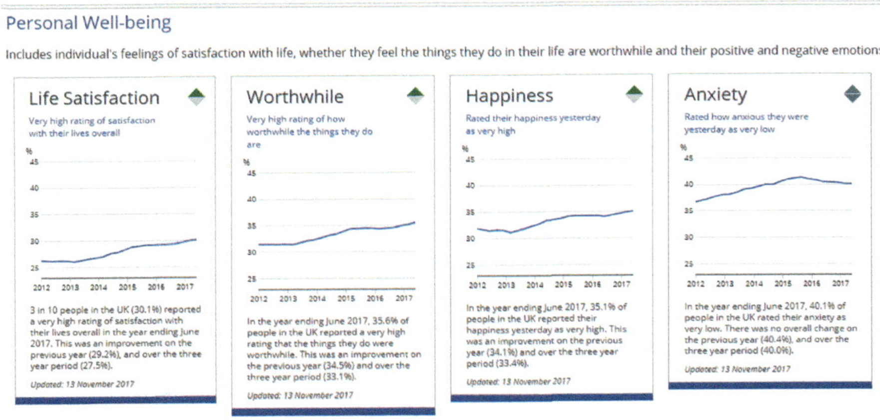

Fig. 10.1 Dashboard measure (UK Office for National Statistics, Measures of National Wellbeing)

For the purpose of this chapter, we advocate the use of existing assessment indices. In Tables 10.1 and 10.2 we list several wellbeing measures that capture how individuals feel about their lives, what they experience in terms of emotion, and how they function on a daily basis as examples. Most of these measures correspond to the theoretical models described earlier and thus reflect aspects of eudaimonic wellbeing rather than financial, physical health, relational, or workplace wellbeing (Cooke et al., 2016). As per Linton et al. (2016), we resist recommending specific measures however, as the appropriate tool should depend on the purpose at hand and the factors of greatest relevance and interest to those conducting the measurements.

In Table 10.3, we include four scales assessing religious faith, beliefs about the fear and fragility of happiness, and individualism/collectivism that can help develop a more nuanced and complete picture of respondents and their wellbeing profiles. Religiosity is a known contributor to wellbeing through its associations with social interaction, a sense of identity and group belonging, rituals that structure time and personal values, opportunities for giving and receiving, and the derivation of a sense of purpose, meaning in life, and a coherent set of goals (Pargament & Raiya, 2007). Religion also fosters a sense of gratitude and appreciation (Wood, Froh, & Geraghty, 2010). In a recent study conducted in the UAE (Thomas, Mutawa, Furber, & Grey, 2016), religiosity was negatively correlated with depressive symptoms. An important point to consider is that, as economic and social conditions improve in society, religiosity commonly tends to decline (Diener, Tay, & Meyers, 2011; Gundlach & Opfinger, 2011) and individualism increases (Ahuvia, 2002; Kitayama & Uskul, 2011). These relationships are vital to consider, as they are one example of how the consequences of greater wellbeing are not always predictable or intended, and thus need repeated assessment over time as societal conditions change.

Beliefs in the fear and fragility of happiness are further dimensions to study. In Islamic cultures, the expression of happiness is sometimes believed to tempt fate, call forth the evil eye, and facilitate a path to sin. Happiness is sometimes thought to make

Table 10.1 Psychological and emotional wellbeing: hedonic scales

Scale	Description
Subjective Happiness Scale (SHS; Lyubomirsky & Lepper, 1999)	This 4-item self-report scale measures subjective happiness. An example of an SHS item is, "Some people are generally very happy. They enjoy life regardless of what is going on, getting the most out of everything. To what extent does this characterization describe you?" to which participants reply on a scale from 1 = "not at all" to 7 = "a great deal". Higher total scores indicate greater subjective happiness. The SHS has demonstrated high internal consistency that is stable across samples, with Cronbach's alpha ranging from 0.79 to 0.94 and test-retest reliability of 0.55–0.90. The SHS scale has been translated into Arabic and has been found to be valid, reliable, and culturally appropriate in Lebanese college students (Moghnie & Kazarian, 2012).
Scale of Positive and Negative Experience (SPANE; Diener et al., 2009)	This 12-item self-report questionnaire includes six items that measure positive feelings and six that measure negative feelings. Respondents rate how often they have experienced the feelings listed (e.g., positive, negative, good, bad) in the past four weeks. Ratings are made on a 5-point scale from 1 = "very rarely or never" to 5 = "very often or always". The SPANE performed well in terms of reliability and convergent validity with other measures of emotion, wellbeing, happiness, and life satisfaction (Diener et al., 2010). The three subscales (SPANE-Positive, SPANE-Negative, and SPANE-Balance) demonstrated high Cronbach's alpha and temporal stability over one month: (respectively) SPANE-P: 0.87, 0.62; SPANE-N: 0.81, 0.63; SPANE-B (affect balance, SPANE-P minus SPANE-B): 0.89, 0.68. The SPANE has been validated in Chinese and Portuguese studies with an internal consistency coefficient of 0.81–0.90 (Li, Bai, & Wang, 2013; Silva & Caetano, 2013). This scale has also been translated into Arabic.
Satisfaction with Life Scale (SWLS; Diener, Emmons, Larsen, & Griffin, 1985)	This 5-item scale assesses an individual's judgement of satisfaction with one's life. Items include: "I am satisfied with my life", "If I could live my life over, I would change almost nothing". Respondents answer on a 7-point scale with endpoints of 1 = "strongly disagree" to 7 = "strongly agree". Higher overall scores indicate greater satisfaction. Existing data suggests that the SWLS has potential to be a cross-cultural index of life satisfaction; it been translated into many languages including Arabic. The scale possesses high internal consistency (0.87), test-retest reliability (0.82), and had demonstrated satisfactory convergent validity. The SWLS captures the stable effects of personality and life-span changes (Pavot & Diener, 1993).

(continued)

Table 10.1 (continued)

Scale	Description
Subjective Wellbeing (SWB; Diener, 1984)	This three-item measure comprises positive and negative affect, as well as life satisfaction. As all reports of wellbeing are subjective, it was proposed that SWB be called hedonic wellbeing (Waterman et al., 2010), although this was never adopted. SWB can be likened to the SPANE (Diener et al., 2009) and SWLS (Diener et al., 1985) combined. It is available in Arabic.
Negative and Positive Affect Scale (NAPAS; Mroczek & Kolarz, 1998)	This 12-item scale provides a measure of both positive and negative affect which can yield an overall affect balance score by subtracting the negative items from the positive items. The NAPAS consists of six positive and six negative affect items and is divided into the positive and negative components with higher scores on the scale indicating a higher frequency of that affect. An item example is: "In the last 30 days, how many times did you feel…so sad nothing could cheer you up?" Participants respond to items on a 5-point scale, ranging from 1 = "none of the time" to 5 = "all of the time". Joshanloo (2017) revised and shortened the NAPAS to ten items and found that it could be used with confidence in American samples. Evidence of cross-cultural validity is needed.
International Wellbeing Index (IWI)	The IWI is composed of two subscales: the Personal Wellbeing Index (PWI; International Wellbeing Group, 2006) and the National Wellbeing Index (NWI; Cummins, Eckersley, Pallant, Van Vugt, & Misajon, 2003). The PWI has seven items measuring satisfaction with: standard of living, health, relationships, achievement in life, safety, community connectedness, and future security. These domains are classified as "satisfaction with life as a whole". The NWI contains six items measuring satisfaction with: economic situation, state of the environment, social conditions, government, business, and national security. Each item is scored on a 10-point scale with greater scores indicating greater satisfaction with the construct being measured. Both subscales show good sensitivity, validity and reliability. In an Algerian sample, Cronbach's alpha for both scales was greater than 0.70 and all items had an item total correlation greater than 0.30 (Tiliouine, Cummins, & Davern, 2006).

individuals appear less serious or responsible. In Iran, sadness is often considered a positive state associated with personal insight and reflection (Joshanloo, 2013). Thus, the fear of happiness revolves around the belief that positive emotions can elicit negative consequences (Joshanloo et al., 2014). Combined, these beliefs cause the pursuit of happiness to be shunned. Alternatively, the fragility of happiness involves the belief that happiness is controlled by an external power (which may be spiritual or include the influence of events and other people), and that happiness can be lost if its pursuit is too motivated (Joshanloo et al., 2015). Hence, the belief that happiness

Table 10.2 Psychological and emotional wellbeing: eudaimonic scales

Scale	Description
Eudaimonic Wellbeing Measure (EWB; Joshanloo, 2018)	This measure is based on a selection of items from the Gallup World Poll (GWP) data set collected from 2005 to 2017. There are seven items which measure the personal and social aspects of EWB (learning, social support, respect, efficacy, freedom, helping strangers, and volunteering). An example item is: "Can people in this country get ahead by working hard, or not?". Response options for all items are 1 = "Yes" or 0 = "No", except for the item assessing 'freedom' for which the options are 1 = "Satisfied" or 0 = "Dissatisfied". The total score is calculated by averaging each item's score, giving a range from 0 to 1. EWB correlates with theoretically relevant variables in the expected direction at the individual and national level and modestly associated with other wellbeing indicators (i.e., life satisfaction, prosperity, quality of life, GDP; Joshanloo, 2018).
Questionnaire for Eudaimonic Wellbeing (QEWB; Waterman et al., 2010)	This 21-item scale measures a range of elements associated with eudaimonic wellbeing across six domains: effort, self-discovery, pleasure, purpose/meaning, fulfillment of potential, and engagement. Respondents rate their agreement to items using a 5-point scale from 0 = "strongly disagree" to 4 = "strongly agree". Items load onto a single factor with high internal consistency (0.85). Waterman et al. (2010) demonstrated sufficient reliability (a = 0.86) and convergent, discriminant, construct, and incremental validity in a diverse American student sample. The QEWB has demonstrated some cross-cultural application by showing reliability and validity in an Indian sample (Areepattamannil & Hashim, 2017).
Flourishing Scale (FS; Diener et al., 2009)	This 8-item scale measures social-psychological prosperity in areas such as a sense of competence, meaning, engagement, interest, optimism, self-acceptance, and relationships. Construct validity is acceptable with moderate to high correlations with other tools. Cronbach's alpha range from 0.81 to 0.87. Items include: "I am engaged and interested in my daily activities" and "I actively contribute to the happiness and wellbeing of others." Participants respond on a 7-point scale from 1 = "strongly disagree" to 7 = "strongly agree". High scores represent strong psychological resources and strengths. Test-retest reliability over one month was 0.71 (Diener et al., 2009). It has been translated into Arabic (Salama-Younes, 2017) and French (Villieux, Sovet, Jung, & Guilbert, 2016).

(continued)

Table 10.2 (continued)

Scale	Description
Meaning in Life Questionnaire (MLQ; Steger, Frazier, Oishi, & Kaler, 2006)	The MLQ is a 10-item scale that measures two dimensions of meaning in life: Presence of Meaning and Search for Meaning. The Presence of Meaning subscale measures how much respondents feel their lives have meaning, while the Search for Meaning subscale measures how motivated they are to find it. An example of an item is "My life has a clear sense of purpose" to which participants respond from 1 = "absolutely untrue" to 7 = "absolutely true". Higher scores on the Presence subscale indicate a greater presence of meaning in participant's life, whereas higher scores on the Search subscale indicate greater motivation to seek it. The MLQ has good internal consistency (0.86), test–retest stability (0.70), and high convergent correlations (0.61–0.74) with similar measures. It is available in multiple languages.
Social Wellbeing Scale (SWBS; Keyes, 1998)	This 15-item scale measures social wellbeing, the extent to which individuals see themselves as thriving in their social lives. Five dimensions of social wellbeing are assessed: social coherence, social integration, social contribution, social actualization, and social acceptance. An example item is: "If you had something to say, you don't think your community would take you seriously." Participants respond on a 7-point scale ranging from 1 = "strongly disagree" to 7 = "strongly agree". Modest Cronbach's alpha scores between 0.60 and 0.76 have been found for the scale (Joshanloo, Rostami, & Nosratabadi, 2006; Keyes, 1998).
The Ryff Scales of Psychological Wellbeing (PWB; Ryff, 1989)	The original questionnaire consisted of 20 items per scale and included 120 items. Shortened versions of the PWB containing 84 items (14 items per scale), 54 items (9 per items per scale), 42 items (7 items per scale), and 18 items (3 items per scale) have been used (Abbott et al., 2006). This measure consists of several statements reflecting the six areas of psychological wellbeing: autonomy, environmental mastery, personal growth, positive relations with others, purpose in life, and self-acceptance. An example item is: "Some people wander aimlessly through life, but I am not one of them." Respondents rate statements on a scale from 1 = "strongly disagree" to 6 = "strongly agree". The full version has a Cronbach's alpha of 0.86–0.93 and test-retest reliability of 0.81–0.88. A version of the PWB has been translated into Urdu and determined to be reliable and valid in a Pakistani sample (Jibeen & Khalid, 2012).

Table 10.3 Culture and religiosity measures

Scale	Description
Brief Version of the Santa Clara Strength of Religious Faith Questionnaire (SCSRFQ; Plante, Vallaeys, Sherman, & Wallston, 2002)	This scale is a shorter version of the original and features five items assessing strength of religious faith. Both the original and brief version of the scale are considered valid and reliable (Cronbach's alpha 0.95). The SCSRFQ is supported by strong correlations with other measures of intrinsic religiosity. An example of the items is: "My religious faith impacts many of my decisions." The SCSRFQ is available in English only.
Fragility of Happiness Scale (Joshanloo et al., 2014, 2015)	This 4-item scale captures the belief in the fleetingness of happiness and is rated on a 7-point scale. The scale has been used, validated, and understood as having a constant meaning across at least 50 national groups and countries; it is considered to have good statistical properties (Joshanloo et al., 2014, 2015). An item example is: "Something might happen at any time and we could easily lose our happiness".
Fear of Happiness Scale (Joshanloo, 2013; Joshanloo et al., 2014)	This 5-item scale captures the stable belief that happiness is a sign of impending unhappiness. The measure is shown to be reliable (Joshanloo, 2013) and has been used and validated across more than 50 national groups and countries; it is considered to have good statistical properties (Joshanloo et al., 2014, 2015). An example item is: "I prefer not to be too joyful, because usually joy is followed by sadness".
Individualism and Collectivism Scale (Triandis & Gelfland, 1998)	This 16-item measure captures aspects of collectivism and individualism and assesses two continuums: vertical collectivism (VC: seeing the self as part of a group and being willing to accept hierarchy and inequality) to horizontal collectivism (HC: perceiving all members as equal) and vertical individualism (VI: seeing the self as independent and accepting that inequality exists) to horizontal individualism (HI: believing that equality between people is the accepted norm). Cronbach's alpha are: 0.81 (HI), 0.82 (VI), 0.80 (HC), 0.73 (VC).

is desirable is not universally shared and may present a stumbling block to greater wellbeing. Assessing the prevalence and change in these beliefs over time and across places may offer useful information in determining whether government efforts are falling on deaf ears, and if efforts to improve wellbeing need to be pre-empted by information about the utility of pursuing such worldly states.

A measure of individualism and collectivism is also presented as it is as yet unclear whether increasing levels of happiness, at least via the standard Western positive psychology interventions currently being promoted, inadvertently bring about cultural change and what effects this increasing level of happiness may have on cultural beliefs (Lambert, Passmore, & Joshanloo, 2018). As individuals focus more on themselves, how they feel, and what they do, they necessarily take a greater "self"-focused orientation. With levels of individualism already rising in the UAE (Whiteoak, Crawford, & Mapstone, 2006), it is imperative that a focus on wellbeing does not come at the expense of the cultural factors that serve to increase it in the first place, i.e., collective family and group support, and foundational religious beliefs and customs (Dwairy, Achoui, Abouserie, & Farah, 2006; Joshanloo, 2013; Lambert D'raven & Pasha-Zaidi, 2015; Layous, Lee, Choi, & Lyubomirsky, 2013). Incorporating measures that focus on such cultural factors can bring about an understanding of what is really being changed when agencies seek to enhance wellbeing. In essence, the goal of any wellbeing initiative should be to increase those terms most relevant for local people's wellbeing. Western norms and practises that were never intended for a global audience, may affect wellbeing components unsuitable in a local context. Such effects may go unnoticed if they are not tracked.

Most wellbeing measures focus on the presence of positive emotions, attributes, experiences and actions conducive to their presence. Wellbeing, nonetheless, also depends on the absence or management of negative emotions which are typically present to varying degrees in daily lives. Thus, measures to specifically assess levels of negative emotions and experiences are necessary. In Table 10.4 we present indices sensitive to the detection of poor mental health. Mental health issues strongly influence wellbeing. Policies targeting both the enhancement of wellbeing and the reduction of poor mental health are necessary. They may do more to boost wellbeing scores than any other policy, given that the ability to fully engage in every aspect of life (e.g., education, work, parenting, health, civic behavior) rests on a foundation of being mentally well and healthy. Physical activity measures (assessing duration, frequency, and intensity) should also be included as physical activity and exercise are strong correlates of wellbeing and depression (see Lambert, D'Cruz, Schlatter, & Barron, 2016 for a review).

Measures relating to time spent in green spaces are included in Table 10.5. The role that contact with nature plays in overall health and wellbeing is increasingly being recognized by governments, and as such is progressively being considered as an important aspect of urban policy planning (Maas, Verheij, Groenewegen, de Vries, & Spreeuwenberg, 2006). This comes on the heels of growing evidence which consistently demonstrates that a feeling of connection with nature and valuing its presence, and spending time in or near nature, can increase emotional, psychological, and social wellbeing (Capaldi, Dopko, & Zelenski, 2014; Capaldi, Passmore, Nisbet, Zelenski, & Dopko, 2015; Cervinka, Röderer, & Hefler, 2012) and can boost physical health outcomes such as greater longevity (Takano, Nakamura, & Watanabe, 2002; Villeneuve et al., 2012), improved quality of sleep (Astell-Burt, Feng, & Kolt, 2013), better birth outcomes (Donovan, Michael, Butry, Sullivan, & Chase, 2011), and increased participation in physical activity (Mytton, Townsend, Rutter, & Foster, 2012; Toftager et al., 2011).

While we have limited ourselves in this chapter to presenting individual psychological scales, we eagerly suggest the inclusion of scales, tools, and methods that capture individuals' experience of life and not only their satisfaction with it. Life is not exclusively carried out in the confines of one's home, but the sidewalk, grocery store, office, health center, tennis court, public park, shopping mall and concert hall as examples. Thus, the influence of the built physical environment and the geographical places in which individuals live must be considered (Ballas & Dorling, 2013; Ballas & Tranmer, 2012). A number of recently developed tools and methods strive to cap-

Table 10.4 Mental health scales

Scale	Description
Mental Health Continuum-Short Form (MCH-SF; Keyes et al., 2008)	This 14-item measure captures three types of wellbeing: social (integration, acceptance, actualization, coherence and contribution), emotional (positive/negative affect), and psychological (based on Ryff's (1989) six factors of autonomy, growth, self-acceptance, relationships with others, purpose in life, and mastery). Estimates of internal consistency for emotional, psychological, and social wellbeing in the short and long forms are over 0.80 (Keyes, 2005), with test-retest reliability over three successive 3-month periods averaging 0.68 and 0.65 at nine months (Lamers, Westerhof, Bohlmeijer, ten Klooster, & Keyes, 2010). Diagnoses range from flourishing, languishing, and moderate mental health. The MCH-SF is available in Arabic (Salama-Younes, 2011) and has been validated for use in diverse cultural contexts.
Beck Depression Inventory (BDI; Beck, Steer & Brown, 1996)	The revised BDI 11-item inventory measures psychological and physical manifestations of major depressive episodes of two-week's duration. The BDI takes less than 10 min to complete. Internal consistency scores range from 0.73 to 0.92 for the original and revised version (Beck, Steer, & Garbin, 1988). The BDI-11 exists in 17 languages and is widely used in the region (see Wang & Gorenstein, 2013 for more).
Depression, Anxiety, and Stress Scale (DASS; Henry & Crawford, 2005)	This 21-item questionnaire measures depression, anxiety, and stress. Participants report how often they experienced the symptoms listed (e.g., "I couldn't seem to experience any positive feeling at all", "I experienced trembling", "I found it hard to wind down") during a specified time period. Items are rated on a scale from 0 (*never*) to 3 (*almost always*), and an aggregate score is calculated by summing the items. The internal consistency coefficient for the DASS is strong (Cronbach alpha = 0.93).

ture these influences, such as: the sustainable neighborhoods for happiness (SNfH) decision tool (Paralkar, Cloutier, Nautiyal, & Mitra, 2017); and the urban emotions mapping movement (Zeile et al., 2015), which combines biometric human sensor technology (wearable devices, microphones, cameras), GPS, crowdsourced data (like Twitter) and subjective wellbeing measures to create a human-sensor network in any given city or region. These measures are already commonly used by developers and urban planners who have a clear commercial advantage in determining how individuals experience a proposed neighborhood park, apartment complex, office pod, or new home. Using virtual reality and other forms of technology can significantly increase our understanding of what makes people feel comfortable, inspired, safe, and well. Thus, expanding the choices of measures and methods to include these aspects can offer a picture of wellbeing overlooked by traditional survey methods.

Table 10.5 Nature scales

Scale	Description
Connectedness to Nature Scale (CNS; Mayer & McPherson Frantz, 2004)	This 14-item scale is rated on a 5-point scale and includes items such as "I often feel a sense of oneness with the natural world around me" and "I think of the natural world as a community to which I belong". The CNS assesses the degree to which people feel part of nature. Scores on this trait scale predict responsible environmental behavior and subjective wellbeing. A Cronbach's alpha of 0.84 is evidenced for the summed scale score; factor analysis consistently yielded a one-factor solution.
Nature Relatedness Scale (NRS; Nisbet, Zelenski, & Murphy, 2009)	This 21-item scale assesses individual differences in people's "appreciation for and understanding of our interconnectedness with all other living things on the earth" (p. 4). Items (e.g., "I enjoy digging in the earth and getting dirt on my hands") are rated on a scale with endpoints 1 = "disagree strongly" and 5 = "agree strongly". An overall score is calculated by summing all items. The NRS has good internal consistency (Cronbach's alpha = 0.87) and good test–retest stability (0.85). Scores correlate positively with experience sampling measures of time spent outdoors and in nature.

10.5 Other Points to Consider

We hope that it is evident that multiple measures are necessary to fully assess wellbeing; a single score or measure cannot do justice to the multiple nuanced facets that comprise wellbeing. Moreover, single scores or single-aspect measures produce data that is, by and large, inadequate as they yield no indication of which domain governments or organizations can most effectively intervene. At the same time, while more and varied data is better, there is a point at which too much data spread across too many domains becomes unhelpful (Nikolova, 2016). Thus, the need for comprehensiveness should be balanced against the practical realities of budgets, time constraints, and utility. As much as possible, only validated scales should be employed; extensive effort should be made to locate existing scales for which there is evidence and which stem from a theoretical model. Models and their scales often go through decades of testing on multiple populations worldwide for reliability (consistency over time), and are confirmed against similar and dissimilar scales for validity, back translation, and empirical robustness. Moreover, it is far easier to compare data with other regions when existing scales have been used. This further allows for determinations of what might account for both similarities and differences across regions. The measures we have noted are freely available without permission other than due citation and, for the most part, are available in Arabic, Farsi, Hindi, Urdu, and other languages.

Data collection relies on the goodwill of individuals to complete. Asking merely one set of questions can lead to a degree of passivity whereby respondents memorize, easily anticipate the questions, or answer out of convenience, overlooking any potential benefits they too could gain from answering such questions. To maintain

Table 10.6 Suggested demographics

Date of birth	Household size (# of people)	Education
Gender	Employment status	Illness or health conditions
Marital status	Number of pets in the house	Commuting time (hours/day)
Nationality	Income	Years in country; residency status
Number of children	Housing quality (satisfied with size, noise, traffic, parking, etc.)	Fitness/health (time in minutes spent exercising in a week)
Hours of sleep per night? Quality of sleep (restful, disrupted, etc.)?	Community (how often do you speak to your neighbors?)	Time lived in current residence? (month, years)
How much time do you spend in nature in any given week? (i.e., parks, desert, sea, green spaces?)	How close do you live to a green/natural space? (i.e., parks, sea, farm, wildlife, zoo, etc.)	How many people would you consider close enough to rely on if you needed help?
How satisfied are you with your salary in comparison to others?	How satisfied are you with your health in comparison to others?	How satisfied are you with your home in comparison to others?

the interest of respondents and ensure that the collected data are accurate, the OECD (2013) offers guidelines for the purpose of data collection and measurement (which we hereby summarize):

- Measures should be treated like an official census and given to all constituents to complete in as many languages and format options as possible (e.g., online, mobile phone apps, over the phone surveys, data collection stations, public kiosks).
- Data should be attached to one's national identification (labor card, passport, etc.) so that socio-demographic changes such as marital status, number of children, and employment status can be tracked over time (see Table 10.6 for suggested items) and with which correlations and trends can be observed.
- Measures should be given annually, with a subset of the population being measured more frequently to see proximal effects of life changes.

The release of such measures should be staggered over all days of the week (including holidays), and responses should be date- and time-stamped to determine mode effects as people report being happier on weekends and during over-the-phone data collection versus face-to-face measures for instance (Dolan & Kavetsos, 2016; Kavetsos, Dimitriadou, & Dolan, 2014; Ryan, Bernstein, & Brown, 2010). The effects of priming should also be monitored as individuals in a good mood are more likely to recall more positive life events and thereby influence their own life assessment (Schwarz & Strack, 1999). Children are considered able to evaluate their own wellbeing from approximately the age of 11 (OECD, 2013), thus appropriately age-related measures may be given to children; these may best be administered by schools. The elderly and non-working population should also be part of this collection.

Both the degree to which people experience wellbeing and sources from which wellbeing springs are important. Assessments should, thus, include both evaluative and experiential measures to gather data regarding how people experience their lives (i.e., the frequency of positive and negative emotions), how people evaluate their lives (i.e., whether their life coincides with their dreams and how their life compares to the lives of others), as well as how individuals function across various life domains (e.g., do they perform well at work and do they parent appropriately?). Supporting these data requirements, both the Experience Sampling Method and the Day Reconstruction Method are additional useful methodological approaches. The Experience Sampling Method (ESM) (Larson & Csikszentmihalyi, 1983) provides real-time self-report data on how individuals feel at any given moment and what they are doing. Although labor intensive, it provides thousands of data points over a short duration (Aan het Rot, Hogenelst, & Schoevers, 2012). ESM is considered highly accurate with ratings correlating with relevant physiological responses (Steptoe, Wardle, & Marmot, 2005). Alternatively, the Day Reconstruction Method (DRM; Kahneman, Krueger, Schkade, Schwarz, & Stone, 2004) asks individuals to reconstruct their past 24 h with the same information. Both the ESM and DRM are less susceptible to recall biases than are subjective wellbeing methods (Tay, Chan, & Diener, 2014).

As for the questions themselves, order is a consideration. Subjective wellbeing measures should always be asked before socio-demographic factors so as not to influence wellbeing responses positively or negatively. Further, it is wise to position the most important measures early on to avoid the effects of survey fatigue. Transition questions or text to break up long segments and indicate that a new category has begun are further methods to refocus respondent attention. Question order should flow from the general to the specific. Positive and negative wording should be alternated (positive-negative-positive-negative) to reduce an "order effect" wherein a long string of negative affect words bias the following string of positive ones or vice versa.

As with all forms of data collection, age is a consideration. Researchers relying on social media, like Tweets for instance should remember that these methods are skewed towards younger users adept in their use (Adler & Seligman, 2016). Yet, in a study conducted by Schwartz et al. (2013), Facebook status updates from 75,000 young volunteers were considered reasonably approximate facsimiles of the settings in which both older and younger age groups are equally present and experienced. This suggests that social media data can still be useful, even if it is not highly representative. Nonetheless, to ensure that a broad population view is captured, the inclusion of qualitative data is recommended, for example from interviews, focus groups, and other ethnographic means that capture cultural or spiritual aspects of wellbeing not elicited by standard measures. Such data collection can be reserved for the elderly, children, or those otherwise not accounted for by current collection methods.

10.6 Conclusion

We feel it necessary to conclude with some thoughts on the implications of collecting data. The temptation to engineer situations or nudge constituents towards greater wellbeing can be great, and this raises ethical questions that must be judiciously considered (Benartzi et al., 2017; Vlaev, King, Dolan, & Darzi, 2016). Every day, governments make decisions to improve the quality of their constituents' lives, decisions like prohibiting smoking, lowering speed limits, and imposing mandatory school attendance. Other measures aim to enrich environments and facilitate opportunities to achieve greater wellbeing (Diener & Tay, 2016). Yet, when nations strive to be ranked first on all indicators of happiness and wellbeing, the pressure on constituents to "be happy" can backfire. Active boycotts of wellbeing and happiness agendas can occur. Worse, happiness and wellbeing levels can actually decline as a consequence of the constant pressure to exhibit and experience a hedonic form of happiness, where positive emotions and experiences become the expected norm (Frey & Stutzer, 2007). Pressure to be happy can be off-putting to less expressive individuals. It can be incongruent with cultures which prioritize other values more highly than happiness, such as religiosity, justice, freedom, or duty to family (Frey & Stutzer, 2007), or where a fear of happiness is the norm (Joshanloo et al., 2014). The promotion of happiness may suggest that negative emotions are dysfunctional or at best, undesirable. However, positive emotionality is in fact not always adaptive nor sufficient for a complete state of mental health and wellbeing (Gruman, Lumley, & Gonzalez-Morales, 2018; Hervás, 2017). Unfortunately, positive psychology, with its focus on individual and social flourishing, has unwittingly contributed to this. Nonetheless, it should be remembered that it did so by addressing professionals in the field in a bid to rebalance psychology away from an exclusive focus on the negative and not because negative emotions were problematic. Second-wave positive psychology (Ivtzan, Lomas, Hefferon, & Worth, 2015), which posits that a true state of wellbeing comes from capitalizing on the positive and managing the negative to achieve a good life, is now gaining strength (see also Wong, 2011).

The measurement of wellbeing is a complex field. We hope to have clarified this somewhat through our presentation of theoretical models and valid measurement tools. We urge researchers to select those which best suit their purposes, but to be explicit in their rationales for doing so. In this manner, and as the field of wellbeing continues to evolve, consensus may emerge as to what tools matter most in the measurement of wellbeing. By taking a multidimensional dashboard approach and relying on an appropriate array of valid and reliable tools, researchers can better determine who is flourishing or languishing. This data can subsequently support policymakers in a concerted response, yielding targeted wellbeing gains and creating better service efficiencies in the process. As such, governments can address higher-order needs of meaning, social relationships, and a sense of personal agency that lead to human excellence and which can drive nations towards their self-actualization goals

(Adler & Seligman, 2016). Treating happiness and wellbeing as a public good and measuring it on par with other indicators of national prosperity is an important aspect of a smart, responsive and civilized government (Kinderman, 2015; Pykett & Cromby, 2017; Thin, 2011) and necessarily relies on the accurate collection of data.

References

Aan het Rot, M., Hogenelst, K., & Schoevers, R. A. (2012). Mood disorders in everyday life: A systematic review of experience sampling and ecological momentary assessment studies. *Clinical Psychology Review, 32*(6), 510–523.

Abbott, R. A., Ploubidis, G. B., Huppert, F. A., Kuh, D., Wadsworth, M. E., & Croudace, T. J. (2006). Psychometric evaluation and predictive validity of Ryff's psychological wellbeing items in a UK birth cohort sample of women. *Health and Quality of Life Outcomes, 4,* 76.

Adler, A., & Seligman, M. E. P. (2016). Using wellbeing for public policy: Theory, measurement, and recommendations. *International Journal of Wellbeing, 6*(1), 1–35.

Ahuvia, A. C. (2002). Individualism/collectivism and cultures of happiness: A theoretical conjecture on the relationship between consumption, culture and subjective wellbeing at the national level. *Journal of Happiness Studies, 3*(1), 23–36.

Alcock, I., White, M. P., Wheeler, B. W., Fleming, L. E., & Depledge, M. H. (2014). Longitudinal effects on mental health of moving to greener and less green urban areas. *Environmental Science and Technology, 48*(2), 1247–1255.

Areepattamannil, S., & Hashim, J. (2017). The Questionnaire for Eudaimonic Wellbeing (QEWB): Psychometric properties in a non-western adolescent sample. *Personality and Individual Differences, 117,* 236–241.

Astell-Burt, T., Feng, X., & Kolt, G. S. (2013). Does access to neighbourhood green space promote a healthy duration of sleep? Novel findings from a cross-sectional study of 259 319 Australians. *British Medical Journal Open, 3,* e003094.

Bakker, A., Burger, M., van Haren, P., Oerlemans, W., & Veenhoven, R. (2015). *Happiness raised by raising awareness: Effect of happiness using the happiness indicator.* EHERO Working Paper 2015/01 310714-01. Retrieved from https://personal.eur.nl/veenhoven/Pub2010s/2015i-full.pdf.

Ballas, D., & Dorling, D. (2013). The geography of happiness. In S. A. David, I. Boniwell & A. Conley Ayers (Eds.), *Oxford handbook of happiness* (pp. 465–481). Oxford, UK: Oxford University Press.

Ballas, D., & Tranmer, M. (2012). Happy people or happy places? A multilevel modeling approach to the analysis of happiness and wellbeing. *International Regional Science Review, 35*(1), 70–102.

Baumeister, R. F., Vohs, K. D., & Funder, D. C. (2007). Psychology as the science of self-reports and finger movements: Whatever happened to actual behavior? *Perspectives on Psychological Science, 2,* 396–403.

Beck, A. T., Steer, R. A., & Brown, G. K. (1996). *Manual for the Beck Depression Inventory-II.* San Antonio, TX: Psychological Corporation.

Beck, A. T., Steer, R. A., & Garbin, M. G. (1988). Psychometric properties of the Beck Depression Inventory: Twenty-five years of evaluation. *Clinical Psychology Review, 8*(1), 77–100.

Benzarti, S., Beshears, J., Milkman, K., Sunstein, C. R., Thaler, R. H., Shankar, M., … Galing, S. (2017). Should governments invest more in nudging? *Psychological Science, 28*(8), 1041–1055.

Binder, M. (2014). Subjective wellbeing capabilities: Bridging the gap between the capability approach and subjective wellbeing research. *Journal of Happiness Studies, 15*(5), 1197–1217.

Black, A. E., & Deci, E. L. (2000). The effects of instructors' autonomy support and students' autonomous motivation on learning organic chemistry: A self-determination theory perspective. *Science Education, 84,* 740–756.

Bronsteen, J., Buccafusco, C., & Masur, J. S. (2014). *Wellbeing and public policy*. Coase-Sandor Working Paper Series in Law and Economics No. 707. Retrieved from http://chicagounbound.uchicago.edu/cgi/viewcontent.cgi?article=2395&context=law_and_economics.

Cacioppo, J. T., Hawkley, L. C., & Berntson, G. G. (2003). The anatomy of loneliness. *Current Directions in Psychological Science, 12*, 71–74.

Canaviri, J. A. (2016). Measuring the concept of "wellbeing": A first approach for Bolivia. *International Journal of Wellbeing, 6*(1), 36–80.

Capaldi, C. A., Dopko, R. L., & Zelenski, J. M. (2014). The relationship between nature connectedness and happiness: A meta-analysis. *Frontiers in Psychology, 5*, 976.

Capaldi, C. A., Passmore, H.-A., Nisbet, E. K., Zelenski, J. M., & Dopko, R. L. (2015). Flourishing in nature: A review of the benefits of connecting with nature and its application as a wellbeing intervention. *International Journal of Wellbeing, 5*, 1–16.

Carlisle, S., Henderson, G., & Hanlon, P. (2009). 'Wellbeing': A collateral casualty of modernity? *Social Science and Medicine, 69*, 1556–1560.

Cervinka, R., Röderer, K., & Hefler, E. (2012). Are nature lovers happy? On various indicators of wellbeing and connectedness with nature. *Journal of Health Psychology, 17*, 379–388.

Chartier, M. J., Finlayson, G., Prior, H., McGowan, K.-L., Chen, H., Walld, R., & De Rocquigny, J. (2014). Are there mental health differences between francophone and non-francophone populations in Manitoba? *Canadian Journal of Psychiatry/Revue Canadienne de Psychiatrie, 59*(7), 366–375.

Coffey, J. K., Wray-Lake, L., Mashek, D., & Branand, B. (2014). A multi-study examination of wellbeing theory in college and community samples. *Journal of Happiness Studies, 17*(1), 187–211.

Cooke, P. J., Melchert, T. P., & Connor, K. (2016). Measuring wellbeing: A review of instruments. *Counseling Psychologist, 44*(5), 730–757.

Cromby, J. (2011). The greatest gift? Happiness, governance, and psychology. *Social and Personality Psychology Compass, 5*(11), 840–852.

Cummins, R. A., Eckersley, R., Pallant, J., Van Vugt, J., & Misajon, R. (2003). Developing a national index of subjective wellbeing: The Australian Unity Wellbeing Index. *Social Indicators Research, 64*(2), 159–190.

Diener, E. (1984). Subjective wellbeing. *Psychological Bulletin, 95*, 542–575.

Diener, E., Emmons, R. A., Larsen, R. J., & Griffin, S. (1985). The satisfaction with life scale. *Journal of Personality Assessment, 49*, 71–75.

Diener, E., Oishi, S., & Lucas, R. E. (2015). National accounts of subjective wellbeing. *American Psychologist, 70*(3), 234–242.

Diener, E., & Ryan, K. (2009). Subjective wellbeing: A general overview. *South African Journal of Psychology, 39*(4), 391–406.

Diener, E., & Seligman, M. E. P. (2004). Beyond money: Toward an economy of wellbeing. *Psychological Science in the Public Interest, 5*(10), 1–31.

Diener, E., & Tay, L. (2016). New frontiers: Societal measures of subjective wellbeing for input to policy. In L. Bruni & P. L. Porta (Eds.), *Handbook of research methods and applications in happiness and quality of life* (pp. 35–52). Northhampton, MA: Edward Elgar Publishing.

Diener, E., Tay, L., & Myers, D. G. (2011). The religion paradox: If religion makes people happy, why are so many dropping out? *Journal of Personality and Social Psychology, 101*(6), 1278–1290.

Diener, E., Wirtz, D., Tov, W., Kim-Prieto, C., Choi, D.-W., Oishi, S., et al. (2009). New measures of wellbeing: Flourishing and positive and negative feelings. *Social Indicators Research, 39*, 247–266.

Diener, E., Wirtz, D., Tov, W., Kim-Prieto, C., Choi, D.-W., Oishi, S., et al. (2010). New wellbeing measures: Short scales to assess flourishing and positive and negative feelings. *Social Indicators Research, 97*, 143–156.

Dolan, P., & Kavetsos, G. (2016). Happy talk: Mode of administration effects on subjective wellbeing. *Journal of Happiness Studies, 17*(3), 1273–1291.

Donovan, G. H., Michael, Y. L., Butry, D. T., Sullivan, A. D., & Chase, J. M. (2011). Urban trees and the risk of poor birth outcomes. *Health Place, 17,* 390–393.

Dwairy, M., Achoui, M., Abouserie, R., & Farah, A. (2006). Parenting styles, individuation, and mental health of Arab adolescents: A third cross-regional research study. *Journal of Cross Cultural Psychology, 37*(3), 262–272.

Epley, D. R., & Mohan, M. (2008). A method of assembling cross-sectional indicators into a community quality-of-life. *Social Indicators Research, 88,* 281–296.

Evans, B. F., Zimmerman, E., Woolf, S. H., & Haley, A. D. (2012). *Social determinants of health and crime in post-Katrina Orleans Parish.* Richmond, USA: Virginia Commonwealth University Center on Human Needs. Retrieved from http://www.societyhealth.vcu.edu/media/society-health/pdf/PMReport_Orleans_Parish.pdf.

Forgeard, M. J. C., Jayawickreme, E., Kern, M., & Seligman, M. E. P. (2011). Doing the right thing: Measuring wellbeing for public policy. *International Journal of Wellbeing, 1*(1), 79–106.

Fortin, N., Helliwell, J. F., & Wang, S. (2015). How does subjective wellbeing vary around the world by gender and age? In J. F. Helliwell, R. Layard, & J. Sachs (Eds.), *World Happiness Report 2015* (pp. 42–71). New York, NY: Sustainable Development Solutions Network.

Frey, B. S., & Stutzer, A. (2007). *Should national happiness be maximized?* Zurich IEER Working Paper No. 306. Retrieved from http://econpapers.repec.org/paper/crawpaper/2006-26.htm.

Frey, B. S., & Stutzer, A. (2017). *Public choice and happiness.* CREMA: Center for Research in Economics, Management and the Arts Working Paper No. 2017-03. Retrieved from http://www.crema-research.ch/papers/2017-03.pdf.

Gagné, M., & Deci, E. L. (2005). Self-determination theory and work motivation. *Journal of Organizational Behavior, 4,* 331–362.

Gallup. (2017). *Gallup 2017 global emotions report.* Retrieved from http://news.gallup.com/reports/212648/gallup-global-emotions-report-2017.aspx.

Gander, F., Proyer, R. T., & Ruch, W. (2016). Positive psychology interventions addressing pleasure, engagement, meaning, positive relationships, and accomplishment increase wellbeing and ameliorate depressive symptoms: A randomized, placebo-controlled online study. *Frontiers in Psychology, 7,* Article 686.

Goodman, F. R., Disabato, D. J., Kashdan, T. B., & Kauffman, S. B. (2018). Measuring wellbeing: A comparison of subjective wellbeing and PERMA. *The Journal of Positive Psychology, 13*(4), 321–332.

Gropper, D. M., Lawson, R. A., & Thorne, J. T., Jr. (2011). Economic freedom and happiness. *The Cato Journal, 31,* 237–255.

Gruman, J. A., Lumley, M. N., & Gonzalez-Morales, M. G. (2018). Incorporating balance: Challenges and opportunities for positive psychology. *Canadian Psychology, 59*(1), 54–64.

Gundlach, E., & Opfinger, M. (2011). *Religiosity as a determinant of happiness.* GIGA, German Institute of Global and Area Studies Working Paper No. 163. Retrieved from http://repec.giga-hamburg.de/pdf/giga_11_wp163_gundlach-opfinger.pdf.

Hart, K. E., & Sasso, T. (2011). Mapping the contours of contemporary positive psychology. *Canadian Psychology, 52*(2), 82–92.

Helliwell, J. F., & Barrington-Leigh, C. P. (2010). Measuring and understanding subjective wellbeing. *Canadian Journal of Economics, 43*(3), 729–753.

Helliwell, J. F., Layard, R., & Sachs, J. (2012). Some policy implications. In J. Helliwell, R. Layard & J. Sachs (Eds.), *World Happiness Report* (pp. 90–107). Retrieved from http://worldhappiness.report/download/.

Henry, J. D., & Crawford, J. R. (2005). The short-form version of the depression anxiety stress scales (DASS-21): Construct validity and normative data in a large non-clinical sample. *The British Journal of Clinical Psychology, 44*(Part 2), 227–239.

Hervás, G. (2017). The limits of positive interventions. *Papeles del Psicólogo/Psychologist Papers, 38*(1), 42–49.

Holt-Lunstad, J., Smith, T. B., Baker, M., Harris, T., & Stephenson, D. (2015). Loneliness and social isolation as risk factors for mortality: A meta-analytic review. *Perspectives on Psychological Science, 10*(2), 227–237.

International Wellbeing Group. (2006). *Personal Wellbeing Index* (4th ed.) Melbourne, Australia: Australian Centre on Quality of Life, Deakin University.

Ivtzan, I., Lomas, T., Worth, P., & Hefferon, K. (2015). *Second-wave positive psychology: Embracing the dark side of life*. London, UK: Routledge.

Jibeen, T., & Khalid, R. (2012). Cross validation of Ryff's Scales of Psychological Wellbeing: Translation into Urdu language. *The International Journal of Educational and Psychological Assessment, 10*(2), 67–91.

Joseph, S., & Wood, A. (2010). Assessment of positive functioning in clinical psychology: Theoretical and practical issues. *Clinical Psychology Review, 30,* 830–838.

Joshanloo, M. (2013). The influence of fear of happiness beliefs on responses to the satisfaction with life scale. *Personality and Individual Differences, 54*(5), 647–651.

Joshanloo, M. (2017). Factor structure and criterion validity of original and short versions of the Negative and Positive Affect Scale (NAPAS). *Personality and Individual Differences, 105,* 233–237.

Joshanloo, M. (2018). Optimal human functioning around the world: A new index of eudaimonic well-being in 166 nations. *British Journal of Psychology, 109*(4), 637–655.

Joshanloo, M., Lepshokova, Z. K., Panyusheva, T., Natalia, A. Poon, W. C., Yeung, V. W., …, Jiang, D. (2014). Cross-cultural validation of the fear of happiness scale across 14 national groups. *Journal of Cross-Cultural Psychology, 45*(2), 246–264.

Joshanloo, M., Rostami, R., & Nosratabadi, M. (2006). Examining the factor structure of the Keyes' comprehensive scale of wellbeing. *Journal of Iranian Psychologists, 9,* 35–51.

Joshanloo, M., Weijers, D., Jiang, D.-Y., Han, G., Bae, J., Pang, J., …, Amerkhanova, N. (2015). Fragility of happiness beliefs across 15 national groups. *Journal of Happiness Studies, 16,* 1185–1210.

Kahneman, D., Krueger, A. B., Schkade, D., Schwarz, N., & Stone, A. A. (2004). A survey method for characterizing daily life experience: The Day Reconstruction Method (DRM). *Science, 306,* 1776–1780.

Kavetsos, G., Dimitriadou, M., & Dolan, P. (2014). Measuring happiness: Context matters. *Applied Economics Letters, 21*(5), 308–311.

Kern, M. L., Waters, L. E., Adler, A., & White, M. A. (2015). A multidimensional approach to measuring wellbeing in students: Application of the PERMA framework. *Journal of Positive Psychology, 10*(3), 262–271.

Keyes, C. L. M. (1998). Social wellbeing. *Social Psychology Quarterly, 61*(2), 121–140.

Keyes, C. L. M. (2002). The mental health continuum: From languishing to flourishing in life. *Journal of Health and Social Behavior, 43,* 207–222.

Keyes, C. L. M. (2005). Mental illness and/or mental health? Investigating axioms of the complete state model of health. *Journal of Consulting and Clinical Psychology, 73,* 539–548.

Keyes, C. L. M., Wissing, M., Potgieter, J., Temane, M., Kruger, A., & Rooy, S. (2008). Evaluation of the Mental Health Continuum-Short Form (MHC-SF) in Swetsana-speaking South Africans. *Clinical Psychology and Psychotherapy, 15,* 181–192.

Kinderman, P. (2015, September 28). *Why are governments interested in our wellbeing?* World Economic Forum. Retrieved from https://www.weforum.org/agenda/2015/09/why-are-governments-interested-in-our-wellbeing/.

Kitayama, S., & Uskul, A. K. (2011). Culture, mind, and the brain: Current evidence and future directions. *Annual Review of Psychology, 62*(1), 419–449.

Kurtz, J. L., & Lyubomirsky, S. (2008). Towards a durable happiness. In S. J. Lopez & J. G. Rettew (Eds.), *The positive psychology perspective series* (Vol. 4, pp. 21–36). Westport, CT: Greenwood Publishing Group.

Lambert, L., D'Cruz, A., Schlatter, M., & Barron, F. (2016). Using physical activity to tackle depression: The neglected positive psychology intervention. *Middle East Journal of Positive Psychology, 2*(1), 42–60.

Lambert D'raven, L., & Pasha-Zaidi, N. (2015). Happiness in the United Arab Emirates: Conceptualizations of happiness among Emirati and Other Arab students. *International Journal of Happiness and Development, 2*(1), 1–21.

Lambert, L., Passmore, H.-A., & Holder, M. (2015). Foundational frameworks of positive psychology: Mapping wellbeing orientations. *Canadian Psychology/Psychologie Canadienne, 56*(3), 311–321.

Lambert, L., Passmore, H.-A., & Joshanloo, M. (2018). A positive psychology intervention program in a culturally diverse university: Boosting happiness and reducing fear. *Journal of Happiness Studies*. https://doi.org/10.1007/s10902-018-9993-z.

Lamers, S. M. A., Westerhof, G. J., Bohlmeijer, E. T., ten Klooster, P. M., & Keyes, C. L. M. (2010). Evaluating the psychometric properties of the Mental Health Continuum-Short Form (MHC-SF). *Journal of Clinical Psychology, 67,* 99–110.

Larson, R., & Csikszentmihalyi, M. (1983). The experience sampling method. *New Directions for Methodology of Social and Behavioral Science, 15,* 41–56.

Layous, K., Lee, H., Choi, I., & Lyubomirsky, S. (2013). Culture matters when designing a successful happiness-increasing activity: A comparison of the United States and South Korea. *Journal of Cross-Cultural Psychology, 44,* 1294–1303.

Li, F., Bai, X., & Wang, Y. (2013). The Scale of Positive and Negative Experience (SPANE): Psychometric properties and normative data in a large Chinese sample. *PLoS ONE, 8*(4), e61137.

Linton, M., Dieppe, P., & Medina-Lara, A. (2016). Review of 99 self-report measures for assessing wellbeing in adults: Exploring dimensions of wellbeing and developments over time. *British Medical Journal Open, 6,* e010641.

Lyubomirsky, S., & Lepper, H. (1999). A measure of subjective happiness: Preliminary reliability and construct validation. *Social Indicators Research, 46,* 137–155.

Maas, J., Verheij, R. A., Groenewegen, P. P., de Vries, S., & Spreeuwenberg, P. (2006). Green space, urbanity, and health: How strong is the relation? *Journal of Epidemiology and Community Health, 60,* 587–592.

Mayer, F. S., & McPherson Frantz, C. (2004). The connectedness to nature scale: A measure of individuals' feeling in community with nature. *Journal of Environmental Psychology, 24,* 503–515.

Mensah, C. A., Andres, L., Perera, U., & Roji, A. (2016). Enhancing quality of life through the lens of green spaces: A systematic review approach. *International Journal of Wellbeing, 6*(1), 142–163.

Moghnie, L., & Kazarian, S. (2012). Subjective happiness of Lebanese college youth in Lebanon: Factorial structure and invariance of the Arabic Subjective Happiness Scale. *Social Indicators Research, 109*(2), 203–210.

Mroczek, D. K., & Kolarz, C. M. (1998). The effect of age on positive and negative affect: A developmental perspective on happiness. *Journal of Personality and Social Psychology, 75*(5), 1333–1349.

Musikanski, L., Polley, C., Cloutier, S., Berejnoi, E., & Colbert, J. (2017). Happiness in communities: How neighborhoods, cities and states use subjective wellbeing metrics. *Journal of Social Change, 9*(1), 32–54.

Mytton, O. T., Townsend, N., Rutter, H., & Foster, C. (2012). Green space and physical activity: An observational study using Health Survey for England data. *Health Place, 18*(5), 1034–1041.

Nikolova, M. (2016). *Happiness and development.* IZA Discussion Paper No. 10088. Retrieved from https://ssrn.com/abstract=2819369.

Nisbet, E. K., Zelenski, J. M., & Murphy, S. A. (2009). The nature relatedness scale: Linking individuals' connection with nature to environmental concern and behavior. *Environment and Behavior, 41,* 715–740.

O'Donnell, G. (2013). Using wellbeing as a guide to policy. In J. Helliwell, R. Layard & J. Sachs (Eds.), *World Happiness Report 2013* (pp. 98–111). Retrieved from http://unsdsn.org/wp-content/uploads/2014/02/WorldHappinessReport2013_online.pdf.

Oishi, S., Schimmack, U., & Diener, E. (2012). Progressive taxation and the subjective wellbeing of nations. *Psychological Science, 23,* 86–92.

Organisation for Economic Co-operation and Development (OECD). (2008). *Handbook on constructing composite indicators: Methodology and Guide*. Paris, France: Organisation for Economic Co-operation and Development.

Organisation for Economic Co-operation and Development (OECD). (2013). *OECD guidelines on measuring subjective wellbeing*. Paris, France: Organisation for Economic Co-operation and Development. Retrieved from http://www.oecd.org/statistics/oecd-guidelines-on-measuring-subjective-wellbeing-9789264191655-en.htm.

Ott, J. C. (2011). Government and happiness in 130 nations: Good governance fosters higher level and more equality of happiness. *Social Indicators Research, 102*(1), 3–22.

Paralkar, S., Cloutier, S., Nautiyal, S., & Mitra, R. (2017). The sustainable neighborhoods for happiness (SNfH) decision tool: Assessing neighborhood level sustainability and happiness. *Ecological Indicators, 74,* 10–18.

Pargament, K. I., & Raiya, H. A. (2007). A decade of research on the psychology of religion and coping: Things we assumed and lessons we learned. *Psyche and Logos, 282,* 742–766.

Pavot, W., & Diener, E. (1993). The affective and cognitive context of self-reported measures of subjective wellbeing. *Social Indicators Research, 28*(1), 1–20.

Pawelski, J. O. (2016). Defining the 'positive' in positive psychology: Part II: A normative analysis. *The Journal of Positive Psychology, 11,* 357–365.

Plante, T. G., Vallaeys, C. L., Sherman, A. C., & Wallston, K. A. (2002). The development of a brief version of the Santa Clara Strength of Religious Faith Questionnaire. *Pastoral Psychology, 50*(2), 359–368.

Pykett, J., & Cromby, J. (2017). Mapping happiness, managing urban emotions. In V. Higgins & W. Larner (Eds.), *Assembling neoliberalism: Expertise, practices, subjects* (pp. 195–216). USA: Palgrave MacMillan.

Ryan, R. M., Bernstein, J. H., & Brown, K. W. (2010). Weekends, work, and wellbeing: Psychological need satisfactions and day of the week effects on mood, vitality, and physical symptoms. *Journal of Social and Clinical Psychology, 29,* 95–122.

Ryan, R. M., & Deci, E. L. (2000). Self-determination theory and the facilitation of intrinsic motivation, social development, and wellbeing. *American Psychologist, 55,* 68–78.

Ryff, C. D. (1989). Happiness is everything, or is it? Explorations on the meaning of psychological wellbeing. *Journal of Personality and Social Psychology, 57*(6), 1069–1081.

Salama-Younes, M. (2011). Validation of the Mental Health Continuum Short Form and Subjective Vitality Scale with Egyptian adolescent athletes. In I. Brdar (Ed.), *The human pursuit of wellbeing: A cultural approach* (pp. 221–234). Springer.

Salama-Younes, M. (2017). Psychometric properties of the Psychological Flourishing Scale in an Egyptian setting. *Journal of Psychology in Africa, 27*(4), 310–315.

Schram, T. (2006). *Conceptualizing and proposing qualitative research* (2nd ed.). Upper Saddle River, NJ: Pearson/Merrill-Prentice Hall.

Schwartz, H. A., Eichstaedt, J. C., Kern, M. L., Dziurzynski, L., Ramones, S. M., Agrawal, M., …, Ungar, L. H. (2013). Personality, gender, and age in the language of social media: The open-vocabulary approach. *PLoS ONE, 8*(9), e73791.

Schwarz, N., & Strack, F. (1999). Reports of subjective wellbeing: Judgmental processes and their methodological implications. In D. Kahneman, E. Diener, & N. Schwarz (Eds.), *Wellbeing: The foundations of hedonic psychology* (pp. 61–84). New York, NY: Russell Sage Foundation.

Seligman, M. E. P. (2002). *Authentic happiness: Using the new positive psychology to realize your potential for lasting fulfillment*. New York, NY: Free Press.

Seligman, M. E. P. (2011). *Flourish: A visionary new understanding of happiness and wellbeing*. New York, NY: Free Press.

Silva, A., & Caetano, A. (2013). Validation of the Flourishing Scale and Scale of Positive and Negative Experience in Portugal. *Social Indicators Research, 110,* 469–478.

Steger, M. F., Frazier, P., Oishi, S., & Kaler, M. (2006). The Meaning in Life Questionnaire: Assessing the presence of and search for meaning in life. *Journal of Counseling Psychology, 53,* 80–93.

Steptoe, A., Wardle, J., & Marmot, M. (2005). Positive affect and health-related neuroendocrine, cardiovascular, and inflammatory processes. *Proceedings of the National Academy of Sciences of the United States of America, 102,* 6508–6512.

Stiglitz, J., Sen, A., & Fitoussi, J.-P. (2009). *The measurement of economic performance and social progress revisited.* Commission on the Measurement of Economic Performance and Social Progress, Paris. Retrieved from http://www.ofce.sciences-po.fr/pdf/dtravail/WP2009-33.pdf.

Takano, T., Nakamura, K., & Watanabe, M. (2002). Urban residential environments and senior citizens' longevity in megacity areas: The importance of walkable green spaces. *Journal of Epidemiology and Community Health, 56,* 913–918.

Tay, L., Chan, D., & Diener, E. (2014). The metrics of societal happiness. *Social Indicators Research, 117,* 577–600.

Tay, L., Herian, M., & Diener, E. (2014). Detrimental effects of corruption and subjective wellbeing: Whether, how, and when. *Social Psychological & Personality Science, 5,* 751–759.

Thin, N. (2011). Socially responsible cheermongery: On the sociocultural contexts and levels of social happiness policies. In R. Biswas-Diener (Ed.), *Positive psychology as a mechanism for social change* (pp. 33–49). Dordrecht: Springer.

Thomas, J., Mutawa, M., Furber, S. W., & Grey, I. (2016). Religiosity: Reducing depressive symptoms amongst Muslim females in the United Arab Emirates. *Middle East Journal of Positive Psychology, 2*(1), 9–21.

Tiliouine, H., Cummins, R. A., & Davern, M. (2006). Measuring wellbeing in developing countries: The case of Algeria. *Social Indicators Research, 75*(1), 1–30.

Toftager, M., Ekholm, O., Schipperijn, J., Stigsdotter, U., Bentsen, P., Grønbæk, M., … Kamper-Jørgensen, F. (2011). Distance to green space and physical activity: A Danish national representative survey. *Journal of Physical Activity and Health, 8*(6), 741–749.

Triandis, H. C., & Gelfland, M. J. (1998). Converging measurement of horizontal and vertical individualism and collectivism. *Journal of Personality and Social Psychology, 74,* 118–128.

Villeneuve, P. J., Jerrett, M., Su, J. G., Burnett, R. T., Chen, H., Wheeler, A. J., et al. (2012). A cohort study relating urban green space with mortality in Ontario, Canada. *Environmental Research, 115,* 51–58.

Villieux, A., Sovet, L., Jung, S.-C., & Guilbert, L. (2016). Psychological flourishing: Validation of the French version of the Flourishing Scale and exploration of its relationships with personality traits. *Personality and Individual Differences, 88,* 1–5.

Vlaev, I., King, D., Dolan, P., & Darzi, A. (2016). The theory and practice of "nudging": Changing health behaviors. *Public Administration Review, 76*(4), 550–561.

Wallace, J., & Schmuecker, K. (2012). *Shifting the dial: From wellbeing measures to policy practice.* Retrieved from https://www.carnegieuktrust.org.uk/carnegieuktrust/wp-content/uploads/sites/64/2016/02/pub1455011624.pdf.

Wang, Y.-P., & Gorenstein, C. (2013). Psychometric properties of the Beck Depression Inventory-II: A comprehensive review. *Revista Brasileira de Psiquiatria, 35*(4), 416–431.

Waterman, A., Schwartz, S., Zamboanga, B. Y., Robert, R., Williams, M., Bede Agocha, V., …, Donnellan, M. B. (2010). The Questionnaire for Eudaimonic Wellbeing: Psychometric properties, demographic comparisons, and evidence of validity. *The Journal of Positive Psychology, 5*(1), 41–61.

Weijers, D. M. (2014). *National accounts that make governments more efficient by making them more accountable.* Retrieved from http://www.danweijers.com/.

Weijers, D. M., & Jarden, A. (2013). The science of happiness for policymakers: An overview. *Journal of Social Research and Policy, 4*(2), 21–40.

White, S. C. (2009). *Analyzing wellbeing: A framework for development practice.* Working paper. Bath: University of Bath/Wellbeing in Developing Countries Research Group. (Wellbeing in

Developing Countries (WeD) Working Papers; WeD Working Paper 09). Retrieved from http://opus.bath.ac.uk/13944/.

Whiteoak, J. W., Crawford, N. G., & Mapstone, R. H. (2006). Impact of gender and generational differences in work values in an Arab culture. *Thunderbird International Business Review, 48*(1), 77–91, 6–25.

Wong, P. T. P. (2011). Positive psychology 2.0: Towards a balanced interactive model of the good life. *Canadian Psychology, 52,* 69–81.

Wood, A., Froh, J., & Geraghty, A. (2010). Gratitude and wellbeing: A review and theoretical integration. *Clinical Psychology Review, 30,* 890–905.

Zeile, P., Resch, B., Exner, J.-P., & Sagl, G. (2015). Urban emotions: Benefits and risks in using human sensory assessment for extraction of contextual emotion in-formation. In S. Geertman, J. Ferreira, R. Goodspeed, & J. Stillwell (Eds.), *Planning support systems and smart cities* (pp. 209–225). Cham, Switzerland: Springer International Publishing.

Part IV
Culture and Religion

Chapter 11
Islamic Perspectives on Wellbeing

Mohsen Joshanloo and Dan Weijers

Abstract The present chapter looks at the Islamic understanding of wellbeing, the good life for the one living it, as reflected in the Quran and the themes commonly recognized in modern Muslim scholarship. The chapter discusses historical and contemporary Islamic interpretations of wellbeing, revealing only slight differences. It also explains how Islam advises one should live in order to achieve wellbeing. Finally, Islamic conceptions of wellbeing are compared to Western ones, revealing that, despite starting out with a similar religious focus, Western views of wellbeing have become much more centered on subjective happiness than Islamic conceptions.

11.1 Introduction

Muslims vary on individual levels of religious commitment, openness to multiple interpretations of Islamic faith, and endorsement of various Islamic sects and movements (Pew Forum, 2011; Pew Research Center, 2012). In particular, there is enormous variation among Muslim communities concerning the interpretation of certain events in the history of Islam (e.g., surrounding succession to Muhammad), religious authority, and the institution of leadership and political power. However, there are also widely accepted beliefs and practices that are considered to be the core of Muslimhood. Central beliefs that unite Muslims include belief in the oneness of Allah, the prophethood of Muhammad, and the Quran as the sacred revelation. Key religious practices that bind Muslims together include *Salat* (daily prayer), *zakat* (annual charity), *sawm* (month-long fasting) during Ramadan , and *hajj*

M. Joshanloo (✉)
Keimyung University, Daegu, South Korea
e-mail: mjoshanloo@hotmail.com

D. Weijers
University of Waikato, Hamilton, New Zealand
e-mail: dan.weijers@waikato.ac.nz

L. Lambert and N. Pasha-Zaidi (eds.), *Positive Psychology in the Middle East/North Africa*, https://doi.org/10.1007/978-3-030-13921-6_11

(pilgrimage to Mecca). Therefore, despite eye-catching disparities in the Islamic world, the basic tenets and practices of Islam are the integrative force behind all Islamic groups and schools of thought.

Although Muslims have been responsive to various historical and cultural developments inside and outside their territories, the overwhelming dominance of the Quranic notion of wellbeing as the prototype of the life well lived is evident in all Islamic eras, and all Islamic schools of thought. Given the absolute and unquestionable authority of the Quran among all Islamic sects and schools, and the fact that the Quran is particularly clear on how a Muslim should live a good, proper, worthy, and admirable life, a rather timeless Quranic account underlies all Islamic formulations of wellbeing throughout Islamic history. The strong influence of the Quranic teachings is obvious in modern Islamic understanding of wellbeing. Representative quotes related to wellbeing from Islamic sources are presented in Tables 11.1, 11.2, and 11.3.

11.2 The Quranic Conception of Human Beings

In order to understand the meaning of wellbeing, the good life for the one living it, one must start with an understanding of what human beings are. Without an understanding of human nature, we might not be able to tell whether the actions and experiences of a person are good for them. So, to understand the meaning of wellbeing in Islam, we first turn to the Islamic conception of human nature. As with everything in Islam, the holiest and least disputed source of information is the Quran. All Muslims believe that the Quran contains all the major Islamic teachings about human life and wellbeing, in this world and the hereafter. In this section, we examine the Quranic conception of wellbeing from which all Islamic schools of thought have derived their particular understandings.

The word Islam literally means "submission" or "surrender". It indicates the believer's absolute submission to the will of Allah. Faith in Allah must be absolute, beyond the least shadow of doubt. It must be deep and enter one's heart (Quran 49:14). In Islam, Allah is of overriding functional importance in all human affairs. He is the creator and sustainer of the world, and the teacher, observer, and evaluator of human beings. Allah is described in the Quran as being omnipresent in every corner of life (57:4), having a close relationship with the world, and being closer to each human being than his or her own jugular veins (50:16). He knows individuals' private feelings and thoughts. Everything in the universe is regarded as a sign of Allah's presence (Leaman & Ali, 2008). The most important thing about Allah is that He is one. Muslims must rely solely upon Allah, which means rejecting Satan's seductive solicitations, never seeking to please other human beings at the cost of disobeying Allah, never following an authority besides Allah, never preferring the will of other human beings over the will of Allah, and never fearing someone more than Allah. To Muslims, Allah is sufficient in all affairs of life, and one's life must be arranged around this unifying principle.

Table 11.1 Quotes from the early Islamic period

Name	Role	Yr. of death	Quote	References
Muhammad	Prophet	632	In comparison with the hereafter this world is nothing more than when you dip your finger in the sea and you look how much water you draw up with it	Juynboll (2007, p. 252)
Muhammad	Prophet	632	Frequently remember the destroyer of pleasures (meaning death)	sunnah.com
Muhammad	Prophet	632	Indifference towards this world does not mean forbidding what is permitted, or squandering wealth, rather indifference towards this world means not thinking that what you have in your hand is more reliable than what is in Allah's Hand, and it means feeling that the reward for a calamity that befalls you is greater than that which the calamity makes you miss out on	sunnah.com
Muhammad	Prophet	632	Whoever focuses all his concerns on one thing, the Hereafter, Allah will relieve him of worldly concerns, but whoever has disparate concerns scattered among a number of worldly issues, Allah will not care in which of its valleys he died	sunnah.com
Ali	The fourth rightly guided caliph	661	The example of the world is like that of a snake which is soft in touch but whose poison is fatal. Therefore, keep yourself aloof from whatever appears to be good to you because of its short stay with you. Do not worry about it because of your conviction that it will leave you and that its circumstances are vicissitudes. When you feel most attracted to it, shun it the most because whenever someone is assured of happiness in it, it throws him into danger, or when he feels secure in it, the world alters his security into fear, and that is the end of the matter	Al-Jibouri (2009, p. 822)

Table 11.2 Quotes from Islamic philosophy and Sufism

Name	Role	Yr. of death	Quote	References
Al-Muhasibi	Sufi	857	The love of God in its essence is really the illumination of the heart by joy because of its nearness to the Beloved, for love, in solitude, rises up triumphant and the heart of the lover is possessed by the sense of its fellowship with Him; and when solitude is combined with secret intercourse with the Beloved, the joy of that intercourse overwhelms the mind, so that it is no longer concerned with this world and what is therein	Vaughan-Lee (1994, p. 131)
Al-Farabi	Philosopher	951	Happiness means that the human soul reaches a degree of perfection in existence where it is in no need of matter for its support, since it becomes one of the incorporeal things … and remains in that state continuously forever	Walker (2005, p. 98)
Abdul Karim Qushayri	Sufi	1074	The servant's love for God is a state too subtle for words. This state brings him to glorify God and to try to gain His pleasure. He has little patience in separation from Him, feels an urgent longing for Him, finds no comfort in anything other than Him, and experiences intimacy in his heart by making continual remembrance of Him. The servant's love for God does not imply affection or enjoyment in the human sense. Describing the lover as annihilated in the Beloved is more fitting than describing him as having enjoyment of Him	Vaughan-Lee (1994, p. 136)
Abdullah Ansari	Sufi	1089	Know that when you learn to lose yourself, you will reach the Beloved. There is no other secret to be learnt, and more than that is not known to me	Vaughan-Lee (1994, p. 18)
Fakhr ad-Din ar-Razi	Philosopher	1209	Induction indicates that perfection is loved in itself. Therefore, it should be said that all that is more perfect will be more deserving of being loved …. The most perfect of things is God, exalted; so He is the most deserving of being loved. The perception of what is loved, *qua* being loved, effects pleasure. And since the perception of the rational soul for the True, exalted, is more perfect than the perception of the physical faculties for their objects of perception, and since the True, exalted, is the most perfect being, the pleasure resulting from perceiving Him will be more perfect than all other pleasures	Shihadeh (2006, p. 112)
Fariduddin Attar	Sufi	1220	If you would glimpse the beauty we revere Look in your heart—its image will appear Make of your heart a looking-glass and see Reflected there the Friend's nobility	Vaughan-Lee (1994, p. 158)

Table 11.3 Quotes from contemporary Muslims

Name	Role	Yr. of death	Quote	References
Amina Wadud	Islamic Modernist	–	The Quran does not promise us a life of ease, while it does give indications of how to live a life of struggle and surrender in order to achieve peace and beauty here on earth as a movement toward the Ultimate	Wadud (2008, p. 6)
Mahmood Ahmadinejad	Political Islamist	–	No purposeful movement is possible without a plan; the Quran provides the plan for moving towards perfection, happiness, and actualizing the divine human potential	president.ir 5 July 2013
Ruhollah Khomeini	Political Islamist	1989	But what is the connection between going to the moon and the laws of Islam? Do they not see that countries having opposing laws and social systems compete with each other in technical and scientific progress and the conquest of space? Let them go all the way to Mars or beyond the Milky Way; they will still be deprived of true happiness, moral virtues and spiritual advancement and be unable to solve their own social problems. For the solution of social problems and the relief of human misery require foundations in faith and morals; merely acquiring material power and wealth, conquering nature and space, have no effect in this regard. They must be supplemented by, and balanced with, the faith, the conviction, and the morality of Islam in order truly to serve humanity instead of endangering it	Khomeini (2002, p. 14)
Sayyid Qutb	Political Islamist	1966	Then came Islam, bringing with it a new, comprehensive, and coherent theory… Islam gave a unity to all powers and abilities, it gave an identity of purposes to all desires and inclinations and leanings, and it gave coherence to all men's efforts. In all these Islam saw one embracing unity which took in the universe, the soul, and all human life. Its aim was to unite earth and Heaven in one world; to join the present world and the world to come in one faith; to link spirit and body in one humanity; to correlate worship… and work… in one life. It sought to bring all these into one path which led to Allah	Khatab (2006, p. 126)

The Quran makes it clear that Allah has created human beings to worship and serve Him: "And I have not created the jinn and the men except that they should serve Me" (51:56). The Quran strongly urges Muslims to fear Allah and His judgment: "Those only are believers whose hearts become full of fear when Allah is mentioned …" (8:2), "…And fear Allah; for Allah is strict in punishment" (59:7). Although Muslims are also discouraged in the Quran from despair and abandoning hope in the "merciful, compassionate" Allah (e.g., Quran 12:92; 16:119), fear of Allah is used as an important motivating force, which intensifies one's devotion. Faith in, and fear of, Allah translates into strict religious practice. Islam "is a law-centred religion rooted in correct practice rather than solely in right belief" (Akhtar, 291). Muslims view the *shari'a*, meaning the path or the way, as a God-given prescription for the right way to live, "the concrete embodiment of the Will of God, how God wants them to act in this life to gain happiness in this world and felicity in the hereafter" (Nasr 2003, p. 75). When the prescriptions of the shari'a are codified into law by human beings, they become shari'a law. The shari'a provides strict rules to govern all aspects of life including personal, social, economic, and political matters, be it walking, talking, eating, sleeping, dressing, laughing, or toileting. Muslims believe that religion cannot be separated from any aspect of life, no matter how insignificant the aspect may seem.

From the Islamic perspective, before great Allah, human beings are no more than slaves and servants. In relation to the rest of creation, however, humankind enjoys a high position. The Quran says "And surely We have honored the children of Adam, and We carry them in the land and the sea, and We have given them of the good things, and We have made them to excel by an appropriate excellence over most of those whom We have created" (Quran 17:70). Humankind is titled as Allah's viceregent on Earth (Quran 2:30). As viceregent, humankind is believed to be an earthly representative of God that exercises powers delegated by God.

Quranic verses confirm the existence of a decent nature for humankind; for example, "We have indeed created man in the best of moulds" (Quran 95:4) and "by nature upright" (Quran 30:30). The Quran states that humankind's unique potential justifies its creation (Quran 2:30–33), and gives it superiority over the rest of creation. What is this positive side to humanity that the Quran finds highly admirable? In the Quranic narrative of creation, we read that Allah breathed His own spirit into the first human being, thus granting it life (Quran, 32:9), and created human beings with an innate inclination for good (*fitrah*). *Fitrah* creates an important motivational force in the human personality, prompting humans to be pious, to devote to the will of Allah and follow the shari'a. Thus, according to Islam, human beings are born with an inclination to surrender to Allah and live a proper life, the right life for God's chosen creations (Joshanloo, 2013). True prophets delivering Allah's revelation are considered an external force that strengthens human beings' God-given internal guidance. Human beings have free will, and so are free to choose to surrender to Allah and follow the shari'a. And if human beings act rightly in this way, they will attain the greatness that is praised in the Quran, they will be rewarded with the great bounties of heaven.

But the dark side of human nature is also acknowledged in Islam. It is recognized in Quranic passages that human beings also possess destructive dispositions, which stem from the carnal or devilish side of human nature. According to the Quran, humans are prone to sinful behavior, having the natural disposition to be forgetful, ignorant, selfish, and disobedient, and even to commit acts of cruelty and murder (Akhtar, 2008). For example, the average human being is described in the Quran as "a tyrant and a fool" (33:72). Islam recognizes external influences that reinforce this wicked internal disposition, including environmental and satanic pressures. Satan is depicted as a powerful omnipresent entity that constantly tries to interfere with divine guidance by seducing human beings into disobeying Allah. In light of human beings' innate negative potential, which is reinforced by external evil influence, they are described in the Quran as having the potential for becoming the lowest of the low, the most despicable beings on Earth (Joshanloo, 2013).

These Quranic teachings can be summarized in two major principles, as summarized below:

1. As clearly stated in the Quran, Allah has created human beings to worship him. Hence, worshiping Allah is the *telos* of humankind, its proper ultimate function. This plays out in a Muslim's life as absolute devotion to the will of Allah, and preferring Him over everything else.
2. In view of the competing carnal and pious inclinations of human nature, and the competing external influences of Satan and true prophets, Islam demands that one's God-given God-seeking nature should be constantly nurtured to avoid a rapid descent into becoming the lowest of the low. The Quran advises that one must always be in active opposition to the carnal dimensions of one's nature. Hence, complete submission to Allah is not a status, or one-off achievement, but a never-ending spiritual work-in-progress. One must constantly keep devilish inclinations in check so that they do not dominate one's personality, rendering one the lowest of the low. Thus, to be a human being is to be constantly attending to an internal combat, with the objective of spiritual self-edification and self-development.

11.3 The Quranic Conception of Wellbeing

Wellbeing, as discussed in the Quran, is quite different a notion of wellbeing to that discussed in secular literature. In Islam, any notions of happiness or wellbeing that are not based on the Quran, such as the achievement of material wealth or an abundance of positive emotions, are considered false conceptions of wellbeing. Indeed, the pursuit of such false goals is exactly the kind of path Satan would recommend.

What, then, is the nature of genuine wellbeing, the only wellbeing worth having, and the ultimate goal for human beings? Islam establishes the good life for humans based on the function of human beings. As stated explicitly in the Quran, worshipping and serving Allah is the specific function and ultimate goal of human beings. So, wellbeing (the good life for the one living it) is a life that is completely devoted to Allah. Human beings' pious inclinations and any true prophetic guidance they encounter are conducive to this function. Following the devilish side of one's nature and giving into satanic temptations, on the other hand, frustrates this function. The process starts from within, from a disposition bestowed by a wise and gracious God to His slaves to assist them in achieving the best within themselves. The ultimate good is only achievable through permanent and absolute devotion to Allah. It requires an enduring pattern of activity in accordance with human beings' spiritual nature as formulated within the shari'a. On this basis, only an objectively well-lived life, a life lived in line with the teaching of the Quran, counts as a good life.

In addition to the objective standard of living in accordance with the prescriptions of the Quran, the Islamic conception of wellbeing also has a subjective side to it. The subjective aspect of wellbeing is not as significant as the objective side for Islam. Nevertheless, the Quran recognizes the importance of subjective mental states in a prudentially good life, a life that is good for the person living it. Joshanloo (2013) argues that the ideal subjective state of mind in Islam is a tranquil and contented state, one that is bestowed by God to a Muslim on the basis of strong religious faith and relentless virtuous activity.

To better understand this tranquil subjective state, one should examine human nature with the objective purpose of life in mind. As already mentioned, there are rival forces in human nature: a devilish force that strongly urges us to do evil, and a pious force that constantly urges human beings to seek Allah. In the Quran, these forces are often referred to as "selves". The devilish self is called the evil-commanding self (*Al-Nafs Al-Ammarah*) (Quran, 12:53). This component of human nature is obviously negative, an unhealthy inclination that is in conflict with both personal and societal wellbeing. The Quran recognizes another aspect of human nature, which is closely connected to *fitrah*: the blaming, reproachful, or self-accusing self (*Al-Nafs Al-Lawwama*). This is the Quranic equivalent of conscience, the inner voice that stands up against the evil-commanding self. This component of human nature counteracts the evil self's destructive power (Akhtar, 2008). The clash between the evil-commanding and self-accusing aspects of human nature often engenders internal imbalance, anxiety, and guilt, as the devilish aspects of human nature are acknowledged and battled against, both before and after improper actions. Without the vigilance of the self-accusing aspect of human nature, human beings would succumb to Satan's seductions and perform improper actions without feeling guilty afterwards. In comparison to following the evil-commanding self without a sense of remorse, the internal state of anxiety and regret caused by the clashes of the evil-commanding self and the self-accusing aspect of human nature are considered spiritually superior. The imbalanced state of battle between the evil-commanding self and the self-accusing aspect of human nature is superior to a life dominated by the evil-commanding self because the battle can ultimately lead to victory over the evil-commanding self. Accordingly, the self-accusing aspect of the self is shown in a positive light in Islamic teachings (Joshanloo, 2013).

To achieve tranquility, the desired subjective state, one must effectively shackle and silence the devilish self. The resulting inaction of a silenced devilish self is immediately followed by the inaction of the self-accusing aspect of human nature; when a person has pious intentions and always acts correctly, no self-accusations need to be made. Then, in the absence of internal clashes between the devilish self and the self-accusing aspect of human nature, tranquility emerges. When a Muslim reaches this state of balance, through absolute devotion to Allah, Allah bestows a highly desirable state of mind on him or her, that is called the peaceful, serene, or tranquil self (*Al-Nafs Al-Mutmainna*) in the Quran. This state is described as an internal assurance resulting from the awareness of one's complete reliance on Allah and having Allah's approval of the life one is living. This subjective state consists of complete harmony within an individual in every realm of functioning, and is regarded to be the highest stage of psycho-spiritual development in Islam (Abu-Raiya, 2012; Joshanloo, 2013). Only someone that has perfected their nature in this way receives this perfect sense of subjective wellbeing. The subjective state of tranquility includes an abiding sense of contentment with whatever God wishes (i.e., whatever happens in life). So, worries about worldly difficulties are said to completely disappear in this state.

11.4 Wellbeing in the Material World and the Hereafter

According to Islam, following the shari'a is the path to wellbeing, and sinning is the path to ill-being. Even those treading the path to wellbeing are regularly disturbed by internal devilish forces that incline them to sin. This existential contradiction necessitates permanent struggle to subjugate the devilish forces. In Islam, this constant struggle is called "the major jihad", the major combat, one not with external enemies but with internal ones. Muslims are urged to constantly engage in this internal battle, with the aim of placing all devilish powers, desires, and instincts under the dictates of God's command (Islami, 2003).

Legitimate pleasures accompanying a genuinely well-lived life are acceptable, whereas pleasures that occur outside the context of a well-lived life are strongly condemned in Islam. Islam associates sinning with the pleasures of attachment to the material world. All sins are pleasurable, and inherently attractive and alluring to humans. However, all sins also indicate a failure to recognize the significance of the afterlife over the material life. If one is not seeking worldly pleasures as an end, and one is not attached to the material world, there remains no incentive for one to commit sin.

The Quran also makes it clear that there is no guarantee that through living a life in accordance with the shari'a, one would enjoy a pleasant and materially prosperous life in this world. In fact, there is no relationship between objective wellbeing and earthly pleasures because Allah may choose to test His servants through pleasant life conditions, or He may choose to test them through adversity and hardship. Therefore, living one's life in accordance with Islam does not guarantee worldly comfort and material blessings. What, then, is the point in bothering to lead an Islamic life, with all the prohibitions and restraints that this pursuit imposes on one's living? The response is, of course, that living such a life will be rewarded with a complete wellbeing, both subjective and objective, both physical and spiritual, in the hereafter.

Quranic passages teach that heavenly pleasures are better in quality and duration than worldly pleasures, and thus a prudent Muslim would prefer them:

> "Fair in the eyes of men is the love of things they covet: Women and sons; Heaped-up hoards of gold and silver; horses branded (for blood and excellence); and (wealth of) cattle and well-tilled land. Such are the possessions of this world's life; but in nearness to Allah is the best of the goals (To return to). Say: Shall I give you glad tidings of things Far better than those? For the righteous are Gardens in nearness to their Lord, with rivers flowing beneath; therein is their eternal home; with companions pure (and holy); and the good pleasure of Allah" (Quran 3:14–15).

Piety and fear of Allah and His punishment in the afterlife are factors that assist Muslims in transcending illegitimate, short, and sometimes harmful pleasures of the material world for the sake of higher pleasures, which are permanent and more intense.

The Quran introduces humans' worldly life as an appealing yet temporary "play and amusement" (6:32). The material world can be problematic for the pursuit of objective wellbeing because it can divert human beings from the remembrance of Allah, and may cost the genuine, permanent, and intense pleasures of the hereafter (Quran 63:9; 87:17). On top of that, life in the material world is plagued by inevitable suffering and hardship, resulting from the inherent limitations and imperfections of matter, the physical constituents of the world. Thus, even if a person chooses to be genuinely and completely happy in a worldly sense, that is not possible.

It is worth mentioning that, although the otherworldly wellbeing overshadows worldly wellbeing, Islam recognizes the possibility of gaining some degree of wellbeing in this world. Islam describes the ideal wellbeing of this world as entailing an absolute devotion to Allah, acting in accordance with the shari'a, enjoying a good personal relationship with Allah, and securing one's happiness in the afterlife, which comes with a feeling of assurance bestowed by Allah. The otherworldly wellbeing, the genuine and unlimited wellbeing of the hereafter, on the other hand, is characterized by the presence of intense and relentless spiritual and material pleasures of all sorts in heaven. The highest pleasure of the hereafter is feeling close to God and gaining His approval. Thus, from a Muslim perspective, one's life in the material world can be good and worthy, but the genuine version of wellbeing is not attainable in this world.

Quranic teachings emphasize that the very reason humans are sent to this world is to demonstrate that they are deserving of genuine wellbeing in the afterlife. Muslims' faith is constantly being tested by Allah in this world via both blessings and hardships: "Who created death and life that He may try you—which of you is best in deeds…" (Quran, 67:2). The hardships test whether Muslims believe in Allah's great knowledge and grace, which would allow them to accept the hardship as part of Allah's great plan. The blessings test whether Muslims truly believe that their purpose on Earth is to serve Allah regardless of the conditions of life. Upon receiving earthly blessings, some people might refocus their efforts on the pursuit of more and better earthly goods, rather than serving Allah. The constant tests reveal a Muslim's depth of faith, which indicates the extent to which they will fully appreciate the genuine happiness of being near to Allah in the afterlife.

11.5 Societal Wellbeing in Islam

Islam puts great emphasis on the social responsibility of each individual Muslim. According to Islamic teachings, the purification of the carnal self must occur in the context of society, not outside of it. Piety in Islam is not supposed to lead to celibacy, monasticism, and seclusion from society:

> "God's Messenger, upon him be peace and blessings, declared: 'There is no monasticism in Islam.' He also declared: 'Monasticism for my Community is striving in God's way.' Islam does not approve of holding aloof from people and life in order to attain self-perfection. Rather, it calls its followers to be among people and to work for their welfare, and to consider self-perfection along with the perfection of others" (Ünal, 2006, p. 1043).

Islam regards social seclusion as turning away from one's social responsibility, and failing to accept the reality of life. To be a Muslim is not only restricted to having personal faith and performing individual acts of worship; being a Muslim also consists of acceptance of one's social responsibility, and having an active presence in society (Islami, 2003). In fact, Islam accentuates the public aspect of religion to complement the private one. According to Islamic teachings:

> "Religion is not only a matter of private conscience, although it certainly includes this dimension; it is also concerned with the public domain, with the social, economic, and even political lives of human beings. There is no division between the Kingdom of God and the kingdom of Caesar in the Islamic perspective. Rather, all belongs to God and must therefore be regulated by Divine Law and moral injunctions that come from Him and are religious in nature" (Nasr, 2003, p. 32).

Islam is concerned with every aspect of human life on earth, including the familial, social, economic, military, and political. It is clear from the earliest phase of Muhammad's teaching in Medina, and the Islamic society he established there, that his purpose was to construct a new nation to be governed by an Islamic constitution. It is a responsibility for Muslims to commit to a structure of law and governance based on the teachings of the Quran and the example of Muhammad (Al-Jibouri, 2009). Using modern terminology, the socio-political theory of Islam (as reflected in the Quran and Muhammad's way of ruling) seems to emphasize social justice, social capital, and the extent to which shari'a laws are respected as the main indicators of societal wellbeing.

11.6 The Islamic Path to Genuine Wellbeing

Islam posits that humanity needs religion to achieve genuine wellbeing. This is because Allah, having created humanity to worship him, has implanted the need to worship into the human soul. Allah has bestowed humankind with a God-seeking *fitrah* that constantly seeks to find Him, and surrender to Him. This God-seeking aspect of human nature creates a strong psychological need to worship a higher power, which should be prioritized over other needs (Joshanloo, 2013). Failure to satisfy this strong need in the correct manner hinders the attainment of genuine wellbeing: "Enjoyments derived from the physical, material, and natural means of life are not sufficient for man's happiness and felicity. A series of spiritual needs are inbuilt in human nature, without whose satisfaction the enjoyment provided by material means of life is not enough to make man truly happy" (Al-Jibouri, 2009). Only satisfying one's spiritual needs through worshipping and serving Allah will lead to genuine wellbeing—being near Allah and gaining His approval in heaven.

The existence of the natural inclination to worship God does not, by itself, assure attainment of the ideal end because this inclination may be suppressed by sinning. Muslims are taught to maintain or rediscover their *fitrah*, and follow its guidance. Walking the path of *fitrah* is only possible through strengthening one's faith in Allah, and following the shari'a. True prophets and revelation, such as in the Quran, are perceived in Islam as God's way of helping those that have lost their way to rediscover their *fitrah*. In other words, the external forces of true prophets and revelation are designed to help channel the inclination to worship towards its rightful target.

In addition to perfect wellbeing in the hereafter, Muslims who maintain their *fitrah* and dedicate their lives to worshipping and serving Allah will be rewarded with a tranquil state of mind, a spiritual kind of pleasure far more intense and enduring than the fleeting pleasures of sin. So, even though the perfect pleasures of heaven would outweigh any amount of earthly suffering, Muslims that observe the shari'a and give their lives completely to Allah get the best possible life in this world and the hereafter.

Before closing this section, it is necessary to comment on the role of human reason and intellect on the path to wellbeing as understood by Islam. An emphasis on reason and intellect independent of religious tradition has never been evident in the history of Islam (Joshanloo, 2013). Abu-Raiya's (2012) in-depth analysis of Quranic verses and Islamic theology indicates that the main functions of human intellect in Islam are to contemplate revelation and Allah, and to discipline devilish inclinations. Thus, according to Islam, human intellect and its exercise in pursuit of any material goals cannot function as an independent means for achieving wellbeing. In other words, wellbeing is not achievable through pure rationality; rationality is just one of many tools that can aid one's servitude to Allah.

11.7 Contemporary Muslim Perspectives on Wellbeing

Some contemporary Muslim scholars take issue with the secularization and hedonism that is growing or already dominant in many parts of the contemporary world (Ahmed, 2002; Joshanloo, 2013; Musawi Lari, 1997). They worry that these material values might creep into Muslim societies, which, in their view, would damage the standing of traditional Islamic values, and possibly lead to a complete breakdown of order in society. Many contemporary Muslim scholars warn about the devastating psychological effects that a lack of religious faith, and the following of hedonic pursuits, can have on people. They argue that a person lacking in religious faith cannot lead a good life. For example, Yahwa (2001) claims that the lives of people who do not have religious faith are undoubtedly afflicted by purposelessness and these people indisputably lack the objective features of a meaningful life. Yahwa (2001) also claims that a lack of faith makes individuals selfish and insensitive to other people's needs. He describes an individual who does not have religious faith and does not fear Allah as one who is likely "to commit any evil and ignore all kinds of immorality when he feels his interests are at stake. Someone, who readily kills a human being, for instance, for no apparent reason or for a worldly interest, does this because he does not fear Allah" (p. 23).

Many contemporary Muslim scholars express similar views: morality, justice, conscience, and societal order are not imaginable without religious faith (e.g., Motahhari, 1992; Musawi Lari, 1997). They regard material striving and the neglect of one's spiritual side as the causes of all vice and all the disorders they recognize in the modern world. These scholars blame the materialistic Western nations for spreading "toxic" values among the people of the world, including any Muslims with a weakness of faith. The general public in Islamic societies tend to agree with Muslim scholars on this. For example, as Hassan (2002) points out, although some positive views on modernization can be found among Muslims, a widespread notion is that Westernization is associated with "promiscuity and all kinds of social problems ranging from latch-key kids to drug and alcohol abuse" (p. 136). As such, Westernization can be considered undesirable by Muslims. Examples of such "toxic" Western ideas for Muslims include gender equality and sexual liberalization. The results of large-scale surveys show that Muslim populations have remained the most traditional societies in the world concerning such values (Inglehart & Norris, 2003). As another example, Muslims have also been found to consider the advertising of sex-related products, such as underwear and contraception, more offensive than Buddhists, Christians, and non-believers do (Shyan Fam, Waller, & Zafer Erdogan, 2004). Therefore, many contemporary scholars and lay Muslim people dismiss Western solutions to contemporary problems.

Muslim writers generally assert that to obtain wellbeing, one needs to know all aspects of humankind, i.e., all its abilities, deficiencies, and needs. Such a complete understanding is beyond human capacity. They assert that modern science and secular worldviews have failed to bring wellbeing to humans' lives, due to an incomplete understanding of human nature and especially its spiritual needs (e.g., Musawi Lari, 1997). Only God can show human beings the way to wellbeing, because He has created them and knows everything about them. Accordingly, Muslim writers argue that human beings should try to find the answer to all their questions in the revealed laws of true religious scriptures. Hence, the core message of modern Islamic scholarship is to solve the existing problems of material striving and spiritual neglect through reviving Islamic values, especially as described in the Quran and the teachings of Muhammad.

Contemporary Muslim writers claim that it is religious faith, rather than hedonic and material motives, that must come to dominate each person. An absolute submission to God and living in accordance with the shari'a are key virtues in contemporary Islamic scholarship (e.g., Motahhari, 1992; Musawi Lari, 1997; Yahwa, 2001). The scholars state that faith helps individuals resist the pressures of carnal desires and inclinations, which are regarded as conducive to ill-being and unhappiness. At the same time, and in line with traditional Islam, contemporary Muslim scholars do not prescribe extreme celibacy or asceticism. Rather, they encourage believers to play their proper role in society, which entails staying connected to this world and to others throughout life (Motahhari, 1992; Musawi Lari, 1997). The scholars assert that individual wellbeing is tied to collective wellbeing, and that a person cannot seek happiness independently of others. In other words, residing within a society that does not collectively live in line with the shari'a makes one's own attainment of wellbeing impossible. Finally, in full conformity with Quranic teachings, contemporary Muslim scholars think that genuine wellbeing can only be experienced in the afterlife, which is generally interpreted as proximity to God in heaven.

The subjective turn in the conceptualization of wellbeing after the enlightenment has prompted contemporary Muslims to pay special attention to subjective and psychological aspects in their accounts of human wellbeing. Contemporary Muslim scholars contend that without spiritual beliefs and strong religious faith, a human being cannot achieve psychological and social wellbeing. They claim that religion gives meaning to the world and human life, and that religion provides us with stronger and more permanent pleasurable experiences, compared to which sensual materialistic pleasures are of little value. An example of these religious pleasures is the serene confidence that one's worshiping and serving Allah will lead to genuine wellbeing in the hereafter. The scholars recognize that life has lots of worries, hardship, and failures, and that human beings cannot overcome all of these on their own. When faced with these maladies, they argue that only religious faith can bring them peace and happiness, the tranquil state that is the most desirable earthly subjective state. The scholars explain that faith helps Muslims to overcome any hardship in life because all earthly experiences, pleasant and painful, are divine trials that will enable unification with Allah in the afterlife. Hence, they argue that a religious believer can find meaning and a spiritual pleasure in any earthly experience, even in apparent hardships.

It is worth noting that the existing reviews of empirical evidence in Muslim samples clearly show that personal religiosity and spirituality are positively correlated with mental wellbeing (Abu-Raiya & Pargament, 2011; Lambert, Pasha-Zaidi, Passmore, & York Al-Karam, 2015; Rao, Donaldson, & Doiron, 2015). For example, religiosity and spirituality have been found to strongly predict various aspects of wellbeing in Iranian Muslims (Joshanloo, 2011; Joshanloo & Daemi, 2015). Positive religious coping and intrinsic religiousness have been found to be particularly strong predictors of wellbeing among Muslims (Abu-Raiya & Pargament, 2011). Some of the contemporary Muslim scholars are aware of these recent scientific findings, and regard these findings as support for their claims about religiosity causing peace of mind, even in a disturbed world. In sum, mainstream Muslim scholars' views on wellbeing can be considered as a contemporary repackaging of the Quranic accounts of wellbeing. Contemporary Muslim scholars emphasize devotion to Allah and living in accordance with the shari'a. However, given the cultural dominance of the West in the contemporary world, and with the aim of giving enough weight to subjective experiences (which are considered very important in the contemporary world), they have paid special attention to the subjective and psychological aspects of wellbeing, introducing religious faith as the ultimate psychological remedy for a myriad of mental disturbances prevalent in the contemporary world. They believe that a life empty of faith is one full of distrust, foreboding and unanswered questions. Thus, contemporary scholars claim that *the* way to wellbeing is through religious faith. However, this new emphasis on the subjective aspects of wellbeing does not mean that they have de-emphasized the objective aspects of wellbeing. Instead, to them, all the subjective and psychological benefits of religious faith are secondary to, and result directly from, submission to Allah and activity in accordance with the shari'a, which are required for objective wellbeing in the hereafter.

11.8 Muslim and Western Conceptions of Wellbeing

In the history of the Western world, conceptions of wellbeing have predominantly been religious (Michalos & Weijers, 2017). Christian philosophers like Saint Augustine and Saint Thomas Aquinas combined aspects of ancient Greek philosophy with the Christian tradition to produce conceptions of wellbeing that shared many central themes with the Muslim conception of wellbeing explained above. Saint Augustine of Hippo (354–430 CE) argued that true wellbeing could only be achieved through true knowledge of God in heaven (Augustine, 1948). In line with Muslim scholars, Augustine advised devotion to God in thought and action during life to ensure entry to heaven in the hereafter. In addition to being the path to heaven, Augustine thought that a devout life on Earth would produce a pleasant spiritual confidence that true wellbeing would be waiting in the hereafter. This pleasant spiritual confidence would not outweigh the many toils and sufferings of life on Earth, but for Augustine it is the best people could hope for during their earthly life. Indeed, Augustine thought that the original sin, when the very first humans disobeyed God, made all human beings guilty and deserving of suffering during their earthly lives (Augustine, 1948).

Nearly one thousand years later, Saint Thomas Aquinas (1225–1274 CE) agreed with Augustine about perfect wellbeing only being available in heaven, but described a much more positive possibility for a devout life on Earth. Inspired by the naturalistic account of wellbeing put forward by Aristotle, Aquinas argued that contemplation of truth was the highest good for intelligent creatures like human beings (McInerny, 1993). Aquinas thought that perfect contemplation of truth was only possible in heaven, but imperfect contemplation of truth is possible on Earth by devoting oneself to the teachings in the Bible (Aquinas, 1955–1957). Furthermore, Aquinas thought that suffering on Earth was not inevitable, and that devotion to God was the best way to avoid suffering and actually live a reasonably decent life on Earth (Aquinas, 1955–1957).

Hundreds of years later again, John Locke (1632–1704 CE) also agreed that the best wellbeing was only available in heaven, but he marked the shifting of the concept of wellbeing in the West away from religious contemplation and towards satisfaction and pleasure. For Locke (1975), the wellbeing of heaven and Earth was happiness—the pleasurable feeling of having one's desires satisfied. In the West, both religious and secular populations are now increasingly embracing the idea that wellbeing consists of a kind of happiness that can be produced by spiritual, but also material means (Ehrenreich, 2009; Michalos & Weijers, 2017). The emerging view is that feeling good and being satisfied is the ultimate goal, as opposed to religious contemplation or service. Indeed, this view continues to strengthen as religious belief declines in the West.

So, although there are similarities between Muslim and historical Western views of wellbeing, contemporary Western views of wellbeing differ considerably from contemporary Muslim views. The main difference between the two sets of views can be understood as a removal of God as the prime focus and ultimate goal of life and the replacement of God with the self. In the West, the ultimate function of human beings is increasingly seen as the pursuit of personal happiness, rather than the devotion to and service of God. Of course, just like some non-Westerners are beginning to pursue personal happiness above all else, there are many in the West that share with the majority of non-Westerners the view that religion is key for genuine wellbeing.

11.9 Implications, Future Research, and Policy

A major tradition of research among Muslim psychologists focuses on investigating Islamic culture to formulate an indigenous psychology for Islam. Those working on this line of research are partly educated in religious and mystical studies. This group generally dismisses Western and modern theories as being alien to Islamic indigenous psychology, and are suspicious of secular quantitative methodologies (e.g., Huq, 2009). This group holds that the postulations, methods, and findings of secular psychology cannot be trusted, and thus, Muslims are in need of a different psychology. However, in this chapter, we showed that Muslim wellbeing can be examined under the scientific frameworks of mainstream psychology. We used dominant concepts of contemporary wellbeing research (such as distinctions between objective, subjective, hedonic, eudaimonic, personal, and social types) to examine the Islamic concept of wellbeing. We showed that Islam is different yet also similar in various ways to other schools of thought.

Therefore, we believe that modern psychology has much to offer in delineating concepts such as wellbeing in populations with various religious affiliations. An emphasis on local texts, along with distrusting mainstream psychology and scientific methodology, may generate an ethnocentric local psychology that is disconnected from mainstream psychology. Such an insular investigation could ultimately result in a distorted and simplistic view of human nature that exaggerates differences and ignores similarities among groups of people. It could also isolate Muslim wellbeing researchers from Western findings that could have benefits for Islamic scholarship on wellbeing and Islamic people. Therefore, indigenous investigations could benefit from staying in touch with advances in international, including Western wellbeing research. This of course does not mean Muslim researchers should ignore indigenous knowledge. Instead, we advocate attempts that aim to develop a bridge between the indigenous psychology of Muslims and a culturally sensitive universal psychology.

Around the world, including in the Middle East, governments and policymakers are considering using conceptions and measures of wellbeing to assess progress and guide public policy. For example, H.H. Mohammed bin Rashid Al Maktoum, Vice-President and Prime Minister of the United Arab Emirates (UAE) and Ruler of Dubai, recently assigned Ohood bint Khalfan Al Roumi as the UAE's new Minister of State for Happiness and Wellbeing. A report in The National (Khaishgi, 2016) stated: During the World Government Summit in Dubai last month, Sheikh Mohammed bin Rashid, Vice President and Ruler of Dubai, announced that Minister of State for Happiness will have the responsibility to "align and drive government policy to create social good and satisfaction… We want a government that works on building the skills of its people, aside from providing services … a government focused on putting the happiness of citizens at the forefront of its priorities". The importance of social cohesion, and perhaps traditional Islamic values, can be seen in the phrase "social good". The inclusion of this in the ambit of the new ministry is to be expected. However, the emphasis on "happiness" also seems to include subjective wellbeing, and possibly even satisfaction with life, which is fairly unexpected. We applaud this approach, as it may have far-reaching beneficial effects that are not immediately obvious.

The Arab Spring, as it is commonly known, was a series of peaceful demonstrations, protests, riots, coups, revolutions, and civil wars that spread across North Africa and the Middle East from 2010 to 2012. Surprisingly, many of the countries in which unrest occurred were stable or progressing well on traditional economic indicators, such as GDP. Why would citizens protest when governments were providing most of the goods that policymakers aimed to provide? Using various data sources, Ianchovichina, Mottaghi, and Devarajan (2015) point out that despite economic growth during the period, subjective wellbeing began dropping shortly before the Arab Spring. Indeed, by 2010 many of the countries that filled the headlines in relation to the Arab Spring, including Egypt, Libya, Syria, Tunisia, and Yemen, were some of the least happy in the world. In particular, the middle class were becoming increasingly dissatisfied with their lives.

By regularly assessing subjective wellbeing, governments can be forewarned about negative public sentiment, and take action, before violence erupts. Furthermore, by aiming to enact public policies that encourage happiness amongst citizens, governments will do their citizens a great service and give them fewer reasons to consider violent actions. So, attending to citizens' mental and social wellbeing seems to be a sensible approach—it stands to benefit everyone. But, as noted above, Islamic governments can be sceptical of Western culture and science, perhaps especially as captured by the often overtly Western-centric field of positive psychology. Some of this scepticism is warranted, as Joshanloo and Weijers (2014, p. 718) point out: "Western culture and psychology also seem to take for granted that happiness is best understood as a personal concept, such that an individual's happiness is not directly constituted (but may be affected) by the success, health, or psychological wellbeing of others." This tension over the importance of social aspects of wellbeing between Western and Islamic views highlights the importance of fully understanding Islamic conceptions of wellbeing (and happiness), and the differences between it and Western views.

In order, then, to enable Islamic governments to use wellbeing research to assess progress and guide policy, we recommend Islamic governments encourage researchers to develop models and measures of wellbeing that draw on the more culturally sensitive research by western scholars, while incorporating Islamic and other local cultural values. Islamic governments might even consider working with international organisations to produce models and measures of wellbeing that capture their specific conception of what it means for life to go well.

11.10 Concluding Remarks

Despite moderate variation across cultures and denominations of Islam, and slight differences over time, the core conception of wellbeing for Muslims is relatively stable. True wellbeing is the most intense and enduring spiritual pleasure, and is only available in the afterlife by being near Allah and gaining His approval. The path to true wellbeing is only available through complete devotion to Allah—a deep faith, and continual worship and service to Him that includes being a positive spiritual influence in one's community. The path to true wellbeing is not easy; the carnal inclinations inherent in human nature, and the materialistic seductions of Satan, encourage Muslims to stray from the path. However, through his grace, Allah has also gifted human beings with a self-criticizing nature, and true prophets and revelation, to help humans resist those negative influences and stay on the path to true wellbeing. Staying on the path to true wellbeing also provides a tranquil kind of subjective wellbeing on Earth. A complete faith in Allah enables Muslims to be relatively unaffected by devilish inclinations and the toils and sufferings of life, as the reward of true wellbeing in the afterlife provides a confident and peaceful state of mind that is more enduring and pleasant than any fleeting pleasure that sin might bring.

References

Abu-Raiya, H. (2012). Towards a systematic Qura'nic theory of personality. *Mental Health, Religion & Culture, 15*(3), 217–233.

Abu-Raiya, H., & Pargament, K. I. (2011). Empirically based psychology of Islam: Summary and critique of the literature. *Mental Health, Religion & Culture, 14*(2), 93–115.

Ahmed, A. S. (2002). *Discovering Islam: Making sense of Muslim history and society*. New York: Routledge.

Akhtar, S. (2008). *The Quran and the Secular Mind: A philosophy of Islam*. New York, USA: Routledge.

Al-Jibouri, Y. T. (Ed.). (2009). *Nahjul-Balagha: Path of eloquence*. New York, USA: Tahrike Tarsile Quran.

Aquinas, T. (1955–1957). *Contra gentiles*. J. Kenny (Ed.), A. Pegis, J. Anderson, V. Bourke, & C. O'Neil (Trans.). New York, USA: Hanover House. Retrieved from http://dhspriory.org/thomas/ContraGentiles.htm.

Augustine (1948). The happy life. In L. Schopp (Ed. & Trans.), *Writings of Saint Augustine* (Vol. 1). CIMA Publishing Co.

Ehrenreich, B. (2009). *Bright-sided: How the relentless promotion of positive thinking has undermined America*. Macmillan.

Hassan, R. (2002). Is Islam a help or hindrance to women's development? In J. Meuleman (Ed.), *Islam in the era of globalization* (pp. 136–151). London, UK: Routledge.

Huq, M. (2009). The heart and personality development. In A. Haque & Y. Mohamed (Eds.), *Psychology of personality: Islamic perspectives* (pp. 159–181). Singapore: Cengage Learning Asia.

Ianchovichina, E., Mottaghi, L., & Devarajan, S. (2015, October). *Inequality, uprisings, and conflict in the Arab World.* Middle East and North Africa, Economic Monitor. Washington, DC: World Bank Group. Retrieved from http://documents.worldbank.org/curated/en/303441467992017147/pdf/99989-REVISED-Box393220B-OUO-9-MEM-Fall-2015-FINAL-Oct-13-2015.pdf.

Inglehart, R., & Norris, P. (2003). The true clash of civilizations. *Foreign Policy, 135,* 63–70.

Islami, S. H. (2003). *Imam Khomeini: Ethics and politics* (Trans. M. Limba). Tehran, Iran: The Institute for Compilation and Publication of Imam Khomeini's Work.

Joshanloo, M. (2011). Investigation of the contribution of spirituality and religiousness to hedonic and eudaimonic wellbeing in Iranian young adults. *Journal of Happiness Studies, 12*(6), 915–930.

Joshanloo, M. (2013). A comparison of Western and Islamic conceptions of happiness. *Journal of Happiness Studies, 14*(6), 1857–1874.

Joshanloo, M., & Weijers, D. (2014). Aversion to happiness across cultures: A review of where and why people are averse to happiness. *Journal of Happiness Studies, 15,* 717–735.

Joshanloo, M., & Daemi, F. (2015). Self-esteem mediates the relationship between spirituality and subjective well-being in Iran. *International Journal of Psychology, 50*(2), 115–120.

Juynboll, G. H. (2007). *Encyclopedia of the Canonical Ḥadīth*. Boston, USA: Brill.

Khaishgi, A. E. (2016, March 20). *'Happiness is a serious job': UAE's Minister of Happiness embraces new role*, The National. Retrieved from https://www.thenational.ae/uae/government/happiness-is-a-serious-job-uae-s-minister-of-happiness-embraces-new-role-1.201750.

Khatab, S. (2006). *The political thought of Sayyid Qutb: The theory of jahiliyyah*. London, UK: Routledge.

Khomeini, R. (2002). *Islamic government: Governance of the jurist* (H. Algar, Trans.). Tehran, Iran: Institute for Compilation and Publication of Imam Khomeini's Work.

Lambert, L., Pasha-Zaidi, N., Passmore, H.-A., & York Al-Karam, C. (2015). Developing an indigenous positive psychology in the United Arab Emirates. *Middle East Journal of Positive Psychology, 1*(1), 1–23.

Leaman, O., & Ali, K. (2008). *Islam: The key concepts*. New York, USA: Routledge.

Locke, J. (1975). *An essay concerning human understanding*. P. H. Nidditch (Ed.). Oxford, UK: Clarendon Press.

McInerny, R. (1993). Ethics. In N. Kretzmann & E. Stump (Eds.), *The Cambridge companion to Aquinas* (pp. 196–216). Cambridge, UK: Cambridge University Press.

Michalos, A. & Weijers, D. (2017). Western historical traditions of wellbeing. In R. Estes & J. Sirgy (Eds.), *The pursuit of human wellbeing: The untold global history* (pp. 31–57). Springer

Motahhari, M. (1992). *Humankind and faith*. Tehran, Iran: Sadra. (in Persian).

Musawi Lari, S. M. (1997). *Ethics and spiritual growth* (A. Quli Qarai, Trans.). Qom, Iran: Foundation of Islamic Cultural Propagation in the World.

Nasr, S. H. (2003). *Islam: Religion, history, and civilization*. New York, USA: HarperCollins.

Pew Forum. (2011). *The future global Muslim population: Projections for 2010–2030*. Washington: Pew Forum on Religion & Public Life. Retrieved from http://www.pewforum.org/files/2011/01/FutureGlobalMuslimPopulation-WebPDF-Feb10.pdf.

Pew Research Center. (2012). The world's Muslims: Unity and diversity. Retrieved from http://www.pewforum.org/files/2012/08/the-worlds-muslims-full-report.pdf.

Rao, M. A., Donaldson, S. I., & Doiron, K. M. (2015). Positive psychology research in the Middle East and North Africa. *Middle East Journal of Positive Psychology, 1*(1), 60–76.

Shihadeh, A. (2006). *The Teleological ethics of Fakhr al-Din al-Razi*. Boston, USA: Brill.

Shyan Fam, K., Waller, D. S., & Zafer Erdogan, B. (2004). The influence of religion on attitudes towards the advertising of controversial products. *European Journal of Marketing, 38*(5/6), 537–555.

Ünal, A. (2006). *The Qur'an with annotated interpretation in modern English*. New Jersey, USA: The Light Inc.

Vaughan-Lee, L. (1994). *Travelling the path of love: Sayings of Sufi masters*. California, USA: The Golden Sufi Center.

Wadud, A. (2008). *Inside the gender jihad: Women's reform in Islam*. Oxford, UK: Oneworld Publications.

Walker, P. E. (2005). Philosophy of religion in al-Fārābī, Ibn Sīnā and Ibn Ṭufayl. In T. Lawson (Ed.), *Reason and inspiration in Islam: Theology, philosophy and mysticism in Muslim thought* (pp. 85–101). London, UK: I. B. Tauris Publishers.

Yahwa, H. (2001). *Solution: The values of the Quran*. Istanbul, Turkey: Ta-Ha Publishers Ltd.

Chapter 12
The Life of PII: Developing a Positive Islamic Identity

Nausheen Pasha-Zaidi and Muna Odeh

Abstract Identity development has been studied from a variety of perspectives within social and developmental psychology, with positive psychology most recently adding to this literature. Finding and moving forward with a unified sense of self has been the primary focus. This search embodies the different social contexts to which we belong—in other words, our group affiliations. Although religion is one factor that provides a sense of belonging and purpose to many people, the development of a religious identity has not been explored as much as other social identities. In this chapter, we begin by providing an overview of Islam and wellbeing, including a mapping of the VIA Classification of Strengths and Virtues to verses from the Quran that form the basis of a framework of Islamic virtues. We review frameworks of identity development, including stages of the development of faith. We also look at the link between religious identity and wellbeing and provide a proposed model of religious identity development for what we term, a "Positive Islamic Identity".

12.1 Introduction

The conceptualization of the "self" has undergone numerous iterations, from focusing on the personal to the social and encompassing a variety of constructs and measures to define its features. In fact, the self-concept is one of the most studied areas in psychology and linked to research in identity development through its focus on questions such as "Who am I?" and "Where do I belong?" (Oyserman, 2001). The earliest studies of identity stemmed from social psychology with Tajfel and Turner's (1979) classic Social Identity Theory, which looks at the ways the self-concept is affected by social groups, and how one's sense of belonging to those groups can be a source of pride and self-esteem. Social identities, however, are also tied to a myriad

N. Pasha-Zaidi (✉)
Houston Community College, University of Houston-Downtown, Houston, TX, USA
e-mail: nausheenpasha@outlook.com

M. Odeh
CARMA, Dubai, UAE
e-mail: muna.odeh@carma.com

L. Lambert and N. Pasha-Zaidi (eds.), *Positive Psychology in the Middle East/North Africa*, https://doi.org/10.1007/978-3-030-13921-6_12

of belief systems that come with each group. Sometimes belief systems overlap, other times, individuals face cognitive dissonance (Festinger, 1957), or psychological discomfort when cross-group belief systems are incongruent. In response, individuals may limit the discomfort by joining groups that support their existing beliefs. Group affiliations offer social support and a sense of belonging (Baumeister & Leary, 1995; Haslam, Jetten, Postmes, & Haslam, 2009); they also help people accomplish goals not done otherwise.

More recently, positive psychology research has also begun investigating the question of identity and its relationship to wellbeing (Ajibade, Hook, Utsey, Davis, & Van Tongeren, 2016; Baron, 2013; Giuliani, Tagliabue, & Regalia, 2018; Ibrahim, 2016; Sumner, Borrow, & Hill, 2015; Wong, 2014). In connecting the domains of positive psychology with social identity, the emphasis is on the ways in which individuals develop a *healthy* identity (Rodrigues, Stobäus, & Mosquera, 2016) and how these negotiated social identities contribute to flourishing. For instance, Ajibade et al. (2016) found that ethnic/racial identity of African Americans is positively associated with meaning and life satisfaction and that these associations are partially mediated by religious commitment. In terms of religious identity, Ysseldyk, Matheson and Anisman (2010) noted that "the uniqueness of a positive social group, grounded in a belief system that offers epistemological and ontological certainty, lends religious identity a twofold advantage for the promotion of wellbeing" (p. 60). As identity can be a major contributor to wellbeing, it is of increasing interest to researchers who may be looking for another route to developing interventions that improve health and wellbeing. Indeed, interventions that strengthen religious and/or cultural identity, especially among minority populations, have shown promise (Bierman, 2006; Rivas-Drake, Umaña-Taylor, Schaefer, & Medina, 2017; Tewari, Khan, Hopkins, Srinivasan, & Reicher, 2012; Zamora, 2017). Yet, less is known about the identity development of majority populations and how this may be linked to different facets of wellbeing.

Of interest to our chapter is the religious identity of Muslims not only in the Middle East/North Africa (MENA) region, but worldwide, given that Islam is practiced in both Muslim-majority and Muslim-minority countries. The study of Islamic identity is of particular relevance in the face of growing discrimination and prejudice against Muslims, as well as the increasing fear among Western populations of the spread of Islamic communities into non-Muslim majority areas as a result of sociopolitical strife, war, and the displacement of Muslims out of the Middle East (Wike, Stokes, & Simmons, 2016). Further, at a time when young Muslims in particular need guidance to become fully functioning adults, the answer is not to remove Islam from the equation, but rather to focus on Islamic values, virtues, and character strengths to help Muslims better identify with their religious group, thus helping them develop what we propose is a *Positive Islamic Identity*.

Topic Box: Identity … A Composite of Images?

Who are you?

If we asked you to describe yourself, what would you say? Are you a doctor? A teacher? A male? A female? A Muslim? Consider your description of a doctor. Words like "hospital", "white coat", "patients", and "stethoscope", are likely to appear and you will probably use male pronouns. If we ask you to describe a teacher, words like "tests", "classroom", and "marks" may be present. Here you may use female pronouns. What about a professor? Are you imagining a male or a female? Does the subject of the course make a difference? Now, if we ask you to describe a Muslim, what would you say? Will you find yourself thinking of a man with an untidy beard? Perhaps carrying a machine gun? Or will you think of a woman wearing a headscarf? Or even a face cover? Or will you think of Ahmad, the person you work with?

In this age of mass media, images are everywhere; in newspapers, billboards, TV shows, online advertisements, You Tube, Instagram posts, and even in shopping mall elevators. Where there is media, there is an overflow of images. Thus, your description of a doctor, a teacher or a Muslim will depend not only on the people you may have met, but the accumulation of images you have seen in the media. Here a question arises; do the images residing within each of us solely influence our perception of others? Or can our perception of *ourselves* also be influenced by the images to which we are exposed? In essence, can the images around us inform our own identity?

As media platforms become increasingly accessible to a wider array of people, these are just a few of the questions that arise from the growing power of the visual element. When reflecting on these questions, it is important to note that images constitute a component, albeit a central one, of today's media culture, which consists of radio and other forms of sound, film (including its different distribution channels), print media, television, and lastly the internet. This culture does not merely fill our leisure time; it goes beyond that to provide us with models for what gender, success, or power mean. It even defines our values as it tells us what is good and bad, and what holds greater prestige, all of which is conveyed through images that we, the audience, can often identify with. Thus, media culture plays an essential role in shaping our identities by influencing our thoughts and behaviors, and as such, it is similar to the myths and rituals of the past. However, it is different in its aims, as media culture is an industrial culture; mass produced for a mass audience. And similar to other industries, its products are aimed at generating profit (Kellner, 2003).

If indeed the media is key in shaping our identities, how is that played out when religion is a core element of how we perceive ourselves? Based on the idea of mediatization, the institution of religion, just like other institutions, has to adapt to the logic of the media so that it can communicate with other institutions and society in general (Hjavard, 2008). In other words, media affects how religion is conveyed, and that in turn shapes how it is perceived and then internalized. However, considering that our identities reflect the social groups to which we belong, it is important to remember that there are a number of identities to which we will adhere over the course of our lives, and media serves as a potent tool for the development of these identities. Globalization, which is one of the products of the proliferation of media around the world, has been criticized as a tool of Western imperialism (Sen, 2002), wherein individualistic norms have begun to change the culture and values of collectivist nations (Zhang, 2009), especially among young people, possibly creating identity crises that were not historically part of non-Western regions. On the other hand, Nisbet and Myers (2010) note that transnational Arab and Muslim identities have strengthened in the MENA region due to a growth in regional media. In fact, Ghoshal (2010) contends that in many parts of Southeast Asia, a "global" Islamic identity is developing that shares many characteristics with the Arab Gulf region.

While we should not overemphasize media's role in identity development, especially when there are regions with limited access to literacy and technology, both of which are important for social media, regional polls indicate that digital media and social networks do contribute to the identity development of the young (Dalacoura, Colombo & Dark, 2017). Thus, the concept of mediatization emphasizes the dominating role of the media in shaping our perceptions, including our faith.

12.2 Islam and Wellbeing

In order to explore the connection between Islam and wellbeing, it is imperative to consider the source of Islamic knowledge, namely the Quran and Sunnah, the Prophetic tradition based on the words and deeds of the Prophet (PBUH), and then investigate how these frameworks impact wellbeing as defined by a variety of positive psychology constructs such as character strengths and virtues. Character strengths are the enduring individual traits that are expressed through thinking, feeling, motivation, and behaviors that are also morally valued across all cultures and beneficial to the self and others (Niemec, 2013). When the Values in Action (VIA) classification system (Peterson & Seligman, 2004) was formally proposed, the strengths were considered universal as they were sourced from broad historical, religious, and literary traditions around the world (Dahlsgaard, Peterson, & Seligman, 2005). Given their varied sources, they are congruent with Islamic notions of good character and supported by examples of religious precepts.

The main difference between a secular and Islamic understanding of virtue is the integration of the divine with the human experience. According to Islamic tradition, human beings are composed of two distinct parts—the body and the soul. The soul resides in the physical body and provides us with consciousness. Briki and Amara (2018) define the Islamic self as a "structured, self-regulated, and evolving phenomenon…driven by a mental tension to develop Islamic virtues" (p. 2). Human nature, or *fitrah* from an Islamic point of view, is inherently connected to God. Our development across the lifespan helps us to either get closer or farther away from the purity of the *fitrah* with which we are born (Rothman & Coyle, 2018). Human beings have free will and a desire to move towards a fulfilling and purposeful life. This is similar to Maslow's (1970) perspective which posits that human beings move up a hierarchy of needs towards self-actualization. In an Islamic framework, positive development is the result of choices that lead one closer to God. Thus, Islamic strengths are those that help us align with our *fitrah*.

Although a comprehensive mapping of positive psychology constructs with Islamic values and beliefs is beyond the scope of this chapter, Table 12.1 proposes a list of 25 Islamic strengths and virtues overlapping with the VIA categories. The bolded Islamic strengths also appear in the VIA Classification Handbook (Peterson & Seligman, 2004). The list below was derived through an online search of the term "Islamic virtues" which were then aligned with the VIA strengths model. Only those virtues that directly appear in the Quran, the primary source of Islamic knowledge, were considered. Thus, the Islamic strengths identified below should not be considered an exhaustive list, but a starting point for further discussion on the ways in which positive psychology constructs may fit with Islamic thought.

Research conducted with Muslim populations worldwide shows that Islam influences wellbeing. In conceptualizing their understanding of happiness, a Muslim sample of Arab students in the United Arab Emirates (UAE) noted morality and religion as major themes (Lambert D'raven & Pasha-Zaidi, 2015). Studies conducted with Muslim populations in Kuwait, Saudi Arabia, Iran, Egypt and Algeria (Abdel-Khalek, 2002, 2007, 2008, 2010, 2011; Abdel-Khalek & Lester, 2006; Abdel-Khalek & Naceur, 2007; Al-Kandari, 2003; Baroun, 2006; Sahraian, Gholami, Javadpour, & Omidvar, 2013) found positive associations between religiosity and self-ratings of happiness, life satisfaction, physical and mental health, and self-esteem and a negative association with psychopathology (anxiety and depression). Of note, Vasegh and Mohammadi (2007) also found a negative correlation between religiosity and anxiety and depression in Iranian Muslim medical students and recently, Thomas, Mutawa, Furber and Grey (2016) found the same among Muslim women in the UAE. In South Asia, religiosity was one factor associated with subjective wellbeing in a group of Pakistani Muslims, although income, marital status, and social class were stronger predictors (Suhail & Chaudhry, 2004). Further positive relationships were found between religiosity and resilience among Muslim adolescents in Kerala (India) (Annalakshmi & Abeer, 2011) and Islamic behaviors and positive affect, emotional ties, and life satisfaction (Parveen, Sandilya, & Shafiq, 2014). The relationship between religion and wellbeing extends to other areas of the world: Lavric and Flere (2008) conducted a study of religiosity and wellbeing across five cultural contexts, Slovenia (Catholic), Serbia (Serbian Orthodox), US (Protestant), Japan (Buddhist), and Bosnia (Muslim), finding a positive correlation between intrinsic religiosity and positive affect.

Table 12.1 Classification of strengths from an Islamic perspective

VIA virtue category	Islamic strength	Select Quranic references
Wisdom & Knowledge: Cognitive strengths that involve getting/using knowledge	1. Tolerance	• "Say: 'O People of the Book! come to common terms as between us and you: That we worship none but Allah; that we associate no partners with Him; that we erect not, from among ourselves, lords and patrons other than Allah.' If then they turn back, say ye: 'Bear witness that we (at least) are Muslims (bowing to Allah's Will)'" (3:64) • "If it had been thy Lord's Will, they would all have believed, all who are on earth! Wilt thou then compel mankind, against their will, to believe!" (10:99)
	2. Love of learning	• "Read. Read in the name of thy Lord who created; [He] created the human being from blood clot. Read in the name of thy Lord who taught by the pen: [He] taught the human being what he did not know" (96: 1–5) • "Are those who have knowledge equal to those who do not have knowledge?!" (39:9)
	3. Moderation, balance	• "Fight in the cause of Allah those who fight you, but do not transgress limits; for Allah loveth not transgressors" (2:190) • "Commit no excess: for Allah loveth not those given to excess" (5:87) • "Seek, with the (wealth) which Allah has bestowed on thee, the Home of the Hereafter, nor forget thy portion in this world: but do thou good, as Allah has been good to thee" (28:77)
Courage: Emotional strengths that involve the will to accomplish goals in the face of difficulties	4. Bravery, dignity	• "(It is) for those who believe… when an oppressive wrong is inflicted on them, (are not cowed but) help and defend themselves" (42:36–39) • "If any do help and defend themselves after a wrong (done) to them, against such there is no cause of blame" (42:41)
	5. Persistence, discipline, patience	• "Ye shall certainly be tried and tested in your possessions and in your personal selves; and ye shall certainly hear much that will grieve you, from those who received the Book before you and from those who worship partners besides Allah. But if ye persevere patiently, and guard against evil, then that will be of great resolution" (3:186) • "Be sure we shall test you with something of fear and hunger, some loss in goods or lives or the fruits (of your toil), but give glad tidings to those who patiently persevere, who say, when afflicted with calamity: 'To Allah We belong, and to Him is our return'. They are those on whom (Descend) blessings from their Lord, and Mercy" (2:155–157)

(continued)

Table 12.1 (continued)

VIA virtue category	Islamic strength	Select Quranic references
	6. Integrity, honesty	• "Fear Allah and make your utterance straight forward: That He may make your conduct whole and sound" (33:70–71) • "Cover not Truth with falsehood, nor conceal the Truth when ye know (what it is)" (2:42) • "Take not your oaths, to practice deception between yourselves" (16:94)
Humanity: Relational strengths that involve tending/befriending others	7. Love	• "We have enjoined on man (to be good) to his parents: in travail upon travail did his mother bear him, and in years twain was his weaning" (31:14) • "It may be that Allah will grant love (and friendship) between you and those whom ye (now) hold as enemies. For Allah has power (over all things); and Allah is Oft-Forgiving, Most Merciful" (60:7) • "And one of His signs is that He has created for you, spouses from amongst yourselves so that you might take comfort in them and He has placed between you, love and mercy. In this there is surely evidence (of the truth) for the people who carefully think" (30:21)
	8. Generosity	• "By no means shall ye attain righteousness unless ye give (freely) of that which ye love" (3:92) • "Those who spend their wealth (for the sake of Allah) night and day, both privately and publicly, will get their reward from their Lord, they shall have no cause to fear nor shall they grieve" (2:274)
	9. Charity	• "Be steadfast in prayer and regular in charity: And whatever good ye send forth for your souls before you, ye shall find it with Allah…" (2:110)
	10. Kindness, courtesy, sincerity	• "Allah loveth those who are kind" (5:13) • "When a (courteous) greeting is offered you, meet it with a greeting still more courteous, or (at least) of equal courtesy. Allah takes careful account of all things" (4:86) • "And (show) kindness to (your) parents and to near relatives, orphans, and the needy and to the neighbour who is your relative and the neighbour who is not your relative…" (4: 36)
	11. Diversity	• "O mankind, indeed We have created you from male and female and made you peoples and tribes that you may know one another. Indeed, the most noble of you in the sight of Allah is the most righteous of you. Indeed, Allah is Knowing and Acquainted" (49:13)
	12. Unity	• "Hold fast, all together, by the Rope which Allah (stretches out for you), and be not divided among yourselves; and remember with gratitude Allah's favor on you; for ye were enemies and He joined your hearts in love, so that by His Grace, ye became brethren" (3:103)

(continued)

Table 12.1 (continued)

VIA virtue category	Islamic strength	Select Quranic references
	13. Respect	• "Enter not houses other than your own, until ye have asked permission and saluted those in them: that is best for you, in order that ye may heed (what is seemly). If ye find no one in the house, enter not until permission is given to you: if ye are asked to go back, go back: that makes for greater purity for yourselves" (24:27–28) • "Avoid suspicion as much (as possible): for suspicion in some cases is a sin: and spy not on each other, nor speak ill of each other behind their backs. Would any of you like to eat the flesh of his dead brother?" (49:12)
Justice: Civic strengths that underlie a healthy community life	14. Citizenship, social responsibility and loyalty	• "Do good to parents, kinsfolk, orphans, those in need, neighbors who are of kin, neighbors who are strangers, the companion by your side, the wayfarer (ye meet), and what your right hands possess" (4:36) • "O' you who believe! Always be upright for Allah, bearing witness in justice, and do not let hatred of a people incite you to be unfair to them. Be fair! That is the nearest to Taqwa (piety). Fear Allah! Indeed, Allah is aware of what you do" (5:8)
	15. Fairness, honesty, trust-worthiness	• "Cover not Truth with falsehood, nor conceal the Truth when ye know (what it is)" (2:42) • "Woe to those that deal in fraud, – Those who, when they have to receive by measure from men, exact full measure, but when they have to give by measure or weight to men, give less than due" (83:1–3) • "Allah loveth those who judge in equity" (5:42)
Temperance: Self-regulation strengths that protect against excess	16. Forgiveness and mercy	• "If the debtor is in a difficulty, grant him time till it is easy for him to repay. But if ye remit it by way of charity, that is best for you if ye only knew" (2:280) • "We ordained therein for them: 'Life for life, eye for eye, nose or nose, ear for ear, tooth for tooth, and wounds equal for equal.' But if any one remits the retaliation by way of charity, it is an act of atonement for himself" (5:45) • "Overlook (any human faults) with gracious forgiveness" (15:85) • "(It is) for those who believe and put their trust in their Lord… when they are angry even then forgive" (42:36-37)
	17. Humility, modesty, frugality	• "Waste not by excess: for Allah loveth not the wasters" (6:141) • "Exult not, for Allah loveth not those who exult (in riches)" (28:76) • "Swell not thy cheek (for pride) at men, nor walk in insolence through the earth; for Allah loveth not any arrogant boaster" (31:18)

(continued)

Table 12.1 (continued)

VIA virtue category	Islamic strength	Select Quranic references
	18. Purity and cleanliness	• "Eat of what is on earth, lawful and good; and do not follow the footsteps of the Satan, for he is to you an avowed enemy" (2:168) • "(Allah) loves those who keep themselves pure and clean" (2:222) • "When ye prepare for prayer, wash your faces, and your hands (and arms) to the elbows; Rub your heads (with water); and (wash) your feet to the ankles. If ye are in a state of ceremonial impurity, bathe your whole body… Allah doth not wish to place you in a difficulty, but to make you clean" (5:6)
	19. Prudence	• "Woe to every (kind of) scandal-monger and backbiter" (104:1) • "When ye deal with each other, in transactions involving future obligations in a fixed period of time reduce them to writing… whether it be small or big; it is just in the sight of Allah, more suitable as evidence, and more convenient to prevent doubts among yourselves" (2:282) • "If a wicked person comes to you with any news, ascertain the truth, lest ye harm people unwittingly and afterwards become full of repentance for what ye have done" (49:6)
	20. Self-regulation, Self-control	• "In no wise covet those things in which Allah hath bestowed His gifts more freely on some of you than on others: to men is allotted what they earn, and to women what they earn: but ask Allah of His bounty" (4:32) • "Fasting is prescribed to you as it was prescribed to those before you, that ye may (learn) self-restraint" (2:183) "(Do not follow) the lust (of thy heart), for it will mislead thee from the Path of Allah" (38:26)
Transcendence: These strengths allow for connections to the universe and offer meaning	21. Appreciation of beauty	• "And the Earth, We spread it out, and cast therein firmly set mountains and We have made to grow therein of all beautiful kinds; to give sight and as a reminder to every servant who turns to Allah" (50:7–8) • "Eat of all the fruits and walk in the ways of your lord submissively. There comes forth from within it a beverage of many colours, in which there is healing for men; most surely there is a sign in this (life of bees) for a people who reflect" (16:69) • "It is Allah Who has made for you the earth as a resting place, and the sky as a canopy, and has given you shape and made your shapes beautiful and has provided for you sustenance" (40:64)
	22. Gratitude	• "Eat of the good things that We have provided for you, and be grateful to Allah, if it is Him ye worship" (2:172) • "And it is He Who made the Night and the Day to follow each other: for such as have the will to celebrate His praises or to show their gratitude" (25:62)

(continued)

Table 12.1 (continued)

VIA virtue category	Islamic strength	Select Quranic references
	23. Hope	• "Here is a plain statement to men, a guidance and instruction to those who fear Allah. So lose not heart, nor fall into despair: For ye must gain mastery if ye are true in Faith" (3:138–139) • "What is with you must vanish: what is with Allah will endure. And We will certainly bestow, on those who patiently persevere, their reward according to the best of their actions" (16:96)
	24. Repentance	• "Seek ye the forgiveness of your Lord, and turn to Him in repentance; that He may grant you enjoyment, good (and true), for a term appointed" (11:3) "Your Lord knoweth best what is in your hearts: If ye do deeds of righteousness, verily He is Most Forgiving to those who turn to Him again and again (in true penitence)" (17:25)
	25. Spirituality, piety	• "Celebrate the praises of thy Lord, and be of those who prostrate themselves in adoration" (15:98) • "Behold! In the creation of the heavens and the earth, and the alternation of night and day, – there are indeed Signs for men of understanding, Men who celebrate the praises of Allah, standing, sitting, and lying down on their sides, and contemplate the (wonders of) creation in the heavens and the earth, (with the thought): 'Our Lord! Not for naught hast Thou created (all) this! Glory to Thee!" (3:190–191) • "Establish regular prayer: for prayer restrains from shameful and evil deeds; and remembrance of Allah is the greatest (thing in life) without doubt" (29:45)

Adapted from "Character Strengths and Virtues: A Handbook and Classification Manual" (Peterson & Seligman, 2004)

Other areas of interest within the realm of religiosity have to do with visible markers of religious identity and belonging. For instance, Jasperse, Ward, and Jose (2012) conducted a study of perceived religious discrimination and Muslim identity in New Zealand that considered three aspects of Muslim identity (psychological, visible, and behavioral). Visible identity in the form of wearing hijab was associated with higher levels of perceived discrimination, but also provided greater psychological benefits for Muslim women. Interestingly, they also found that a strong affiliation with the Islamic faith was associated with increased susceptibility to psychological distress in response to perceived discrimination. Religious affiliation, which is mere identification with a religious group and thus constitutes the lowest level of involvement, may not be enough to develop a positive Islamic identity. Studies show that being involved in the social practices of a religion is strongly correlated with subjective wellbeing. In fact, social participation is stronger than private participation in religion. While this research suggests there is a link between religiosity and wellbeing, it nonetheless does not explore religious identity itself. How is it formed and based on what? Does it look different for Muslims in majority or minority status cultures?

12.3 Frameworks of Identity Development

Identity development is a process through which personal identity evolves over time as a result of social interactions (Hogg, Terry, & White, 1995). Erikson's (1963) influential theory of psychosocial development paved the way for numerous studies on the topic. According to Erikson, the search for identity begins in adolescence through the exploration of social roles. Identity is developed from a lifetime of choices and opportunities that are afforded throughout adolescence and into early adulthood. Those who are able to successfully resolve the crisis of adolescence forge a sense of identity, while others may continue to experience role confusion. Consider Amina graduating from secondary school. For perhaps the first time in her life, she will have greater influence over the choices she makes. Deciding which college to attend or with which groups to socialize may be the beginning of her search for identity. If she is able to make decisions that help define her self-concept, she may succeed in forging an identity. On the other hand, if she is unable to come to terms with such issues, she may remain in a state of role confusion wherein she experiences doubt about who she is and where she wants to go in life.

Marcia (1966, 1976, 1980) later expanded Erikson's theory by identifying four identity statuses. Each was determined by the presence or absence of active exploration and commitment to a particular identity. The first status is *diffusion*, where no identity is formed and no identity exploration has occurred. The next, according to Marcia, is *foreclosure*. Here, an identity is chosen, but without exploration, often as a result of taking on an identity prescribed by one's family or society. If Amina accepts a path decided upon by her parents, like getting married instead of going to college, she is in foreclosure. Next, *moratorium* occurs when exploration has taken place, but no identity has formed. Individuals in this stage may be in a continuing state of psychosocial conflict as they look at different options, but do not commit. If Amina is torn between following her parent's wishes, contemplating her dreams of becoming an engineer and the financial constraints her family faces, she may not be able to come to a decision and remain in a state of moratorium. The final stage is *identity achievement* where an identity is chosen after exploration. If Amina realizes she wants to go to college to study engineering and convinces her parents she will marry after her degree, she has consciously decided on her future and reached this stage.

It is evident from Amina's example that in collectivist cultures, the notion of choice and who one can or will become is different than in individualistic cultures. In fact, most of the theories explored in this chapter are based on individualistic cultural norms, which may not fit with identity development in non-Western cultures. The lack of identity frameworks for collectivist and non-Western populations is a concern given that Western industrialized nations only account for about 12% of the global population (Henrich, Heine, & Norenzayan, 2010), yet they put forward the majority of psychological models used around the world. To illustrate, Table 12.2 provides an overview of some of the influential models of cultural identity development in Western, particularly American, majority contexts. It is worthy to note that the White Racial Identity framework may be applicable to other cultural models where power, privilege, or social class form the basis for one's identity development, a notion that was espoused by the famed French social theorist, Michel Foucault (1977, translated 1995).

12.3.1 Ethnic Identity Development

Whereas personal identity development answers the question, "Who am I?" from an individualistic perspective, ethnic or cultural identity development reflects both an internal sense of self as well as the integration of cultural norms and values derived from a collective group into a cohesive self-concept (Jensen, 2003). This notion underlies the relative importance or priority given to an individual versus the group. Many models (Berry, 1997; Cross, 1991; Helms, 1990; Nadal, 2011; Poston, 1990) explore identity from racial and ethnic perspectives and many consider identity development as a reflection of one's place in the minority or majority culture, with the underlying assumption that those who are a part of a minority group are likely to deal with forms of oppression that may be invisible to those in a majority group. As a result, experiences of oppression are integral to the identity development of minority groups whereas the notion of privilege is more reflective of majority cultures (Berry, 1997; Helms, 1990).

Phinney (1993) applied Marcia's identity statuses to the development of an ethnic identity that focuses on the process of acculturation; that is, the cultural and psychological changes that occur following contact between cultures (Berry, 2003). To Phinney (1993), ethnic minority adolescents go through three stages. In Stage 1, ethnic identity is unexplored and the values and customs of the majority are accepted.

Table 12.2 Additional identity development frameworks

Framework	Levels of Identity development
Berry's Ethnic Minority Model (1984)	**Assimilation**: choosing to belong to the majority culture other than one's own **Separation**: withdrawing from the majority culture in order to focus on the preservation of one's own culture **Marginalization**: withdrawing from both the majority culture and one's own; loss of identification with both cultures **Integration**: valuing and identifying with majority culture and one's own
Nadal's Filipino American Identity Development (2004)	**Ethnic Awareness**: positive or neutral feelings towards all ethnic groups, little exposure to racism **Assimilation to Dominant Culture**: valuing White culture while holding negative views of other ethnic groups **Social Political Awakening**: anger towards White culture and positive attitudes towards other ethnic groups triggered by event(s) **Pan-Ethnic Asian American Consciousness**: taking ownership of Asian identity and developing a preference towards Asian Americans **Ethnocentric Realization**: feeling empowered as a person of color with a quest to empower others; develops identity as a Filipino and may develop a negative view towards other Asian Americans **Incorporation**: pride and appreciation of one's own culture and other cultures, including White culture
Cross' Black American Racial Identity (1971)	**Pre-Encounter**: lacking knowledge of racial differences, reflecting beliefs of the dominant White culture, de-emphasizing racial group membership **Encounter**: forced to deal with racial inequities in one's life as a result of event(s) **Immersion/Emersion**: actively seeking out ways of exploring one's history and culture while simultaneously rejecting symbols of White culture **Internalization**: being secure in one's Black identity, resulting in less defensiveness towards White culture **Internalization-Commitment**: having comfort with one's own race and development of action plans to address community needs
Helms' White Racial Identity Model (1990)	**Contact**: a belief in "colorblindness" where race is not considered salient; instead racism is believed to result from discussion and acknowledgment of race **Disintegration**: experiences promote an awakening of the disparities associated with racial categories resulting in feelings of shame and guilt **Reintegration**: intense "blame the victim" attitudes develop where whatever White privilege is considered a reflection of the higher aptitude or superiority of Whites in society **Pseudo-independence**: first stage of positive White identity where White privilege is no longer considered automatically deserved; the onus for changing racial inequities is still thought to be on the shoulders of minorities. Emotional support is provided to minorities in an effort to validate one's desire to be non-racist **Immersion/Emersion**: effort is taken to actively connect with one's racial group and be non-racist, including a deep concern for other Whites who have been dealing with racism **Autonomy**: positive connection with White identity has been established and an active role in pursuing social justice has developed

Consider Amir, an Indian student in a secondary school in Dubai that is largely European. He may act and think more like a European because that is his majority peer group. When his parents want him to participate in Indian activities outside of school, he is embarrassed and refuses. He may even hold negative views about his heritage. In Stage 2, ethnic identity exploration is triggered by a situation. In the case of Amir, while playing football, one of his friends makes fun of his Indian accent, which makes the rest of the team howl with laughter. Now, he may decide that he does not fit with his European peers and begins to explore his own ethnicity. This may trigger the identity crisis theorized by Erikson (1963), prompting Amir to engage in exploratory activities such as reading about alternative perspectives, speaking with different people, and experimenting with new lifestyles (Waterman, 1985). In Stage 3, ethnic identity is achieved when one's ethnicity is accepted and internalized. After taking time to understand his cultural heritage, Amir can be proud and feel a sense of belonging to it. In doing so, he also learns to appreciate other ethnicities and belong to several groups without relinquishing his own. In terms of wellbeing, adolescents who have gone through the exploration process and reached an understanding of their ethnic identities are likely to show better adjustment than those who have not or who are uncertain about the role it plays in their lives (Phinney, 1993).

12.3.2 Religious Identity Development

One of the most common ways of exploring religion and identity has been through the concept of intrinsic and extrinsic religiosity (Allport & Ross, 1967), the former of which has been shown to be correlated with Marcia's identity achievement status (Markstrom-Adams & Smith, 1996). People with an extrinsic orientation toward religion tend to use religion to achieve a purpose such as social status, belonging or self-justification (Allport & Ross, 1967). Religious values are utilitarian and perhaps even superficial. People with an intrinsic religious orientation, on the other hand, internalize the values of their faith and *live* it so their practices embody a harmonious unification of the self. These concepts have typically been defined as opposite ends of a continuum with an intrinsic orientation considered a positive religious identity.

Fowler's (1981) stages of faith are an important theoretical framework to consider in regards to the development of a religious identity. According to Fowler (1981), the *Intuitive-Projective Stage (Stage 1)* occurs in early childhood, where faith is a reflection of the impressions that children make based on what they see their parents and other adults do. The *Mythic-Literal stage (Stage 2)* develops in middle childhood, but may be representative of adults as well, and is characterized by concrete, literal thinking. In this stage, children appropriate beliefs and moral guidelines, accepting the stores told to them by their faith communities but generally understanding them in literal ways. Later, children begin to understand that not everyone shares the same beliefs. The *Synthetic-Conventional Stage (Stage 3)* emerges in adolescence and is initiated by the clash of narratives that leads individuals to reflect on meaning. During this process, literalism comes to an end and one's world extends beyond family. Faith becomes more of an ideology that organizes values, but conforms to the expectations of significant others. Beliefs may be deeply felt, but not subjected to explicit examination.

The fourth stage, *Individuative-Reflective,* is associated with questioning the assumptions of faith, as well as its associated authority figures. In this stage, people may leave their religion if their concerns are not adequately addressed. In either case, Stage 4 represents an active commitment and personal responsibility for the chosen faith. The *Conjunctive-Postformal (Stage 5)* stage is generally not reached until middle age. Here, the struggles and questions of Stage 4 give way to a greater comfort in the answers that have been received as well as a greater understanding that not all questions have an answer. Individual reflection is replaced with a greater commitment to community development and characterized by a commitment to justice that surpasses social constraints such as tribe or religious community (Fowler, 1996). Finally, *Universalizing, which* is difficult to achieve for most, describes those who see faith as a common feature of all religions and can integrate many teachings. They can look beyond the norms of any specific religion and find harmony across faith systems, as well as look for ways to put it into action (Fowler, 1981).

12.3.3 Islamic Identity Development

Although many of the models presented here appear to be linear and are often interpreted as such, identity development is a flexible, spiraling process that occurs over the lifespan through interactions between contexts and individual experience. As self-concepts differ based on participation and identification with varied groups, it is critical to look at the multiplicity of identities to which one ascribes and how these interact within social spaces that come with their own sets of norms and challenges. This may be particularly relevant for Muslims living in non-Muslim contexts as their religious identity is not supported within the mainstream culture. In fact, given the increasing Islamophobia in non-Muslim majority countries, an Islamic identity may be created in opposition to mainstream cultural norms.

Peek's (2005) qualitative study of 127 Muslim students in the United States provides an identity framework that is applicable to Muslims living in non-Muslim majority contexts. She notes three categories of Islamic identity development following a model based on identity as a social and developmental process: (1) ascribed, (2) chosen, and (3) declared identity. In the first (*Religion as Ascribed Identity*), being Muslim is a part of everyday life as a child and is not consciously considered. In Stage 2 (*Religion as Chosen Identity*), reflection on one's religious identity begins to occur as a part of entering adolescence and young adulthood. Entering college was mentioned as the most important time for reflection and peer groups such as Muslim Student Associations on college campuses played a major role in this reflection as associations offered a space to learn common narratives about beliefs. For second-generation immigrants, the awareness of belonging to a minority also played a role in reinforcing an Islamic identity. Another factor contributing to an

Islamic identity was the rejection of other identities as holding other cultural, ethnic or national identities was viewed as un-Islamic. Finally, Stage 3 (*Religion as a Declared Identity*) develops as a result of a crisis. In Peek's (2005) study, this was 9/11; individuals reported how their Islamic identities were reinforced due to the need for stronger spiritual safety or the desire to change the negative perception of Islam by engaging in further study to answer others' questions, which served to strengthen their own Islamic identities. It appeared that as Muslims became increasingly associated with terrorism and violence in a non-Muslim majority environment, the impetus for presenting a positive public identity may have become more salient.

Peek's (2005) model suggests that the social context of adolescent Muslims can offer more or less support for the development of a religious identity. For example, if an Islamic identity is chosen in Stage 2 as a result of the exploration of religious conceptualizations that are supported by a strong peer group, what does this mean for young Muslims who do not have access to other Muslims during adolescence and young adulthood? Conversely, if one is living in a Muslim majority country where Islam is integrated into the mainstream culture, what does that imply for the notion of choice in Islamic identity development? It is possible that in the latter case, the norms of society may provide a context where Islamic identity formation remains in the ascribed state as adherents may not perceive a need to actively choose an Islamic identity. In fact, the notion of choosing identity is more in line with adolescent development in individualistic countries and may not fit with adolescent development in Muslim majority countries.

While not specifically addressing the development of an Islamic identity, Rothman and Coyle (2018) emphasize the cosmology of an Islamic worldview and thus provide an alternative model that incorporates the metaphysical aspects of Islamic thought with lifespan development. In defining self-concept, they join others within the Islamic psychology movement in discussing the structure of the soul according to the four aspects (the *nafs* or ego, the *aql* or intellect, the *qalb* or heart and the *ruh* or spirit) as described by the 12th century scholar Al-Ghazali (Haque, 2018). In brief, the *nafs* is the part of the self that leans towards worldly desires and thus may lead a person away from God; the *aql* is the intellect and works together with the heart (*qalb*) to develop knowledge, which encompasses both rational thought and a deeper spiritual intelligence. Finally, the *ruh* is the spirit, or the part of the soul that is directly connected to God and through which a person can find divine guidance and healing (Rothman & Coyle, 2018). Within this framework, the main stages in the development of the self are focused on the changes to the *nafs* with the goal of purifying oneself and thus returning to the natural state of *fitrah* in which human beings are believed to be born.

As religious identity is also influenced by historical and cultural elements founded upon shared rituals, symbols, and faith-based spaces, the interplay of non-religious factors in the development of a religious identity must also be explored. Thus, in considering the development of an Islamic identity, the diversity of the *Ummah,* or Muslim nation, which consists of approximately 1.8 billion Muslims and constitutes 24% of the global population, only 20% of whom live in the Middle East, must also be considered (Pew Research Center, 2015). Although the MENA region has the highest concentration of Muslims in one region, Muslims make up a majority of the population in 49 countries around the world. The diversity of cultures that make up the global Islamic community is broad, yet, as noted by Peek's (2005) study, for many Muslims, culture is secondary to religion in terms of group affiliation. As most of the work on psychological processes has been conducted in Western industrial countries, a fact that is being increasingly given consideration as a limitation in the general psychology literature, studies of Muslim identity have generally focused on the intersection of ethnic identity and religious identity as well as on the politics of identity for Muslims living in non-Muslim (often Western) contexts (Ajrouch, 2004; Bartowski & Read, 2003; Bozorgmehr, 2000; Khan & Uneke, 2000; Naber 2000). Abu Rayya and Abu Rayya (2009), for example, found that both the ethnic identity and religious identity of indigenous Muslim and Christian Palestinians in Israel contributed to wellbeing. Yet, when ethnic identity was parceled out of the model, religious identity showed a greater relationship to wellbeing than ethnic identity.

12.4 A "Positive Islamic Identity"

Intrinsic religiosity and participation in faith-based activities have a relationship with wellbeing in different countries around the world; an achieved identity that entails pride in one's ethnic practices and a commitment to one's cultural group is also related (Mossakowski, 2003; Phinney & Ong, 2007). Similarly, studies of Muslims suggest that an Islamic identity may be linked to subjective wellbeing if it is accompanied by active participation in positive faith-based activities. Given that an Islamic model of the self joins the physical and metaphysical realms through the connection of body and soul, we offer the following definition as a starting point for discussion:

> **A Positive Islamic Identity (PII)** is the alignment of the *nafs* with the innate purity of the *fitrah*, which results in an integrated self-concept that reflects the salience of an Islamic group affiliation such that identifying as a Muslim would be positively associated with measures of wellbeing. Achievement of a PII would reflect both private religious activities and public or social engagement, resulting in greater pride and commitment to the group and realization of Islamic virtues.

The following proposed model of Islamic Identity development is based on existing models of faith and identity development discussed in this chapter and may be worth exploring empirically within Islamic contexts, both in Muslim majority and Muslim minority regions (Table 12.3).

Although the model is presented in a linear fashion, the trajectory of identity development may be different depending on the context within which one becomes, or exists as a Muslim. For example, a person born into a Muslim family in a Muslim majority culture may only experience Emergent and Accepted Identities and be able to find wellbeing within homogenous cultural groups that define one's identity as a Muslim. Participation in public forms of worship would reflect cultural norms, particularly for women. There would be little incentive to change such cultural norms as they are accepted and viewed through the lens of one's social norms. On the other

Table 12.3 Proposed model of Islamic identity development

Identity level	Description
Emergent identity	Religion is taught by parents and/or other authority figures. There is little discussion or reflection on the information provided by authority figures as these shape a child's worldview of what is right and wrong
Accepted identity	Islamic values, as taught during childhood, are accepted. There is a reliance on authority figures and historical, generally patriarchal, interpretations of text. Islam and culture are integrally connected and questioning of norms may be discouraged
Threatened identity	Accepted Identity is threatened by repeated exposure to opposing, dominant ideas. A retreat to religious authority figures, a strict, literal, and dogmatic approach, and increased attachment to historical anecdotes follows. In this stage, a constant feeling of being targeted by a hostile environment is present, resulting in an increased sense of isolation. Differentiation of "us" versus "others" is salient, and negative feelings toward "others" are encouraged
Quest identity	Reflection on Islamic teachings is triggered by significant experiences or cognitive dissonance due to many factors, including disillusionment with traditionally religious figures who do not appear to live up to Islamic norms or lack of coherence between Islamic concepts of justice and the reality of injustices committed in the name of Islam or in Muslim communities. This stage represents an identity crisis, and the inability to resolve the conflicting ideas means that the individual remains in a state of constant uncertainty. Leaving Islam and/or Islamic communities may be seriously considered
Consolidated identity	A coherent and inclusive identity develops as a result of critical analysis and personal reflection of historical, cultural, and sociopolitical factors involved in the ideology of Islam. People at this stage are cognizant of the ways in which Islam is used and misused in different contexts. This is the stage where activism may be seen as a way to improve the state of affairs within Muslim communities as well as between Muslims and non-Muslims around the world

hand, converts to Islam may begin their journey through Quest Identity and move towards either an Accepted Identity or Consolidated Identity depending on their level of social activism and comfort with Islamic cultural traditions in their area of residence. Additionally, many Muslims may go through a period of Threatened Identity, especially in contexts where affiliation with any religion (but Islam in particular) is not supported by the mainstream (Pew Research, 2015).

This model does not imply that all Muslims who experience a Threatened Identity become a danger to the societies in which they live! We believe it is important to reiterate this point as the model should not be used to further Islamophobic rhetoric. In fact, despite the increase in Islamophobia in many Muslim minority countries, such as the United States, statistics show that the majority of terrorism in such contexts is committed by nationalist extremists. For example, the FBI reported that most terrorist attacks in the US from 1980 to 2005 were carried out by non-Muslims (US Department of Justice, 2005), and The Center for Investigative Reporting noted that from 2008 to 2016, right-wing extremists in the US (often White supremacists) accounted for twice as many terrorist plots than those identified as domestic Islamist terrorists (Neiwert, Ankrom, Kaplan, & Pham, 2017). It is also important to note that a Threatened Identity does not only categorize non-Muslims as "others", but also Muslims who follow approaches that are deemed incorrect. In fact, the number of terrorism-related deaths has affected more people in the MENA region, with 75% of terror-related activities occurring there (Roser, Nagdy, & Ritchie, 2018). As terrorism has political causes, whose discussion goes beyond the scope of this chapter, a Threatened Identity may only be one factor in the larger scheme. Finally, the proposed model should not be viewed as hierarchical with the Consolidated Identity most applicable to positive identity development. Instead, it should serve as a model for future empirical work to investigate Islamic identity in Muslim majority and Muslim minority contexts with the aim of developing a religious identity that correlates with wellbeing. Consideration of this framework with the structure and stages of the soul in Islamic tradition would provide another avenue of discussion for Islamic identity development.

12.5 Challenges to a Positive Islamic Identity

The relationship between wellbeing and religiosity is not straightforward. Individuals who are involved in social participation for extrinsic religious purposes (seeing religion as a means to an end—for social recognition or advancement) do not reap the benefits of subjective wellbeing (Dezutter, Soenens, & Hutsebaut, 2006). Additionally, people who have a quest religious orientation, or one in which they are searching for answers to existential questions may have both positive and negative psychological characteristics. For instance, they may show traits like flexibility and self-acceptance, but also experience worry, guilt, and have higher rates of mental distress (Kojetin, McIntosh, Bridges, & Spilka, 1987). Interestingly, Green and Elliot (2010) found that people with a liberal religious affiliation were healthier but less happy than people with a fundamentalist religious affiliation.

Although religious affiliation and practice brings a host of wellbeing factors, it is imperative to consider that extremist versions of religious ideology have taken a central role in international relations. "Despite several theoretical and empirical advances, the struggle to understand how or why religious identification become extreme in nature continues" (Ysseldyk, Matheson, & Anisman, 2010, p. 64). The interaction of socio-political factors with religious identity as well as religious group discrimination may be perceived as greater threats for highly religious individuals given the sacred ideals of religion and its place as a revered system of belief within their social group. Religious zeal may also provide a psychological buffer to personal uncertainty and the salience of one's own mortality (McGregor, Haji, Nash, & Teper, 2008). Additionally, the diversity of thought and experiences reflected in the ways in which different cultures approach Islamic practices could lead to intragroup conflict. In situations where groups feel they are being persecuted, there is a tendency for highly identified individuals to be intolerant of intragroup differences as these may be seen as lending support to the out-group (Matheson, Cole, & Majka, 2003). The current international climate of Islamophobia provides fodder for both intergroup and intragroup tensions, which may promote conditions where fundamentalist versions of Islam can take root.

Although fundamentalism is not limited to Islamic ideology, nor is terrorism a new form of violent resistance to power structures that are deemed oppressive to certain segments of the population (Oberschall, 2004), Islam has unfortunately become the face of terrorism in Western media. Based on qualitative responses from a pilot study conducted in the UAE and Turkey (Pasha-Zaidi, in progress), Western media coverage of Islam can have both a negative and positive effect on being Muslim. It may be particularly harmful for the disenfranchised who are unable to find a sense of belonging in existing social groups as well as those who are looking for simple answers to complex questions (Lynch, 2013; McDonald, 2011). Further, the Al-Yaqeen Institute (Chouhoud, 2018) noted the following areas that cause Muslims to doubt Islam: intolerance of some Muslims towards other people and other faiths, the nonreligious behavior of religious individuals, the insistence by some that there is only one “right” way to practice Islam, teachings about the role of women, the nature of suffering in the world, and questionable and indeed, terrible things done in the name of religion. Thus, the ideology of Islam versus the reality of Muslim behaviors may become areas of contention in the development of a PII. However, initiatives that focus on training new Islamic scholars to reach out to the disenfranchised youth to counter the messages and interpretations of the Quran used by extremist groups are making a positive impact in countries such as Morocco. Interestingly, it is the female graduates of that particular program that are leading the way (Temple-Raston, 2018).

12.6 Recommendations

Islamic identity development programs and policies need to be put in place to link religious identity development with positive behaviors and internal states of contentment. As Muslims consider this world to be a temporary place where happiness is neither guaranteed nor necessary for having a fulfilled life, it is important to remember that positive states of being for Muslims are the result of good works in this life that allow one to have the opportunity for everlasting peace and wellbeing in the hereafter. Of necessity, a PII requires one to follow the pillars of Islam, engage in positive social activities as well as remember that God is the provider of all experiences, both positive and negative. The present life is considered a trial, and one must remember that “with every hardship comes ease” (Al-Quran, 94:5). Keeping these ideas in mind, the following suggestions are offered to forge a stronger link between Islamic identity development and wellbeing.

12.6.1 Positive Youth Development

Positive Youth Development (PYD) is a framework that views young people as resources to be developed (Lerner, von Eye, Lerner, & Lewin-Bizan, 2009). PYD focuses on five traits (the Five C's)—competence, confidence, connection, character, and caring—that, when taken together, indicate the presence of PYD. Competence includes a positive view of one's abilities and actions across social, academic, health, and vocational development. Confidence involves positive self-worth and self-efficacy. Connection refers to positive bonds with peers, family and community, while character focuses on morality and positive standards of conduct based on social and cultural norms. Finally, caring is having a sense of compassion for others. Lerner, Almerigi, Theokas, and Lerner (2005) note that adolescents who develop along the Five C's tend to make positive contributions (the sixth C) to themselves, their families, communities and society.

Research on PYD has shown a relationship between religiosity and positive behaviors and attitudes among adolescents (Crystal & DeBell, 2002; King & Furrow, 2004). Interestingly, King and Furrow (2004) found that religious practices in themselves did not lead to prosocial behavior. Instead, the social interactions in which these were performed, like the religious community, is what mattered. Developing a PII would likely emerge from positive interactions with other Muslims. Community programs and spaces that focus on positive interactions and the exercise of character may be best suited for this purpose. Focusing on the positive traits that embody an Islamic identity, such as those reflected in the five pillars of faith (belief, prayer, charity, fasting, and pilgrimage) as well as the Islamic virtues and character strengths listed in Table 12.1, would provide young Muslims the opportunity to integrate a religious identity into a personal one.

12.6.2 Positive Islamic Psychology Interventions

Positive psychology interventions (PPIs) may provide another route to developing a PII. PPIs are intentional activities that aim to improve wellbeing and can include gratitude activities such as counting one's blessings and writing letters of thanks (Emmons & McCullough, 2003; Lyubomirsky, Sheldon, & Schkade, 2005), savoring interventions such as revisiting positive memories, noticing positive aspects of one's present, and anticipating positive future events (Bryant & Veroff, 2007; Bryant, Chadwick, & Kluwe, 2011; Bryant, Ericksen, & DeHoek, 2008), creative activities like expressive writing and art (Wilkinson & Chilton, 2013), or mindfulness and meditation (Sedlmeier et al., 2012) as examples. As PPIs improve wellbeing (Sin & Lyubomirsky, 2009), they may be useful in the development of a PII, especially when "other-oriented" interventions are used (Shin & Lyubomirsky, 2017). A qualitative study of young Muslim adults in the UAE (Lambert D'raven & Pasha-Zaidi, 2014) noted that many of the factors associated with happiness reflected the collectivist nature of the culture. Yet, not all Muslims are part of a collectivist culture. Some may not have access to a welcoming family or community, whereas others may be introverted and less inclined to participate in other-oriented activities. Thus, self-oriented PPIs such as personal prayer (salat) are valuable. In fact, EEG studies have shown that performing the four stages of salat increases mental concentration (especially during prostration) and improves focused attention and relaxation (Doufesh, Faisal, Lim, & Ibrahim, 2012; Doufesh, Ibrahim, Ismail, & Wan Ahmad, 2014). Further, engaging in behaviors that reflect the five pillars of Islam may be considered Islamic PPIs as they reflect the same types of activities that positive psychology researchers have linked to wellbeing. Integrating Islamic practices into one's personal routine may help Muslims develop a stronger sense of identity and belonging to the larger Muslim community, thus promoting a PII.

12.6.3 Eudaimonic Wellbeing

In designing programs to increase wellbeing among Muslims, it is also important to keep in mind the understandings Muslims have towards "happiness". Islamic cultures in general are wary of excessive displays of happiness as these are subject to the evil eye, a concept reflecting the Quranic reference to the dangers of envy, whereby it is believed that an emphasis on overt or superficial exhibition of happiness can invite jealousy or negative energy, which can lead to personal loss or harm. Joshanloo (2013) notes that this fear of happiness may be associated with lower life satisfaction, a key indicator of wellbeing, among Muslims. Yet, how can Muslims develop a PII if they fear being (too) happy? Focusing on eudaimonic wellbeing (Waterman, 1990), which is based on activity, meaning and purpose rather than on hedonic wellbeing, which is a reflection of one's personal state of happiness and maximization of pleasurable states (Ryan & Deci, 2001), may be an approach. As Islam emphasizes improving oneself and society, focusing on prosocial behaviors may minimize an emphasis on the sole pursuit of positive emotions.

12.6.4 A Moderate Life

Finally, another way to promote a PII would be to seek wellbeing in moderation. Moderation is an important concept in Islam and has been discussed within the positive psychology literature. Grant and Schwartz (2011) note the inverted-U relationship between positive and negative states and behaviors. "Indeed, in disparate domains of research, psychologists have increasingly discovered that at high levels, positive effects begin to turn negative" (Grant & Schwartz, 2011, p. 62). A number of studies confirm the notion that it is possible to have too much of a good thing, whether it is too much happiness (Martin et al., 2002; Oishi, Diener, & Lucas, 2007), too much self-efficacy or self-esteem (Baumeister, Campbell, Krueger, &

Vohs, 2003; Vancouver & Kendall, 2006), too much empathy (Galinsky, Maddux, Gilin, & White, 2008; Gino & Pierce, 2009) or too much of a justice virtue (Bolino & Turnley, 2005). In developing a PII, it would therefore be important to consider moderation as a key component in whatever one does.

12.7 Conclusion

This chapter looked at the relationship between identity development, religion, and wellbeing and how these may play a role in promoting what we have put forward as a PII. Given the increase in Islamophobia around the world and the need for young adults to be guided in navigating this landscape, it is imperative to investigate how Islam can provide a positive influence on the development of a Muslim identity. Just as Islamic virtues fit well within and add to the VIA Classification of Character Strengths and Virtues (Peterson & Seligman, 2004), other ways of connecting positive psychology with Islamic beliefs and practices can help to create a uniquely indigenous Islamic positive psychology wherein the proposed model of PII development can be further explored and refined. As much of the research on wellbeing fits with Islamic notions of community, compassion, gratitude, prosocial behavior, and moderation, integrating these ideas is an important step in helping Muslims gain the benefits that a PII may be able to provide.

References

Abdel-Khalek, A. M. (2002). Age and sex differences for anxiety in relation to family size, birth order, and religiosity among Kuwaiti adolescents. *Psychological Reports, 90*(3), 1031–1036.

Abdel-Khalek, A. M. (2007). Assessment of intrinsic religiosity with a single-item measure in a sample of Arab Muslims. *Journal of Muslim Mental Health, 2*(2), 211–215.

Abdel-Khalek, A. M. (2008). Religiosity, health, and wellbeing among Kuwaiti personnel. *Psychological Reports, 102*(1), 181–184.

Abdel-Khalek, A. M. (2010). Quality of life, subjective wellbeing, and religiosity in Muslim college students. *Quality of Life Research, 19*(8), 1133–1143.

Abdel-Khalek, A. M. (2011). Subjective wellbeing and religiosity in Egyptian college students. *Psychological Reports, 108*(1), 54–58.

Abdel-Khalek, A., & Lester, D. (2006). Optimism and pessimism in Kuwaiti and American college students. *International Journal of Social Psychiatry, 52*(2), 110–126.

Abdel-Khalek, A. M., & Naceur, F. (2007). Religiosity and its association with positive and negative emotions among college students from Algeria. *Mental Health, Religion & Culture, 10*(2), 159–170.

Abu-Rayya, H. M., & Abu-Rayya, M. H. (2009). Acculturation, religious identity, and psychological wellbeing among Palestinians in Israel. *International Journal of Intercultural Relations, 33*(4), 325–331.

Ajibade, A., Hook, J. N., Utsey, S. O., Davis, D. E., & Van Tongeren, D. R. (2016). Racial/ethnic identity, religious commitment, and wellbeing in African Americans. *Journal of Black Psychology, 42*(3), 244–258.

Ajrouch, K. J. (2004). Gender, race, and symbolic boundaries: Contested spaces of identity among Arab American adolescents. *Sociological Perspectives, 47*(4), 371–391.
Al-Kandari, Y. Y. (2003). Religiosity and its relation to blood pressure among selected Kuwaitis. *Journal of Biosocial Science, 35*(3), 463–472.
Allport, G. W., & Ross, J. M. (1967). Personal religious orientation and prejudice. *Journal of Personality and Social Psychology, 5*(4), 432–443.
Annalakshmi, N., & Abeer, M. (2011). Islamic worldview, religious personality and resilience among Muslim adolescent students in India. *Europe's Journal of Psychology, 7*(4), 716.
Baron, J. G. (2013). *Curating the self: A proposed intervention for positive identity crafting through self-presentation and clothing (Capstone Project)*. University of Pennsylvania, Philadelphia, PA.
Baroun, K. A. (2006). Relations among religiosity, health, happiness, and anxiety for Kuwaiti adolescents. *Psychological Reports, 99*(3), 717–722.
Bartowski, J. P., & Read, J. G. (2003). Veiled submission: Gender, power, and identity among Evangelical and Muslim women in the United States. *Qualitative Sociology, 26,* 71–92.
Baumeister, R. F., & Leary, M. R. (1995). The need to belong: Desire for interpersonal attachments as a fundamental human motivation. *Psychological Bulletin, 117*(3), 497–529.
Baumeister, R. F., Campbell, J. D., Krueger, J. I., & Vohs, K. D. (2003). Does high self-esteem cause better performance, interpersonal success, happiness, or healthier lifestyles? *Psychological Science in the Public Interest, 4,* 1–44.
Berry, J. W. (1984). Multicultural policy in Canada: A social psychological analysis. *Canadian Journal of Behavioural Science/Revue canadienne des sciences du comportement, 16*(4), 353–370.
Berry, J. W. (1997). Immigration, acculturation, and adaptation. *Applied Psychology, 46*(1), 5–34.
Berry, J. W. (2003). Conceptual approaches to acculturation. In K. Chun, P. Balls-Organista, & G. Martin (Eds.), *Acculturation: Advances in theory, measurement, and applied research* (pp. 17–37). Washington DC: American Psychological Association Press.
Bierman, A. (2006). Does religion buffer the effects of discrimination on mental health? Differing effects by race. *Journal for the Scientific Study of Religion, 45*(4), 551–565.
Bolino, M. C., & Turnley, W. H. (2005). The personal costs of citizenship behavior: The relationship between individual initiative and role overload, job stress, and work–family conflict. *Journal of Applied Psychology, 90,* 740–748.
Bozorgmehr, M. (2000). Does host hostility create ethnic solidarity? The experience of Iranians in the United States. *Bulletin of the Royal Institute for Inter-Faith Studies, 2*(1), 159–178.
Briki, W., & Amara, M. (2018). Perspective of Islamic self: Rethinking Ibn al-Qayyim's three-heart model from the scope of dynamical social psychology. *Journal of Religion and Health*, 1–13.
Bryant, F. B., & Veroff, J. (2007). *Savoring: A new model of positive experience*. Mahwah, NJ: Lawrence Erlbaum Associates.
Bryant, F. B., Ericksen, C. L., & DeHoek, A. H. (2008). Savoring. In S. J. Lopez (Ed.), *Encyclopedia of positive psychology* (Vol. 2, pp. 857–859). New York, NY: Wiley/Blackwell.
Bryant, F. B., Chadwick, E. D., & Kluwe, K. (2011). Understanding the processes that regulate positive emotional experience: Unsolved problems and future directions for theory and research on savoring. *International Journal of Wellbeing, 1,* 107–126.
Chouhoud, Y. (2018). *What causes Muslims to doubt Islam? A quantitative analysis*. Dallas, TX: Al-Yaqeen Institute. Retrieved from https://yaqeeninstitute.org/en/youssef-chouhoud/what-causes-muslims-to-doubt-islam-a-quantitative-analysis/.
Cross, W. E. (1971). The negro-to-black conversion experience. *Black world, 20*(9), 13–27.
Cross, W. (1991). *Shades of black: Diversity in African-American identity*. Philadelphia, USA: Temple University Press.
Crystal, D. S., & DeBell, M. (2002). Sources of civic orientation among American youth: Trust, religious valuation, and attributions of responsibility. *Political Psychology, 23*(1), 113–132.
Dahlsgaard, K., Peterson, C., & Seligman, M. E. P. (2005). Shared virtue: The convergence of valued human strengths across culture and history. *Review of General Psychology, 9*(3), 203–213.
Dalacoura, K., Colombo, S., & Dark, G. (2017). *Global identities: Embedding the Middle East and North Africa region in the wider world.* Working Papers No. 2, Middle East and North

Africa Regional Architecture: Mapping Geopolitical Shifts, Regional Order and Domestic Transformations. European Union's Horizon 2020 Research and Innovation Programme.

Dezutter, J., Soenens, B., & Hutsebaut, D. (2006). Religiosity and mental health: A further exploration of the relative importance of religious behaviors vs. religious attitudes. *Personality and individual Differences*, *40*(4), 807–818.

Doufesh, H., Faisal, T., Lim, K. S., & Ibrahim, F. (2012). EEG spectral analysis on Muslim prayers. *Applied Psychophysiology and Biofeedback, 37*(1), 11–18.

Doufesh, H., Ibrahim, F., Ismail, N. A., & Wan Ahmad, W. A. (2014). Effect of Muslim prayer (Salat) on α electroencephalography and its relationship with autonomic nervous system activity. *The Journal of Alternative and Complementary Medicine, 20*(7), 558–562.

Emmons, R. A., & McCullough, M. E. (2003). Counting blessings versus burdens: An experimental investigation of gratitude and subjective wellbeing in daily life. *Journal of Personality and Social Psychology, 84,* 377–389.

Erikson, E. H. (1963). *Childhood and society* (2nd ed.). New York, NY: Norton.

Festinger, L. (1957). *A theory of cognitive dissonance*. Stanford, CA: Stanford University Press.

Foucault, M. (1995 [1977]). *Discipline and punish: The birth of the prison* (Alan Sheridan, Trans.). New York, NY: Vintage Books.

Fowler, J. W. (1981). *Stages of faith*. New York, NY: HarperCollins.

Fowler, J. W. (1996). Pluralism and oneness in religious experience: William James, faith-development theory, and clinical practice. *Religion and the Clinical Practice of Psychology, 1,* 165–186.

Galinsky, A. D., Maddux, W. W., Gilin, D., & White, J. B. (2008). Why it pays to get inside the head of your opponent: The differential effects of perspective taking and empathy in negotiations. *Psychological Science, 19,* 378–384.

Ghoshal, B. (2010). Arabization: The changing face of Islam in Asia. *India Quarterly, 66*(1), 69–89.

Gino, F., & Pierce, L. (2009). Dishonesty in the name of equity. *Psychological Science, 20,* 1153–1160.

Giuliani, C., Tagliabue, S., & Regalia, C. (2018). Psychological wellbeing, multiple identities, and discrimination among first and second generation immigrant Muslims. *Europe's Journal of Psychology, 14*(1), 66–87.

Grant, A. M., & Schwartz, B. (2011). Too much of a good thing: The challenge and opportunity of the inverted U. *Perspectives on Psychological Science, 6*(1), 61–76.

Green, M., & Elliott, M. (2010). Religion, health, and psychological wellbeing. *Journal of Religion and Health, 49*(2), 149–163.

Haque, A. (2018). A brief overview of Islamic psychology. In L. Lambert & N. Pasha-Zaidi (Eds.), *An introduction to psychology for the Middle East (and beyond)* (pp. 40–51). Newcastle upon Tyne: Cambridge Scholars.

Haslam, S. A., Jetten, J., Postmes, T., & Haslam, C. (2009). Social identity, health and wellbeing: An emerging agenda for applied psychology. *Applied Psychology: An International Review, 58*(1), 1–23.

Helms, J. E. (Ed.). (1990). *Contributions in Afro-American and African studies, No. 129. Black and White racial identity: Theory, research, and practice*. New York, NY: Greenwood Press.

Henrich, J., Heine, S. J., & Norenzayan, A. (2010). Most people are not WEIRD. *Nature, 466*(7302), 29.

Hjarvard, S. (2008). The mediatization of society. *Nordicom Review, 29*(2), 102–131.

Hogg, M. A., Terry, D. J., & White, K. M. (1995). A tale of two theories: A critical comparison of identity theory with social identity theory. *Social Psychology Quarterly, 58*(4), 255–269.

Ibrahim, M. H. (2016). *Religion and wellbeing: Differences by identity and practice* (Psychology Honors Project). Macalester College, St. Paul, MN. Retrieved from http://digitalcommons.macalester.edu/cgi/viewcontent.cgi?article=1039&context=psychology_honors.

Jasperse, M., Ward, C., & Jose, P. E. (2012). Identity, perceived religious discrimination, and psychological well-being in Muslim immigrant women. *Applied Psychology, 61*(2), 250–271.

Jensen, L. A. (2003). Coming of age in a multicultural world: Globalization and adolescent cultural identity formation. *Applied Developmental Science, 7*(3), 189–196.

Joshanloo, M. (2013). The influence of fear of happiness beliefs on responses to the satisfaction with life scale. *Personality and Individual Differences, 54*(5), 647–651.

Kellner, D. (2003). *Media culture: Cultural studies, identity and politics between the modern and the post-modern*. London, UK: Routledge.

Khan, S., & Uneke, O. (2000). Muslim women: Crafting a North American identity [Book Review]. *Canadian Woman Studies, 20*(3), 115–118.

King, P. E., & Furrow, J. L. (2004). Religion as a resource for positive youth development: Religion, social capital, and moral outcomes. *Developmental Psychology, 40*(5), 703–713.

Kojetin, B. A., McIntosh, D. N., Bridges, R. A., & Spilka, B. (1987). Quest: Constructive search or religious conflict? *Journal for the Scientific Study of Religion, 26*(1), 111–115.

Lambert D'raven, L., & Pasha-Zaidi, N. (2014). Happiness strategies among Arab university students in the United Arab Emirates. *The Journal of Happiness & Wellbeing*, 2(1), 1–15.

Lambert D'raven, L., & Pasha–Zaidi, N. (2015). Happiness in the United Arab Emirates: Conceptualisations of happiness among Emirati and other Arab students. *International Journal of Happiness and Development*, 2(1), 1–21.

Lavrič, M., & Flere, S. (2008). The role of culture in the relationship between religiosity and psychological wellbeing. *Journal of Religion and Health, 47*(2), 164–175.

Lerner, R. M., Almerigi, J. B., Theokas, C., & Lerner, J. V. (2005). Positive youth development a view of the issues. *The Journal of Early Adolescence, 25*(1), 10–16.

Lerner, R. M., von Eye, A., Lerner, J. V., & Lewin-Bizan, S. (2009). Exploring the foundations and functions of adolescent thriving within the 4-H study of positive youth development: A view of the issues. *Journal of Applied Developmental Psychology, 30*(5), 567–570.

Lynch, O. (2013). British Muslim youth: Radicalisation, terrorism and the construction of the "other". *Critical Studies on Terrorism, 6*(2), 241–261.

Lyubomirsky, S., Sheldon, K. M., & Schkade, D. (2005). Pursuing happiness: The architecture of sustainable change. *Review of General Psychology, 9*, 111–131.

Marcia, J. E. (1966). Development and validation of ego-identity status. *Journal of Personality and Social Psychology, 3*, 551–558.

Marcia, J. E. (1976). Identity six years after: A follow-up study. *Journal of Youth and Adolescence, 5*, 145–160.

Marcia, J. E. (1980). Identity in adolescence. In J. Adelson (Ed.), *Handbook of adolescent psychology* (pp. 149–173). New York, NY: Wiley.

Markstrom-Adams, C., & Smith, M. (1996). Identity formation and religious orientation among high school students from the United States and Canada. *Journal of Adolescence, 19*(3), 247–261.

Martin, L. R., Friedman, H. S., Tucker, J. S., Tomlinson-Keasey, C., Criqui, M. H., & Schwartz, J. E. (2002). A life course perspective on childhood cheerfulness and its relation to mortality risk. *Personality and Social Psychology Bulletin, 28*, 1155–1165.

Maslow, A. H. (1970). *Motivation and personality*. New York: Harper & Row.

Matheson, K., Cole, B., & Majka, K. (2003). Dissidence from within: Examining the effects of intergroup context on group members' reactions to attitudinal opposition. *Journal of Experimental Social Psychology, 39*(2), 161–169.

McDonald, L. Z. (2011). Securing identities, resisting terror: Muslim youth work in the UK and its implications for security. *Religion, State and Society, 39*(2–3), 177–189.

McGregor, I., Haji, R., Nash, K. A., & Teper, R. (2008). Religious zeal and the uncertain self. *Basic and Applied Social Psychology, 30*(2), 183–188.

Mossakowski, K. N. (2003). Coping with perceived discrimination: Does ethnic identity protect mental health? *Journal of Health and Social Behavior, 44*(3), 318–331.

Naber, N. (2000). Ambiguous insiders: An investigation of Arab American invisibility. *Ethnic and Racial Studies, 23*(1), 37–61.

Nadal, K. L. (2004). Pilipino American Identity Development Model. *Journal of Multicultural Counseling and Development, 32*(1), 45–62.

Nadal, K. L. (2011). *Filipino American psychology: A Handbook of theory, research, and clinical practice*. New York, NY: Wiley.

Neiwert, D., Ankrom, D., Kaplan, E., & Pham, S. (2017). *Homegrown terror.* Reveal from the Center for Investigative Reporting. Retrieved from https://apps.revealnews.org/homegrown-terror/.

Niemiec, R. M. (2013). VIA character strengths: Research and practice (the first 10 years). In H. H. Knoop & A. Delle Fave (Eds.), *Cross-cultural advancements in positive psychology: Vol. 3. Wellbeing and cultures: Perspectives from positive psychology* (pp. 11–29). New York, NY: Springer Science+Business Media.

Nisbet, E. C., & Myers, T. A. (2010). Challenging the state: Transnational TV and political identity in the Middle East. *Political Communication, 27*(4), 347–366.

Oberschall, A. (2004). Explaining terrorism: The contribution of collective action theory. *Sociological Theory, 22*(1), 26–37.

Oishi, S., Diener, E., & Lucas, R. E. (2007). The optimum level of wellbeing: Can people be too happy? *Perspectives on Psychological Science, 2,* 346–360.

Oyserman, D. (2001). Self-concept and identity. In A. Tesser & N. Schwarz (Eds.), *The Blackwell handbook of social psychology* (pp. 499–517). Malden, MA: Blackwell.

Parveen, S., Sandilya, G., & Shafiq, M. (2014). Religiosity and mental health among Muslim youth. *Indian Journal of Health and Wellbeing, 5*(3), 316–319.

Peek, L. (2005). Becoming Muslim: The development of a religious identity. *Sociology of Religion, 66,* 215–242.

Peterson, C., & Seligman, M. E. P. (2004). *Character strengths and virtues: A handbook and classification.* New York, NY: Oxford University Press/American Psychological Association.

Pew Research Center. (2015). *The future of world religions: Population, growth projections, 2010–2050,* Washington, DC.

Phinney, J. S. (1993). A three-stage model of ethnic identity development in adolescence. In M. E. Bernal & G. P. Knight (Eds.), *Ethnic identity: Formation and transmission among Hispanics and other minorities* (pp. 61–80). Albany, NY: State University of New York Press.

Phinney, J. S., & Ong, A. D. (2007). Conceptualization and measurement of ethnic identity: Current status and future directions. *Journal of Counseling Psychology, 54*(3), 271–281.

Poston, W. C. (1990). The biracial identity development model: A needed addition. *Journal of Counseling & Development, 69*(2), 152–155.

Rivas-Drake, D., Umaña-Taylor, A. J., Schaefer, D. R., & Medina, M. (2017). Ethnic-racial identity and friendships in early adolescence. *Child Development, 88*(3), 710–724.

Rodrigues, A. B. G. C., Stobäus, C. D., & Mosquera, J. J. M. (2016). Identity as study object of positive psychology. *Creative Education, 7,* 1119–1125.

Roser, M., Nagdy, M., & Ritchie, H. (2018). *Terrorism.* Our World in Data, Oxford Martin Programme on Global Development, University of Oxford. Retrieved from https://ourworldindata.org/terrorism.

Rothman, A., & Coyle, A. (2018). Toward a framework for Islamic psychology and psychotherapy: An Islamic model of the soul. *Journal of Religion and Health,* 1–14.

Ryan, R. M., & Deci, E. L. (2001). On happiness and human potentials: A review of research on hedonic and eudaimonic wellbeing. *Annual Review of Psychology, 52*(1), 141–166.

Sahraian, A., Gholami, A., Javadpour, A., & Omidvar, B. (2013). Association between religiosity and happiness among a group of Muslim undergraduate students. *Journal of Religion and Health, 52*(2), 450–453.

Sedlmeier, P., Eberth, J., Schwarz, M., Zimmermann, D., Haarig, F., Jaeger, S., et al. (2012). The psychological effects of meditation: A meta-analysis. *Psychological Bulletin, 138*(6), 1139–1171.

Sen, A. (2002). How to judge globalism. *The American Prospect, 13*(1), 1–14.

Shin, L. J., & Lyubomirsky, S. (2017). Increasing wellbeing in independent and interdependent cultures. In M. A. Warren & S. I. Donaldson (Eds.), *Scientific advances in positive psychology* (pp. 11–36). Santa Barbara, CA: Praeger.

Sin, N. L., & Lyubomirsky, S. (2009). Enhancing well-being and alleviating depressive symptoms with positive psychology interventions: A practice-friendly meta-analysis. *Journal of Clinical Psychology, 65*(5), 467–487.

Suhail, K., & Chaudhry, H. R. (2004). Predictors of subjective wellbeing in an Eastern Muslim culture. *Journal of Social and Clinical Psychology, 23*(3), 359–376.

Sumner, R., Burrow, A. L., & Hill, P. L. (2015). Identity and purpose as predictors of subjective wellbeing in emerging adulthood. *Emerging Adulthood, 3*(1), 46–54.

Tajfel, H., & Turner, J. C. (1979). An integrative theory of intergroup conflict. In W. G. Austin & S. Worchel (Eds.), *The social psychology of intergroup relations* (pp. 33–37). Monterey, CA: Brooks/Cole.

Temple-Raston, D. (2018). The female Quran experts fighting radical Islam in Morocco. *The Atlantic.* Retrieved from https://www.theatlantic.com/international/archive/2018/02/the-female-quran-experts-fighting-radical-islam-in-morocco/551996/.

Tewari, S., Khan, S., Hopkins, N., Srinivasan, N., & Reicher, S. (2012). Participation in mass gatherings can benefit wellbeing: Longitudinal and control data from a North Indian Hindu pilgrimage event. *PLoS ONE, 7*(10), e47291.

Thomas, J., Mutawa, M., Furber, S. W., & Grey, I. (2016). Religiosity: Reducing depressive symptoms amongst Muslim females in the United Arab Emirates. *Middle East Journal of Positive Psychology, 2*(1), 9–21.

US Department of Justice. (2005). *Terrorism 2002–2005*. Federal Bureau of Investigation Counterterrorism Division. Retrieved from https://www.fbi.gov/stats-services/publications/terrorism-2002-2005.

Vancouver, J. B., & Kendall, L. N. (2006). When self-efficacy negatively relates to motivation and performance in a learning context. *Journal of Applied Psychology, 91,* 1146–1153.

Vasegh, S., & Mohammadi, M. R. (2007). Religiosity, anxiety, and depression among a sample of Iranian medical students. *The International Journal of Psychiatry in Medicine, 37*(2), 213–227.

Waterman, A. S. (1985). *Identity in adolescence: Processes and contents*. San Francisco, CA: Jossey-Bass.

Waterman, A. S. (1990). The relevance of Aristotle's conception of eudaimonia for the psychological study of happiness. *Theoretical and Philosophical Psychology, 10,* 39–44.

Wike, R., Stokes, B., & Simmons, K. (2016). Europeans fear wave of refugees will mean more terrorism, fewer jobs. *Pew Research Center, 11*. Retrieved from http://www.pewglobal.org/2016/07/11/europeans-fear-wave-of-refugees-will-mean-more-terrorism-fewer-jobs/.

Wilkinson, R. A., & Chilton, G. (2013). Positive art therapy: Linking positive psychology to art therapy theory, practice, and research. *Art Therapy, 30*(1), 4–11.

Wong, J. L. (2014). *A structural model of religious identity as a predictor of wellbeing.* Masters thesis, California State University, Sacramento, CA.

Ysseldyk, R., Matheson, K., & Anisman, H. (2010). Religiosity as identity: Toward an understanding of religion from a social identity perspective. *Personality and Social Psychology Review, 14*(1), 60–71.

Zamora, A. L. (2017). *Promoting racial and ethnic identity: Academic intervention to support scholastic success of Latinos*. Doctoral dissertation, Northwest Nazarene University, Nampa, Idaho, USA.

Zhang, Y. (2009). Individualism or collectivism? Cultural orientations in Chinese TV commercials an analysis of some moderating factors. *Journalism & Mass Communication Quarterly, 86*(3), 630–653.

Chapter 13
Advances in Wellbeing in the MENA Region: Accentuating the Positive

Richard J. Estes and M. Joseph Sirgy

Abstract While positive psychology is a relatively new science, the notion of wellbeing itself is not novel and has always existed across all societies throughout history. In this chapter, we trace the origins of contemporary civilizations across the Middle East/North Africa (MENA) region from ancient (c. 9200 BCE) to modern times (2018 CE) and explore their notions of social and political wellbeing. The region's past is characterized by remarkable intellectual and past social accomplishments, especially during the "Islamic Golden Age" (8th–14th centuries CE). Coming up to the modern era, we then highlight original data spanning the period of 1970–2011 to summarize the major drivers of the region's social development and wellbeing as well as the challenges it confronts, particularly considering new political and military developments emerging in the region.

13.1 Introduction

The notion of wellbeing is not new despite its scientific investigation taking a serious turn in the social sciences in the past few years with quality of life studies and more recently, positive psychology, leading the way. All civilizations have had various conceptualizations of what a good life or society should comprise, and these scientific investigations have allowed for the emergence of what these wellbeing notions might have been. Such wellbeing accounts are informed by multiple sources, such as historical, social, and scientific accounts and include the investigation of religious influences, social or tribal affiliations, peaceful relations with neighbors, or sound political and governing structures and practices as major drivers of wellbeing (Estes & Sirgy, 2017). These recipes for wellbeing across time and history provide interesting trajectories of how civilizations developed and can help to explain or

R. J. Estes (✉)
University of Pennsylvania, Philadelphia, PA, USA
e-mail: restes@upenn.edu

M. J. Sirgy
Virginia Tech, Blacksburg, VA, USA
e-mail: sirgy@vt.edu

L. Lambert and N. Pasha-Zaidi (eds.), *Positive Psychology in the Middle East/North Africa*, https://doi.org/10.1007/978-3-030-13921-6_13

contextualize present-day circumstances. By using a multi-disciplinary approach to the investigation of wellbeing, we explore the major influences on the Middle East/North Africa (MENA) region from ancient civilization to the modern era and conclude with insights from our previous investigation of contemporary social, political, and economic trends that characterize the region's social and wellbeing development from 1970 to the present time (Estes & Sirgy, 2014; Sirgy, Estes, & Rahtz, 2017; Sirgy, Joshanloo, & Estes, 2018).

13.2 The MENA Region Defined

The countries of the MENA region include many of the world's most ancient and influential civilizations, encompassing all the Arab (Arabic) countries, as well as Turkey (Turkic), Iran (Persian), and Israel (Hebrew). Given the recent split of Sudan into North Sudan and South Sudan, geographers and political scientists consider North Sudan part of the MENA region because it is mostly Arab in character. The region's population exceeds 411 million people residing in 26 countries and, in all, account for 6% of the world's total or approximately 23% of all persons of Arabic extraction worldwide (Organization of Islamic Cooperation, 2018; United Nations Department of Economic and Social Affairs, 2017). The region's countries are located primarily in North Africa and West Asia, but when defined more broadly, they include portions of Central and South-Central Asia as well.

High fertility rates, dramatic increases in the region's population aging, and advances in population health have contributed to tremendous population growth accounting for the region's longer years of average life expectancy, reductions in formerly high levels of infant and child mortality and declines in maternal mortality. Educational levels are also on the increase and, today, new opportunities for skilled employment in the technology, financial, and social infrastructures have emerged (International Labour Organization, 2018). None of these profound changes in the region's development were expected as recently as 1990 given the limited financial resources available to the region's recently independent countries. Today, the MENA region's countries are predominately youthful with more than half of their population aged 25 years and younger, a pattern that is expected to continue throughout much of the 21st century (UNDESA, 2017).

13.3 Ancient Civilizations of the MENA Region and the Emergence of Wellbeing and Happiness

The region's multiple civilizations are ancient and date back to at least 9200 BCE including those of: Sumeria, including the City of Ur (a major Sumerian city-state located in Mesopotamia); the Akkadian Empire, centered in the city of Akkad and the

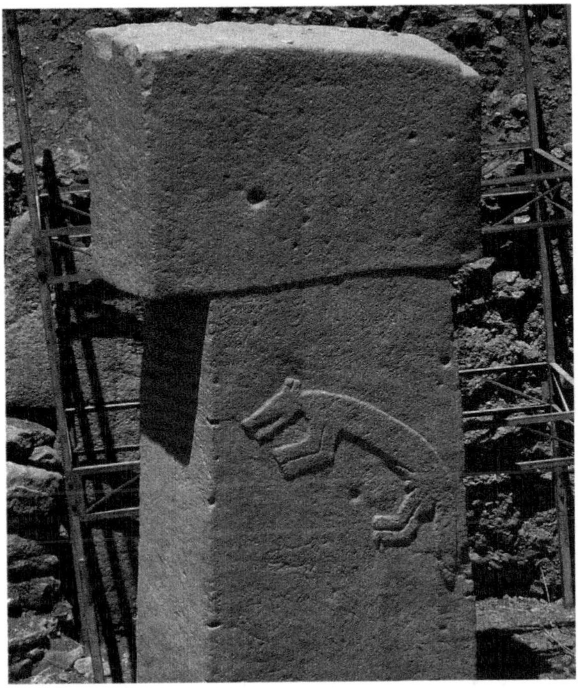

Fig. 13.1 10,000–12,000 year old stele with carving at Gobekli Tepi, Turkey. These and other carvings have readjusted the date of human civilization back by as much as 5000 years to approximately 12,000 BCE. Photo taken by Zhengan, Own work, CC BY-SA 4.0. Reprinted under license granted to Wikicommons

first Semitic-speaking people of the region which united the Akkadian and Sumerian speakers under one rule; the Babylonians with their rich history of legal and commercial activities; pre-dynastic and dynastic Egyptians with their centuries-long megalithic building activities that included the Sphinx and the pyramids; Lebanon, with its long history of geographic expansion and the country's emergence as the center of economic growth concentrated around Ba'albek, among others (Donner, 2014; Fagan, 2009; New World Encyclopedia, 2018a). Many approximations of the dates of the region's earliest civilizations should be regarded as tentative and are based on re-reassessments of the age of the enormous megalithic structures that exist in Egypt, Iran, and Iraq. In recent years, Turkey has also been added to this list, which includes the recently discovered megaliths of Gobekli Tepi, a series of circular and oval-shaped structures set atop a hill, of which there are at least 20 and thought to collectively represent a temple (see Fig. 13.1). The age of these megaliths is believed to exceed the revised age of the Sphinx and pyramids which were earlier estimated to have been constructed around 2500 BCE but are now are widely believed to date back to as far as 9500 BCE, or earlier (Albright, 2018; New World Encyclopedia, 2018b; Schoch, 2018).

Even while the great civilizations of the MENA states were developing, they also were engaged in formulating seminal ideas concerning the nature of "humanness" and the prerequisites for attaining quality of life, wellbeing and, for a precious few, genuine happiness (Albright, 2018; Andrews, 2012; Cleveland & Bunton, 2016; Estes & Sirgy, 2016; Pew Research Center, 2013; Remina et al., 2016a, b). These contributions included not only the development of an advanced written script but also the transfer of poetry, stories, and myths across at least five millennia, which served to promote notions of good character. They also developed a foundational legal system, the *Code of Hammurabi* (reign 1792–1750 BCE), with its carefully formulated set of legal principles including 282 laws carved in stone on a stele that governed nearly all aspects of collective life (King, 2015). The *Code's* preamble emphasized the importance of wellbeing in society and the importance of laws to provide the foundation for attaining personal and collective wellbeing. The *Code* was not rediscovered until 1901–1902 by the French archeologist, Jacques de Morgan. During its functioning, the *Code* served as the foundation for a comprehensive legal system which was subsequently refined by the Greeks and Romans and carried forward into the Western Middle Ages (5th–15th centuries) and throughout the period of European enlightenment (Andrews, 2012; Lambert, 1990). Thus, many of today's fundamental legal principles had their origins in the ancient Middle East but, over the centuries, became refined and consistent with the cultures in which these laws were enforced.

Without the region's ancient clay tablets and stele like the one shown in Fig. 13.2, information concerning humanity's earliest civilizations would have been unlikely. Of importance, too, are still other megaliths used to preserve messages for the ages from ancient peoples. Most have not yet been fully interpreted. Translated myths from some of these recordings, however, continue to inspire even modern generations of scholars, including the *Epic of Gilgamesh* (12 Sumerian Cuneiform tablets, c. 2750 and 2500 BCE), which shares ancient conceptions of leadership, perseverance, personal sacrifice, and generosity. These contributions from the past influenced the story telling of other civilizations including Homer's *Iliad* (c.750 BCE) and the *Odyssey* (c.725 BCE).

13.4 Ancient Philosophies of Wellbeing and Happiness

A core belief in ancient Mesopotamia, the political and cultural center of the MENA region, was based on the philosophy of "eye for an eye" in response to local conflict. Referred to in Latin as *lex talionis* or "the law of talion" (retaliation), this principle persisted in various forms as a source of recurrent diversity-related social conflict. Within the MENA and Gulf States region, the principle was conveyed in the carvings from above and expressed in the *Code of Hammurabi*, which was promulgated as far back in time as 1754 BCE, in order "to bring about the rule of righteousness in the land, to destroy the wicked and the evil-doers; so that the strong should not harm the weak; so that I (Hammurabi and his successors) should rule…and enlighten the

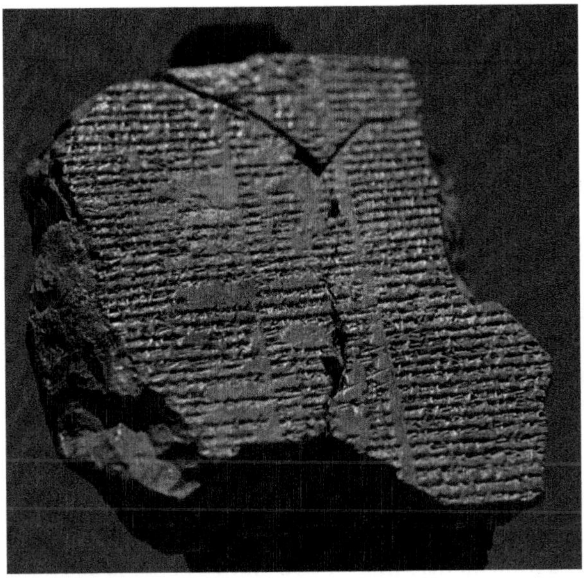

Fig. 13.2 The newly discovered tablet V of the Epic of Gilgamesh, The Sulaymaniyah Museum, Iraq.jpg. The tablet dates to the Old-Babylonian Period, 2003–1595 BCE. Licensed under the Creative Commons Attribution-Share Alike 4.0 International license

land, to further the wellbeing of mankind" (King, 2015). This statement places the ultimate source of wisdom in the hands of a single person; in this case, a powerful and expansive ruler. Yet, the mandate also speaks to the reciprocal relationships that existed between rulers and the ruled, as well as those that existed between individuals and various social collectives.

The "eye for an eye" principle is found in the political and military cultures of many societies, both ancient and modern (Miller, 2006). The notion of reconciliation, however, is nearly, but not entirely, absent from the recorded past for many societies of the MENA and Gulf States whereas the concept of retaliation persisted and often was generalized to entire populations and not just those who committed the original infraction (Abu-Nimer & Said, 2001). The concept of forgiveness for past infractions was not to emerge in the broader region for many centuries and, in the context of Islam, not before the Prophet explicitly instructed followers to show tolerance and forgiveness toward those who committed infractions against them, albeit selected exceptions to the admonition for tolerance were made.

From analysis of the legal principles summarized in the *Code of Hammurabi*, the ethical guidance provided in *The Advice of an Akkadian Father to His Son* (Arkenberg, 1998) contains beliefs that are central to both past and contemporary understanding of "wellbeing." These teachings were associated with the underlying philosophical assumptions of ancient Babylonian and Sumerian cultures as well as those of the Egyptian and other cultures that flourished in the region for thousands of years. Other propositions included (1) no act of ill-will is to go unpunished, nor should acts of good-will go unrewarded; (2) punishments in response to these acts should be consistent with the magnitude of the acts committed against the aggrieved; (3) the community as a whole not the individual, is the target of acts of wellbeing (this principle is covered in depth on the stele and clay tablets); and (4) enemies, including those already defeated, need to be treated with respect or, at a minimum, with caution lest they or others associated with them re-emerge as more threatening enemies in the future.

Individuals were further encouraged to attain a state of wellbeing via a dedicated attention to family and community values. Gender roles on the other hand, reflected the prevailing norm found in many parts of the world at the time in that girls and women were second to males, although this changed with the emergence of Islam through the teachings of the Prophet which sought to elevate and preserve women and girls' rights to property, inheritance, work, marriage and education. Personal happiness was also thought to emerge through the harmony achieved with the values, norms, and laws of the larger community—an idea that Plato, Aristotle, and other major Greek philosophers also taught, as did the Sumerian (c. 4500 BCE–c.1900 BCE) and Akkadian (2300 BCE–2100 BCE) civilizations. What also distinguished the pre-Islamic era from modern times was a limited belief in an afterlife, whereby all positive and negative transactions directed at other people needed to take place within one's own lifetime (Fagan, 2009). The only exception to this principle were those held by the ancient Egyptians who, through their god of the underworld, Osiris, used a feather to determine the relative "goodness" or "badness" of a person depending on the relative weight of the individual's heart. "Good lives" and "bad lives," as measured by the scale of life, rewarded or punished a person's life and no exceptions to that final assessment could be substituted (Mark, 2012).

13.5 Islamic Conceptions of the Good Life, Wellbeing, and Happiness

With the advent of Islam in 632 CE as a unifying political and spiritual force, philosophical principles that contribute to a sense of wellbeing are found in the region's monotheistic teachings. From its earliest inception following the death of the Prophet in 632 CE, Islam expressed tolerance for the adherents to other monotheistic religions in the MENA and Gulf States region, including Jews and Christians, who, like the various Muslim sects, were also recognized as being "Peoples of the Book" and as such, followers of Abrahamic values. These practices were established during the lifetime of the Prophet who welcomed people of different faiths into his tent for social occasions and, most importantly, for the resolution of conflicts between people both within their own group and those between people of multiple religions (Abu-Nimer & Said, 2001). "People of the book" brought complex land, marital and other conflicts to the Prophet for resolution. His wisdom on such matters was readily accepted and often contributed to a successful resolution.

The wisdom imparted by the Prophet to his followers and non-followers eventually was codified into Islam's second sacred book, the *Hadith,* which in Sunni Islam denotes the words, actions, and the silent approval of the Prophet. The Quran instructs Muslims to emulate, obey, and abide by the judgement of the Prophet Muhammad. It was in accordance with this Quranic stricture that the Companions recorded all of his words, advice, practices and actions, and the daily rituals and events of his life. The writing of the *Hadith* took several centuries to complete with many of its principles transferred into *Shari'a* law. Shari'a is the religious legal system governing the members of the Islamic faith. It is derived from the religious precepts of Islam, particularly based on the Quran and the *Hadith*. Historically, the scholars of the *Hadith*, as narrated by Abdur-Rahman bin Ghanm Al-Ash'ari (who died 697 CE), also recorded a set of principles that guided interactions with non-Muslims, like Christians and Jews. These were put into writing by Ibn-Kathir (1301–1373) in collaboration with a leader of the Christian community of Ash-Sham (Syria).

Interpretations of Islam's two sacred texts—the *Quran* and the *Hadith*, which record the daily life experiences and teachings of the Prophet (Lucas, 2002), as well as Shari'a law (Tibi, 2008), provide guidance on how to live a meaningful and good life with, and for, others. Virtually no aspect of personal behavior is left out of these texts, which many countries of the region retain as a source of primary influence. While some countries, such as Saudi Arabia, seek to modernize their judicial systems (Bassiouni, 2016; Keshavjee, 2016; Rivers, 2017; Warner, 2010), in other nations, such as the United Arab Emirates (UAE), a combination of civil, common, customary and Shari'a law is practiced. These three sources form the essence of individual and collective guidance (Leaman, 2004; Tiliouine & Estes, 2016) associated with Islam's five pillars, which include (1) *Shahada* (Faith) and (2) *Salah* (prayer); (3) *Zakāt* (charity); (4) *Sawm* (fasting); and (5) *Hajj* (pilgrimage to Mecca) (Joshanloo, 2017). Faith is the central pillar of all Islamic belief and practice, but the other pillars are of fundamental significance as well. Only the fifth pillar, that relating to the *Hajj*, may be deemed discretionary should the individual not have the financial means, be in poor health, or otherwise limited in making the journey.

Islam was established as a formal religion following the death of the Prophet and was focused on unifying the highly diverse peoples of the MENA region, disavowing polytheism and the idolatry associated with those times (Renima et al., 2016a, b). The intellectual and technological innovations that resulted from collaborations among Islamic interfaith scholars during these centuries resulted in many achievements that continue to influence humanity today (Atiyeh & Hayes, 1992). Today, Islam is the world's second largest religion after Catholicism but is the most rapidly expanding with a membership of more than 1600 million (De Silver & Masci, 2017; Rogan, 2017). Only about 20%, or one-fifth of the world's Muslim population reside in the MENA and Gulf Cooperation Council (GCC) (Bahrain, Kuwait, Qatar, Oman, UAE, and Saudi Arabia) nation region, most of whom are people of Berber, Arabic or Persian extraction (Central Intelligence Agency, 2018).

13.6 Contemporary Conceptions of the Good Life, Wellbeing, and Happiness

Development on what the good life entails continues to this day from a religious perspective. For instance, Gordon (2008), Joshanloo (2013, 2014, 2017), Leaman (2004), and Saeed (2006) explore the basic tenets of Islam as it relates to quality of life, wellbeing, and happiness. Their analyses provide insights into the intersection between religion and philosophy as well as instructions for daily life in a manner consistent with the teachings of Allah as reported by the Prophet Mohammed (PBUH). Joshanloo (2013) has focused on quality of life and wellbeing issues within the context of an Islamic tradition, noting that,

> "…happiness should be formulated in such way that it guarantees the satisfaction of the individual's need for worship (which is considered inherent) and his or her happiness both in this life and the hereafter. The key to achieving this is an Islamic-based virtuous life-style accompanied by religious faith" (p. 1868).

Joshanloo (2013) further suggests that one of the biggest distinctions between Islamic wellbeing and that of Western conceptualizations for instance, is that Islamic wellbeing focuses on the attainment of non-earthly pleasure for a life lived in conformity with the teachings of good as revealed through the Prophet. Thus, earthly pleasure in and of itself carries little lasting value and the postponement of immediate gratification for richer rewards that will accrue in the afterlife is preferable. It is not that the faithful never seek pleasure in the here and now but, rather, that true pleasure comes from living a life of justice and community. Filial respect, fulfilling duty to one's family and parents in particular, and to the extent possible, engaging in daily acts of charity directed to the poor are also expected towards living a good life. Thus, the accumulation of wealth and in particular, how it is used to improve the lives of others can significantly enhance the wellbeing of people in the eyes of Allah (Joshanloo, 2014). All "People of the Book" share these basic tenets, having a long list of charitable giving starting with setting aside a parcel of land and harvest for use by the poor, and engaging in acts of philanthropy and kindness, which count heavily in people's judgment before their maker.

Further to the development of an Islamic conceptualization of the good life is the development of scientific models and their investigation. Positive psychology, the science of wellbeing, was introduced in 2000 (Seligman & Csikszentmihalyi, 2000), but is concurrently evolving under Islamic scientific inquiry as well. Much work has been done to this effect including Khodayarifard et al.'s (2016) attempts at viewing positive psychology from an Islamic perspective, the use of positive psychology interventions with an Islamic approach in medical patients (Saeedi, Nasab, Zadeh, & Ebrahimi, 2015), the development of character virtues from an Islamic ethical viewpoint (Abdullah, 2014), the portrayal of positive psychological capital in the Quran (Riaz, 2015), and the use of positive psychology interventions such as gratitude as examples of this work (Al-Seheel & Noor, 2016). This is in addition to the work being done on the role of religion and wellbeing overall, of which there are many examples that relate to Islam (e.g., Abdel-Khalek, 2014; Rizvi & Hossain,

2017; Thomas, Mutawa, Furber, & Grey, 2016; Tiliouine & Belgoumidi, 2009), as well as the philosophical meaning of happiness from an Islamic perspective and its policy and development implications (Abde & Salih, 2015; Askari, Iqbal, Krichene, & Mirakhor, 2014; Ismail & Haron, 2014). Wellbeing and its definitions, practises, and implications are part of a serious and active body of inquiry in the region.

Topic Box: A Look at Regional Young Adults and Wellbeing

The 2018 ASDA'A Burson-Masteller Arab Youth Survey (AYS) paints both an optimistic and pessimistic future for young adults, squarely divided between the have and have not nations of the MENA region. Undisputedly, young adults in the GCC region are overwhelmingly positive and 82% feel their best days are ahead of them, while only 26% in the Levant region agree. This figure is not a surprise given the continued bloodshed in Syria and resulting effects on migration, jobs, education, and social cohesion across that region, while the GCC nations, apart from hosting job-seeking migrants, have been spared these effects. Faith in government is also split between the three emerging sub-regions of the MENA area. A mere 7% of young adults in the GCC feel their governments are heading in the wrong direction. This stands in contrast to 87% in the Levant region that disapproves of the current direction taken by their governments, while 46% in North Africa feel the same.

Support for greater female participation in society is most highly supported by young Saudi men across the region, with 92% reporting that more needs to be done in this area for their mothers, sisters, wives, aunts, and daughters. Women have tremendous political and social support who in June (2018) took the driver's seat for the first time, and are also enjoying a number of positive workplace legislative changes. As a result of sweeping changes happening across the Kingdom, Saudi Crown Prince Mohammed Bin Salman received top marks as the GCC region's biggest influencer in the context of increased participation of women and young people.

Finally, "civilian investigations" of the good life for lack of a better term, also are taking place via social media. Increasingly, young adults have access to the internet and mobile phones and can readily see how their regional neighbors are faring, and not only what their governments provide but, how their governments treat them. The region surpasses Western and European nations with the highest global internet and smartphone penetration rates in the world (McKinsey, 2016). Specifically, Qatar and the UAE have the highest social media penetration worldwide, while Saudi Arabia has seen the largest growth with a 73% rise accounting for 59% of Saudis using social media channels (We Are Social/Hootsuite, 2017). The notion of wellbeing and the good life is shaping itself through social media discourse and transforming itself in line with the concerns of youths under the age of 18 who represent over half the region's entire population (Khan, 2018). This is propelling high expectations for greater government accountability towards the provision of jobs, quality education, entertainment, and freedoms (Arab Youth Survey; ASDA'A Burson Marsteller, 2017).

Topic Box: Human Development and National Progress—A View of the MENA Region

The role of governments is implicated in the ability of people to live lives of dignity, equality, safety, and security. Human capital, the skills and knowledge that facilitates the ability to generate economic value, is a determinant of a nation's success. How well nations harness education to meet the needs of changing global economies ensures their long-term competitiveness and sustainability. The role of technology in what has been called the "Fourth Industrial Revolution" makes the ability of human capital to withstand change and transition, as well as seize opportunities, all the more salient. Thus, human capital is not only about having good schools; it also includes the ability of that education to produce real social and economic value across all ranks of society. The *Human Capital Index* ranks nations on how well they deploy and develop that potential, and assesses learning and employment outcomes across five age groups. The index focuses on educational attainment, how education and skills are used in the workplace, continued learning and employment quality, whether and how senior members of the labor force continue to attain and be engaged at work, and the continued opportunity and health of the oldest workers of a nation.

Of 130 nations, the MENA region is one that spans high, medium, and low levels of development. Bahrain (47th), Qatar (55th), and the UAE (45th) outperform the 15 MENA nations covered in the index, which places them midway in the rankings and on par with European nations. Yet, compared to other nations and relative to their income, there is room to grow as these same three report low skill diversity, as well as tertiary and vocational enrolment. At the other end is Morocco (118th), Tunisia (115th) and Algeria (112th), while Yemen (130th) is last for various reasons, one of which is its current political instability. In 2016, Egypt (86th) and Saudi Arabia (87th) were tied, with Egypt ranking better on vocational enrolment, despite the quality of Saudi Arabia's education system perceived to be superior to Egypt's. In 2017, they moved in opposing directions with Saudi Arabia reaching 82nd position and Egypt sliding to 97th. Both have high youth unemployment rates and large employment gender gaps, and Saudi Arabia a GDP far higher than Egypt's. Kuwait with a GDP almost eight times that of Egypt, ranks at 96, lending credence to the fact that money does not buy capacity.

Human capital determines, along with government efforts, the business community and civil society, a nation's competitiveness, as well its ability to finance innovation and adopt technology, provide for labor market flexibility and protect workers. It also involves productivity and the quality of public institutions and their regulations around investment, labor and business operations. Also important is infrastructure that allows productivity to ensue, i.e., roads, telecommunications, as well as the health and education of workers. Of 137 nations on the *Global Competitiveness Index 2017–2018*, the UAE ranks 17th, Qatar 25th, Saudi Arabia 30th, Bahrain 44th, Kuwait 52nd and Oman 62nd. It should be said that these GCC countries are host to millions of expatriates, which comprise over 70% of these nations. At the lower end of the scale is Egypt in 100th position, Lebanon at 105th, and Yemen last.

There remain significant gender gaps, as well as reports of child labor which limit children's ability to attend school. In 2016, youth unemployment was prominent among the 15–24 year group, with Jordan's (86th in 2017) young adults in that category unemployed at a rate of almost 33%, reaching 38% in Tunisia (115th in 2017). Still, Tunisia was identified as an achiever with good growth the previous year and dedicated efforts to implement a culture of entrepreneurship, an example of which is Innajim (www.commententreprendre.tn), a program aiming to help young adults develop their own start-ups, which offers legal support, business registration, and other help. Other groups offer mentoring, start-up funds and innovation hubs (i.e. http://www.intilaq.tn/).

13.7 Social Development, Social Progress, and Wellbeing of the MENA Countries

How well are the nations of the MENA region performing from the perspective of social, political, economic, and related areas of development? Progressively higher levels of social development are associated with increased levels of wellbeing and are important questions with respect to contemporary development both within the region and vis-à-vis other major world regions. Thus, this section of the chapter provides an empirical profile of changing patterns of development relative to that of the world-as-a-whole and makes the necessary link between the region's past, present and future. The data that follow summarize 40 years of social development and wellbeing progress for the 26 nations of the region. The data are fundamentally objective and, as such, can be used to compare the region's social performances with that of other major geopolitical regions worldwide (Estes, 2015a, b; Tiliouine & Estes, 2016). We relied on the *Weighted Index of Social Progress* (*WISP*), a well-established instrument that has been extensively used in conducting social development analyses in many regions of the world (Estes & Sirgy, 2017; Tiliouine & Estes, 2016). The *WISP* consists of 41 social indicators that are divided across 10 sectors of social development, which can be used to inform wellbeing policy at various levels of analysis. The category sectors and their indicators include:

- **Educational Status**: Public expenditure on education as % of GDP; Primary school completion rate; Secondary school enrollment rate; Adult literacy rate
- **Health Status**: Life expectation at birth; Infant mortality rate; Under-5 child mortality rate; Physicians per 100,000 population; % of population undernourished; Public expenditure on health as % of GDP
- **Women's Status**: Female adult literacy as % of male literacy; Contraceptive prevalence among married women; Maternal mortality ratio; Female secondary school enrollment as % of male enrolment; Seats in Parliament held by women as % of total
- **Defense Effort**: Military expenditures as % of GDP
- **Economic Status**: Per capita gross national income as measured by PPP; % growth in GDP; Unemployment rate; Total external debt as % of GDP; GINI Index score (most recent year)
- **Demographic Trends**: Average annual rate of population growth; % of population aged <15 Years; % of population aged >64 Years
- **Environmental Status**: Percent of Nationally Protected Area; Average annual number of disaster-related deaths; Per capita metric tons of carbon dioxide emissions
- **Social Chaos**: Strength of political rights; Strength of civil liberties; Number of internally displaced persons per 100,000 population; Number of externally displaced persons per 100,000 population; Estimated number of deaths from armed conflicts (lowest estimate); Perceived corruption index
- **Cultural Diversity**: Largest % of population sharing the same or similar racial/ethnic origins; Largest % of population sharing the same or similar religious beliefs; Largest share of population sharing the same mother tongue
- **Social Welfare Effort**: Age first national law for: Old age, invalidity and death; Sickness and maternity; Work injury; Unemployment; Family allowance.

The *WISP* has been used extensively in studies of socio-economic development, including in the MENA region and functions as a proxy measure for assessing subjective levels of quality of life and wellbeing (Estes, 2015a, b; Estes & Tiliouine, 2016a; Tiliouine & Estes, 2016). Below, regional data are reported that compare social gains and net social losses in the MENA region over a 41-year period. These data are important in assessing the context of the quality of life of the region's citizens since they identify the major drivers that can impede or facilitate the development capacity of the region. Readers are referred to more in-depth analyses of these patterns to obtain a fuller understanding of the nature and drivers of wellbeing in the region (see Estes 2000; Estes & Sirgy, 2018 for selected resources).

Topic Box: Gender Gaps in the Region

The *Global Gender Gap Index* measures gender-based disparities in economic participation and opportunity (including wage equality), educational attainment (enrolment and attainment), health and survival (life expectancy), and political empowerment (women as head of state or in ministerial positions). The MENA region's gap remains large. However, there is progress: The region's best-performing nations for 2017 are Tunisia, the UAE and Bahrain, having closed more than 60% of their overall gender gaps. Of 144 countries, the MENA nations all figure at 117th (Tunisia) or below, with the nations ranking as follows: UAE, 120; Bahrain, 116; Algeria, 127; Kuwait, 129; Qatar, 130; Egypt, 134; Jordan, 135; Morocco, 136; Lebanon, 137; Saudi Arabia, 138, Syria, 142 and Yemen, 144.

The sub-index gives more information. Bahrain is the highest scoring nation of the region when it comes to economic participation, followed by Qatar (122), Kuwait (125) and the UAE (130), with Saudi Arabia coming in below Yemen in 142nd position. Yet, MENA countries score far higher than most of the world when it comes to educational attainment, with Jordan taking first place in the region at 51st place, Kuwait (52), UAE (62), and Bahrain at 75, as examples. Access to health care and longevity also show significant gaps, with Egypt taking first regional place in 98th position, followed by Algeria (106), Lebanon (109), Jordan (113), Kuwait (117), and Yemen (119). When it comes to empowerment, Lebanon, Qatar and Yemen have the lowest rankings worldwide, having closed under 2% of their political gender gap, while the UAE scores quite high in 67th position, recently passing a law, similar to one in Iceland, outlawing gender pay discrimination and deliberately nominating and supporting women in high-ranking government ministerial positions.

13.8 WISP Scores: Member States of Organization of Islamic Cooperation (OIC)

The 26 countries of the MENA region are part of the larger 57, previously 53, member-states of the *Organization of Islamic Cooperation* (OIC), an international governmental and non-governmental organization devoted to the advancement of Islamic countries worldwide (https://www.oic-oci.org/). More specifically, the OIC has adopted a 10-year plan to address the overall development of its members, including efforts to reduce factors that contribute to ill-being like weak or inadequate governance systems (Estes & Tiliouine, 2014; Freedom House, 2017; Tiliouine & Estes, 2016), chronic poverty combined with intractable joblessness (Haas & Lesch, 2016), and weak social safety nets (Estes, 2015a; International Social Security Association, 2017; Tiliouine & Estes, 2016). Further, the OIC has become active in

Table 13.1 OIC 10-year plan outlined

I. Moderation in Islam	1. Condemn extremism in all its forms and manifestations, as it contradicts Islamic and human values; and address its political, economic, social, and cultural root-causes, which are to be faced with rationality, persuasion, and good counsel 2. Strive for the teaching of Islamic education, culture, civilization, and the jurisprudence and literature of difference; call on member states to co-operate amongst themselves to develop balanced educational curricula that promote values of tolerance, human rights, openness, and understanding of other religions and cultures; reject fanaticism and extremism and establish pride in the Islamic identity
II. Human rights	1. Seriously endeavor to enlarge the scope of political participation, ensure equality, public liberties, social justice, transparency, and accountability, and eliminate corruption in the OIC member states 2. Call upon the Islamic Conference of Foreign Ministers to consider the possibility of establishing an independent permanent body to promote human rights in the member states, in accordance with the provisions of the Cairo Declaration on Human Rights in Islam
III. Conflict resolution and peace building	1. Strengthen the role of the OIC in confidence-building, peacekeeping and conflict resolution in the Muslim world
IV. Reform of the OIC	1. Reform the OIC through restructuring, and consider changing its name, review its Charter and activities and provide it with highly qualified manpower, in such a manner as to promote its role, reactivate its institutions and strengthen its relations with NGOs in the OIC member states; empower the secretary-general to discharge his duties and provide him with the necessary powers and sufficient flexibility and the resources that enable him to carry out the tasks assigned to him

Retrieved from http://www.sciencedev.net/Docs/OIC%2010%20year%20plan.htm

humanitarian assistance and in 2008 established the *Islamic Cooperation Humanitarian Affairs Department* (ICHAD) for coordinating humanitarian activities throughout the region. The OIC is the most influential Islamic organization regionally and internationally. The goals associated with the OIC's 10-year development plan are found on their website. We summarize those relevant to this discussion in Table 13.1.

Figure 13.3 summarizes the *WISP* scores for all 53 member states of the OIC over an 11-year period (2000–2011) with a focus on the countries of the MENA region. More particularly, *WISP* scores for the OIC member states are reported for: (1) each of the OIC's nine sub-regions; (2) OIC average *WISP* scores for the OIC-as-a-group (N = 53) and for the world-as-a-whole (N = 162); and (3) the percentage change in *WISP* rank score position for each of the nine sub-regions for the 11-year period, 2000–2011. The countries with the most favorable *WISP* scores in 2011 are reported at the top of the table whereas those with the least favorable scores are reported at the bottom. The bars reported in the figure represent net changes in *WISP* rank positions for the period 2000–2011, several of which are dramatic in terms of net social gains (North Africa and West Asia) and losses (Southern Europe, South America, and Southeast Asia).

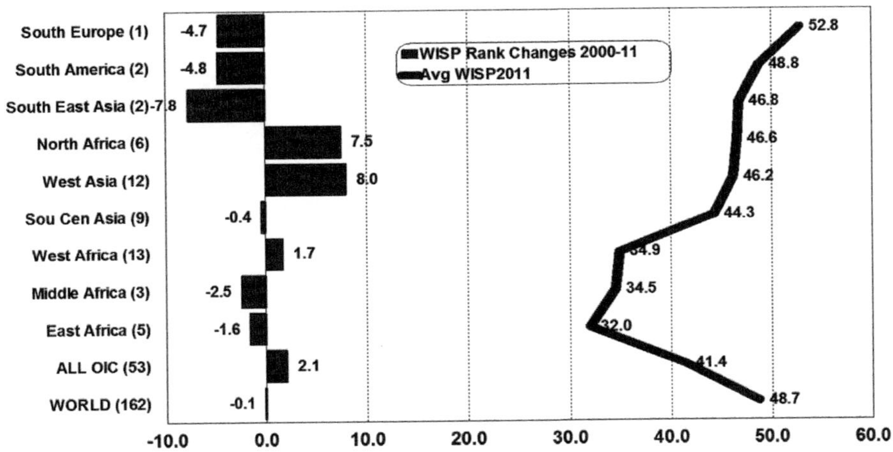

Fig. 13.3 Rank ordered average OIC subregional WISP 2011 scores (N = 9 Regions)

13.9 WISP Scores for the OIC Member States of North Africa and West Asia

The most significant 11-year gains in overall socio-political-economic development took place among the 18 nations of North Africa (N = 6, *WISP* Rank Change = + 7.5%) and West Asia (N = 12, *WISP* Rank Change = + 8.0%). In every case, these gains were substantial and differ dramatically from those reported during earlier decades of development (Estes, 2015b). The gains also suggest that the external factors that impede the attainment of wellbeing are being steadily addressed in OIC subregions where, during past decades, such gains have proven difficult to achieve (Joshanloo, 2014, 2017). The pattern has now changed and, barring unforeseen political or economic turbulence in the near-term, it is likely that social and subjective progress will continue to increase at a steady rate over the decade ahead for most of these countries (United Nations Development Programme; Arab Human Development Report, 2002). More modest gains in *WISP* scores also occurred for the 13 nations of West Africa (*WISP* Rank Change = −1.7). In all cases, a more positive attitude toward the future of these countries now exists, an attitude that is expected to deepen as these countries achieve progressively higher levels of social, political, economic, and technological development (UNDP-AHDR, 2016).

Overall though, and examining the data more closely, all member states of the OIC (N = 53), on average, experienced a net loss in *WISP* rank positions by −2.1% relative to the world-as-a-whole of −0.1%. The most significant losses occurred in the Islamic nations of South East Asia (N = 2, −7.8%), South America (N = 2, −4.8%), and Southern Europe (N = 1, −4.7%). Smaller net rank losses in *WISP* rank positions occurred in Islamic countries of Middle Africa (N = 3, −2.5%) and East Africa (N = 5, −1.6%). The net losses in levels of social progress for these Islamic subregions over an 11-year period, though small in a comparative sense to

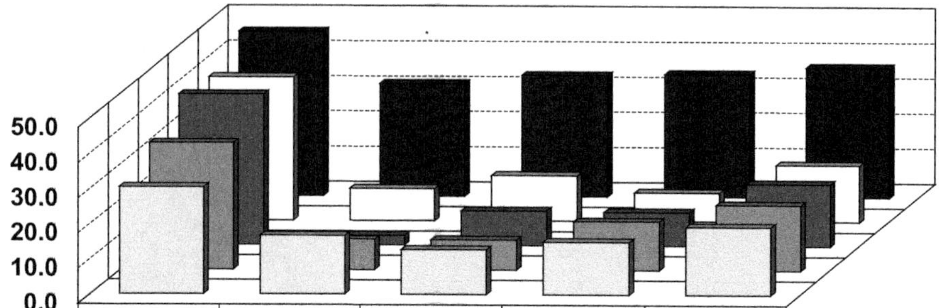

	North (6)	East (5)	Middle (3)	West (13)	ALL (27)
1970	30.5	16.7	12.7	15.0	19.4
1980	36.0	8.7	8.6	13.9	18.7
1990	42.7	2.9	9.9	9.6	17.7
2000	40.7	9.1	12.9	8.2	16.1
2011	46.7	32.0	34.5	34.9	36.9

Fig. 13.4 Average WISP scores for African members of the OIC by subregion 1970–2011 (N = 27)

both the larger OIC and world-as-a-whole, support the need for greater subregional investments to avoid comparative social stagnation. These and other data suggest that even greater investments are needed in the subregions for which average *WISP* social resources have been less than adequate. These investments must be strategic and targeted toward very discrete goals of advancing the wellbeing of women and girls, more investments in at least basic health and educational services, job development and promotion, and increasing levels of participatory political development (Baldawi, 2018; Guzman, 2018). Increased levels of press and internet freedom also are critical to social and interpersonal development.

13.9.1 Social Progress in the African Member States of the OIC

The Islamic nations of North Africa (Fig. 13.4) have a long history of comparative stagnation vis-à-vis the pace of social development occurring in other countries of nearby regions, including those of other countries in sub-Saharan Africa (Estes & Tiliouine, 2016b). Yet, the reported data provide empirical evidence that the levels of social development and wellbeing of the 27 member states of the OIC have begun to increase and in time, can attain comparable levels of social development relative to other continental nations. They are also attaining progress in levels of social development at a faster rate than in other Islamic nations of Africa and the larger community of Muslims worldwide.

Average *WISP* scores for the 27 African member states of the OIC are reported in Fig. 13.4 along the four major African subregions and for the region-as-a-whole.

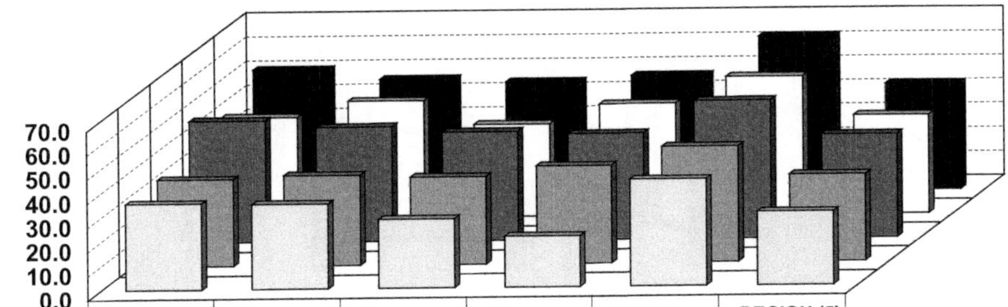

	Algeria	Egypt	Morocco	Libya	Tunisia	REGION (5)
1970	35.6	35.2	28.6	21.2	44.2	30.5
1980	35.8	37.2	36.2	40.4	47.9	36.0
1990	50.3	47.3	44.9	43.8	57.0	42.7
2000	41.9	48.3	38.1	46.3	57.2	40.7
2011	51.8	47.5	46.0	48.1	63.9	44.0

Fig. 13.5 Country WISP scores for the North African segion, 1970–2011

The figure reports data for the 41-year period 1970–2011 and tracks social progress over the entire period. The most impressive changes reflected in this figure are those reported for North Africa (N = 6 countries), which have been consistently the most developed of the continent and, as reflected in Fig. 13.4, continue to be its most rapidly developing. Social development and wellbeing trends are comparable for the countries of the remaining three subregions and these countries, too, share a profound movement forward in overall level of social progress. The countries of North Africa, though, represent the most developed of the continent. At least part of it can be attributed to very active trade patterns between these countries of the Mediterranean and other countries in the subregion, especially trade and commerce with the countries of Southern Europe.

The Islamic countries of North Africa (Fig. 13.5), which led social development over the full 41-year period, include Tunisia (*WISP* M2011 = 63.9) and Algeria (*WISP* M2011 = 51.8). The remaining three countries of the North African subregion (Egypt, Morocco, and Libya) have *WISP* scores in 2011 ranging from 46.0 to 47.5. These latter scores closely approximate those reported for the world-as-a-whole and indicate a substantial level of increase in social progress and wellbeing in the MENA region between 2000 and 2011.

13.9.2 Social Progress in the Asian Islamic Member States of the OIC

Figure 13.6 groups *WISP* scores for Asian Islamic OIC member states by each of the Asia region's three subregions, i.e., West Asia (N = 12), South Central (N = 12), and Southeast Asia (N = 2) (Estes, 2015b). The data summarized in Fig. 13.6 confirm that the average social development and wellbeing performances of each

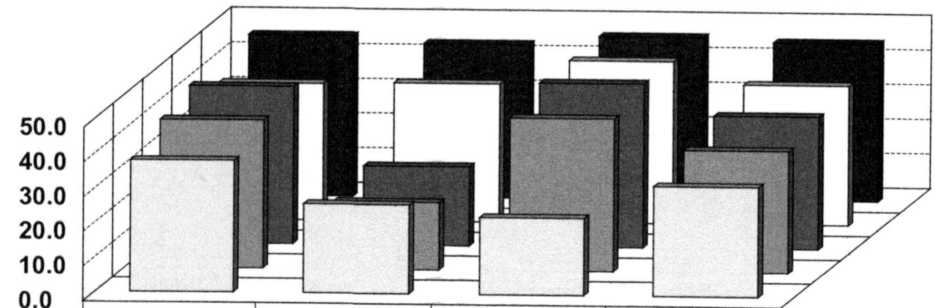

	West (12)	South Central (9)	South East (2)	ALL (23)
1970	37.9	25.7	22.3	31.7
1980	42.6	19.5	43.9	35.1
1990	45.4	22.8	47.3	38.2
2000	39.4	39.9	46.7	40.2
2011	46.2	44.3	46.8	45.5

Fig. 13.6 Average WISP scores for Asian members of the OIC 1970–2011 (N = 23)

of the three Asian Islamic subregions achieved parity by the year 2011. The most significant changes that made this possible were the significant gains in wellbeing achieved by the nine nations of South Central Asia since regaining independence in 1991. These successor states to the Former Soviet Union (FSU) reorganized their social and political systems to compete more successfully in the global community (Lipovsky, 2016). While they achieved this goal as a region at a rapid pace, they did so at varying rates of social progress. Nevertheless, they outpaced other world regions. These findings imply an optimistic perspective.

This pattern is further reinforced in Fig. 13.7, which rank orders the development performances of 16 Islamic and non-Islamic countries of West Asia. The nations with the most significant positive changes on the *WISP* for the 9-year period from 2000 to 2009 are Turkey (+17), Jordan (+10), Bahrain (+9), and Yemen (+8). Their gains in development and wellbeing are especially impressive given the short time period over which this progress has been achieved. Nations that lost social ground, in several cases with very significant drops, are countries associated with high levels of social chaos including war. The development and wellbeing of Iraq, for example, dropped 28 ranks during the same 11-year period.

13.10 Development and Wellbeing of Countries of the Fertile Crescent

The countries of the Fertile Crescent are among the oldest and most influential nations in the MENA region. Yet many of these are characterized by high levels of political instability and a tendency toward authoritarian regimes (Cuoto, 2010). Accordingly, Fig. 13.8 presents both *WISP* scores and changes in *WISP* order position for each

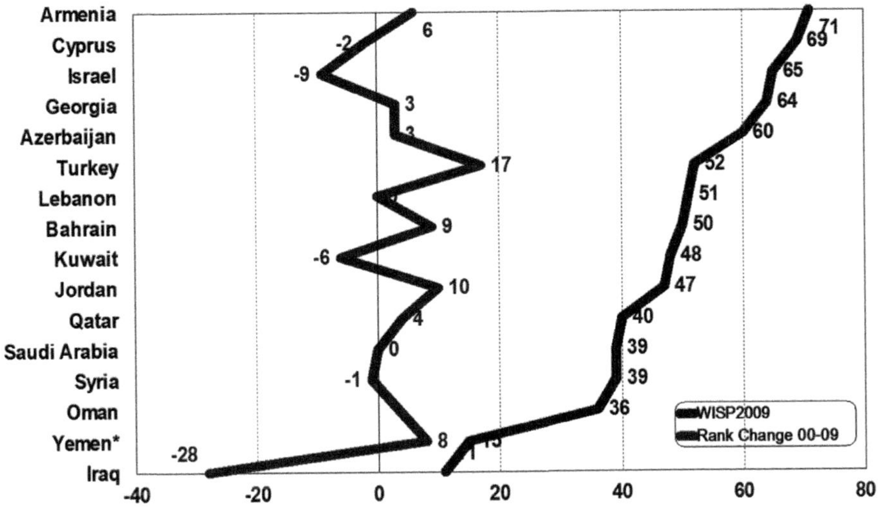

Fig. 13.7 Rank ordered WISP scores and net rank changes for West Asia, 2000–2009 (N = 16)

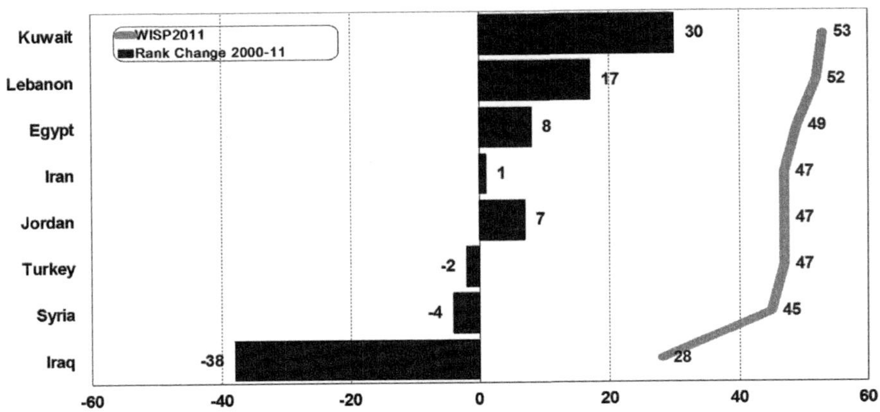

Fig. 13.8 Islamic countries with territories in the Fertile Crescent 2000–2011 (N = 8)

of the eight countries that make up the Fertile Crescent subregion for the 11-year period of 2000–2011 (Estes & Tiliouine, 2016b).

Fortunately, the *WISP* scores for all eight countries increased over the period, albeit only five of the eight were able to increase their rank order position relative to other nations in the MENA region. The net period increases in development and wellbeing performance were especially impressive for Kuwait (*WISP*2011 = 53, Rank Increase = + 30), Lebanon (*WISP*2011 = 52, Rank Increase = + 17), Egypt (*WISP*2011 = 49, Rank Increase = + 9), and Jordan (*WISP*2011 = 47, Rank Increase = + 7). The most significant social losses occurred for Iraq (*WISP*2011 = 28, Rank Decrease = −38), Syria (*WISP*2011 = 45, Rank Decrease = −4), and Turkey

(*WISP*2011 = 47, Rank Decrease = −2). However, two of these countries, Iraq and Syria, are engaged in civil wars, and Turkey is experiencing considerable economic problems in combination with a shift toward an autocratic government. The social situation in Turkey is deteriorating, however, and requires considerable restructuring of its economy and political systems to regain its previously higher levels of social development and wellbeing (Zürcher, 2017). The social situation for Iran has remained mostly constant over the 11-year period despite their large oil reserves and substantial levels of human resources.

The profound changes occurring in many of these countries are impacting the wellbeing of not only their citizens but those of other world regions. This turmoil is especially reflected in the mounting numbers of deaths and serious disabilities associated with the conflicts occurring within their borders (Estes & Tiliouine, 2016a; International Federation of Red Cross and Red Crescent Societies, 2016). Substantial numbers of citizens in these societies have become either internally displaced (United Nations High Commissioner for Refugees, 2018) or have fled their countries in search of safety and economic opportunities elsewhere, especially in nearby European nations, which are increasingly unable or unwilling to receive the hundreds of thousands of people seeking entry (UNHCR, 2018). Recurring Sunni-Shia conflicts has resulted in violence between the two groups and have contributed to undermining social developments (Estes & Sirgy, 2016) in and beyond the region as well.

13.11 Conclusion

A limitation of our assessment refers to the fact that the data only covers the years up to 2011 and thus, fails to capture much of the present-day growth as well as losses taking place in the region. In the next round of analyses we will focus in considerable depth on overall patterns of socio-economic development as well as political developments. We anticipate that poverty will continue to be a challenge in the region in combination with weak, ineffective, or absent social welfare systems intended to eliminate poverty. These issues, in combination with fragile educational and health care systems, exacerbate the regional challenges associated with poverty, albeit most of the region's nations have attained highly favorable outcomes in each of these sectors since at least the year 2000.

An additional issue that is closely associated with the region's development has been the emergence of conflict including Jihadism and Jihadist-inspired terrorism, which has now spread beyond the region to major capitals and financial centers located in Europe and North America (Moore, 2014; Sirgy et al., 2018). Nearly all these conflicts are related to one another and more particularly, are focused on prior European colonizing powers and the US, perceived to be using their financial and military resources to undermine the legitimacy of many of the region's governments. These conflicts have and will continue to result in thousands of people being killed, injured, and rendered socially insecure—often resulting in large numbers of the region's peoples seeking safety in other nearby and distant countries (IFRC,

2016; UNHCR, 2018). In some situations, these conflicts are expected to result in region-wide instability. These long-standing conflicts have slowed the region's overall pattern of development. While our data is only available in 5-year periods and ends in 2011, the conflicts have unfortunately been predicted to destabilize the region even more with the current proxy battles emerging between Syria, Russia, Qatar, the Gulf States, Iran, the US and respective allies—this despite the important social gains made possible through the Arab Spring of 2010–2012 (Haas & Lesch, 2016). Nevertheless, the reality is that most of the subregions and the OIC region as a whole are making progress in achieving major social outcomes, especially in the health, education, job development, international trade, and social welfare sectors (Estes & Sirgy, 2017; Tiliouine & Estes, 2016; UNDP-AHDR, 2016). These gains have been impressive, and the future prognosis for the region is positive, provided it can maintain enough stability and resolve its long-standing as well as emerging conflicts currently brewing.

Steady progress in attaining peace through development, including the promotion of happiness and positive approaches to quality of life in the region, will also depend on the attainment of co-equal status between all members of the region, but especially the attainment of women and girls' equality (Baldawi, 2018). Additional social gains are needed, however, and these will be possible only through the realization of major social, political and economic development objectives over the long-term. We are optimistic that such outcomes will be attained as the region's governments continue to make the critical social investments needed to achieve the multidimensional goals and objectives outlined by the OIC in its multi-decade plans focused on the advancement of Muslim people residing both in the region and other regions of the world (OIC, 2018).

References

ASDA'A Burson Marsteller. (2017). *Arab Youth Survey 2017*. Retrieved from http://arabyouthsurvey.com/findings.html.

ASDA'A Burson Marsteller. (2018). *Arab Youth Survey 2018: A decade of hopes & fears*. Retrieved from http://arabyouthsurvey.com/findings.html.

Abde, A. N. Y., & Salih, K. (2015). The literature of happiness "with reference of the philosophy of happiness in Islam". *Journal of Islamic Studies and Culture, 3*(2), 179–194.

Abdel-Khalek, A. M. (2014). Religiosity, health and happiness: Significant relations in adolescents from Qatar. *International Journal of Social Psychiatry, 60*(7), 656–661.

Abdullah, F. (2014). Virtues and character development in Islamic ethics and positive psychology. *International Journal of Education and Social Science, 1*(2), 69–77.

Abu-Nimer, M., & Said, A. A. (2001). *Reconciliation, justice, and coexistence: Theory and practice*. New York, NY: Lexington Books.

Albright, W. F. (2018). Ancient Middle East. *Encyclopedia Britannica*. Retrieved from https://www.britannica.com/place/ancient-Middle-East.

Al-Seheel, A. Y., & Noor, N. M. (2016). Effects of an Islamic-based gratitude strategy on Muslim students' level of happiness. *Mental Health, Religion & Culture, 19*(7), 686–703.

Andrews, W. (2012). *Mesopotamian religion and philosophy*. Retrieved from https://prezi.com/nd1nvoawlud0/mesopotamian-religion-and-philosophy/.

Arkenberg, J. S. (1998). *Ancient history sourcebook: The advice of an Akkadian father to his son, c. 2200 BCE.* Retrieved from https://sourcebooks.fordham.edu/halsall/ancient/2200akkad-father.asp/.

Askari, H., Iqbal, Z., Krichene, N., & Mirakhor, A. (2014). Understanding development in an Islamic framework. *Islamic Economic Studies, 22*(1). Retrieved from https://ssrn.com/abstract=3158589.

Atiyeh, G. N., & Hayes, J. R. (1992). *The genius of Arab civilization*. New York, NY: New York University Press.

Baldawi, J. (2018). *The status of women in Islam*. Retrieved from http://islamswomen.com/articles/status_of_women_in_islam.php.

Bassiouni, C. M. (2016). Islam and contemporary radicalized violence: A historic turning point. In H. Tiliouine & R. J. Estes (Eds.), *The state of social progress in Islamic Societies: Social, political, economic, and ideological challenges* (pp. 547–573). Dordrecht, NL: Springer.

Central Intelligence Agency (CIA). (2018). *World factbook, 2017*. New York, NY: Skyhorse Publishing.

Cleveland, W. L., & Bunton, M. (2016). *A history of the modern Middle East* (6th ed.). Boulder, CO: Westview Press.

Cuoto, R. A. (2010). The politics of terrorism: Power, legitimacy, and violence. *Integral Review, 6*(1), 1–20. Retrieved from http://integral-review.org/documents/Couto,%20Politics%20of%20Terrorism,%20Vol.%206%20No.%201.pdf.

De Silver, D., & Masci, D. (2017, January 31). World's Muslim population more widespread than you might think. *Pew Research Center News*. Retrieved from http://www.pewresearch.org/fact-tank/2017/01/31/worlds-muslim-population-more-widespread-than-you-might-think/.

Donner, F. M. (2014). *The early Islamic conquests*. Princeton, NJ: Princeton University Press.

Estes, R. J. (2000). Social development trends in the Middle East, 1970–1995: Implications for social policy reform. In L. Belkacem (Ed.), *Building and sustaining the capacity for social policy reforms* (pp. 17–46). Aldershot, UK: Ashgate Publishers.

Estes, R. J. (2015a). Development trends among the world's socially least developed countries: Reasons for cautious optimism. In B. Spooner (Ed.), *Globalization in progress: Understanding and working with world urbanization*. Philadelphia, USA: University of Pennsylvania Museum Press.

Estes, R. J. (2015b). Trends in world social development: The search for global wellbeing. In W. Glatzer (Ed.), *The global handbook of wellbeing: From the wealth of nations to the human wellbeing of nations*. Dordrecht, NL: Springer.

Estes, R. J., & Sirgy, M. J. (2014). Radical Islamic militancy and acts of terrorism: A quality-of-life analysis. *Social Indicators Research, 117*(2), 615–652.

Estes, R. J., & Sirgy, M. J. (2016). Is quality of life related to radical Islamic militancy and acts of terrorism? In H. Tiliouine & R. J. Estes (Eds.), *The state of social progress in Islamic societies: Social, political, economic, and ideological challenges* (pp. 575–605). Dordrecht, NL: Springer.

Estes, R. J., & Sirgy, M. J. (2017). *The pursuit of human wellbeing: The untold global history*. Dordrecht: Springer.

Estes, R. J., & Sirgy, M. J. (2018). Global advances in quality of life and wellbeing: Past, present, and future. *Social Indicators Research*. Retrieved from https://doi.org/10.1007/s11205-018-1869-4.

Estes, R. J., & Tiliouine, H. (2014). Islamic development trends: From collective wishes to concerted actions. *Social Indicators Research, 116*(1), 67–114.

Estes, R. J., & Tiliouine, H. (2016a). Social development trends in the countries of the Fertile Crescent: Jordan, Iraq, Lebanon and Syria. In H. Tiliouine & R. J. Estes (Eds.), *The state of social progress in Islamic societies: Social, political, economic, and ideological challenges* (pp. 179–210). Dordrecht, NL: Springer.

Estes, R. J., & Tiliouine, H. (2016b). Social progress in Islamic societies: Achievements and challenges. In H. Tiliouine & R. J. Estes (Eds.), *The state of social progress in Islamic societies: Social, political, economic, and ideological challenges* (pp. 69–106). Dordrecht NL: Springer.

Fagan, B. M. (2009). *People of the earth: An introduction to world pre-history* (13th ed.) London, UK/Washington, DC: Pearson Publishing Company.

Gopin, M. (2005). *Holy war, holy peace: How religion can bring peace to the Middle East*. Oxford, UK: Oxford University Press.

Gordon, M. S. (2008). *The rise of Islam*. Indianapolis, IN: Hackett Publishing Company.

Guzman, A. (2018). *The role of women in Islam: The role of women in Islam is often misunderstood*. Retrieved from http://www.beliefnet.com/faiths/islam/the-role-of-women-in-islam.aspx#D2YpXlLut2AIG0Qh.99.

Haas, M. L., & Lesch, D. W. (2016). *The Arab spring: The hope and reality of the uprisings*. New York, NY and London, UK: Routledge.

House, F. (2017). *Freedom throughout the world*. New York, NY: Freedom House.

Ibn-Kathir. (1373/2013). *Tafseer: The status of non-Muslims under Muslim rule (circa. 700 years after Mohammed)*. Retrieved from http://4freedoms.com/group/theology/forum/topics/the-status-of-non-muslims-under-muslim-rule.

International Federation of Red Cross and Red Crescent Societies (IFRC). (2016). *IFRC annual report, 2016*. Retrieved from http://www.ifrc.org/.

International Labour Organization (ILO). (2018). *Statistics and data bases*. Retrieved April 1, 2018, from http://www.ilo.org/global/statistics-and-databases/lang--en/index.htm.

International Social Security Association (ISSA). (2017). *Social security programs throughout the world*. Geneva, Switzerland: ISSA.

Ismail, A. G., & Haron, N. (2014). Happiness in economics as understood across Ism and religion. *SAGE Open, 4*(4). https://doi.org/10.1177/2158244014560543.

Joshanloo, M. (2013). A comparison of Western and Islamic conceptions of happiness. *Journal of Happiness Studies, 14,* 1857–1874.

Joshanloo, M. (2014). Eastern conceptions of happiness: Fundamental differences with Western views. *Journal of Happiness Studies, 15,* 475–493.

Joshanloo, M. (2017). Islamic conceptions of wellbeing. In R. J. Estes & M. J. Sirgy (Eds.), *The pursuit of human wellbeing: The untold global history* (pp. 109–131). Dordrecht, NL: Springer.

Keshavjee, M. M. (2016). Alternative dispute resolution (ADR) and its potential for helping Muslims reclaim the higher ethical values (Maqasid) underpinning the Sharia. In H. H. Tiliouine & R. J. Estes (Eds.), *The state of social progress in Islamic societies: Social, political, economic, and ideological challenges* (pp. 607–621). Dordrecht, NL: Springer.

Khan, S. (2018, February 4). *MENA's youth bulge is a regional security challenge*. Retrieved from https://thearabweekly.com/menas-youth-bulge-regional-security-challenge.

Khodayarifard, M., Ghobari-Bonab, B., Akbari-Zardkhaneh, S., Zamanpour, E., Zandi, S., & Derakhshan, M. (2016). Positive psychology from Islamic perspective. *International Journal of Behavioural Science, 2*(10), 1–7.

King, L. W. (2015). *The code of Hammurabi*. Various: CreateSpace Independent Publishing Platform.

Lambert, W. G. (1990). Ancient Mesopotamian gods: Superstition, philosophy, theology. *Revue de l'histoire des religions, 207–2,* 115–130. English version: http://www.persee.fr/doc/rhr_0035-1423_1990_num_207_2_1735.

Leaman, O. (2004). *An introduction to classical Islamic philosophy*. Cambridge, UK: Cambridge University Press.

Lipovsky, I. (2016). Central Asian Islamic state: The challenges of independence. In H. Tiliouine & R. J. Estes (Eds.), *The state of social progress of Islamic nations: Social, political, economic, and ideological challenges* (pp. 303–318). Dordrecht, NL: Springer.

Lucas, S. (2002). *The arts of Hadith compilation and criticism*. Chicago, IL: University of Chicago.

Mark, J. J. (2012). The Egyptian afterlife and the feather of truth. *Ancient History Encyclopedia*. Retrieved from https://www.ancient.eu/article/42/.

McKinsey. (2016, October). *Digital Middle East: Transforming the region into a leading digital economy*. Retrieved from https://www.mckinsey.com/global-themes/middle-east-and-africa/digital-middle-east-transforming-the-region-into-a-leading-digital-economy.

Miller, L. (2006). The terrorist mind: I. A psychological and political analysis. *International Journal of Offender Therapy and Comparative Criminology, 50*(2), 121–138.

Moore, J. (2014). The evolution of Islamic terrorism: An overview. *Frontline USA*. Retrieved March 6, 2018, from https://www.pbs.org/wgbh/pages/frontline/shows/target/etc/modern.html.

Rivers, C. (Ed.). (2017). *Sharia law: The history and legacy of the religious laws that governed Islamic societies*. Various: Amazon Digital Services.

New World Encyclopedia. (2018a). *Sumerian civilization.* Retrieved from http://www.newworldencyclopedia.org/entry/Sumerian_Civilization.

New World Encyclopedia. (2018b). *Cuneiform script.* Retrieved from http://www.newworldencyclopedia.org/entry/Cuneiform_script.

Organization of Islamic Cooperation (OIC). (2018). Homepage. Retrieved from https://www.oic-oci.org/.

Pew Research Center. (2013). *The world's Muslims: Religion, politics and society.* Washington: Pew Research Center's Forum on Religion & Public Life. Retrieved from http://www.pewforum.org/2013/04/30/the-worlds-muslims-religion-politics-society-overview/.

Renima, A., Tiliouine, H., & Estes, R. J. (2016a). The Islamic golden age: A story of the triumph of the Islamic civilization. In H. Tiliouine & R. J. Estes (Eds.), *The state of social progress in Islamic societies: Social, political, economic, and ideological challenges* (pp. 25–52). Dordrecht, NL: Springer.

Renima, A., Tiliouine, H., & Estes, R. J. (2016b). The changing map of the Islamic world: From the Abbasid Era to the Ottoman Empire of the 20th Century. In H. Tiliouine & R. J. Estes (Eds.), *The state of social progress in Islamic societies: Social, political, economic, and ideological challenges* (pp. 53–68). Dordrecht, NL: Springer.

Riaz, M. N. (2015, December). Portrayal of positive psychological capital in Quran. *Al-Idah, 31*, 37–73. Retrieved from https://www.szic.pk/journal/dec2015/4.pdf.

Rizvi, M. A. K., & Hossain, M. Z. (2017). Relationship between religious belief and happiness: A systematic literature review. *Journal of Religion and Health, 56*(5), 1561–1582.

Rogan, E. (2017). *The Arabs: A history.* New York, NY: Basic Books, Hachette Book Group.

Saeed, A. (2006). *Islamic thought: An introduction.* New York, NY/London, UK: Routledge.

Saeedi, H., Nasab, S. M. H. M., Zadeh, A. M., & Ebrahimi, H. A. (2015). *The effectiveness of positive psychology interventions with Islamic approach on quality of life in females with multiple sclerosis. Biomedical and Pharmacology Journal, 8*(2), 965–970.

Schoch, R. (2018). *The great sphinx of Egypt (at Giza).* Retrieved from http://www.robertschoch.com/sphinx.html.

Seligman, M. E. P., & Csikszentmihalyi, M. (2000). Positive psychology: An introduction. *American Psychologist, 55*(1), 5–14.

Sirgy, M. J., Estes, R. J., & Rahtz, D. R. (2017). Combatting jihadist terrorism: A quality-of-life perspective. *Journal of Applied Research in Quality of Life.* https://doi.org/10.1007/s11482-017-9574-z.

Sirgy, M. J., Joshanloo, M., & Estes, R. J. (2018). The global challenge of jihadist terrorism: A quality-of-life model. *Social Indicators Research.* https://doi.org/10.1007/s11205-017-1831-x.

Thomas, J., Mutawa, M., Furber, S. W., & Grey, I. (2016). Religiosity: Reducing depressive symptoms amongst Muslim females in the United Arab Emirates. *Middle East Journal of Positive Psychology, 2*(1), 9–21.

Tibi, B. (2008). The return of the sacred to politics as a constitutional law the case of the Shari'atization of politics in Islamic civilization. *Theoria, 55*(115), 91–119.

Tiliouine, H., & Belgoumidi, A. (2009). An exploratory study of religiosity, meaning in life and subjective wellbeing in Muslim students from Algeria. *Applied Research in Quality of Life, 4*(1), 109–127.

Tiliouine, H., & Estes, R. J. (Eds.). (2016). *The state of social progress in Islamic societies: Social, political, economic, and ideological challenges.* Dordrecht, NL: Springer.

United Nations Department of Economic and Social Affairs (UNDESA). (2017). *World population prospects, 2017.* New York, NY: UNDESA, Population Division. Retrieved from https://esa.un.org/unpd/wpp/.

United Nations Development Programme-Arab Human Development Report (UNDP-AHDR). (2002). Creating opportunities for future generations. *Arab Human Development Report, 2002.* New York, NY: UNDP. Retrieved from http://www.arab-hdr.org/publications/other/ahdr/ahdr2002e.pdf.

United Nations Development Programme-Arab Human Development Report (UNDP-AHDR). (2016). *Arab Human Development Report, 2016: Enabling youth to shape their own future key to progress on development and stability in Arab region.* Retrieved from http://www.undp.org/content/undp/en/home/presscenter/pressreleases/2016/11/29/arab-human-development-report-2016-enabling-youth-to-shape-their-own-future-key-to-progress-on-development-and-stability-in-arab-region-.html.

United Nations High Commissioner for Refugees (UNHCR). (2018). *Data sources.* Retrieved from http://www.unhcr.org/en-us/data.html.

Warner, B. (2010). *Sharia law for non-Muslims (A taste of Islam)*. Lowell, MA: CSPI Press.

We are Social/Hootsuite. (2017). *Digital in 2017 global overview.* Retrieved from https://wearesocial.com/special-reports/digital-in-2017-global-overview.

World Bank. (2018). *World development report, 2018: Learning to realize education's promise.* Washington, USA: World Bank Group. Retrieved from http://hdl.handle.net/10986/28340.

Zürcher, E. J. (2017). *Turkey: A modern history*. London, UK/New York, NY: I. B. Tauris.

Part V
Physical and Psychological Health

Chapter 14
"It Brings Out the Best": Incorporating Positive Health into Health Promotion Initiatives from the UAE's Physically Active

Louise Lambert and Lily O'Hara

Abstract Traditional health promotion efforts focus on reducing factors that contribute to ill-health, such as sedentary behavior or smoking. Yet, this focus on negative or deficit behaviors overlooks those who engage in positive health activities and their reasons for doing so, as well as the positive health assets they gain as a result. Focusing on the absence of health promoting attitudes does little to shed light on why and how individuals successfully build states of good health and wellbeing. However, this information is useful for the development of health promotion initiatives. Consequently, this study investigates the experiences of ten physically active Emirati nationals and the psychosocial assets they have developed through their various activities. We also explore the relevancy of positive psychology and of positive health in particular, for health promotion efforts.

14.1 Introduction

The field of health promotion involves working with people to address the social, economic, environmental and personal factors that contribute to health and wellbeing at the individual, community and population levels (Cottrell, Girvan, & McKenzie, 2012; Taylor, O'Hara, & Barnes, 2014). As part of the health promotion process, it is imperative to first assess the assets and needs that contribute to physical, mental, spiritual, social and environmental health and wellbeing. Physical activity (PA) is an issue high on the agenda of health authorities, particularly in countries with higher levels of socio-economic development, due to its contribution to reducing the risk of chronic degenerative diseases such as cardiovascular disease, type 2 diabetes and cancer. However, rather than the presence of PA as a positive behavior, it is the absence of PA and the presence of sedentary lifestyles (O'Keefe, Vogel, Lavie, & Cordain,

L. Lambert (✉)
United Arab Emirates University, Al Ain, UAE
e-mail: ltlamber@yahoo.com

L. O'Hara
Qatar University, Doha, Qatar
e-mail: lohara@qu.edu.qa

L. Lambert and N. Pasha-Zaidi (eds.), *Positive Psychology in the Middle East/North Africa*, https://doi.org/10.1007/978-3-030-13921-6_14

2010) that have been the dominant focus of health promotion efforts. This emphasis on the deficit or lack of PA and its contribution to pathogenesis or disease creation, is consistent with the biomedical-behavioral public health paradigm (Gregg & O'Hara, 2014). Studies on physical activity in the Gulf Cooperation Council (GCC) nations (United Arab Emirates (UAE), Saudi Arabia, Kuwait, Oman, Qatar, and Bahrain) and the Middle East/North Africa (MENA) region are consistent with this paradigm and focus on physical inactivity.

For instance, in a cross-sectional study in Saudi Arabia (Amin, Alkhoudair, Al-Harbi, & Al Ali, 2012), rates of physical inactivity reached 48% in a group of 2176 individuals ranging from 18 to 64 years. In another, the average daily step count of Saudi Arabian women aged 19–44 years was the same as those aged 65 years and older (Al-Eisa & Al-Sobayel, 2012). Almost half of a sample of 800 Kuwaiti college students self-reported engaging in no PA (Al-Isa, Campbell, Desapriya, & Wijesinghe, 2011). The authors of this study noted that this age group should be in their prime for PA, and that without a standardized measure to capture actual minutes of PA, it is likely that the self-reported active group may not have met recommended levels of PA either. In the UAE, the Dubai Health Authority (2010) found that 81% of national citizens did not attain the World Health Organization (WHO) standard of 30 min of moderate PA a day, five days per week. Only 7% of men aged 40–59 years attained the WHO standard, while only 5% of national women 60 years and over met the standard. Althoff et al. (2017) reviewed the daily smartphone application recorded steps taken by a minimum of 1000 individuals in 46 nations, finding low levels of activity in the region, with residents of Qatar recording an average of 4158 steps per day, the UAE 4516, and Saudi Arabia at the lowest level of 3807 steps per day.

Youngsters are no different. Haroun, El Saleh and Wood (2016) conducted a cross-sectional study on over 1000 students (915 of which were Emirati nationals) aged 12–16 years across 17 government schools in Dubai and found that only 37% reported playing sport or exercising. This number differed greatly by gender: 52% for boys and 19% for girls. Yammine's (2017) meta-analysis of over 12,000 UAE adolescents similarly found that one quarter reported no PA at all. Assessing existing data and devising a scorecard for the UAE with respect to youths meeting the recommended activity guidelines (60 min daily), Al Zaabi et al. (2016) found that rates between 2005 and 2010 actually declined from 19.9 to 17.2%.

While these numbers serve to highlight the extent of physical inactivity, there has been limited research on individuals in the Middle East who do engage in physical activity and their reasons for it, providing little insight into how to increase physical activity. To address this gap, we examine the experiences of ten UAE nationals who enjoy high levels of physical activity, and reflect upon the importance of using a positive lens in health promotion by introducing the emerging field of positive health (Kobau et al., 2011; Seligman, 2008; Seligman et al., 2010) and its intersection with positive psychology (Seligman & Csikszentmihalyi, 2000).

14.2 A Shift Toward the Positive

Despite the 1946 WHO Constitution's (amended in 2006) definition of health as "a state of complete physical, mental and social wellbeing and not merely the absence of disease or infirmity," health promotion efforts often neglect health enhancing behaviors, focusing instead on trying to reduce behaviors that increase disease or injury risk. As such, traditional research paradigms used in medicine, health promotion and psychology focus predominantly on behaviors regarded as problematic and states of ill-health, despite rhetoric claiming to prioritize states of health and wellbeing (Bolier et al., 2013). These traditional paradigms fail to recognize the utility of positive health behaviors, treating them as an anomaly with little value for building states of good health for individuals, and even less for health promotion or public health efforts (Bolier et al., 2013). The dominance of the negative or deficit biomedical-behavioral health paradigm is evident in a review of the published scientific literature (Salanova, 2008) which showed that from 1907 to 2007, there were 77,614 articles published on stress, 44,667 on depression and 24,814 on anxiety compared to a mere 6434 on wellbeing. Within medical journals specifically, the propensity towards negative topics was just as strong with six times as many studies focused on negative factors (i.e., depression, stress, anxiety) as those with a positive focus (i.e., satisfaction, wellbeing, happiness).

In fact, a negative view of health is so ingrained that it influences the entire research process, to the extent that researchers themselves no longer recognize this inherent negative bias (Rozin & Royzman, 2001). For instance, Amin et al.'s (2012) study aimed to establish prevalence rates of physical activity in Saudi women, yet did not address the fact that "10.4% (of participants) were in the high activity category" (p. 357). Beyond this mention, the active group was entirely disregarded and questions like how or why they were active remained unexplored. This example shows that a dominant focus on negative health obscures the positive health behaviors, diverting resources away from an understanding of how individuals increase their levels of wellbeing (Bermant, Talwar, & Rozin, 2011).

To counter this, positive psychology, a new branch of psychology, was introduced in 2000, presuming that individuals have a propensity for growth and the skills with which to mobilize and actualize themselves towards greater wellbeing (Linley, Joseph, Maltby, Harrington, & Wood, 2009). In contrast with the more traditional biomedical-behavioral approaches, positive psychology provides a lens through which to study the processes and conditions that contribute to human flourishing (Seligman & Csikszentmihalyi, 2000). From a research perspective, inquiry questions and methodologies differ significantly between traditional and positive psychology. For instance, in traditional psychology, researchers focus on mental illness and emotional distress, while in positive psychology, researchers focus on flourishing states of mental health (Keyes, 2007), self-determination (Deci, Ryan, & Guay, 2013), purpose (Steger, 2012), passion (Vallerand, 2008) or flow (Csikszentmihalyi, 1990) as examples.

Intersecting with the field of positive psychology is the concept of positive health, which focuses on "promoting people's positive health assets" (University of Pennsylvania, 2015), including psychological and physical strengths that prolong life, promote better disease prognosis and predict health outcomes (Park et al., 2014; Seligman et al., 2010). Assets include locus of control, recuperative ability, cardiorespiratory strength, optimism, a sense of meaning, positive emotions, self-regulation, relationships, and physical activity (Boehm & Kubzansky, 2012; Calado & Young, 2009; Cohen & Janicki-Deverts, 2009; Kim, Park, & Peterson, 2011; Park et al., 2014; Seligman et al., 2010; Sone et al., 2008). Thus, positive health is focused on individuals who exhibit health assets in order to understand the mechanisms that allow for their expression and translation into health promoting strategies for the broader population. Positive health is an integral component of critical health promotion (Gregg & O'Hara, 2014; Park et al., 2014). It values a holistic health paradigm which includes mental, physical, spiritual and social health and wellbeing, and a salutogenic approach (Antonovsky, 1996). In contrast to the pathogenic approach, it focuses on the factors that build and facilitate health and wellbeing rather than those that lead to pathology.

14.3 Physical Activity

Long recognized as a contributor to physical and psychological wellbeing (Ekkekakis, 2013) and also considered a positive psychology strategy (Faulkner, Hefferon, & Mutrie, 2015; Hefferon & Mutrie, 2012; Lambert, D'Cruz, Schlatter, & Barron, 2016), PA confers multiple benefits. Studies report positive mood induction, minimization of workplace stress (Hyde, Conroy, Pincus, & Ram, 2011; Josefsson, Lindwall, & Archer, 2014; Schneider & Graham, 2009), anxiety, negative emotions (Bhui, 2002; Johansson, Hassmén, & Jouper, 2011; Nguyen-Michel, Unger, Hamilton, & Spruijt-Metz, 2006) and insomnia (Al-Eisa, Buragadda, & Melam, 2014). Symptoms of depression also decrease with greater PA, with research suggesting that its efficacy rivals that of antidepressants (Al-Eisa et al., 2014; Conn, 2010; Cooney et al., 2013; Mura, Moro, Patten, & Carta, 2014; Pinto Pereira, Geoffroy, & Power, 2014; Wegner et al., 2014). Reducing physiological reactivity to stress and allowing the body to recover more quickly (Wipfli & Ramirez, 2013; Rimmele et al., 2009; Spalding, Lyon, Steel, & Hatfield, 2004), PA protects against disability, the risk of premature death (Anderson, Seib, & Rasmussen, 2014) and physiological aging (Pollock et al., 2015).

PA also contributes to meaning (Haverly & Davison, 2005) by offering the opportunity to distract one's self from problems and attend to positive stimuli such as positive emotions, relationships, and achievements (Sonnentag, 2012; Tian & Smith, 2011). Put forward as a strength in positive psychology, physical assets build confidence and improve self-esteem as well as perceptions of the physical self (Armstrong & Oomen-Early, 2009; Feuerhahn, Sonnentag, & Woll, 2014; Mutrie & Faulkner, 2004). Active individuals report greater wellbeing (Netz & Wu, 2005), life satisfaction (Piko & Keresztes, 2006), and self-efficacy (McAuley et al., 2006). A daily diary study also showed that on days when individuals took part in PA, they were more likely to experience other positive events and emotions, as well as next-day increases in positive social events (Young, Machell, Kashdan, & Westwater, 2018). PA offers the opportunity to use one's strengths as evidence of achievements with which to approach challenges with confidence and competence (Gavin, Mcbrearty, & Harvey, 2013; Whitehead & Biddle, 2008) as individuals surpass their limits, control their body's abilities, and make meaning of what they do (Kimiecik & Newburg, 2009; Mulholland, 2008).

These and other positive emotional responses are useful for the continued adherence to PA with studies reporting participation up to one year later (Schneider, Dunn, & Cooper, 2009; Williams, Dunsinger, Jennings, & Marcus, 2012; Williams et al., 2008), a finding important in light of the fact that attrition rates in exercise regimens are typically in the 25–50% range (see Linke, Gallo, & Norman, 2011). Positive responses to activity also allow individuals to build psychosocial resources (Hogan, Catalino, Mata, & Fredrickson, 2015), such as self-acceptance, environmental mastery, purpose in life, autonomy, positive relations with others, social contribution, social integration and social actualization. Several experiments have demonstrated a positive relationship between PA and these resources, and an inverse association between sedentary behavior and positive emotions and resources. Explained by the Broaden and Build Theory (Fredrickson, 2006), positive emotions immediately provide broader thought-action repertoires which result in individuals being more motivated, engaged, open, intellectually flexible, and playful (Fredrickson & Branigan, 2005; Kok, Catalino, & Fredrickson, 2008) and over time, these lead to the construction of social, physical, psychological and cognitive resources responsible for individual growth (Cohn, Fredrickson, Brown, Mikels, & Conway, 2009). Thus, the transformations that PA can help achieve over time can be used to generate change, allowing individuals to reach greater versions of themselves by helping them to accumulate positive psychosocial outcomes.

14.4 The Present Study

Knowing what PA means to individuals can be useful for health initiatives; yet, research often focuses on negative health behaviors, barriers to participation, prevalence rates, or on the prevention of disease (Sleap & Wormald, 2001). In contrast, a positive view highlights immediate, tangible rewards like fun, energy and strength, as well as opportunities for self-development and empowerment (Kimiecik, 2002). Learning about positive health behaviors from active individuals and understanding why they engage in activity and what it generates can offer insight into how these behaviors can be strengthened. As PA is a positive health asset (Seligman et al., 2010), the present study aimed to determine why a sample of UAE nationals engaged in it and what implications could be derived for health promotion efforts.

14.4.1 Participants

The study's participants were UAE nationals (male n = 4; female n = 6) ranging in age from 19 to 42 years. Respondents were from the emirate of Dubai and all took part in PA, such as aerobics, running, triathlon, weight lifting, cycling, endurance horseracing, and soccer. Participants were informed of the study's purpose and given the option to not participate and withdraw their responses at any time. No identifying information beyond demographic data (age, gender, activity, and city) was requested.

14.4.2 Study Design

This study involved an exploration of experience and novel understanding of PA participation, meriting a qualitative design (Bernard & Ryan, 2010), which, recently called for in positive psychology (Hefferon, Ashfield, Waters, & Synard, 2017; Rich, 2017; Yardley, 2017), posits that experiences can be understood by how they are described and exist as a source of authority for knowledge. These assumptions are consistent with those put forward regarding the validity of self-report and subjective experience (Baumeister et al., 2007; Diener & Ryan, 2009). A semi-structured protocol was used to guide interviews, drawing on Kobau et al.'s (2011) positively-framed asset-focused questions. Examples of questions included: What does physical activity mean to you? What do you appreciate about its experience?

14.4.3 Procedure

A snowball sampling technique was used to recruit participants through social networks. The inclusion criteria were that participants were UAE nationals, took part in regular PA, and were open to discussing their experiences. In qualitative studies, it is assumed that experiences share common features making sample diversity and sample size less relevant as it is the experience under study rather than the settings or participants that is vital; consequently, samples of up to 10 participants are considered standard (Creswell, 2007; Starks & Brown-Trinidad, 2007).

Interviews were audio-recorded and transcribed. Participants were given their transcript to approve with analysis following suit. Ethics approval was granted for the study by the primary author's former institution and all participants gave written consent to participate. Thematic analysis (Braun & Clarke, 2006; Clarke & Braun, 2017) was used to analyze the data as it is independent of any theoretical model, makes no assumptions about the nature of data, and has been used successfully in other open-ended methodologies (Bulley, Donaghy, Payne, & Mutrie, 2009; Delle Fave, Brdar, Freire, Vella-Brodrick, & Wising, 2011; Pflug, 2009; Takkinen, Ruoppila, & Suutama, 2001). This type of analysis involves the examination of recurring themes important to the description of experiences, which were then noted, tentatively grouped and solidified into themes. This inductive process involves relying on the data for themes to become clear, as opposed to deductive forms of analysis, which run the risk of interpreting data to fit researcher-derived categories (Braun & Clarke, 2006; Clarke & Braun, 2017).

14.4.4 Results

Participants conveyed many themes across their narratives, including group belonging, the importance of social support, a sense of achievement, physical activity as a lifestyle, the experience of positive emotions, and the accrual of social and psychological resources, meaning, and growth. Each theme is discussed and supported by excerpts of verbatim statements. Participants are indicated by their participant (PPT) number, as well as gender and activity in Table 14.1. Quotations from participants have been edited for clarity and grammar; identifying information and names have also been removed for confidentiality. The quotations have been selected to provide a representation of the reported themes.

- **Belonging and support**: Being with like-minded people who shared activities, values, and energy was noted as a benefit of PA. For example, "[If] anyone says, I don't want to go the gym, we say no, but sometimes, we tell her to rest. Otherwise, it's been three days, we tell her to come" (5); "I was new, I had a few friends, but the family I made was at the cross-fit gym. I like the whole community aspect" (3); "I need a group. I won't cycle alone, always with others" (10).
  - Another joined a running program and encouraged others. "I started putting running on my Instagram. I want them to enjoy it. I know many ladies, they hated

Table 14.1 Participant demographics

Participant #	Sport	Gender
1	Running	Female
2	Aerobics	Female
3	Weight lifting	Female
4	Endurance riding	Male
5	Cross-fit	Female
6	Cycling	Female
7	Triathlon	Male
8	Endurance riding	Female
9	Soccer	Male
10	Cycling	Male

running, but now, they are in. I didn't expect so many. Usually, it's everyone else, now, it's us Emiratis" (1).

- Being the only Emirati in a group of cyclists, participant 6 felt she belonged. "When I met the women, I felt they were welcoming and wanted me to improve. It makes you keep going even if you're not feeling good, others push you."
- Coaches helped too. "My trainer is supportive. Some days, I'm going to be in a bad mood and I don't want to do it, but you're there to push me; some days, you're going to need to stop me from pushing myself too much" (3).
- New movements brought excitement. "When I started, I was the only local. I was in an all-guys gym. My trainer insisted I coach with him. His attitude is there has to be a woman at the gym to motivate ladies. We started getting more ladies. Now, we see their statuses on Instagram with Cross-Fit, it makes me happy to see this" (3).
- For others, the prestige attached to a sport was attractive. "I heard people talking about it. Sheikh Mohammed and Sheikh Hamdan, they are all into it. You see the pictures; it's attractive, it's big, important. So, I tried. It was brilliant and I loved it. A year after, a trainer said, I want you to ride for me. I did well and they told me to stay so, I did" (4).

- **Success and recognition**: Participants expressed satisfaction with their PA achievements, especially those they did not think possible. A rider explained, "In Royal Windsor, it was the first endurance timed race. Bahrainis, the Sheikh of Bahrain, they were sponsors. The Queen was there, the Shaikha; it was the first race in Europe. I won. I was so nervous, I met the Queen! It was getting better and better. I was trying hard, doing my best, training every day. That was a big step" (4); "I never thought that exercise could change so many things; I knew I had potential, but did not know how to express what I had" (2).

  - Accomplishments also led to independence and mastery. "When people see a woman, they underestimate her and try to help with boxes and stuff. I say, do you know how much I lift? This is nothing! I like the independence it gives you. You can do it yourself, that feels good" (3); "There is equipment I need them to bring. I go by myself and pick it up and they say no, that's too heavy! I say, no, it's fine, I lift, bro!" (5)!
  - What also emerged was the recognition of their efforts. For example, "An instructor told me you can be more, you have more. I was like, why not? I kept pushing, going to all the classes. Finally, I am at the same level. I never thought this would happen. The members started giving feedback, 'you are inspiring us! You are the reason I come to the gym. You have no idea how proud you make us since you are local.' It's really an achievement" (2); "The girls say you inspire me, I want to do so much. When they see people do this, they say we can too" (5); "People look at me, 'that's impressive, she's young and horse rides like guys;' this makes me feel good" (8); "I want to do something good so I get a good name, so they say, Mash'Allah, he is a good rider. This is what you want, a good name" (4). One was recognized by a very important other, "I want to be a good

role model for Emiratis. I might not be that good, but when I was at the Dubai Tour, His Excellency said 'we're proud of you', I was very proud" (6).

- **Personal growth**: The feeling of accomplishment extended to one's ability to control, transform, and push limits. They explain: "It's like, wow, how far can I push my body? It's nice to see how far it's going" (3); "There are moments where you test yourself. Three months ago I was squatting this, now I'll try again. It's important to see how I've progressed" (5); "Every time I break a personal best, it's like winning an Oscar. I'll be running and wow, I got a personal best again. Even if it's a second; I sometimes push for 5. You see the bar increasing, your potential is increasing, you believe in your capability" (7); "I love to make it a goal. This week, 4 km, then I have a challenge, 5 km. Even when I am tired, I go because I want to reach more; I don't want to stay the same" (1); "I don't mind finishing last but I always challenge myself to be better" (6).
- **Changing motivations**: Most identified external reasons for their early participation and found that their motivations changed. For instance, "I wanted to be thin, but then I wanted to be in shape. I wanted to build muscles. Now, I want to be stronger!" (1); "My goal was to look better; I started going three days a week, then five… I started for the purpose of a good body, now I'm continuing to maintain a good body and good performance. It's not because I have to go to the gym, I want to" (5); "At first, you're there to have fun and then with time you put a challenge. I remember when I first started cycling; my goal was to go for the 50 km loop. Then I started to look for speed, then I did 85. It changed" (6). "At first, I wanted to lose weight, but then I saw there is more to exercise than losing weight. Emotionally I felt good, so I kept going. It's become not about losing weight, but the emotional feeling" (2). "I moved to weight lifting and the trigger was to put on weight because I was skinny. Now, I'm not fussed about how I look, never look at the scale, never watch my food. It became a lever to drive other things, to be a better man, father, professional" (7).
- **A lifestyle**: The word "lifestyle" was common as activities were done not for a time, but as a way of life and something from which to obtain joy and structure time. "When my friends, my family visit, I tell them, you people, fix your schedule to suit mine. My mom is like, you're always at the gym, it became your life, give us time. I said, mom, I'm 30, it's time for me now. I have something great; I want to do it. It's not temporary, it's part of my life" (2); "You get used to it, you commit, make it work. If there is a dinner, you put gym time before. Even if I have to study, I'll go to the gym and stay later at university. There is gym time and everything else" (5). "Sometimes I have exams, projects, you need to sacrifice something, maybe sleep, friends, but I don't sacrifice training" (6); "It becomes a lifestyle. What are you doing this weekend? I am going to do a half Ironman" (7). "I cancel university to go riding. I'm not ashamed; it's something I enjoy. If it's a race, I can't cancel; it's a commitment. If I don't, something is missing" (8). "My Master's classes were from 4 to 8 and our gym was open from 4 to 8. So, I pushed our coach to start a 6am class. I started waking up at 5, having a coffee, driving

to the gym, working out at 6… it was never a matter of 'I have to stop because of university', it was 'I have to make this work while in university'" (3).

- **Happiness**: Participants identified the generation of positive emotions and the decrease of negative ones. "After I finish, I am really happy. I love to run in the morning before work. When you are stressed, you want this (stress) to go. I sleep early when I exercise, when I don't, I sleep late, feel depressed, like I don't want to talk, not sad, just not in the mood. When I exercise, I feel relaxed" (1); "Excited. inspired, motivated. When I play good and score, the whole match is good" (9); "I come back happy every time and use sport to reverse stress, convert that negative energy to physical output" (7); "When I am depressed or feel bad, I get all my emotions out, all the tension goes; you go as a negative person and come back positive" (8). "I had issues, like anger, I was moody. [Then], I forgot how to get angry, I was happy all the time. When I had my injury, I stopped going for two months and was super depressed. The second I went back, I went back up. It's the emotional effects" (2); "It gave me a rush like nothing else did. I love to dance, I love yoga, but nothing gave me happiness like heavy weights. When you land it; you stand up and drop the weight—that rush—it's very difficult to replicate in other parts of life. It definitely helped psychologically" (3). "It makes happiness. When I don't do sports, I don't feel well, it's not me. I get angry and don't focus" (6); "If I fail something or fight with my girlfriend, my parents, whatever, and I'm mad, the second I sit on a horse, I forget. After riding, if I did something wrong, I call them, say I'm sorry; it brings me back to normal" (4).

  - Many found they were not themselves in the absence of activity and noted better mood upon resumption. "I had to stop because I travelled. I felt that my sleep was heavier, I ate a lot of junk, I get tired really fast, I can't concentrate, so many bad things happened. I thought oh, I didn't exercise. Once I started, everything went away" (10); "After the season, okay guys, you did a good job, take a month until we go again. I sat at home, eating, doing nothing, not exercising, no running, nothing. In one week, I was sick, actually sick. I went to the hospital, but I realized it was because I was doing nothing. I went to run, by the second day, I was fine" (4).

- **Resources**: Participants were rewarded with resources like confidence, sociability, self-acceptance, and knowledge. They also learned to deal with criticism.

  - **Information**: "I know what to eat. I changed from full to low fat, brown bread, cow milk to camel. I changed portions" (1); "Healthier of course; I started taking care of my body. I want to know what happens" (5).
  - **Habits**: "I sleep early and wake early. Before, I sleep at 3am. I wake up at 1 pm. I didn't like to work. I liked to watch TV. Now, I don't like to sit" (1); "I eat good, sleep good. If I didn't play soccer, I would sleep at 3am" (9); "I used to sleep 14 h a day, that much! I used to walk when I travelled and I was tired and would look for a chair. My friends were having coffee and I would sit and say, 'Yes, it's good to sit'. Now, it's the opposite" (10).

- **Psychological**: "I am more confident. I accept myself, my body" (1); "I used to take care of people 100% and forgot myself" (2); "It made me look at life more positively. It makes you stronger, like 'I can do it if I want to'" (6); "Sport gave me self-confidence. My mother would say before he cared about what people say, but now I don't. She says 'Everybody is doing this, why don't you?' I say 'No, if everybody doing it, I'm not'. I don't follow" (9).
- **Cognitive resources**: "When I run, I come up with ideas. Your body is on that status, everything is on a high, your emotions, blood pressure, energy, muscles, you think very clearly when you run. You think of many things" (7); "That's the only hour I get to myself, I know what I want. I like to figure out my goals in one hour and decide everything I want" (8).
- **Resilience**: "People say, you have stretch marks and you are not married. 'What is it?' I say, 'What do you want to say? Say something good or don't say it'. I tell them that. That is your body, this is mine" (1). "You get comments that you have to be more feminine, you have to wear lipstick. I don't reply. It's okay to be different" (6). "I say, you are laughing at me? You have a sheesha in your hand … and I become the center of fun? One guy, I told him, I did an Ironman this morning and you don't even have the patience to watch it on YouTube" (7). "I don't quit things anymore. Now, if I get a project, I want it done as soon as possible. At university, I'd start something and leave it. You can't do that in a workout" (3); "It's not easy to do 120 kms in one day. It's tough and needs fitness. Sometimes you ride horses that do crazy things, you have to handle that. You have to be fit, ride every day, race every week, exercise, gym, running. You get to a point where your horse is tired and you have 10kms left. You go down with him and walk. It [also] taught me to control my anger; sometimes you get through the race and your horse is fine, but the vet thinks he's lame. I used to fight, are you kidding me, check the horse again! Then you realize there is no point, you need to be nice" (4).
- **People skills**: "Endurance racing has given me good English. I stay in summer in the UK training, so I have to talk. I try to be friends and nice to everyone because in races, everyone wants to win and sometimes people say, he was cheating… if you're not friends and they don't know you, they talk bad. But, if everyone knows you as a good person, you don't have problems" (4). "I am more social. I used to be a very shy person. I got to know girls at the gym, different ages, nationalities. I am with you here. Two years back, I wouldn't have" (5).

- **Meaning**: Participants became philosophical about their activities. "I want Emirati ladies to feel what is running, what it is to be active. I want them to feel what it is to join, see the other side of life" (1); "My life changed from doing nothing and now I have a sport. I'm so into it. I can't live without it. It's a way to make you better in life" (4); "Sleeping and eating, watching TV is not what a human being is made for. We're meant to do something fun and feeling happy while doing it and keeping up with your health" (6); "Real things matter. It brings the best out of me" (7); "You need to have a goal or purpose in life; you need to have something other than things like work or studying. You need to find something to lose yourself in, something you have passion for. You need to have something that makes you special" (8). "My friends, they can't run; they can't play or do anything. He is living without sport. He is not happy because he is not doing anything. How come you don't have anything, why do you live? What do you want to be? You need to do something in life" (9).

- **Family and culture**: Participants identified critical family support. "My mom sees it as a good thing. She says, 'I'm happy she's going to the gym instead of wasting her time, at least she found something healthy to do.' (After an article appeared): My mom said, 'what are your uncles going to say?' I said, 'Mom, I'm covered, you saw the photo.' The second the paper came, she almost cried! She was proud. Even my uncle, 'I'm so proud; bring the magazine'" (2); "My mom was against me going cause females and stuff…but now my mom is supportive when she saw how I'm getting 2nd and 3rd places" (8); "My family allows me to go any time. They never say no; I'm lucky" (6). Families began being active. "I've motivated my Dad because he's like 'I'm not going to let my daughter get more muscular than me!' There's a bit of a competition between us. He'll ask, 'What's that protein shake you're having? No, I don't want any.' Next day, I see him putting it in the blender" (3); "My Dad supports. My Mom also because when she was my age she was doing gymnastics and marathon stuff, she loves when I bring certificates or medals. She started going back to the gym" (5); "My uncle is forcing his son to go. He says, 'Look at your cousin, she is super fit and healthy!'" (2); "When I hurt myself, my mother said, 'who is going to carry our suitcases?' I was like, 'I can't walk and you're asking who is going to carry your bags?!' She's proud that I don't need a man to carry things, but she'll never admit it" (3).
  - Participants perceived no cultural barriers. "They put in obstacles that are not there just to get themselves an excuse to not go to the gym. I've heard it. I cannot go to the gym, my parents won't allow me. I say, you travel outside without your abaya and sheila, but you cannot work out? This doesn't make sense" (2); "That is people making excuses. We have so many women options. For example, there's a sheikha who holds tennis tournaments for ladies; they're not a joke where you show up and win. Sheikh Majid holds a fitness competition for ladies. There is a ladies only cross-fit gym, ladies only beach. Religion does not prevent an active lifestyle" (3).
- **Health promotion**: Participants were favorable towards competitions organized by the municipality, local sheikhs as well as members of the royal family and their offerings. "It might sound greedy, but I started competing with those. They brought in a lot of people because they knew that they if they could do really well, they could get 5000 AED. That is how he motivated them; it worked. Now, it's intense, a lot of people attend" (3); "Sheikh Mohammed and Sheikh Hamdan, they give it big support. They put prize money for everyone who finishes. That's why people are doing well" (4); "There's no way other than if you make prizes, money. Sheikh Hamdan has a prize in Nad Al Sheba; number 1 gets 500,000 AED with a car, number 2 gets 300,000 AED, third gets 100,000 and, and, and… That's for 80 K; you'll see 1000 people" (10).

- They were less favorable about messages about the duty to exercise, i.e., "It's not a chore, you're not doing this because you have to, you're doing this because you want to. We need to promote it in a different way" (3); "I encourage people to do something enjoyable. I cycle with a bunch of people, they chat, compete, draft, they move, you move! I say to people when you go out, make it fun. Register for events, you go in the morning, there is people, music, everybody is there. The second it's an obligation, it becomes a burden. Do it for the sake of enjoying it" (7).
- Members of the royal family acting as role models made an impact. "Sheikha Maitha, she's doing Taekwondo and was an Olympic flag bearer. She's a good role model. When the royal family is out there competing, it's really good" (6); "You saw the paper? The Crown Prince participated and his father went to cheer. You know what's going to happen, the next Spartan, everybody's going to do it! Role models" (7); "We have Sheikh Hamdan who's very active. He tells us never give up. I really love him. I love how this country supports us, it's not all money and business; we focus on things that make you happy" (8).

14.5 Discussion

The reasons for which participants took part in PA included a sense of achievement, belonging, the experience of positive emotions and overall happiness. These findings are aligned with those in the research literature suggesting that motivations do change over time, often from extrinsic to intrinsic orientations (Gavin, Keough, Abravanel, Moudrakovski, & Mcbrearty, 2014; Havenar & Lochbaum, 2007), and that individuals tend to stick with PA not for attempted weight loss, but for benefits like positive mood induction and the minimization of stress (Josefsson et al., 2014; Hyde et al., 2011; Schneider, & Graham, 2009) as well as reductions in negative emotion and depression (Johansson et al., 2011; Mura et al., 2014; Pinto Pereira et al., 2014; Wegner et al., 2014). Participants also reported greater meaning (Kimiecik & Newburg, 2009), self-esteem and more positive perceptions of the self (Armstrong & Oomen-Early, 2009; Feuerhahn et al., 2014; Mutrie & Faulkner, 2004), as well as greater wellbeing (Netz & Wu, 2005), confidence and competence (Gavin et al., 2013). These reasons contributed to their continued engagement (Schneider et al., 2009; Williams et al., 2012).

Their participation in PA also afforded them several health, psychological, social, and cognitive resources (Fredrickson, 2006; Hogan et al., 2015), such as learning English, becoming more social, dealing with criticism, developing resilience, getting better sleep, managing time and prioritizing themselves. These resources were of immediate and long-term benefit and identified as being useful in work and family life, too (Cohn et al., 2009). Like the Hogan et al. (2015) study, there appeared to be a positive relationship between PA and the resources listed, and equally, that imposed sedentary behavior was associated with less frequent positive emotions and fewer psychosocial resources. The results also give credence to the upward spiral theory of lifestyle change (Van Cappellen, Rice, Catalino, & Fredrickson, 2018), which states that positive affect can strengthen adherence to PA and build resources that, in turn, boost the positive emotions generated during such activity, reinforcing future motives to engage in it. All the same, our conclusions are limited by the fact that the group was small and participants were limited to the emirate of Dubai, known to be more liberal than other areas. Thus, our results do not claim to be representative of the UAE or GCC region.

14.6 Implications and Conclusions

A focus on the presence of positive health behaviors like PA can expand the understanding of why and more importantly, how individuals increase their levels of wellbeing (Bermant et al., 2011). These understandings can offer clues to the mechanisms of change, which can then be translated into successful health promotion efforts in ways that focusing on the absence of health promoting behaviors cannot (Seligman et al., 2010). Thus, by using a positive health framework (Kobau et al., 2011; Seligman, 2008), this study revealed that PA was not something sustained for instrumental reasons, despite it sometimes beginning that way, but for reasons of happiness, belonging, and achievement, as well as the psychosocial resources that accrued from it. We contend that these themes, emerging from a positive health lens, can and should be used to inform health promotion efforts.

For instance, many national health promotion initiatives encourage individuals to partake in PA for the purpose of attempted weight loss, as part of the global "war on obesity" (O'Hara et al., 2015). The findings of this study suggest that this is misguided as participants were motivated to take part in PA to experience a range of positive outcomes. Shifting the focus from weight to wellbeing is consistent with the Health at Every Size® approach, which is trademarked by the Association for Size Diversity and Health, a non-profit professional organisation with the aim of maintaining the meaning and purpose of the approach (Bacon, 2010; Bacon & Aphramor, 2014; O'Hara et al., 2015). The approach advocates helping people find joyful and individually-appropriate physical movement for the purpose of positive mental, physical, and social health outcomes. Thus, health promotion policies and programs should adopt the Health at Every Size® approach and promote PA as a source of wellbeing, positivity and human striving and not as a form of remedial action one is obliged to do. Shifting health promotion efforts from a narrow view of illness and disease prevention to one of daily success, excellence, belonging and happiness is not only fruitful in increasing PA levels, but may yield greater results for health promotion efforts overall (Segar, Eccles, & Richardson, 2011). Further, listening to those who are successful in strengthening their state of health must be encouraged rather than trying to encourage participants to take on agendas set forth by those health promotion experts who operate from a negative, disease prevention paradigm.

That so many participants identified members of the royal family as instrumental in their PA regimes may be a worthwhile avenue to pursue in terms of strategic partnerships. Given their nonofficial, yet voluntary roles in health promotion efforts due to their reach, influence, popularity, and esteem, their involvement in the organization of competitions, prizes, sponsorships, and even venue creation should be fostered and officially solidified. Contrary to research suggesting that external rewards may decrease one's internal motivation (Deci, Koestner, & Ryan, 2001), money, cars and other prizes nonetheless appeared to contribute to individuals taking the first steps to becoming more active and has been noted in the research literature with success (Charness & Gneezy, 2009; Patel et al., 2016; Promberger, Dolan, & Marteau, 2012). Further, health promotion efforts may want to take direction from participants who noted that social media (Instagram, Facebook, etc.) channels about health, fitness, excellence and happiness were more effective in getting them to begin and continue with PA compared to posters, public health announcements and medical advice centered on illness and disease prevention.

While traditional health promotion efforts emphasize health gain through disease prevention as the ultimate goal (Gregg & O'Hara, 2007), for the participants in this study, the most important benefits of PA were health gain through experiencing joy, growth, success and positivity (Kimiecik, 2002). Perhaps by listening more to the success stories of participants, made possible by using a qualitative lens that is increasingly encouraged in positive health psychology (Hefferon et al., 2017; Ruch, 2017; Yardley, 2017), health promotion can reorient its aims towards increasing health and wellbeing rather than decreasing ill-being. We propose that using the lens of positive health psychology (Kobau et al., 2011; Seligman, 2008; Seligman et al., 2010) is indispensable for the task and will drive the field of health promotion forward in the region and in a way that is most locally relevant (Lambert, Pasha-Zaidi, Passmore & York Al-Karam, 2015), achieving its aims of discovering what leads to better health and how to make those a reality for individuals and communities alike (Cottrell et al., 2012; Taylor et al., 2014).

References

Al-Eisa, E., Buragadda, S., & Melam, G. R. (2014). Association between physical activity and psychological status among Saudi female students. *BMC Psychiatry, 14,* 238.

Al-Eisa, E., & Al-Sobayel, H. I. (2012). Physical activity and health beliefs among Saudi women. *Journal of Nutrition and Metabolism,* Article ID 642187. Retrieved from http://www.hindawi.com/journals/jnme/2012/642187/.

Al-Isa, A. N., Campbell, J., Desapriya, E., & Wijesinghe, N. (2011). Social and health factors associated with physical activity among Kuwaiti college students. *Journal of Obesity,* Article ID 512363.

Althoff, T., Sosič, R., Hicks, J. L., King, A. C., Delp, S. L., & Leskovec, J. (2017). Large-scale physical activity data reveal worldwide activity inequality. *Nature, 547,* 336–339.

Al Zaabi, M., Shah, S. M., Sheek-Hussein, M., Abdulle, A., Al Junaibi, A. A., & Loney, T. (2016). Results from the United Arab Emirates' 2016 report card on physical activity for children and youth. *Journal of Physical Activity and Health, 13*(11, Suppl. 2), S299–S306.

Amin, T. T., Al Khoudair, A. S., Al Harbi, M. A., & Al Ali, A. R. (2012). Leisure time physical activity in Saudi Arabia: Prevalence, pattern and determining factors. *Asian Pacific Journal of Cancer Prevention, 13*(1), 351–360.

Anderson, D., Seib, C., & Rasmussen, L. (2014). Can physical activity prevent physical and cognitive decline in postmenopausal women?: A systematic review of the literature. *Maturitas, 79*(1), 14–33.

Antonovsky, A. (1996). The salutogenic model as a theory to guide health promotion. *Health Promotion International, 11*(1), 11–18.

Armstrong, S., & Oomen-Early, J. (2009). Social connectedness, self-esteem, and depression symptomatology among collegiate athletes versus nonathletes. *Journal of American College Health, 57*(5), 521–526.

Bacon, L. (2010). *Health at every size: The surprising truth about your weight*. Dallas, TX: BenBella Books.

Bacon, L., & Aphramor, L. (2014). *Body respect: What conventional health books get wrong, leave out, and just plain fail to understand about weight*. Dallas, TX: BenBella Books.

Baumeister, R., Vohs, K., Funder, D. (2007). Psychology as the science of self-reports and finger movements: Whatever happened to actual behavior? *Perspectives on Psychological Science, 2*(4), 396–403.

Bhui, K. (2002). Physical activity and stress. In S. A. Stanfeld & M. G. Marmot (Eds.), *Stress and the heart: Psychosocial pathways to coronary heart disease* (pp. 158–167). Williston, VT: BMJ Books.

Bermant, G., Talwar, C., & Rozin, P. (2011). To celebrate positive psychology and extend its horizons. In K. M. Sheldon, T. B. Kashdan, & M. F. Steger (Eds.), *Designing positive psychology: Taking stock and moving forward* (pp. 430–438). Oxford: Oxford University Press.

Bernard, H. R., & Ryan, G. W. (2010). *Analyzing qualitative data: Systematic approaches*. Thousand Oaks, CA: Sage Publications.

Boehm, J. K., & Kubzansky, L. D. (2012). The heart's content: The association between positive psychological wellbeing and cardiovascular health. *Psychological Bulletin, 138*(4), 655–691.

Bolier, L., Haverman, M., Westerhof, G. J., Riper, H., Smit, F., & Bohlmeijer, E. (2013). Positive psychology interventions: A meta-analysis of randomized controlled studies. *BMC Public Health, 13,* 119.

Braun, V., & Clarke, V. (2006). Using thematic analysis in psychology. *Qualitative Research in Psychology, 3,* 77–101.

Bulley, C., Donaghy, M., Payne, A., & Mutrie, N. (2009). Personal meanings, values and feelings relating to physical activity and exercise participation in female undergraduates: A qualitative exploration. *Journal of Health Psychology, 14*(6), 751–760.

Calado, R. T., & Young, N. S. (2009). Telomere diseases. *New England Journal of Medicine, 361*(24), 2353–2365.

Charness, G., & Gneezy, U. (2009). Incentives to exercise. *Econometrica: Journal of the Econometric Society, 77*(3), 909–931.

Clarke, V., & Braun, V. (2017). Thematic analysis. *Journal of Positive Psychology, 12*(3), 297–298.

Cohen, S., & Janicki-Deverts, D. (2009). Can we improve our physical health by altering our social networks? *Perspectives on Psychological Science, 4*(4), 375–378.

Cohn, M. A., Fredrickson, B. L., Brown, S. L., Mikels, J. A., & Conway, A. M. (2009). Happiness unpacked: Positive emotions increase life satisfaction by building resilience. *Emotion, 9*(3), 361–368.

Conn, V. (2010). Depressive symptom outcomes of physical activity interventions: Meta-analysis findings. *Annals of Behavioral Medicine, 39,* 128–138.

Cooney, G. M., Dwan, K., Greig, C. A., Lawlor, D. A., Rimer, J., Waugh, F. R., ... & Mead, G. E. (2013). Exercise for depression. *Cochrane Database Systematic Review, 19*, CD004366.

Cottrell, R. R., Girvan, J. T., & McKenzie, J. F. (2012). *Principles and foundations of health promotion and education*. Boston, USA: Benjamin Cummings.

Creswell, J. (2007). *Qualitative inquiry and research design: Choosing among five traditions*. Thousand Oaks, CA: Sage Publications.

Csikszentmihalyi, M. (1990). *Flow: The psychology of optimal experience*. New York, NY: Harper and Row.

Deci, E. L., Koestner, R., & Ryan, R. M. (2001). Extrinsic rewards and intrinsic motivation in education: Reconsidered once again. *Review of Educational Research, 71*(1), 1–27.

Deci, E. L., Ryan, R. M., & Guay, F. (2013). Self-determination theory and actualization of human potential. In D. McInerney, H. Marsh, R. Craven, & F. Guay (Eds.), *Theory driving research: New wave perspectives on self processes and human development* (pp. 109–133). Charlotte, NC: Information Age Press.

Delle Fave, A., Brdar, I., Freire, T., Vella-Brodrick, D., & Wissing, M. P. (2011). The eudaimonic and hedonic components of happiness: Qualitative and quantitative findings. *Social Indicators Research, 100*(2), 185–207.

Diener, E., & Ryan, K. (2009). Subjective wellbeing: A general overview. *South African Journal of Psychology, 39*(4), 391–406.

Dubai Health Authority. (2010). *Dubai Household Health Survey 2009*. Dubai, UAE: Dubai Government.

Ekkekakis, P. (2013). Pleasure from the exercising body: Two centuries of changing outlooks in psychological thought. In P. Ekkekakis (Ed.), *Routledge handbook of physical activity and mental health* (pp. 35–56). New York, USA: Routledge.

Faulkner, G., Hefferon, K., & Mutrie, N. (2015). Positive psychology in motion. In S. Joseph (Ed.), *Positive psychology in practice* (2nd ed., pp. 207–221). Hoboken, USA: Wiley.

Feuerhahn, N., Sonnentag, S., & Woll, A. (2014). Exercise after work, psychological mediators, and affect: A day-level study. *European Journal of Work and Organizational Psychology, 23,* 62–79.

Fredrickson, B. L. (2006). Unpacking positive emotions: Investigating the seeds of human flourishing. *Journal of Positive Psychology, 1,* 57–60.

Fredrickson, B. L., & Branigan, C. (2005). Positive emotions broaden the scope of attention and thought-action repertoires. *Cognition and Emotion, 19,* 313–332.

Gavin, J., Keough, M., Abravanel, M., Moudrakovski, T., & Mcbrearty, M. (2014). Motivations for participation in physical activity across the lifespan. *International Journal of Wellbeing, 4*(1), 46–61.

Gavin, J., Mcbrearty, M., & Harvey, W. (2013). Involvement in physical activity: Adolescents' perceptions of outcomes. *SAGE Open, 3*(2). Retrieved from https://doi.org/10.1177/2158244013485094.

Gregg, J., & O'Hara, L. (2007). Values and principles evident in current health promotion practice. *Health Promotion Journal of Australia, 18*(1), 7–11.

Gregg, J., & O'Hara, L. (2014). Health promotion: A critical salutogenic science. *International Journal of Social Work and Human Services, 2*(6), 283–290.

Haroun, D., ElSaleh, O., & Wood, L. (2016). Dietary and activity habits in adolescents living in the United Arab Emirates: A cross-sectional study. *Arab Journal of Nutrition and Exercise, 1*(2), 119–141.

Havenar, J., & Lochbaum, M. (2007). Differences in participation motives in first-time marathon finishers and pre-race dropouts. *Journal of Sport Behavior, 30,* 270–279.

Haverly, K., & Davison, K. K. (2005). Personal fulfillment motives adolescents to be physically active. *Archives of Pediatrics and Adolescent Medicine, 159,* 1115–1120.

Hefferon, K., Ashfield, A., Waters, L., & Synard, J. (2017). Editorial: Understanding optimal human functioning: The 'call for qual' in exploring human flourishing and wellbeing. *The Journal of Positive Psychology, 12,* 211–219.

Hefferon, K., & Mutrie, N. (2012). Physical activity as a "stellar" positive psychology intervention. In E. O. Acevedo (Ed.), *Oxford handbook of exercise psychology* (pp. 117–128). Oxford, UK: Oxford University Press.

Hogan, C. L., Catalino, L. I., Mata, J., & Fredrickson, B. (2015). Beyond emotional benefits: Physical activity and sedentary behavior affect psychosocial resources through emotions. *Psychology & Health, 30,* 354–369.

Hyde, A. L., Conroy, D. E., Pincus, A. L., & Ram, N. (2011). Unpacking the feel-good effect of free-time physical activity: Between- and within-person associations with pleasant-activated feeling states. *Journal of Sport & Exercise Psychology, 33*(6), 884–902.

Johansson, M., Hassmén, P., & Jouper, J. (2011). Acute effects of Qigong exercise on mood and anxiety. *Sport, Exercise, and Performance Psychology, 1,* 60–65.

Josefsson, T., Lindwall, M., & Archer, T. (2014). Physical exercise intervention in depressive disorders: Meta-analysis and systematic review. *Scandinavian Journal of Medicine and Science in Sports, 24*(2), 259–272.

Keyes, C. L. M. (2007). Promoting and protecting mental health as flourishing: A complementary strategy for improving national mental health. *The American Psychologist, 62*(2), 95–108.

Kim, E. S., Park, N., & Peterson, C. (2011). Dispositional optimism protects older adults from stroke: The health and retirement study. *Stroke, 42*(10), 2855–2859.

Kimiecik, J. C. (2002). *The intrinsic exerciser: Discovering the joy of exercise*. Boston, MA: Houghton Mifflin.

Kimiecik, J., & Newburg, D. (2009). *Runner as hero: The inner quest of becoming a runner or athlete or just about anything…at any age*. Lanham, MA: University Press of America.

Kobau, R., Seligman, M. E. P., Peterson, C., Diener, E., Zack, M. M., Chapman, D., & Thompson, W. (2011). Mental health promotion in public health: Perspectives and methods from positive psychology. *American Journal of Public Health, 101*, e1–e9.

Kok, B. E., Catalino, L. I., & Fredrickson, B. L. (2008). The broadening, building, buffering effects of positive emotions. In S. J. Lopez (Ed.), *Positive psychology: Exploring the best of people* (Vol. 3, pp. 1–19). Westport, CT: Greenwood Publishing Company.

Lambert, L., D'Cruz, A., Schlatter, M., & Barron, F. (2016). Using physical activity to tackle depression: The neglected positive psychology intervention. *Middle East Journal of Positive Psychology, 2*(1), 42–60.

Lambert, L., Pasha-Zaidi, N., Passmore, H.-A., & York Al-Karam, C. (2015). Developing an indigenous positive psychology in the United Arab Emirates. *Middle East Journal of Positive Psychology, 1*(1), 1–23.

Linke, S. E., Gallo, L. C., & Norman, G. J. (2011). Attrition and adherence rates of sustained vs. intermittent exercise interventions. *Annals of Behavioral Medicine: A Publication of the Society of Behavioral Medicine*, *42*(2), 197–209.

Linley, P., Joseph, S., Maltby, J., Harrington, S., & Wood, A. M. (2009). Positive psychology applications. In C. R. Snyder & S. J. Lopez (Eds.), *Oxford handbook of positive psychology* (2nd ed., pp. 35–47). Oxford, UK: Oxford University Press.

McAuley, E., Konopack, J. F., Motl, R. W., Morris, K. S., Doerksen, S. E., & Rosengren, K. R. (2006). Physical activity and quality of life in older adults: Influence of health status and self-efficacy. *Annals of Behavioral Medicine, 31*(1), 99–103.

Mulholland, E. (2008). *What sport can do.* Retrieved from True Sport Foundation: http://www.truesportpur.ca/files/tsreport/TS_report_EN_webdownload.pdf.

Mura, G., Moro, M. F., Patten, S. B., & Carta, M. G. (2014). Exercise as an add-on strategy for the treatment of major depressive disorder: A systematic review. *CNS Spectrums, 19*(6), 496–508.

Mutrie, N., & Faulkner, G. (2004). Physical activity: Positive psychology in motion. In A. Linley & S. Joseph (Eds.), *Positive psychology in practice* (pp. 146–164). Hoboken, NJ: Wiley.

Netz, Y., & Wu, M. J. (2005). Physical activity and psychological wellbeing in advanced age: A meta-analysis of intervention studies. *Psychology and Aging, 20*(2), 272–284.

Nguyen-Michel, S. T., Unger, J. B., Hamilton, J., & Spruijt-Metz, D. (2006). Associations between physical activity and perceived stress/hassles in college students. *Stress and Health: Journal of the International Society for the Investigation of Stress, 22*(3), 179–188.

O'Hara, L., Taylor, J., & Barnes, M. (2015). The extent to which the public health 'war on obesity' reflects the ethical values and principles of critical health promotion: A multimedia critical discourse analysis. *Health Promotion Journal of Australia, 26*(3), 246–254.

O'Keefe, J. H., Vogel, R., Lavie, C. J., & Cordain, L. (2010). Achieving hunter-gatherer fitness in the 21st century: Back to the future. *The American Journal of Medicine, 123*(12), 1082–1086.

Park, N., Peterson, C., Szvarca, D., Vander Molen, R. J., Kim, E. S., & Collon, K. (2014). Positive psychology and physical health: Research and applications. *American Journal of Lifestyle Medicine, 10*(3), 200–206.

Patel, M. S., Asch, D. A., Rosin, R., Small, D. S., Bellamy, S. L., & Volpp, K. G. (2016). Framing financial incentives to increase physical activity among overweight and obese adults: A randomized, controlled trial. *Annals of Internal Medicine, 164*(6), 385–394.

Pflug, J. (2009). Folk theories of happiness: A cross-cultural comparison of conceptions of happiness in Germany and South Africa. *Social Research Indicators, 92*(3), 551–563.

Piko, B. F., & Keresztes, N. (2006). Physical activity, psychosocial health, and life goals among youth. *Journal of Community Health, 31*(2), 136–145.

Pinto Pereira, S. M., Geoffroy, M., & Power, C. (2014). Depressive symptoms and physical activity during 3 decades in adult life: Bidirectional associations in a prospective cohort study. *JAMA Psychiatry, 71*(12), 1373–1380.

Pollock, R. D., Carter, S., Velloso, C. P., Duggal, N. A., Lord, J. M., Lazarus, N. R., & Harridge, S. D. R. (2015). An investigation into the relationship between age and physiological function in highly active older adults. *The Journal of Physiology, 593*(3), 657–680.

Promberger, M., Dolan, P., & Marteau, T. M. (2012). "Pay them if it works": Discrete choice experiments on the acceptability of financial incentives to change health related behaviour. *Social Science and Medicine, 75*(12), 2509–2514.

Rich, G. J. (2017). The promise of qualitative inquiry for positive psychology: Diversifying methods. *Journal of Positive Psychology, 12*(3), 220–231.

Rimmele, U., Seiler, R., Marti, B., Wirtz, P. H., Ehlert, U., & Heinrichs, M. (2009). The level of physical activity affects adrenal and cardiovascular reactivity to psychosocial stress. *Psychoneuroendocrinology, 34,* 190–198.

Rozin, P., & Royzman, E. B. (2001). Negativity bias, negativity dominance, and contagion. *Personality and Social Psychology Review, 5*(4), 296–320.

Salanova, M. (2008). Organizaciones saludables: Una aproximación desde la psicología positiva. In C. Vázquez & G. Hervás (Eds.), *Psicología positiva aplicada* (pp. 403–427). Madrid, Spain: Desclée de Brouwer.

Schneider, M., Dunn, A., & Cooper, D. (2009). Affect, exercise, and physical activity among healthy adolescents. *Journal of Sport and Exercise Psychology, 31,* 706–723.

Schneider, M., & Graham, D. (2009). Personality, physical fitness, and affective response to exercise among adolescents. *Medicine and Science in Sports and Exercise, 41*(4), 947–955.

Segar, M. L., Eccles, J. S., & Richardson, C. R. (2011). Rebranding exercise: Closing the gap between values and behavior. *The International Journal of Behavioral Nutrition and Physical Activity, 8,* 94.

Seligman, M. E. P. (2008). Positive health. *Applied Psychology: An International Review, 57,* 3–18.

Seligman, M. E. P., & Csikszentmihalyi, M. (2000). Positive psychology: An introduction. *American Psychologist, 55*(1), 5–14.

Seligman, M. E. P., Peterson, C., Barsky, A. J., Boehm, J. K., Kubzansky, L. D., Park, N., & Labarthe, D. (2010). *Positive health and health assets: Re-analysis of longitudinal data sets.* University of Pennsylvania, White Paper. Retrieved from http://www.sas.upenn.edu/psych/seligman/positivehealthassetspub.pdf.

Sleap, M., & Wormald, H. (2001). Perceptions of physical activity among young women aged 16 and 17 years. *European Journal of Physical Education, 6,* 26–37.

Sone, T., Nakaya, N., Ohmori, K., Shimazu, T., Higashiguchi, M., Kakizaki, M.,..., Tsuji, I. (2008). Sense of life worth living (ikigai) and mortality in Japan: Ohsaki study. *Psychosomatic Medicine, 70*(6), 709–715.

Sonnentag, S. (2012). Psychological detachment from work during leisure time: The benefits of mentally disengaging from work. *Current Directions in Psychological Science, 22,* 114–118.

Spalding, T. W., Lyon, L. A., Steel, D. H., & Hatfield, B. D. (2004). Aerobic exercise training and cardiovascular reactivity to psychological stress in sedentary young normotensive men and women. *Psychophysiology, 41,* 552–562.

Steger, M. F. (2012). Making meaning in life. *Psychological Inquiry, 23,* 381–385.

Starks, H., & Brown-Trinidad, S. (2007). Choose your method: A comparison of phenomenology, discourse analysis, and grounded theory. *Qualitative Health Research, 17*(10), 1372–1380.

Takkinen, S., Ruoppila, I., & Suutama, T. (2001). More meaning by exercising? Physical activity as a predictor of a sense of meaning in life and of self-rated health and functioning in old age. *Journal of Aging and Physical Activity, 9*(2), 128–141.

Taylor, J., O'Hara, L., & Barnes, M. (2014). Health promotion: A critical salutogenic science. *International Journal of Social Work and Human Services Practice, 2,* 283–290.

Tian, Q., & Smith, J. C. (2011). Attentional bias to emotional stimuli is altered during moderate but not high intensity exercise. *Emotion, 11,* 1415–1424.

University of Pennsylvania. (2015). *What is positive health?* Retrieved from https://www.authentichappiness.sas.upenn.edu/learn/positivehealth.

Vallerand, R. (2008). On the psychology of passion: In search of what makes people's lives most worth living. *Canadian Psychological Association, 49*(1), 1–13.

Van Cappellen, P., Rice, E. L., Catalino, L. I., & Fredrickson, B. L. (2018). Positive affective processes underlie positive health behavior change. *Psychology & Health, 33*(1), 77–97.

Wegner, M., Helmich, I., Machado, S., Nardi, A., Arias-Carrion, O., & Budde, H. (2014). Effects of exercise on anxiety and depression disorders: Review of meta-analyses and neurobiological mechanisms. *CNS & Neurological Disorders: Drug Targets, 13*(6), 1002.

Whitehead, S., & Biddle, S. (2008). Adolescent girls' perceptions of physical activity: A focus group study. *European Physical Education Review, 14*(2), 243–262.

Williams, D. M., Dunsiger, S., Ciccolo, J. T., Lewis, B. A., Albrecht, A. E., & Marcus, B. H. (2008). Acute affective response to a moderate-intensity exercise stimulus predicts physical activity participation 6 and 12 months later. *Psychology of Sport and Exercise, 9,* 231–245.

Williams, D. M., Dunsiger, S., Jennings, E. G., & Marcus, B. H. (2012). Does affective valence during and immediately following a 10-min walk predict concurrent and future physical activity? *Annals of Behavioral Medicine, 44,* 43–51.

Wipfli, B., & Ramirez, E. (2013). Stress reactivity in humans and animals: Two meta-analyses. *International Journal of Exercise Science, 6,* 144–156.

World Health Organization (2006). *Constitution of the World Health Organization.* Retrieved from http://www.who.int/governance/eb/who_constitution_en.pdf.

Yammine, K. (2017). The prevalence of physical activity among the young population of UAE: A meta-analysis. *Perspectives in Public Health, 137*(5), 275–280.

Yardley, L. (2017). Demonstrating the validity of qualitative research. *Journal of Positive Psychology, 12*(3), 295–296.

Young, K. C., Machell, K. A., Kashdan, T. B., & Westwater, M. L. (2018). The cascade of positive events: Does exercise on a given day increase the frequency of additional positive events? *Personality and Individual Differences, 120,* 299–303.

Chapter 15
Positive Psychotherapy: Clinical and Cross-cultural Applications of Positive Psychology

Tayyab Rashid and Mohammed K. Al-Haj Baddar

Abstract This chapter offers a review of what is called positive psychotherapy (PPT) and the existing positive psychology clinical interventions (PPIs) currently being used in the field. We examine their efficacy and use within clinical and non-clinical populations. We further review the 24 character strengths, also used in PPT, as an adjunct to therapy and their corresponding over- and underuse. The chapter is further supplemented by the work of a Jordanian positive psychologist currently using PPIs and the principles of positive community development in different refugee hosting areas in Jordan. The lessons provided will be of value to clinicians in the region and elsewhere.

15.1 Introduction

Many people read self-help books, attend retreats, take courses, and use alternative health remedies to feel happier, and many forms of psychotherapies exist to alleviate symptoms of psychological stress. The focus of these is generally on symptom remittance and habit remediation as individuals experience significantly more negatives than positives when needing help (Schwartz et al., 2002; Wong, 2012). When their emotions feel acutely negative, they opt for treatment. There, they feel fragile and see themselves as flawed, and psychological help or psychotherapy becomes a process where bottled emotions are vented, tangled relationships sorted, and secrets disclosed—all to restore a tattered self-concept with an empathic therapist. Clinicians of all descriptions (i.e., psychotherapists, counsellors, mental health practitioners, etc.) dispense the bulk of their efforts and expertise in making such clients less depressed or anxious by uncovering traumas, untwisting faulty thinking, or fixing dysfunction. Clients and clinicians focus almost exclusively on negatives as the function of

T. Rashid (✉)
Positive Clinical Psychologist, Toronto, ON, Canada
e-mail: tayyab.rashid@utoronto.ca

M. K. Al-Haj Baddar
Jannati Clinics, Amman, Jordan
e-mail: moh.baddar@gmail.com

L. Lambert and N. Pasha-Zaidi (eds.), *Positive Psychology in the Middle East/North Africa*, https://doi.org/10.1007/978-3-030-13921-6_15

psychological treatment has, at least traditionally, been to unpack the negatives, but also because the negative invariably carries more weight, is quicker to form, harder to undo and lasts far longer (Baumeister, Bratslavsky, Finkenauer, & Vohs, 2001; Lyubomirsky, Caldwell & Nolen-Hoeksema, 1998; Rozin & Royzman, 2001).

Of late, there are also positive psychology interventions (PPIs) to help people feel more positive (Baños et al., 2017; Bolier et al., 2013; Khazaei, Khazaei, & Ghanbari, 2017). One form applied in clinical settings is Positive Psychotherapy (PPT; Rashid, 2008, 2013, 2015). PPT, the focus of this chapter, is a protocoled, sequential and systematic set of 14 PPIs and the therapeutic arm of positive psychology, which integrates symptoms and strengths, risks and resources, weaknesses and values, delights and despairs, and set-backs with successes. Without dismissing, minimizing or hastily replacing negatives with positives, PPT dispenses equal effort on the positives, as most clients wish not to be merely less sad, anxious, or angry, but happy, kind, interested, and optimistic. They want lives that are meaningful and worth living. PPT addresses that desire beyond its rhetoric. Thus, it is a treatment approach, which systematically amplifies the positive resources of clients—specifically positive emotions, character strengths, meaning, positive relationships, and intrinsically motivated accomplishments—with the aim of undoing psychopathology. PPT is not only about the positive, nor does it suggest that other treatments are negative. The "positive" merely focuses on increasing and maintaining the presence of the preferred and the absence of the dispreferred (Pawelski, 2016). It is also not an alternative to established treatments for severe clinical conditions.

PPT is based on the premise that psychological treatment presents an opportunity for accentuating positive aspects of human experience as well as ameliorating the negatives. Focusing exclusively on negatives or positives might be simpler, but the challenge is to understand the complexity of life which includes both negative and positive experience. Psychotherapy and counselling have done well in assessing and intervening with psychopathology (Castonguay, 2013; Lambert, 2017). However, the next frontier for treatment is to consider clients' distress, deficits, dysfunctions, and disorders along with their assets, abilities, strengths, and skills. This integration opens additional therapeutic avenues for therapists. PPT is an attempt to translate this integration from abstraction into concrete application. It is important to expand the horizons of psychological treatments, especially when their use is on the decline and psychotropic medications have become the most prescribed class of medication (Olfson & Marcus, 2010), and when so many unsubstantiated self-help remedies are accessible. Psychotherapy, on the other hand, has a solid scientific foundation that is effective and in most cases, works equally, or better than medication (Castonguay, 2013; Leykin & DeRubeis, 2009). There is also a need to make the therapeutic process attractive and accessible. Many do not seek treatment due to stigma (Corrigan, 2004) and for cyber-savvy, urban and culturally diverse millennials, psychotherapy also needs to be innovative, de-stigmatizing, focused, short-term and compatible with technological interfaces (Smith & Aaker, 2013).

15.2 Assumptions of PPT

PPT has three assumptions regarding the nature, cause, course and treatment of behavior. First, PPT assumes that psychopathology follows when capacities for growth, fulfillment, and wellbeing are thwarted. Wellbeing and psychopathology are not entirely endogenous processes, rather a complex interplay between clients' responses and environmental factors. Psychotherapy can initiate or restore human potential through the transformative power of human connection and presents an interaction in which an empathetic and nonjudgmental therapist is privy to client's emotions, desires, aspirations, thoughts, beliefs, actions and habits. If this gives way to only processing the negatives, the opportunity to nurture growth is lost. Venting anger may be cathartic (and necessary at times), but mustering the will to forgive may be more therapeutic. Deliberate exposure to feared stimuli may be necessary for anxiety, but experiences that yield genuine positive emotion could in fact, take the edge off anxiety. Thus, assessing and enhancing strengths towards growth is as important as assessing and alleviating symptoms to ward off distress. Focusing on strengths enables clients to learn skills to be more spontaneous, playful, creative and grateful, rather than learning skills for how *not* to be rigid, boring, conventional and complaining.

Indeed, emerging evidence shows that strengths play a role in growth even in dire circumstances. In a multiyear longitudinal study, people with a history of some lifetime adversity reported better mental health and wellbeing outcomes than not only people with a high history of adversity but also people with none (Seery, Holman, & Silver, 2010). Likewise, the presence of character strengths such as optimism, appreciation of beauty, and spirituality facilitates recovery from depression (Huta & Hawley, 2008). Individuals who use their strengths are more likely to achieve their goals (Linley, Nielsen, Wood, Gillett, & Biswas-Diener, 2010), whereas those high on positive characteristics are buffered from the impact of negative life events and psychopathology (Johnson, Wood, Gooding, Taylor, & Tarrier, 2011). These suggest that resilience to withstand psychological stressors, and recovery to adaptively deal with them, two features of psychological growth and maturity, may not be possible without attention to the positive.

Second, PPT considers positive emotions and strengths to be as valid as symptoms and disorders, and valued in their own right. Strengths are neither defenses, nor illusions and by-products of symptom relief. If resentment, jealousy, greed, and worry are real, so are attributes like honesty, cooperation, contentment, gratitude, and serenity. Much research has shown that the absence of symptoms is not the presence of mental wellbeing (Fink, 2014; Keyes & Eduardo, 2012; Wood & Joseph, 2010). When therapists work to restore and nurture courage, kindness, modesty, or emotional intelligence, the lives of clients are likely to become fulfilling. In contrast, when a counselor focuses on the amelioration of symptoms, clients' lives can only become less miserable. A focus on symptoms overlooks strengths with an underlying assumption that a cluster of symptoms explains a coherently constructed diagnosis. In doing so, therapy inevitably becomes a process of exploring client's clinical issues

(Boisvert & Faust, 2003). Considering strengths as authentic and active therapeutic ingredients is vital as distressed clients are likely to accept without reservation whatever diagnosis therapists formulate. Some may even define themselves through diagnostic labels, "I am so OCD!" (Obsessive Compulsive Disorder). Incorporating strengths along with symptoms expands the self-perception of clients and offers the therapist additional pathways in which to intervene.

PPT's third and last assumption is that effective therapeutic relationships can be built on the exploration of positive characteristics and experiences (e.g., positive emotions, strengths, and virtues). This contrasts with the traditional approach where therapists analyse and explain the constellation of symptoms to clients in the form of a diagnosis. The role of therapist is further reinforced by the portrayal of psychotherapy in the popular media, where the therapeutic relationship is marked by "problem-talk", socializing clients with the belief they are flawed and the only way out being long and painful discussions of childhood trauma, dissatisfaction, and unmet needs. The reinforcement of stereotypes may increase the dispositional negative bias among therapists who have pre-existing knowledge of psychiatric labels and conditions to draw negative inferences about the client's support systems and subsequently overvalue the therapeutic relationship (Boisvert & Faust, 2003). Clients, already vulnerable due to psychiatric distress, are more likely to adopt a "sick" role consistent with such labels. For some, the role offers a socially sanctioned relief, but to others it brings shame and isolation, which may lead to a premature termination of therapy. Some clients become fixated by the diagnosis and use it as an excuse to avoid responsibility.

15.3 PPT: From Theory to Application

PPT is based on Seligman's conceptualization of happiness and wellbeing (Seligman, 2002, 2011), which operationalized unwieldy concepts into five measurable, manageable and malleable components: (1) Positive emotion, (2) Engagement, (3) Relationships, (4) Meaning and (5) Accomplishment. The first letter of each corresponds to the mnemonic PERMA (Seligman, 2011), which is a revised version of the authentic happiness theory that included positive emotions, engagement and meaning (Seligman, 2002). Research has shown that fulfillment in three elements is associated with lower rates of depression and higher life satisfaction (Headey, Schupp, Tucci, & Wagner, 2010; Lamont, 2011; Sirgy & Wu, 2009; Vella-Brodrick, Park, Peterson, 2009). PPT was originally based on these three elements but its exercises also encapsulate relationships and accomplishment.

PPT can be divided into initial, middle and final phases, although the sequence can be tailored. The initial phase focuses on establishing rapport and understanding clients' narratives to instill hope and enhance self-efficacy and allows clients to hear that they are more than the sum of their symptoms. Clients then assess their strengths from multiple sources and set goals connected to their presenting problems as well as towards their wellbeing. The middle phase focuses on helping clients apply strengths adaptively and deal with grudges, crippling negative memories or traumas. They are invited to explore potential growth from their adversities. Clients develop awareness about the allocation of their attentional resources and learn skills to simplify their lives and savor good experiences to improve wellbeing. The final phase focuses on restoring or fostering positive relationships and the search and pursuit of meaning and purpose. Throughout therapy, clients journal on a daily basis about good things, small or large, that happen to offset the impact of negativity-bent. Although PPT exercises appear well planned in Table 15.1, flexibility in sequence and structure is recommended to accommodate clients best. Also given in Table 15.1 are cultural considerations which should be kept in mind while administrating the treatment protocol.

From the onset, therapists empathically listen to clients' concerns to establish and maintain a trusting therapeutic relationship, while looking for opportunities to help them identify and own their strengths. Attending to their concerns, the therapist encourages clients to discuss events, experiences and anecdotes which brought out the best of them such as handling challenge, learning constructively from mistakes, or helping others. The goal of the Positive Introduction is to expand clients' fractured, fragmented, and fragile self-concept and draw parallels to the current situation. Without giving any descriptors of strengths, clients are invited to identify strengths shown in their Introduction. Connected meaningfully with the current situation, this becomes a dynamic narrative, an internal positive anchor for clients to start the process of healing and growth. This personal, uplifting, yet authentic representation enhances self-efficacy. Many clients seek therapy after hearing from others and themselves that they are inadequate. Yet, the recall of positive memories influences mood regulation (Joormann, Siemer, & Gotlib, 2007), and facilitating such emotions in the early phase of therapy predicts therapeutic change (Fitzpatrick & Stalikas, 2008).

Following this, participants complete an online measure, the Values in Action survey (VIA; Peterson & Seligman, 2004; 240 items) and are coached to use their top five strengths more often in life. In PPT, as clients are part of complex interpersonal dynamics which contain both resources and risks, they are guided to complete a comprehensive process that incorporates multiple self-report measures and collateral reports from significant others identifying their strengths (Rashid & Ostermann, 2009). For self-report, PPT uses a briefer, equally valid and reliable 72-item self-report measure, Signature Strength Questionnaire (Rashid et al., 2013) based on the Classification of Strengths and Virtues (CSV; Peterson & Seligman, 2004). To keep signature strengths front and center throughout the course of PPT, clinicians nudge clients to share memories, experiences, stories, accomplishments, and skills that illustrate their use.

Collaboratively, clients set specific, attainable goals that are meaningful to them, and which target their concerns and adaptive use of strengths. For example, if the goal is for clients to use more curiosity, an optimal balance through concrete action is discussed so that it does not become intrusiveness (overuse) or boredom (underuse). A description of the 24 character strengths and their under- and overuse is presented in Table 15.2. While setting goals, clients are encouraged to use their strengths in a calibrated way (Biswas-Diener, Kashdan, & Minhas, 2011; Schwartz

Table 15.1 Overview of PPT: sessions, themes, skills, practice and cultural considerations

Session & theme	Skill description	Skill practice	Cultural considerations
1. Orientation to PPT: Positive emotions	Discuss client-clinician role/responsibilities; Discuss role of practicing skills within/after therapy	***Positive Introduction***: Client recalls, reflects and writes 1 page Positive Introduction sharing a full story, which called for the best in the client	Clients may consider this self-congratulation and not culturally desirable; encourage significant others to share a story
2. Gratitude (ongoing exercise): Positive emotions	Honing gratitude skills from developing awareness, acknowledging and appreciating everyday events and experiences	***Gratitude Journal***: Client starts ongoing journal to record three good things and what made these happen	Clients may be distressed from forced immigration, famine, oppression, or abuse. It may be hard to find things for which to be grateful. Keep timing in mind
3. Character strengths: Engagement	Understand that strengths are intrinsically valued attributes that can be used, refined and developed towards self-development; Exploring strengths is as real as exploring weakness	***Character Strengths***: Client compiles strengths profile by collecting information from multiple sources including self-report, online measure, a family member and a friend	Explore cultural/religious expressions of strengths including actions, habits, customs, rituals, with which client identifies
4. Signature strengths action plan (A Better Version of Me): Accomplishment	Integrate strengths from many views to determine signature strengths; Learn/practice wisdom to use signature strengths in a balanced and adaptive way, especially in the context of one's presenting concerns	***A Better Version of Me***: Client writes a self-development plan "A Better Version of Me" which uses strengths adaptively through specific, measurable and achievable goals	Explore whether individualized, autonomous and independent Better Self is preferred for clients from cultures that expect communal, interdependent, and socially harmonious Better Self

(continued)

Table 15.1 (continued)

Session & theme	Skill description	Skill practice	Cultural considerations
5. Open vs. Closed memories: Meaning	Reflect and explore consequences of holding open (bitter) memories including those that perpetuate distress	***Positive Cognitive Appraisal***: After practicing relaxation, the client writes bitter memories, and learns ways to deal with them better	Client may find it hard to recall negative memories, especially if these involve a family member with whom they interact often
6. Forgiveness: Positive relationships	Discern forgiveness as a process of deceasing negative resentment-based emotions, motivation and thoughts; Learn how forgiveness can heal and empower; Learn what forgiveness is	***Forgiveness***: Client learns about REACH—a process of forgiveness and/or writes a letter of forgiveness but not necessarily delivers it	Explore if the client feels forgiveness is forced as socially desirable; are they prepared for it? Explore the culturally appropriate meaning of forgiveness for the client
7. Gratitude: Positive emotions & relationships	Attuning awareness towards the good; Explore gratitude as process of enduring thankfulness; Broaden perspective and build positive emotions	***Gratitude Letter & Visit***: Client writes a letter of gratitude to someone whom they never properly thanked; Client writes a draft and makes arrangements to deliver it in person	Clients from interdependent cultures may find writing/reading a gratitude letter uncomfortable and against cultural value of modesty
8. Therapeutic progress: Accomplishment	Discuss motivation and therapeutic progress, elicit and offer feedback; Discuss potential barriers and generate strength-based solutions	Client completes the Forgiveness and Gratitude exercises; Client discusses the experience regarding *A Better Version of Me*	Explore with the client the impact (or lack) of change within a cultural context; discuss needed changes to maintain motivation

(continued)

Table 15.1 (continued)

Session & theme	Skill description	Skill practice	Cultural considerations
9. Satisficing vs. Maximizing: Positive emotions & meaning	Learn about maximizing, i.e., getting the best possible option, decision or product, while satisficing entails opting for good enough; Understand the cost of maximizing	***Satisficing***: Client explores in which domains of life they maximize or satisfice. Client drafts a plan to boost satisficing	Maximizing may be related to a family's financial situation; it may be adaptive for families who experienced impoverishment
10. Hope & Optimism: Positive emotions	Develop the ability to see the best, yet realistic side of most things; Believe that challenges faced are temporary and can be overcome; Hoping goals are attainable	***One Door Closed, One Door Opened***: Client reflects and writes of three doors that closed and three that opened	Pessimism, instead of hope and optimism, may be more important in preserving cultural norms of prudence and risk aversion
11. Post-traumatic Growth (PTG): Meaning	Explore that Post-Traumatic Growth (PTG) can occur even after trauma; PTG is accompanied by renewed life philosophy, resolve to prevail, commitment to improve relationships	***Reflection & Writing about PTG***: Clients complete an optional exercise of transporting traumatic experiences on paper and kept in a secure place. This is done after the client develops healthy coping skills and is less affected by stressors	Discuss with the client culturally adaptive ways of coping and responding to trauma; mind that meaning is almost always steeped in cultural dynamics and religious ethos
12.Slowness & Savooring: Positive emotions & engagement	Learn about psychological hazards of being fast and apply ways to slow down; Awareness of savoring; Attend mindfully to features of the event, experience or situation	***Slow & Savor***: Client selects one slowness and one savoring technique that fits their personality and life circumstance	Explore cultural, social, or economic barriers that prevent a client from slowness and savoring. Explore which aspects of a client's culture may benefit

(continued)

Table 15.1 (continued)

Session & theme	Skill description	Skill practice	Cultural considerations
13. Positive relationships: Relationships	Learn that connecting with others is a need and motivates us to achieve and maintain wellbeing; Learn about Capitalization, a process of being seen, felt and valued	***Active-Constructive Responding (ACR)***: Client explores strengths of significant others and practices active-constructive responding	Mind disclosure of emotions; cultures differ in celebration of positive emotion, which may be more or less desirable given cultural/relational dynamics
14. Altruism: Meaning	Learn about belonging to and serving something larger than oneself as antidote to distress	***Gift of Time***: Client plans to give the gift of time, doing something that also uses the client's signature strengths	Explore if altruism is part of a client's cultural or religious tradition; adapt practice within the client's embedded altruistic practices
15. Positive legacy: Meaning & accomplishment	Integrate elements of wellbeing and reflect on group exercises; Maintain client therapeutic progress	***Positive Legacy***: Client writes personal actions and how they would like to be remembered: what would be the client's positive legacy	Explore ways in which meaning is constructed/pursued in the client's culture; explore circumstances and what provides a sense of purpose that fulfils cultural needs

Table 15.2 Character strengths: definitions and usage (lacking/excess)

Character strength	Description	Lacking/underuse	Excess/overuse
Appreciation of beauty & excellence	Being moved deeply by beauty in nature, in art (painting, music, theatre, etc.) or in excellence in any field of life	Oblivion	Snobbery
Authenticity & honesty	Not pretending to be someone one is not; coming across as a genuine and honest person	Shallowness, phoniness	Righteousness
Bravery & valour	Overcoming fears to do what needs to be done; not give up in face of a hardship or challenge	Fears, easily scared	Foolhardiness, risk-taking
Creativity & originality	Thinking of new and better ways to do things; not being content with doing things conventionally	Conformity	Eccentricity
Curiosity, interest in world & open to experience	Being driven to explore things; asking questions, not tolerating ambiguity easily; being open to different experiences and activities	Disinterest, boredom	Nosiness
Fairness, equity & justice	Standing up for others when they are treated unfairly, bullied or ridiculed; daily actions show sense of fairness	Prejudice, partisanship	Detachment
Forgiveness & mercy	Forgiving easily those who offend; not holding grudges	Mercilessness	Permissive
Gratitude	Expressing thankfulness for good things through words and actions; not take things for granted	Entitlement	Ingratiation
Hope, optimism & future-mindedness	Hoping and believing that good things will happen; recovering from setbacks and taking steps to overcome them	Present orientation	Unwarranted Optimism
Humour & playfulness	Being playful, funny and uses humour to connect with others	Humourless	Buffoonery
Kindness & generosity	Doing kind deeds for others without asking; helping others regularly; being known as a kind person	Indifference	Intrusiveness
Leadership	Organizing activities that include others; being someone others like to follow; being chosen to lead	Compliance	Despotism
Capacity to love and be loved	Having warm/caring relationships with family/friends; showing genuine love and affection through actions	Isolation, detachment	Emotional promiscuity
Love of learning	Loving to learn many things, concepts, ideas, facts in school or on one's own	Complacency, smugness	"Know-it-all"
Modesty & humility	Not liking to be the center of attention; admitting shortcomings; knowing what one cannot do	Groundless self-esteem	Self-depreciation

(continued)

Table 15.2 (continued)

Character strength	Description	Lacking/underuse	Excess/overuse
Open-mindedness & critical thinking	Thinking through and examining all sides before deciding; consulting with others; being flexible to change one's mind when necessary	Unreflective	Cynicism, scepticism
Perseverance, diligence & industry	Finishing most things; able to refocus when distracted and complete task without complaining; overcoming challenges to complete the task	Slackness, laziness	Obsession, pursuing impossible goals
Perspective (wisdom)	Putting things together to understand underlying meaning; settling disputes among friends; learning from mistakes	Superficiality	Obscure and Esoteric
Prudence, caution & discretion	Being careful and cautious; avoid taking undue risks; not easily yielding to external pressures	Recklessness	Prudishness, stuffiness
Religiousness & spirituality	Believing in God or higher power; like to participate in religious/spiritual practice, i.e., prayer, meditation	Anomie	Fanaticism
Self-regulation & self-control	Managing feelings and behaviour well most of the time; following gladly rules and routines	Self-indulgence	Inhibition
Social intelligence	Easily understanding others' feelings; managing oneself well in social situations; displaying interpersonal skills	Obtuseness, cluelessness	Over- emotional association
Teamwork, citizenship & loyalty	Relating well with teammates or group members; contributing to the success of the group	Selfishness & rebelliousness	Mindless obedience
Zest, enthusiasm & energy	Being energetic, cheerful and full of life; being liked by others to hang out with	Passivity, restraint	Hyperactivity

& Sharpe, 2006), otherwise, actions or habits are identified that may explain troubles as either lack of, or excess of strengths. Illustrations include depressed mood, feeling hopeless or low as a lack of zest and playfulness, worrying excessively as lack of gratitude or inability to let go, or indecision as lack of determination. Progress towards goals is monitored and therapists provide and elicit feedback (Lambert, 2010), continuously exploring the nuances of strengths. Clients identify troubling emotions and memories by harnessing social intelligence, toning down grudges by accessing positive memories of situations, individuals or experiences, and instead of avoiding difficult situations, muster courage and self-regulation to face them. The following scenarios are from clients seen by the first author (Rashid) at a university counselling center. All three are self-identified Muslim students and depict their goal-directed use of strengths in overcoming presenting problems.

- **Case 1:** Saba, a 22-year-old female international student from the MENA region sought therapy for depressive symptoms. She had been seeing a Caucasian male, also a student, for two years, but had not shared this information with her parents, who are conservative Muslims. She returned home during break with intentions of disclosing this information. However, before she could do so, her mother revealed that her father had been diagnosed with cancer. Being very close to her father and family, Saba opted not to disclose the relationship and returned to university. Her mood became low, she lost her appetite, and stopped enjoying things. She blamed herself for keeping her relationship a secret. After validating her feelings, we discussed her strengths and ways she could use them to let her parents know about her relationship. Rather than assume her parents would reject it, she aimed for an optimal yet realistic outcome and began working towards it, blending hope with social intelligence. Although it took time to convince her parents, after several months of reluctance, they appeared open to acceptance. This case illustrates, without dismissing symptomatic stress, that strengths were used in culturally respectful ways; that is, involving her family, rather than isolating or ignoring them.
- **Case 2:** Mustafa, a 24-year male and undergraduate university student, whose parents immigrated to Canada from the MENA region about 15 years ago, sought psychotherapy for symptoms of anxiety and perfectionism. Mustafa, despite a solid academic achievement record, expected the worst in the future and believed he would not achieve his goal of getting into a graduate school. This precipitated symptoms of anxiety and panic, as well as experimentation with illicit drugs. He felt that he would be "worthless" if he couldn't get into medical school. Several family members were doctors, and he was expected to follow suit. Through individual PPT, he discovered his signature strengths were love of learning, spirituality, authenticity, persistence, appreciation of beauty and kindness. Over the course of the therapy, he started using his strengths, specifically, kindness towards self, i.e., self-compassion. This helped Mustafa become more attuned to his intrinsic motivation, to articulate his interests and aspirations. Instead of becoming a physician, he opted to pursue a career in animation. He was pleasantly surprised when his parents did not object to his career choice.
- **Case 3:** The signature strength profile of a 20-year old, single client from a conservative Muslim and South Asian cultural background showed that kindness, authenticity, humility, social intelligence and spirituality were core parts of her personality. An introvert by disposition, she presented with symptoms consistent with dysthymic depression disorder. Although PPT exercises helped her to improve her mood somewhat, her interpersonal challenges did not improve. Her family responded negatively when she started using strengths (e.g., expressing her emotions; social intelligence), asking for more gender-based equality (fairness), standing up for her rights (courage), and not being humble and kind when someone violated her rights. Although the client felt empowered, at the same time, friction between her and her family increased. The client dealt with this friction with kindness but success was moderate.

Conflicts arising from cultural values are better handled using and enhancing strengths than trying to eliminate weaknesses and vulnerabilities that are embedded in complex ways. Further, inherent bias towards negativity and symptomatic distress may obscure client strengths. PPT brings strengths to the forefront and offers therapists and clients multiple avenues to deal with problems. As such, PPT never dismisses, avoids, nor trivializes negatives and as such, negative emotions in PPT are not inherently undesired. Sadness, anxiety, anger, embarrassment, shame, guilt, jealousy, and envy can be beneficial in some cultural and social interactions and in maintaining or restoring balance in relationships. Further, negative emotions are valued and expressed differently in different cultures (Parrott, 2014). For example, anger in specific cultural and sociopolitical contexts, especially against cruelty, discrimination, injustice and wrongdoing, is preferred over unconditional forgiveness.

Many clients seek therapy to manage the stressors associated with living in fast-paced and complex urban environments. PPT exercises such as satisficing versus maximizing (Schwartz, Ward et al., 2002) and savoring (Bryant & Veroff, 2007) teach clients to deliberately slow down and enjoy small pleasures (e.g., eating a meal, taking a shower, walking to work). Clients also keep a daily gratitude journal and write three good things that happened and why, directing their attention deliberately to good experiences, otherwise missed in the hustle of life. In this sense, PPT integrates fast paced urban Western cultural norms and brings an antidote from Eastern traditions (i.e., Buddhism, Sufism, Confucianism), which all prioritize connecting with others to slow things down. For example, in the gratitude letter and visit exercise, clients recall someone who has done something positive and supportive for them and write a draft in the session. They describe specifics of the kindness and its consequences. Clients are then encouraged to read the letter to the recipient in person or by phone. In person, this exercise generates powerful positive emotions on both ends—often described by clients as a deeply moving experience in which they were initially reluctant to engage. In group PPT, the exercise on slowness and savoring introduces clients to be aware of how speed and multi-tasking nullifies appreciation and enjoyment.

According to the Broaden and Build Theory (Fredrickson, 2001), the goal is to change clients' mindsets, expanding attention, broadening behavioral repertoires and enhancing creativity. Positive emotions build resilience by "undoing" the effects of negative emotions (Fredrickson, Mancuso, Branigan, & Tugade, 2000). Positive emotions such as joy, amusement and awe, if cultivated systematically, intentionally, in a culturally contextual way, buffer against and undo the deleterious effects of psychological distress. When we experience positive emotions, contextual cues are better incorporated; that is, individuals notice others more readily and consider alternative explanations for complex situations. The more positive emotional experiences, the more durable are changes in neuro-functioning and gene expression (Fredrickson et al., 2013; Garland & Howard, 2009). The goal is not to cultivate decontextualized positive emotions, but adaptively use positive and negative emotions. Notwithstanding the value of positive emotions, clients presenting for therapy often experience at least twice the negative emotions as non-depressed individuals (Schwartz et al., 2002). In the middle phase of PPT, clients are thusly encouraged to write grudges, bitter memories, or resentments and discuss the effects of holding these.

Positive appraisal, shown to build resilience and healthy coping, helps clients unpack resentments (Luyten, Boddez, & Hermans, 2015) and includes the following strategies:

- **Psychological space**: Clients write or describe bitter memories from a third person's view (Ayduk & Kross, 2010; Joormann, Dkane, & Gotlib, 2006).
- **Reconsolidation**: Clients recall a troubling memory and look for positives, learning that memory recall offers a chance for revision and new meaning (Alberini & Ledoux, 2013; Sandler, 2007).
- **Mindful focus**: Clients mindfully observe, rather than react to negative memories and develop greater awareness about cues, situations and experiences that trigger them (Gockel, 2010).
- **Diversion/Intentional forgetting**: As clients develop awareness of triggers, they inventory alternative, adaptive behaviors to stop the recollection of negative memories, which are often triggered by external cues. Engaging in alternative activities to divert attentional resources away from these can stop downward affective spirals (Hertel & McDaniel, 2010; Van Dillen & Koole, 2007).

In addition to positive appraisal, clients are invited to consider forgiveness. In PPT, forgiveness is considered a process of change, not an event or exercise to willingly forsake one's right (perceived or real) or take revenge (Worthington, Witvliet, Pietrini & Miller, 2007). Clients, especially from cultures where forgiveness may be rushed to uphold cultural norms, are educated that forgiveness is not condoning or pardoning the offender, lowering the demands for justice, forgetting a wrong, or ignoring the consequence of an offense. It is about replacing negative thoughts or emotions with neutral or positive ones (Enright & Fitzgibbons, 2014). Forgiveness may generate negative and uncomfortable emotions—some of which can be associated with trauma or traumatic memories. While empathetically attending to pain associated with traumatic experiences, PPT encourages clients to explore psychological growth (Bonanno & Mancini, 2012; Calhoun & Tedeschi, 2006; McKnight & Kashdan, 2009). An example is *One Door Closes, One Door Opens,* which focuses on exploring growth, exploration and meaning that might have opened after opportunities, attachments and expressions closed. Therapists should avoid finding positive outcomes too quickly. Emphasis is on the integration of strengths with symptoms to help clients encounter negative experiences with a more positive mindset and reframe those experiences helpfully.

The final PPT exercises (positive relationships, positive communication, gift of time, positive legacy) continue to use strengths but their use is focused on belonging and serving higher values. For instance, positive communication teaches clients ways to validate and capitalize upon precious moments when close others share their good news (Gable, Reis, Impett, & Asher, 2004). Others, such as *Gift of Time,* help clients search and pursue purpose by using their strengths. Almost all cultures endorse the pursuit of meaning and purpose via the strengthening of close interpersonal and communal relationships, or via the pursuit of artistic, intellectual or scientific innovations, philosophical or religious contemplation (Frankl, 1963; Hicks & King, 2009; Stillman & Baumeister, 2009; Wrzesniewski, McCauley, Rozin, & Schwartz, 1997).

There is evidence that having a sense of meaning and purpose helps individuals recover quickly from adversity and buffer against feelings of hopelessness and lack of control (Graham, Lobel, Glass, & Lokshina, 2008; Lightsey, 2006).

15.4 Caveats of PPT Use

In conducting PPT, caveats are important to note. First, despite emphasizing strengths, PPT is not prescriptive. Rather, it is a descriptive approach based on converging scientific evidence indicating that benefits accrue when individuals attend to the positive aspects of experience. With time, specific lines of evidence will also accumulate to show that positives and strengths play a causal role measured by biological and genetic markers. For example, doing well, not simply feeling good, is associated with stronger expression of antibody and antiviral genes (Fredrickson et al., 2013). Studies have even tracked heart disease risk through the social media Twitter expressions of individual's negative emotions such as anger, stress, and fatigue, with positive emotions signaling lower risk (Eichstaedt et al., 2015).

Further, PPT is beneficial for some psychological concerns and not others. PPT was initially validated with adults experiencing symptoms of severe depression (Seligman, Rashid, & Parks, 2006) and replicated in studies (Asgharipoor, Farid, Arshadi, & Sahebi, 2010; Bay & Csillic, 2012; Cuadra-Peralta, Veloso-Besio, Pérez, & Zúñiga, 2010). It is also effective with symptoms of anxiety (Kahler et al., 2014) and more recently with symptoms of borderline personality disorder (Uliaszek, Rashid, Williams, & Gulamani, 2016) and psychosis (Riches, Schrank, Rashid, & Slade, 2016; Schrank et al., 2016). Since its initial validation, eight peer reviewed studies of manualized PPT have found it equally effective or better when compared to active treatments such as cognitive-behavioral therapy and dialectical behavior therapy. Yet, it would be imprudent to use PPT with clients experiencing acute symptoms of panic disorder, selective mutism, or paranoid personality disorder as there is no evidence of efficacy for these.

Some clients feel that their symptoms, not strengths ought to be the focus of treatment, but fear the expression or articulation of their weaknesses may invoke judgment. For others, the identification of strengths may exaggerate narcissistic tendencies. Therefore, it is important that strengths are discussed in specific situational contexts. Similarly, clients with a history of abuse and with a strengths profile of humility, kindness or forgiveness may not benefit from PPT until they develop the strength of perspective and critical thinking to understand their situations. Clients with a history of unresolved trauma and symptoms of post-traumatic stress may respond better to symptom focused treatments for a time. In short, PPT is not a panacea nor is it completely irrelevant. Its fit has to be explored and monitored, and may not be appropriate for all clients in all contexts. A therapist using PPT also should not expect a linear progression of improvement because the motivation to change long-standing patterns fluctuates during the course of therapy, and the progress of one client should not bias therapists about the likely progress of another. The mechanisms of change in PPT have not been explored systematically, but changes brought by positive interventions are moderated by level of symptom severity, individual personality variables (motivation, effort), flexibility in completing and practicing the exercises and skills and overall client-intervention fit (Lyubomirsky & Layous, 2013). Finally, cultural sensitivities in assessing strengths should be considered. An emotive style of communication, interdependence on extended family members or avoiding direct eye contact may convey zest, love, and respect (Pedrotti, 2011) and possible interpretations of the kind should be on the top of therapist's minds to consider.

15.5 Empirical Evidence and Future Directions

Initially, individual PPI exercises were validated through a randomized control trial (RCT; Seligman, Steen, Park, & Peterson, 2005) with participants in the positive intervention condition showing a significant decrease in symptoms of depression and increase in wellbeing. These findings have since been independently replicated with somewhat similar results (Giannopoulos & Vella-Brodrick, 2011; Mongrain & Anselmo-Matthews, 2012; Senf & Liau, 2013). Subtle aspects such as preference for specific exercises and its relation to adherence have been explored (Schueller, 2010). Table 15.3 lists 22 studies that explicitly used the PPT manual as treatment (Rashid & Seligman, 2018; Seligman et al., 2006). Mostly group treatments, eight of the 20 are randomized controlled studies, nine are published in peer reviewed journals and three are dissertations. Seven of these treated community samples from Canada, China, Chile, France, Iran, and USA addressing depression, anxiety, borderline personality disorder, psychosis, and nicotine dependence. Of these, the most rigorous was completed at the Institute of Psychiatry, London, UK, where the randomized study WELLFOCUS PPT used an adapted version to compare with treatment as usual (Riches et al., 2016). Results showed that PPT groups experienced significant improvement in symptoms of depression, whereas changes in wellbeing were found on PPT related measures but not on a second measure of wellbeing (Schrank et al., 2016). A further five of the 22 studies compared PPT with two other manualized treatments: dialectical behavior therapy (DBT) and cognitive-behavioral therapy (CBT). In these, PPT lowered symptoms of distress and enhanced wellbeing on post-treatment outcome measures when compared to control or pre-treatment scores, with medium to large effect sizes (see Rashid, 2015). Compared to CBT or DBT, PPT performed equally well or better on wellbeing measures (e.g., Asgharipoor et al., 2010; Cuadra-Peralta et al., 2010; Uliaszek et al., 2016).

The study results are consistent with two meta-analyses on positive interventions. A meta-analysis of 51 interventions by Sin and Lyubomirsky (2009) found that positive interventions are effective, with moderate effect sizes in significantly decreasing symptoms of depression (mean $r = 0.31$) and enhancing wellbeing (mean $r = 0.29$). Positive interventions, including PPT are beginning to establish that positives can reduce symptoms of depression and enhance wellbeing. The second meta-analysis by Bolier et al. (2013), reviewed 39 randomized published studies totaling 6139 participants and found that such interventions reduced depression (mean $r = 0.23$) with a small effect size but enhanced wellbeing with a moderate effect size ($r = 0.34$).

Table 15.3 Positive psychotherapy: summary of studies

Authors	Study description	Key findings
Seligman, Rashid, and Parks (2006), published	Individual PPT; $n = 11$; 12–14 sessions with clients diagnosed with major depressive disorder, compared with treatment as usual (TAU; $n = 9$) and treatment as usual plus medication (TAUMED; $n = 12$)	Undergraduate/graduate students at university counselling center in USA. Clients completing PPT fared significantly better on measures of depressive symptoms, overall psychiatric distress and wellbeing
Seligman, Rashid, and Parks (2006), published	Group PPT ($n = 21$) with clients at university counselling center with mild to moderate depressive symptoms compared to no-treatment control ($n = 21$) in six sessions	PPT did better on measure of depression at 3, 6, and 12-month follow-up with rate of change significantly greater than that of the control group
Parks-Sheiner (2009), dissertation	Individuals ($n = 52$) who completed six PPT exercises were compared with no-treatment control group ($n = 69$)	Individuals completing PPT exercises reported significantly less depression at post-treatment, 3- and 6-month follow-ups
Lü, Wang, and Liu (2013), published	Group PPT ($n = 16$), (2 h, 16 weekly sessions), university students in China compared with no-treatment control group ($n = 18$). Study explored impact of positive affect on vagal tone	Participants completing PPT exercises reported significantly fewer depressive symptoms, less negative emotion and more positive emotions
Rashid and Anjum (2008) published	Group PPT ($n = 9$) was offered in eight sessions to 6th and 7th grade students at a public school in Canada and compared with no-treatment control ($n = 9$)	Participants improved their social skills as rated by parents and teachers
Reinsch (2012), dissertation	Group PPT ($n = 9$) was compared with a no-treatment control group ($n = 8$) with adults seeking psychotherapy through employee assistance program in Canada	Compared to controls, treatment group showed significant decreases in depression at a rate of 45%. Gains held 1 month post intervention
Uliaszek, Rashid, Williams, and Gulamani (2016), published	Group PPT ($n = 27$) compared group DBT ($n = 27$) with undergraduate students diagnosed with symptoms of borderline personality disorder at a university counselling center in Canada	PPT and DBT differed from pre- to post-treatment on almost all measures (e.g., depression, anxiety, distress tolerance, emotional regulation, coping, mindfulness, life satisfaction, wellbeing). PPT had higher dropout rate
Asgharipoor et al. (2010), published	Group PPT ($n = 9$) compared with CBT for 12 weeks. Each group comprised adults diagnosed with major depressive disorder seeking treatment at a hospital/psychological treatment center in Iran	At post-intervention, PPT group showed significantly higher level of happiness, whereas no differences between the two treatments were found on measures of depression

(continued)

Table 15.3 (continued)

Authors	Study description	Key findings
Schrank et al. (2016), published	Group PPT adapted for psychosis called WELLFOCUS PPT was completed ($n = 43$) for 11 weeks vs. treatment as usual (TAU; $n = 41$) with community adults diagnosed with psychosis	At post-intervention and follow-up, PPT group showed improvement in wellbeing on three measures as well as symptoms of depression, hope, self-esteem, and sense of coherence
Dowlatabadi et al. (2016), published	36 women with concerns over infertility and showing signs of mild to moderate depression were randomly placed into: control ($n = 18$) or intervention ($n = 18$)	Compared to control, the women in the intervention group showed significant increases in life satisfaction
Dowlatabadi et al. (2016), published	Patients with breast cancer were randomized to PPT ($n = 21$) and a control group ($n = 21$) at the Oncology Center in Kermanshah, Iran	PPT group at post-intervention showed significant decreases in depression and a significant increase in happiness
Carr, Finnegan, Griffin, Cotter, and Hyland (2017), published	$n = 82$ diagnosed with MDD assigned to Say Yes to Life (SYTL), PPT integrated with CBT ($n = 40$), or treatment as usual ($n = 42$), which included CBT, client-centered therapy, psychodynamic and integrative psychotherapy. Both had 2-h weekly sessions over 20 weeks	Effect sizes favored SYTL group and ranged from small- to medium-sized effects. A cost-consequence analysis showed that the average total cost of service usage in euros per case in the SYTL group was significantly lower than that of the TAU group
Furchtlehner and Laireiter (2016); presentation	Group PPT ($n = 44$) was compared with group CBT ($n = 44$) with patients diagnosed with depression in small groups in 2-h sessions for 14 weeks	PPT fared better than CBT on all measures with moderate- to large-sized effects on depression, life satisfaction, happiness, and symptom reduction
Hwang, Kwon, and Hong (2017); published	University students in Busan, South Korea randomly assigned to: individual modified (PPTm; $n = 8$), group neurofeedback-aided meditation therapy (NFB; $n = 8$), or no treatment ($n = 8$)	Both PPTm and NFB-aided therapy showed positive effects on psychological wellbeing and positive and negative emotions compared to no-treatment group.
Cullen et al. (2018)	Individual PPT and Treatment as Usual to 27 individuals with Acquired Brain Injury. Used Depression & Anxiety Scale (DASS); Authentic Happiness Inventory (AHI)	Due to small sample size, statistical significance was not achieved but PPT group showed drop in depression and anxiety scores

(continued)

Table 15.3 (continued)

Authors	Study description	Key findings
Ochoa, Casellas-Grau, Vives, Font, and Borràs (2017), published	126 female adult survivors of breast cancer with emotional distress assigned to PPT for cancer (PPC; $n =$ 73) in group or wait-list control ($n =$ 53). PPC conducted in 12 sessions of 90–120 min; each group had 8–12 members	PPC group obtained significantly better results after treatment than control group, showing reduced distress, decreased posttraumatic symptoms, increased PTG. Benefits held at 3- and 12-month follow-up
Cuadra-Peralta, Veloso-Besio, Pérez, and Zúñiga (2010), published	Group PPT ($n = 8$) in nine sessions, with clients diagnosed with depression, compared with behavioral therapy ($n =$ 10) at a community center in Chile	Compared to behavior therapy, PPT showed significant increases in happiness and decreases in symptoms of depression
Csillik, Aguerre, and Bay (2012), published	Group PPT ($n = 10$) compared with group CBT ($n = 8$) and medication (n $= 8$)	PPT fared better than CBT and medication group on measures of depression, optimism, emotional intelligence, and wellbeing
Meyer, Johnson, Parks, Iwanski, and Penn (2012), published	Group PPT with two cohorts recruited from hospital/community mental health, diagnosed with schizophrenia or schizoaffective disorder over ten sessions	At post-treatment, PPT fared better on depression, happiness, optimism, and life satisfaction. In most cases, PPT and CBT fared better than the medication group
Kahler et al. (2014), published	Individual PPT ($n = 19$) in eight sessions was integrated with smoking cessation counselling and nicotine patches at a community medical center	Attendance and treatment satisfaction were high. Nearly one third (31.6%) sustained smoking abstinence for 6 months after quit date
Goodwin (2010), dissertation	Group PPT ($n = 11$) in a pre- to post-group design explored relationship satisfaction among anxious and stressed individuals at a community center	Individuals who experienced a reduction in perceived stress and anxiety also showed improvement in relationship functioning

Positive interventions could also benefit non-clinical patrons as wellbeing enhancing strategies can prevent or reduce the risk of future disorders.

Additional links between clinical conditions and strengths as well as wellbeing have also been explored including creativity and bipolar disorder (Murray & Johnson, 2010), positive psychology and brain injury (Evans, 2011), positive emotions and social anxiety (Kashdan, Julian, Merritt, & Uswatte, 2006), social relationships and depression (Oksanen, Kouvonen, Vahtera, Virtanen, & Kivimäki, 2010), as well as various aspects of wellbeing and psychosis (Schrank et al., 2013), positive psychology and war trauma (Al-Krenawi et al., 2011), school-based positive psychology interventions (Waters, 2011), neuroscience (Kapur et al., 2013), and character strengths (Niemiec, Rashid, & Spinella, 2012). A number of online studies have effectively used PPT-based interventions with good results (e.g., Mitchell, Stanimirovic, Klein, & Vella-Brodrick, 2009; Parks, Della Porta, Pierce, Zilca, &

Lyubomirsky, 2012; Schueller & Parks, 2012), offering a cost effective means of providing mental health services as a preventative strategy. In addition to these, single positive interventions have been applied to examine their effectiveness for clinical conditions such as gratitude (Wood, Maltby, Gillett, Linley, & Joseph, 2008), the best possible self and three good things for depression (Pietrowsky & Mikutta, 2012), hope as a treatment of posttraumatic stress disorder (Gilman, Schumm, & Chard, 2012), the therapeutic role of spirituality and meaning in psychotherapy (Steger & Shin, 2010), positive psychology interventions to treat drug abuse (Akhtar & Boniwell, 2010), cultivation of positive emotions in treating symptoms of schizophrenia (Johnson et al., 2009), and forgiveness to devolve anger (Harris et al., 2006). The role of positive interventions to complement and supplement traditional clinical work is also being explored (e.g., Frisch, 2006; Harris, Thoresen, & Lopez, 2007; Karwoski, Garratt, & llardi, 2006; Moeenizadeh & Salagame, 2010; Ruini & Fava, 2009).

15.5.1 Local Studies

There have been notable works showing how positivity is already part of the Arabic Islamic culture. Although the word "positivity" is not mentioned in the Holy Quran, it is a fundamental concept in Quranic discourse (Al-Namrat, 2017). Tajdin (2015) showed some of the Muslim thinkers' contributions to the issue of happiness from a moderate cultural relativist approach. Islam, as a comprehensive religion, opened spaces for approaching happiness from both hedonic and eudaimonic perspectives, although historical scholarship enriched the philosophical or theological perspectives if not experimental human psychology. Yet, religiosity in Muslim communities is a positive contributing component of many positive psychology concepts. For example, Abdel-Khalek (2010) found positive correlations between quality of life, subjective wellbeing, and religiosity in Muslim college students in Kuwait. Abdel-Khalek (2016) returned with the Arabic Scale of Religiosity that significantly correlated with positive psychology variables in Arab male and female university students in Algeria, Kuwait, and Egypt. Moreover, Thomas, Mutawa, Furber, and Grey (2016) showed that religiosity had negative correlations with depressive symptoms in Muslim females in the UAE and that those experiencing severe depressive symptoms reported lower levels of religiosity compared to their asymptomatic counterparts.

Topic Box: Positive Psychology in Action by Mohammad Al-Haj Baddar

After my training in positive psychology, I decided that I needed to act locally. One pressing concern in Jordan is the ongoing strife in neighboring Syria and the influx of refugees. One organization, CARE International, is working alongside many others to lend a hand. CARE International is a humanitarian organization that works around the globe to save lives, defeat poverty and achieve social justice. Its primary work is protection and it aims to enhance the resilience of populations impacted by regional conflict. In Jordan, on a daily basis, people are coming into our country, needing support, food, shelter, as well as jobs and schools for their children. These people also need to be heard and given hope. I decided this was where I wanted to spend my energy.

I got the chance with CARE International to conduct seven psychosocial support programs for several groups of adolescents and adults that ranged from Syrian refugees to local Jordanian community members. I decided to develop a positive psychology-based psychosocial support program to build the level of resilience amongst participants in the regions of Mafraq and Azraq, where large communities of Syrian refugees are based. These participants are from disenfranchised areas, often unemployed and lack coping techniques in the wake of their recent hardships.

To meet these needs, I developed a program of 8–10 sessions based on three ideas; time perspective, character strengths and the PERMA model. This involves Zimbardo's (Boniwell & Zimbardo, 2004) time perspective theory so participants can have a balanced time perspective and adaptive orientations towards savoring the positive and coping with the negative whether from today, yesterday or coming tomorrow. While contemplating the past, the trauma of leaving Syria, they learn to become frustration tolerant, and focus on how they used their character strengths to survive and continue to do so. Reframing the past to something more positive can be a good way to live less in the past focusing on regret and sadness, or future with much anxiety and worry and not enough in the present with a measure of hope and acceptance.

Character strengths like persistence, courage, and forgiveness as examples were also used and stem from Peterson and Seligman's (2004) classification. I use Seligman's (2011) PERMA model, which posits that wellbeing is possible through the pathways of positive emotion, engagement, relationships, meaning and achievement. For positive emotions, techniques are done based on Fredrickson's (2013a) Broaden and Build Theory. For engagement, techniques are taken from Kabat-Zinn's (1990) mindfulness, Bryant and Veroff's (2007) savoring, and flow theory (Nakamura & Csikszentmihalyi, 2009). I focus on love and kindness for relationships (Fredrickson, 2013b) and refer to Steger, Kashdan and Oishi's (2008) work on meaning and purpose. Finally, I use Oettingen's (2014) Wish-Outcome-Obstacles-Plan (WOOP) technique where wishes can not only be dreamed of, but steps developed for them to become a reality. That alone makes participants feel in control and less anxious.

Partaking in these activities has helped participants to improve resilience across their daily lives. Our post-program interviews using the Connor and Davidson Resilience Scale (CD-RISC) (Alsheikh Ali, 2014; Campbell-Sills & Stein, 2007; Connor & Davidson, 2003) revealed that participants had become closer to people around them, used their strengths more often and in different contexts, and were more grateful and optimistic. CARE International in particular was pleased that participants were functioning better in different contexts as employees at work, mothers at home, or students at school.

In terms of the Arabic PPT literature, Al-Sabwah (2010) introduced the role of positive psychology activating prevention procedures and psychotherapy in comparison with those of classical psychology. Salama-Younes (2015) included it as a main part of his introduction to positive psychology as one of the most important applications. Younis (2017) also introduced to the Arab world a group of PPT principles and techniques in his book "The Power of Positive Psychology." A total of four Arabic PPT studies (Table 15.4) delivered intervention programs in Egypt, Kuwait, and Jordan using positive psychology interventions, techniques, or counselling to improve subjective wellbeing in a variety of groups, such as learning disabled females, injured military personnel, and diabetics (Al-Hattab, 2017; Al-Wakeel, 2010; Al-Yamani, Al-Adel & Hussein, 2014; Ramadan, 2014). They did not follow PPT exactly, but adapted principles and techniques. Another (Elsayed, 2016) showed a negative correlation between aggressiveness and optimism, hope, love of life, and satisfaction with life, recommending PPT programs for the reduction of aggression. While the positive psychology literature in the region is still young, studies are growing in number, with Rao, Donaldson and Doiron (2015) reporting that 53 studies had already been conducted by 2014.

15.6 Conclusion

Establishing the effectiveness of interventions takes decades of research, including open trial, case reports, and then moving into controlled pilots and finally multi-site studies. While we are well on our way, PPT nonetheless has a long journey to travel in order to establish its efficacy and the discovery of change mechanisms, especially relative to other longer-standing programs. PPT must also answer sophisticated questions about specific aspects of the treatment over and beyond a symptoms-focused approach. Moving forward, longitudinal and multi-method (e.g., experiential sampling, physiological and neurological indices) research designs may uncover the effectiveness of PPT for specific disorders. There is a dearth of knowledge about epistemology of wellbeing, especially in clinical settings and these questions will hopefully be answered through more rigorous and refined studies, helping to boost the relevancy of positive psychology overall around the world.

Table 15.4 Arabic positive psychotherapy: summary of studies

Authors	Study description	Key findings
Ramadan (2014), published	Group PPI ($n = 30$) (12 sessions/12 weeks) with Egyptian university students experiencing low subjective wellbeing compared with no-treatment control ($n = 30$)	Students completing PPIs fared significantly better on measures of subjective wellbeing
Al-Yamani, Al-Adel, and Hussein (2014), published	Two groups; Positive psychology techniques ($n = 11$; $n = 12$), (16 sessions/4 weeks) with learning disabled females from 5th (n = 394) and 7th (n = 384) grade in Kuwait experiencing low scholastic adjustment compared to no-treatment equivalent control groups	The 5th and 7th grade students fared significantly better on scholastic adjustment
Al-Hattab (2017), dissertation	Group Positive Psychology Counseling ($n = 20$), (14 sessions in 7 weeks) with injured military in Jordan experiencing anxiety and depression amongst 1790 peer injured military persons compared to no-treatment controls	Injured military Jordanians reported significantly reduction of anxiety and depression and quality of life improvement
Al-Wakeel (2010), published	Group Positive Psychology Techniques ($n = 40$), (7 sessions/3 weeks) with Egyptian diabetics (30–45 years) experiencing low psychological adjustment	Participants completing program reported better psychological adjustment (personal, emotional, social and family) at post-test
Elsayed (2016), published	Egyptian university male and female students ($n = 395$) and employees ($n = 266$) tested on aggression scale, self rating scale, adult dispositional hope scale, Arabic scale of optimism and pessimism, satisfaction with life scale, and love of life scale	Positive correlation between self general satisfaction and measures of optimism, hope, love of life, and satisfaction with life; negative correlation between aggressiveness and optimism, hope, love of life, and satisfaction with life

References

Abdel-Khalek, A. M. (2010). Quality of life, subjective wellbeing, and religiosity in Muslim college students. *Quality of Life Research, 19,* 1133–1143.

Abdel-Khalek, A. M. (2016). The Arabic Scale of Religiosity: Its development, psychometric parameters, and relation with positive psychology variables. *Journal of Psychological Studies, Egypt, 26*(2), 159–182.

Akhtar, M., & Boniwell, I. (2010). Applying positive psychology to alcohol-misusing: A group intervention. *Groupwork, 20,* 7–23.

Al-Hattab, A. M. (2017). *The effectiveness of group counselling program on positive psychology to reduce anxiety and depression and to improve the quality of the life for a sample of the injured Jordanian military.* Unpublished dissertation, The World Islamic Science and Educational University, Amman, Jordan.

Al-Krenawi, A., Elbedour, S., Parsons, J. E., Onwuegbuzie, A. J., Bart, W. M., & Ferguson, A. (2011). Trauma and war: Positive psychology/strengths approach. *Arab Journal of Psychiatry, 22,* 103–112.

Al-Namrat, M. (2017). The role of Quranic story in building the value of positivity: Surat Yusuf as a model. *Jordanian Journal of Islamic Studies, 13*(2), 413–440.

Al-Sabwah, M. N. (2010). The role of positive psychology in activating prevention procedures and psychotherapy. *Arabic Studies in Psychology, 9*(1), 1–25.

Al-Wakeel, S. A. (2010). Efficacy of using some techniques of positive psychology in improving level of the psychological adjustment for a sample of diabetic patients. *Journal of Education, Borsaeed University, 2*(7), 118–156.

Al-Yamani, S. A., Al-Adel, A. M., & Hussein, Z. H. (2014). The effectiveness of some positive psychology techniques on increasing the level of scholastic adjustment of learning disabled female students in the primary and intermediate stages in the state of Kuwait. *Journal of Special Education, Zaqazeeq Faculty of Education, 9,* 1–65.

Alberini, C. M., & Ledoux, J. E. (2013). Memory reconsolidation. *Current Biology, 23,* R746–R750.

Alsheikh Ali, A. (2014). Resilience levels and their relationship to academic adjustment and achievement among graduates of orphanages. *Jordan Journal of Educational Sciences, 10*(4), 411–430.

Asgharipoor, N., Farid, A. A., Arshadi, H., & Sahebi, A. (2010). A comparative study on the effectiveness of positive psychotherapy and group cognitive-behavioral therapy for the patients suffering from major depressive disorder. *Iranian Journal of Psychiatry and Behavioral Sciences, 6,* 33–41.

Ayduk, Ö., & Kross, E. (2010). From a distance: Implications of spontaneous self-distancing for adaptive self-reflection. *Journal of Personality and Social Psychology, 98,* 809–829.

Baños, R. M., Etchemendy, E., Mira, A., Riva, G., Gaggioli, A., & Botella, C. (2017). Online positive interventions to promote wellbeing and resilience in the adolescent population: A narrative review. *Frontiers in Psychiatry, 8,* 10.

Baumeister, R. F., Bratslavsky, E., Finkenauer, C., & Vohs, K. D. (2001). Bad is stronger than good. *Review of General Psychology, 5*(4), 323–370. https://doi.org/10.1037/1089-2680.5.4.323

Bay, M., & Csillic, A. (2012). *Comparing positive psychotherapy with cognitive behavioral therapy in treating depression.* Unpublished manuscript. Paris West University Nanterre La Défense (Université Paris Ouest Nanterre La Défense).

Biswas-Diener, R., Kashdan, T. K., & Minhas, G. (2011). A dynamic approach to psychological strength development and intervention. *The Journal of Positive Psychology, 6*(2), 106–118.

Boisvert, C. M., & Faust, D. (2003). Leading researchers' consensus on psychotherapy research findings: Implications for the teaching and conduct of psychotherapy. *Professional Psychology: Research and Practice, 34,* 508–513.

Bolier, L., Haverman, M., Westerhof, G., Riper, H., Smit, F., & Bohlmeijer, E. (2013). Positive psychology interventions: A meta-analysis of randomized controlled studies. *BMC Public Health, 13* (119).

Bonanno, G. A., & Mancini, A. D. (2012). Beyond resilience and PTSD: Mapping the heterogeneity of responses to potential trauma. *Psychological Trauma: Theory, Research, Practice, and Policy, 4*(1), 74–83.

Boniwell, I., & Zimbardo, P. G. (2004). Balancing time perspective in pursuit of optimal functioning. In P. A. Linley & S. Joseph (Eds.), *Positive psychology in practice* (pp. 165–178). Hoboken, NJ: Wiley.

Bryant, F. B., & Veroff, J. (2007). *Savoring: A new model of positive experience*. Mahwah, NJ: Erlbaum.

Calhoun, L. G., & Tedeschi, R. G. (Eds.). (2006). *Handbook of posttraumatic growth: Research and practice*. Mahwah, NJ: Erlbaum.

Campbell-Sills, L., & Stein, M. B. (2007). Psychometric analysis and refinement of the Connor-Davidson Resilience Scale (CD-RISC): Validation of a 10-Item measure of resilience. *Journal of Traumatic Stress, 20*(6), 1019–1028.

Carr, A., Finnegan, L., Griffin, E., Cotter, P., & Hyland, A. (2017). A randomized controlled trial of the say yes to life (SYTL) positive psychology group psychotherapy program for depression: An interim report. *Journal of Contemporary Psychotherapy, 47*(3), 153–161.

Castonguay, L. G. (2013). Psychotherapy outcome: An issue worth re-revisiting 50 years later. *Psychotherapy, 50*(1), 52–67.

Connor, K. M., & Davidson, J. R. (2003). Development of a new resilience scale: The Connor-Davidson Resilience Scale (CD-RISC). *Depression and Anxiety, 18*(2), 76–82.

Corrigan, P. (2004). How stigma interferes with mental health care. *American Psychologist, 59*, 614–625.

Csillik, A., Aguerre, C., & Bay, M. (2012). Psychothérapie positive de la dépression: Spécificités et apports cliniques. *Annales médico-psychologiques, 170*(8), 541–546.

Cuadra-Peralta, A., Veloso-Besio, C., Pérez, M., & Zúñiga, M. (2010). Resultados de la psicoterapia positiva en pacientes con depresión [Positive psychotherapy results in patients with depression.]. *Terapia Psicológica, 28*, 127–134.

Cullen, B., Pownall, J., Cummings, J., Baylan, S., Broomfield, N., Haig, C., et al. (2018). Positive psychotherapy in ABI Rehab (PoPsTAR): A pilot randomised controlled trial. *Neuropsychological Rehabilitation, 28*(1), 17–33.

Dowlatabadi, M. M., Ahmadi, S. M., Sorbi, M. H., Beiki, O., Razavi, T. K., & Bidaki, R. (2016). The effectiveness of group positive psychotherapy on depression and happiness in breast cancer patients: A randomized controlled trial. *Electronic Physician, 8*(3), 2175–2180.

Eichstaedt, J. C., Schwartz, H. A., Kern, M. L., Park, G., Labarthe, D. R., Merchant, R. M., et al. (2015). Psychological language on Twitter predicts county-level heart disease mortality. *Psychological Science, 26*(2), 159–169.

Elsayed, H. S. (2016). Aggressiveness and its relationship to some variables in positive psychology among samples of university students and employees. *Journal of Psychological Counseling, Center of Psychological Counseling, Egypt, 1*(46), 433–477.

Enright, R. D., & Fitzgibbons, R. P. (2014). *Forgiveness therapy: An empirical guide for resolving anger and restoring hope*. Washington, DC: American Psychological Association.

Evans, J. (2011). Positive psychology and brain injury rehabilitation. *Brain Impairment, 12*, 117–127.

Fitzpatrick, M. R., & Stalikas, A. (2008). Integrating positive emotions into theory, research, and practice: A new challenge for psychotherapy. *Journal of Psychotherapy Integration, 18*, 248–258.

Frankl, V. E. (1963). *Man's search for meaning: An introduction to logotherapy*. New York, NY: Washington Square Press.

Fredrickson, B. L. (2001). The role of positive emotions in positive psychology. *American Psychologist, 56*, 218–226.

Fredrickson, B. L. (2013a). Positive emotions broaden and build. In E. A. Plant & P. G. Devine (Eds.), *Advances in experimental social psychology* (pp. 47–53). San Diego, CA: Academic Press.

Fredrickson, B. L. (2013b). *Love 2.0: How our supreme emotion affects everything we feel, think, do, and become*. New York, NY: Hudson Street Press.

Fredrickson, B. L., Mancuso, R. A., Branigan, C., & Tugade, M. M. (2000). The undoing effect of positive emotions. *Motivation and Emotion, 24*(4), 237–258.

Fredrickson, B. L., Grewen, K. M., Coffey, K. A., Algoe, S. B., Firestine, A. M., Arevalo, J. M. G., et al. (2013). A functional genomic perspective on human wellbeing. *Proceedings of the National Academy of Sciences of the United States of America, 110*(33), 13684–13689.

Fink, J. E. (2014). Flourishing: Exploring predictors of mental health within the college environment. *Journal of American College Health, 62,* 380–388.

Frisch, M. B. (2006). *Quality of life therapy: Applying a life satisfaction approach to positive psychology and cognitive therapy*. Hoboken, NJ: Wiley.

Furchtlehner, L. M., & Laireiter, A.-R. (2016, September). *Comparing positive psychotherapy (PPT) and cognitive behavior therapy (CBT) in the treatment of depression. Preliminary ITT-results from a RCT-study*. Paper presented at the 1st Conference on Positive Psychology of DACH PP (German-language Association of Positive Psychology), Berlin, Germany.

Gable, S. L., Reis, H. T., Impett, E. A., & Asher, E. R. (2004). What do you do when things go right? The intrapersonal and interpersonal benefits of sharing positive events. *Journal of Personality and Social Psychology, 87,* 228–245.

Garland, E. L., & Howard, M. O. (2009). Neuroplasticity, psychosocial genomics, and the biopsychosocial paradigm in the 21st century. *Health and Social Work, 34*(3), 191–199.

Giannopoulos, V. L., & Vella-Brodrick, D. (2011). Effects of positive interventions and orientations to happiness on subjective wellbeing. *The Journal of Positive Psychology, 6,* 95–105.

Gilman, R., Schumm, J. A., & Chard, K. M. (2012). Hope as a change mechanism in the treatment of posttraumatic stress disorder. *Psychological Trauma: Theory, Research, Practice, and Policy, 4,* 270–277.

Gockel, A. (2010). The promise of mindfulness for clinical practice education. *Smith College Studies in Social Work, 80,* 248–268.

Goodwin, E. M. (2010). *Does group positive psychotherapy help improve relationship satisfaction in a stressed and/or anxious population?* (Order No. 3428275, Palo Alto University). *ProQuest Dissertations and Theses,* 166. Retrieved from http://search.proquest.com/docview/822195958?accountid=14707 (822195958).

Graham, J. E., Lobel, M., Glass, P., & Lokshina, I. (2008). Effects of written constructive anger expression in chronic pain patients: Making meaning from pain. *Journal of Behavioral Medicine, 31,* 201–212.

Harris, A. H. S., Luskin, F., Norman, S. B., Standard, S., Bruning, J., Evans, S., et al. (2006). Effects of a group forgiveness intervention on forgiveness, perceived stress, and trait-anger. *Journal of Clinical Psychology, 62,* 715–733.

Harris, A. S. H., Thoresen, C. E., & Lopez, S. J. (2007). Integrating positive psychology into counseling: Why and (when appropriate) how. *Journal of Counseling & Development, 85,* 3–13.

Headey, B., Schupp, J., Tucci, I., & Wagner, G. G. (2010). Authentic happiness theory supported by impact of religion on life satisfaction: A longitudinal analysis with data for Germany. *The Journal of Positive Psychology, 5,* 73–82.

Hertel, P. T., & McDaniel, L. (2010). The suppressive power of positive thinking: Aiding suppression-induced forgetting in repressive coping. *Cognition and Emotion, 24,* 1239–1249.

Hicks, J. A., & King, L. A. (2009). Meaning in life as a subjective judgment and lived experience. *Social and Personality Psychology Compass, 3,* 638–658.

Huta, V., & Hawley, L. (2008). Psychological strengths and cognitive vulnerabilities: Are they two ends of the same continuum or do they have independent relationships with wellbeing and ill-being? *Journal of Happiness Studies, 11,* 71–93.

Hwang, K., Kwon, A., & Hong, C. (2017). A preliminary study of new positive psychology interventions: Neurofeedback-aided meditation therapy and modified positive psychotherapy. *Current Psychology, 36*(3), 683–695.

Johnson, D. P., Penn, D. L., Fredrickson, B. L., Meyer, P. S., Kring, A. M., & Brantley, M. (2009). Loving-kindness meditation to enhance recovery from negative symptoms of schizophrenia. *Journal of Clinical Psychology, 65,* 499–509.

Johnson, J., Wood, A. M., Gooding, P., Taylor, P. J., & Tarrier, N. (2011). Resilience to suicidality: The buffering hypothesis. *Clinical Psychology Review, 31*(4), 563–591.

Joormann, J., Dkane, M., & Gotlib, I. H. (2006). Adaptive and maladaptive components of rumination? Diagnostic specificity and relation to depressive biases. *Behavior Therapy, 37*, 269–280.

Joormann, J., Siemer, M., & Gotlib, I. H. (2007). Mood regulation in depression: Differential effects of distraction and recall of happy memories on sad mood. *Journal of Abnormal Psychology, 116*(3), 484–490.

Kabat-Zinn, J. (1990). *Full catastrophe living: Using the wisdom of your body and mind to face stress, pain, and illness*. New York, NY: Dell.

Kahler, C. W., Spillane, N. S., Day, A., Clerkin, E. M., Parks, A., Leventhal, A. M., et al. (2014). Positive psychotherapy for smoking cessation: Treatment development, feasibility, and preliminary results. *The Journal of Positive Psychology, 9*(1), 19–29.

Kapur, N., Cole, J., Manly, T., Viskontas, I., Ninteman, A., Hasher, L., et al. (2013). Positive clinical neuroscience: Explorations in positive neurology. *The Neuroscientist, 19*, 354–369.

Kashdan, T. B., Julian, T., Merritt, K., & Uswatte, G. (2006). Social anxiety and posttraumatic stress in combat veterans: Relations to wellbeing and character strengths. *Behaviour Research and Therapy, 44*, 561–583.

Karwoski, L., Garratt, G. M., & Ilardi, S. S. (2006). On the integration of cognitive-behavioral therapy for depression and positive psychology. *Journal of Cognitive Psychotherapy, 20*, 159–170.

Keyes, C. L. M., & Eduardo, J. S. (2012). To flourish or not: Level of positive mental health predicts ten-year all-cause mortality. *American Journal of Public Health, 102*, 2164–2172.

Khazaei, F., Khazaei, O., & Ghanbari, H. B. (2017). Positive psychology interventions for internet addiction treatment. *Computers in Human Behavior, 72*(C), 304–311.

Lambert, M. J. (2010). *Prevention of treatment failure: The use of measuring, monitoring, and feedback in clinical practice*. Washington, DC: American Psychological Association.

Lambert, M. J. (2017). Maximizing psychotherapy outcome beyond evidence-based medicine. *Psychotherapy and Psychosomatics, 86*(2), 80–89.

Lamont, A. (2011). University students' strong experiences of music: Pleasure, engagement, and meaning. *Music and Emotion, 15*, 229–249.

Leykin, Y., & DeRubeis, R. J. (2009). Allegiance in psychotherapy outcome research: Separating association from bias. *Clinical Psychology: Science and Practice, 16*, 54–65.

Lightsey, O. (2006). Resilience, meaning, and wellbeing. *The Counseling Psychologist, 34*, 96–107.

Linley, P. A., Nielsen, K. M., Wood, A. M., Gillett, R., & Biswas-Diener, R. (2010). Using signature strengths in pursuit of goals: Effects on goal progress, need satisfaction, and wellbeing, and implications for coaching psychologists. *International Coaching Psychology Review, 5*, 8–17.

Lü, W., Wang, Z., & Liu, Y. (2013). A pilot study on changes of cardiac vagal tone in individuals with low trait positive affect: The effect of positive psychotherapy. *International Journal of Psychophysiology, 88*, 213–217.

Luyten, L., Boddez, Y., & Hermans, D. (2015). Positive appraisal style: The mental immune system? *Behavioral and Brain Sciences, 38*, e112.

Lyubomirsky, S., & Layous, K. (2013). How do simple positive activities increase wellbeing? *Current Directions in Psychological Science, 22*, 57–62.

Lyubomirsky, S., Caldwell, N. D., & Nolen-Hoeksema, S. (1998). Effects of ruminative and distracting responses to depressed mood on retrieval of autobiographical memories. *Journal of Personality and Social Psychology, 75*(1), 166–177. https://doi.org/10.1037/0022-3514.75.1.166

McKnight, P. E., & Kashdan, T. B. (2009). Purpose in life as a system that creates and sustains health and wellbeing: An integrative, testable theory. *Review of General Psychology, 13*, 242–251.

Meyer, P. S., Johnson, D. P., Parks, A., Iwanski, C., & Penn, D. L. (2012). Positive living: A pilot study of group positive psychotherapy for people with schizophrenia. *Journal of Positive Psychology, 7*(3), 239–248.

Mitchell, J., Stanimirovic, R., Klein, B., & Vella-Brodrick, D. (2009). A randomised controlled trial of a self-guided internet intervention promoting wellbeing. *Computers in Human Behavior, 25*, 749–760.

Moeenizadeh, M., & Salagame, K. K. K. (2010). Wellbeing therapy (WBT) for depression. *International Journal of Psychological Studies, 2,* 107–115.

Mongrain, M., & Anselmo-Matthews, T. (2012). Do positive psychology exercises work? A replication of Seligman et al. (2005). *Journal of Clinical Psychology, 68,* 382–389.

Murray, G., & Johnson, S. L. (2010). The clinical significance of creativity in bipolar disorder. *Clinical Psychology Review, 30,* 721–732.

Nakamura, J., & Csikszentmihalyi, M. (2009). Flow theory and research. In S. J. Lopez & C. R. Snyder (Eds.), *Oxford handbook of positive psychology* (pp. 195–206). New York, NY: Oxford University Press.

Niemiec, R. M., Rashid, T., & Spinella, M. (2012). Strong mindfulness: Integrating mindfulness and character strengths. *Journal of Mental Health Counseling, 34,* 240–253.

Ochoa, C., Casellas-Grau, A., Vives, J., Font, A., & Borràs, J. M. (2017). Positive psychotherapy for distressed cancer survivors: Posttraumatic growth facilitation reduces posttraumatic stress. *International Journal of Clinical and Health Psychology, 17*(1), 28–37.

Oettingen, G. (2014). *Rethinking positive thinking: Inside the new science of motivation*. New York, NY: Penguin Group.

Oksanen, T., Kouvonen, A., Vahtera, J., Virtanen, M., & Kivimäki, M. (2010). Prospective study of workplace social capital and depression: Are vertical and horizontal components equally important? *Journal of Epidemiology and Community Health, 64,* 684–689.

Olfson, M., & Marcus, S. C. (2010). National trends in outpatient psychotherapy. *American Journal of Psychiatry, 167,* 1456–1463.

Parks-Sheiner, A. C. (2009). *Positive psychotherapy: Building a model of empirically supported self-help.* Dissertation Abstracts International: Section B: *The Sciences and Engineering, 70(6-B),* 3792.

Parks, A., Della Porta, M., Pierce, R. S., Zilca, R., & Lyubomirsky, S. (2012). Pursuing happiness in everyday life: The characteristics and behaviors of online happiness seekers. *Emotion, 12,* 1222–1234.

Parrott, W. G. (Ed.). (2014). *The positive side of negative emotions*. New York, NY: Guilford.

Pawelski, J. O. (2016). Defining the 'positive' in positive psychology: Part II. A normative analysis. *The Journal of Positive Psychology, 11*(4), 357–365.

Pedrotti, J. T. (2011). Broadening perspectives: Strategies to infuse multiculturalism into a positive psychology course. *Journal of Positive Psychology, 6*(6), 506–513.

Peterson, C., & Seligman, M. E. P. (2004). *Character strengths and virtues: A handbook and classification.* New York/Oxford: Oxford University Press/Washington, DC: American Psychological Association.

Pietrowsky, R., & Mikutta, J. (2012). Effects of positive psychology interventions in depressive patients—A randomized control study. *Psychology, 3,* 1067–1073.

Ramadan, H. A. (2014). The effectiveness of a therapeutic program to promote subjective wellbeing by using multi-components of positive psychology interventions. *Journal of Arabic Studies in Education and Psychology, KSA, 54,* 251–280.

Rao, M. A., Donaldson, S. I., & Doiron, K. M. (2015). Positive psychology research in the Middle East and North Africa. *Middle East Journal of Positive Psychology, 1*(1), 60–76.

Rashid, T. (2008). Positive psychotherapy Positive psychology: Exploring the best in people, Vol 4: *Pursuing human flourishing* (pp. 188–217). Westport, CT: Praeger

Rashid, T. (2013). Positive psychology in practice: Positive psychotherapy. *The Oxford handbook of happiness* (pp. 978–993). New York, NY: Oxford University Press.

Rashid, T. (2015). Positive psychotherapy: A strength-based approach. *The Journal of Positive Psychology, 10*(1), 25–40.

Rashid, T., & Anjum, A. (2008). Positive psychotherapy for young adults and children. In J. R. Z. Abela & B. L. Hankin (Eds.), *Depression in children and adolescents: Causes, treatment and prevention* (pp. 250–287). New York, NY: Guilford Press.

Rashid, T., & Ostermann, R. F. O. (2009). Strength-based assessment in clinical practice. *Journal of Clinical Psychology, 65,* 488–498.

Rashid, T., & Seligman, M. E. (2018). *Positive psychotherapy: A manual*. Oxford, UK: Oxford University Press.

Rashid, T., Anjum, A., Lennex, C., Quinlin, D., Niemiec, R., Mayerson, D., et al. (2013). In C. Proctor & A. Linley (Eds.), *Research, applications, and interventions for children and adolescents: A positive psychology perspective*. New York, NY: Springer.

Reinsch, C. (2012). *Adding science to the mix of business and pleasure: An exploratory study of positive psychology interventions with teachers accessing employee assistance counselling*. Master's thesis, University of Manitoba, Winnipeg, Manitoba, Canada. Retrieved from http://hdl.handle.net/1993/14436.

Riches, S., Schrank, B., Rashid, T., & Slade, M. (2016). WELLFOCUS PPT: Modifying positive psychotherapy for psychosis. *Psychotherapy, 53*(1), 68–77.

Rozin, P., & Royzman, E. (2001). Negativity bias, negativity dominance, and contagion. *Personality and Social Psychology Review, 5*(4), 296–320. https://doi.org/10.1207/S15327957PSPR0504_2

Ruini, C., & Fava, G. A. (2009). Wellbeing therapy for generalized anxiety disorder. *Journal of Clinical Psychology, 65*, 510–519.

Salama-Younes, M. (2015). Positive psychology: Applications, concepts and future perspectives in Arab countries. *Middle East Journal of Positive Psychology, 1*(1), 45–59.

Sandler, S. (2007). The reunion process: A new focus in short-term dynamic psychotherapy. *Psychotherapy (Chicago, IL), 44*, 121–136.

Schrank, B., Bird, V., Tylee, A., Coggins, T., Rashid, T., & Slade, M. (2013). Conceptualising and measuring the wellbeing of people with psychosis: Systematic review and narrative synthesis. *Social Science and Medicine, 92*, 9–21.

Schrank, B., Brownell, T., Jakaite, Z., Larkin, C., Pesola, F., Riches, S., et al. (2016). Evaluation of a positive psychotherapy group intervention for people with psychosis: pilot randomised controlled trial. *Epidemiology and Psychiatric Sciences, 25*(3), 235–246.

Schueller, S. (2010). Preferences for positive psychology exercises. *The Journal of Positive Psychology, 5*, 192–203.

Schueller, S. M., & Parks, A. C. (2012). Disseminating self-help: Positive psychology exercises in an online trial. *Journal of Medical Internet Research, 14*(3), e63.

Schwartz, B., & Sharpe, K. E. (2006). Practical wisdom: Aristotle meets positive psychology. *Journal of Happiness Studies, 7*, 377–395.

Schwartz, B., Ward, A., Monterosso, J., Lyubomirsky, S., White, K., & Lehman, D. R. (2002a). Maximizing versus satisficing: Happiness is a matter of choice. *Journal of Personality and Social Psychology, 83*, 1178–1197.

Schwartz, R. M., Reynolds, C. F., III, Thase, M. E., Frank, E., Fasiczka, A. L., & Haaga, D. A. F. (2002b). Optimal and normal affect balance in psychotherapy of major depression: Evaluation of the balanced states of mind model. *Behavioral and Cognitive Psychotherapy, 30*, 439–450.

Seery, M. D., Holman, E. A., & Silver, R. C. (2010). Whatever does not kill us: Cumulative lifetime adversity, vulnerability, and resilience. *Journal of Personality and Social Psychology, 99*(6), 1025–1041.

Seligman, M. E. P. (2002). *Authentic happiness: Using the new positive psychology to realize your potential for lasting fulfillment*. New York, NY: Free Press.

Seligman, M. E. P. (2011). *Flourish: A visionary new understanding of happiness and wellbeing*. New York, NY: Simon & Schuster.

Seligman, M. E., Rashid, T., & Parks, A. C. (2006). Positive psychotherapy. *American Psychologist, 61*, 774–788.

Seligman, M. E., Steen, T. A., Park, N., & Peterson, C. (2005). Positive psychology progress: Empirical validation of interventions. *American Psychologist, 60*, 410–421.

Senf, K., & Liau, A. K. (2013). The effects of positive interventions on happiness and depressive symptoms, with an examination of personality as a moderator. *Journal of Happiness Studies, 14*, 591–612.

Sin, N. L., & Lyubomirsky, S. (2009). Enhancing wellbeing and alleviating depressive symptoms with positive psychology interventions: A practice-friendly meta-analysis. *Journal of Clinical Psychology, 65,* 467–487.

Sirgy, M. J., & Wu, J. (2009). The pleasant life, the engaged life, and the meaningful life: What about the balanced life? *Journal of Happiness Studies, 10,* 183–196.

Smith, E. E., & Aaker, J. L. (2013, November 30). *Millennial searchers (Sunday Review).* Retrieved from http://www.nytimes.com/2013/12/01/opinion/sunday/millennial-searchers.html?_r=0.

Steger, M. F., & Shin, J. Y. (2010). The relevance of the meaning in life questionnaire to therapeutic practice: A look at the initial evidence. *International Forum for Logotherapy, 33,* 95–104.

Steger, M. F., Kashdan, T. B., & Oishi, S. (2008). Being good by doing good: Eudaimonic activity and daily wellbeing correlates, mediators, and temporal relations. *Journal of Research in Personality, 42,* 22–42.

Stillman, T. F., & Baumeister, R. F. (2009). Uncertainty, belongingness, and four needs for meaning. *Psychological Inquiry, 20,* 249–251.

Tajdin, M. (2015). The concept of happiness in medieval Islamic thought: From philosophy to religion. *Middle East Journal of Positive Psychology, 1*(1), 36–44.

Thomas, J., Mutawa, M., Furber, S. W., & Grey, I. (2016). Religiosity: Reducing depressive symptoms amongst Muslim females in the United Arab Emirates. *Middle East Journal of Positive Psychology, 2*(1), 9–21.

Uliaszek, A. A., Rashid, T., Williams, G. E., & Gulamani, T. (2016). Group therapy for university students: A randomized control trial of dialectical behavior therapy and positive psychotherapy. *Behaviour Research and Therapy, 77,* 78–85.

Van Dillen, L. F., & Koole, S. L. (2007). Clearing the mind: A working memory model of distraction from negative mood. *Emotion, 7,* 715–723.

Vella-Brodrick, D. A., Park, N., & Peterson, C. (2009). Three ways to be happy: Pleasure, engagement, and meaning: Findings from Australian and U.S. samples. *Social Indicators Research, 90,* 165–179.

Waters, L. (2011). A review of school-based positive psychology interventions. *The Australian Educational and Developmental Psychologist, 28*(2), 75–90.

Wong, W. J. (2012). Strength-centered therapy: A social constructionist, virtue-based psychotherapy. *Psychotherapy, 43,* 133–146.

Wood, A. M., & Joseph, S. (2010). The absence of positive psychological (eudemonic) wellbeing as a risk factor for depression: A ten year cohort study. *Journal of Affective Disorders, 122,* 213–217.

Wood, A. M., Maltby, J., Gillett, R., Linley, P. A., & Joseph, S. (2008). The role of gratitude in the development of social support, stress, and depression: Two longitudinal studies. *Journal of Research in Personality, 42,* 854–871.

Worthington, E. L., Witvliet, C. V. O., Pietrini, P., & Miller, A. J. (2007). Forgiveness, health, and wellbeing: a review of evidence for emotional versus decisional forgiveness, dispositional forgivingness, and reduced unforgiveness. *Journal of Behavioral Medicine, 30*(4), 291–302.

Wrzesniewski, A., McCauley, C., Rozin, P., & Schwartz, B. (1997). Jobs, careers, and callings: People's relations to their work. *Journal of Research in Personality, 31,* 21–33.

Younis, I. (2017). *The power of positive psychology: In your life and with your children.* Alexandria, Egypt: Houras.

Chapter 16
Repercussions of Individual and Societal Valuing of Happiness

Paul K. Lutz and Holli-Anne Passmore

Abstract Western culture has developed an obsession with happiness. At first glance, the premium placed on happiness seems warranted given that a large body of research has highlighted its benefits. Yet, emerging lines of research suggest that the outcomes of being happy are very different from the outcomes of seeking to be happy. Whereas the former is often linked to, and in some cases even causes, positive outcomes, the latter seems to do the opposite. This chapter first reviews research examining the negative effects of pursuing happiness at the individual level. We then highlight a number of important differences between Western and Eastern notions of happiness while also considering how these notions are beginning to change. Next, we examine the consequences stemming from valuing happiness at the societal level. We discuss prominent cultural emotion norms tied to happiness and the implications that these norms have for individual emotional functioning. Throughout, we note that the downsides of pursuing happiness may spread to other Eastern societies, such as the Middle East/North Africa region, through increased exposure to Western values, norms, and practices via globalization. Lastly, we highlight a number of important social determinants of happiness that can inform governments in their mandate to boost the happiness, life satisfaction, and overall wellbeing of their citizens.

16.1 Repercussions of Individual and Societal Valuing of Happiness

What does a happy person look like? For many of us, the first feature we think of when envisioning a happy person is a smile. Indeed, the smile is a universal sign of happiness that is deeply rooted in our evolution (Burgoon, Guerrero, & Floyd, 2016). Yet, despite the smile's extended history, it did not become a cultural icon until the mid 20th century with the advent of the famous smiley. In 1963, the State Mutual

---

P. K. Lutz (✉) · H.-A. Passmore
University of British Columbia, Kelowna, BC, Canada
e-mail: paul.k.lutz@alumni.ubc.ca

H.-A. Passmore
e-mail: passmoreh@alumni.ubc.ca

L. Lambert and N. Pasha-Zaidi (eds.), *Positive Psychology in the Middle East/North Africa*, https://doi.org/10.1007/978-3-030-13921-6_16

Life Insurance Company hired American commercial artist Harvey Ball to design an image that would boost the morale of company employees (Stamp, 2013). In less than ten minutes, Ball designed a stylized smiley face that would earn him 45 dollars (Savage, 2009). Ball's image soon became an international icon. Today, the smiley and its various renditions are but one of the many cultural artifacts that signify our growing obsession with happiness.

The premium placed on happiness appears to be inescapable in Western cultures, such as America (Tamir & Ford, 2012), where individuals think about it at least once a day (Freedman, 1978). This premium, however, is not limited to the West; happiness is desired around the world (Diener, 2000). Recognizing this, in 2011, the United Nations General Assembly adopted a resolution that positioned happiness as a "fundamental human goal" (United Nations, 2011). The following year, the Assembly embraced a resolution that declared the 20th of March the International Day of Happiness (United Nations, 2012). These are not the only efforts aimed at promoting happiness. Initiatives such as the *Happiness Alliance* (Happiness Alliance, 2010) and most notably, *Action for Happiness* (Action for Happiness, 2010), a non-profit movement involving individuals from over 160 countries, are making strides to enhance happiness within and across countries. Happiness is a growing topic of interest among policymakers and governing bodies (Dolan & Metcalfe, 2012), a goal of education and counselling (Harper, Guilbault, Tucker, & Austin, 2007; Suissa, 2008), and an aim of organizations seeking to boost employee productivity (Diener et al., 2017). Unsurprisingly, happiness receives a great deal of attention from researchers and academics. The positive psychology movement has fueled scientific inquiry into happiness; at the same time, this area of study has attracted researchers from diverse fields such as economics, sociology, and political science (Diener et al., 2017). This growing interest among scholars has resulted in an exponential increase in the number of happiness articles published each year (Myers & Diener, 2018), and this research is often more likely to be picked up by media platforms than alternative research produced by the social sciences (De Vos, 2012).

Happiness is inescapable in popular media: It is a regular topic discussed on talk shows and podcasts; it seems to be mentioned endlessly on social media sites such as Facebook and Twitter; it is a common theme depicted in television and film, and editors of magazines and newspapers frequently choose to feature happiness content. Over the past few decades a happiness industry has emerged with motivational speakers, websites, and self-help books claiming to provide the secrets to the good life. Unfortunately, many of these resources, with some notable exceptions (e.g., Lyubomirsky, 2013), lack an empirical foundation that may limit their effectiveness (Parks, Schueller, & Tasimi, 2013). Happiness has also become a powerful tool in the world of advertising with global brands employing happiness-based campaigns to sell their products (e.g., McDonald's Happy Meal). In sum, happiness has developed into a cultural obsession. As McGuirk, Kuppens, Kingston, and Bastian (2018) conclude: "Rather than being the by-product of a life well lived, feeling happy has become a goal in itself…" (p. 755).

Our preoccupation with happiness has prompted many criticisms and concerns from scholars. For instance, Held (2002) observes that the cultural focus on promoting positivity has become tyrannical, resulting in immense societal pressure to be happy. Even more concerning, emerging evidence suggests that the relentless pursuit of happiness can negatively affect wellbeing (e.g., Mauss, Tamir, Anderson, & Savino, 2011). These criticisms stem not only from academia. Citing an oversaturation of happiness within contemporary culture, Coca-Cola has recently replaced their famous "Open Happiness" slogan with the less emotionally driven "Taste the Feeling" (Ghosh, 2016). Together, these criticisms raise a number of questions, including: What are the potential repercussions of placing such extreme value on happiness? The aim of the present chapter is to address this question. We first review research examining the consequences of individual and societal valuing of happiness. We then broaden this discussion by highlighting a number of important social determinants of happiness that might be fruitful for governments, intent on boosting the happiness of their citizens, to measure and address.

16.2 Clarification of Key Terms

Before reviewing the literature on the harmful effects of pursuing happiness, we wish to clarify and define some important terms. Borrowing from Ford and Mauss (2014), we use the terms *wanting*, *valuing*, *pursuing*, and *seeking happiness* interchangeably throughout this chapter. As noted by Ford and Mauss, wanting and valuing happiness can be considered an emotional goal (i.e., a goal in which one aims to experience more happiness), while pursuing and seeking happiness involves not only possessing this emotional goal, but actively engaging in behaviours to achieve it. Therefore, although these terms entail different processes, they are highly related and when taken to excess, seem to be linked to negative outcomes. Another important concept to define is happiness itself. In the social sciences, happiness is often replaced with the term subjective wellbeing (Diener, 1984), which includes both affective and cognitive evaluations of one's life. The affective component is comprised of high positive affect and low negative affect, while the cognitive component consists of a judgment of one's overall satisfaction with life. Much of the research discussed below defines happiness as the emotional component of subjective wellbeing. Therefore, we use the term *happiness* to refer to increased positive emotion and decreased negative emotion. For the sake of simplicity, life satisfaction will be referred to separately; nonetheless, we remain cognizant that life satisfaction is still a key component of happiness.

16.3 Repercussions of Individual Valuing of Happiness

It seems perplexing that the pursuit of happiness can be potentially maladaptive given that happiness itself is linked to a number of beneficial outcomes. For instance, happy individuals enjoy greater career success (Walsh, Boehm, & Lyubomirsky,

2018), more fulfilling and stable social relationships (De Neve, Diener, Tay, & Xuereb, 2013), and enhanced physical health and longevity (Chida & Steptoe, 2008; Diener & Chan, 2011) when compared to their less happy peers. Additionally, at a fundamental level, happiness simply feels good; it is an enjoyable experience (Brülde, 2007). Thus, it is easy to see why happiness is a goal held by individuals around the world (Diener, Sapyta, & Suh, 1998). Yet, a growing body of research suggests that a critical difference exists between being happy and wanting to be happy. Whereas being happy is linked to, and in some cases even causes, beneficial outcomes (Diener, Oishi, & Lucas, 2015), wanting or striving to be happy appears to do the opposite (Ford & Mauss, 2014).

Reservations expressed against seeking happiness are not new. Theorists dating as far back as Aristotle have posited that the pursuit of happiness can be counterproductive. Only recently, however, has this proposition been empirically tested. Some of the earliest evidence of this phenomenon comes from an experiment examining the ironic effects of mental control. Wegner, Erber, and Zanakos (1993, Experiment 1) tested the ironic process theory, which posits that attempting to exert mental control while under conditions of diminished mental capacity can result in outcomes that run counter to those desired (see Wegner, 1994 for a review). In the case of mood control, this theory predicts that those attempting to be happy will be successful so long as there is sufficient cognitive capacity to achieve control. However, when under conditions of mental load, those striving to feel happy will ironically experience a mood that is the opposite of one's intentions, that is, sadness. To test this, Wegner and colleagues asked participants to recall either a happy or sad experience and to write down their thoughts as they reflected on the event. Those thinking about happy experiences were either asked to attempt to be happy, to not be happy, or were given no unique instructions. Similarly, individuals thinking about sad experiences were either asked to attempt to be sad, to not be sad, or were given no instructions. Some participants were placed under cognitive load by having to remember a 9-digit number during the study. Observer ratings of the written responses along with participant self-ratings were used to measure participant mood. Results indicated that those participants who tried to be happy under conditions of limited cognitive load did indeed become happier. The same was true for those attempting to be sad. However, when faced with a cognitively distracting task, individuals who tried to be happy became sad and those who tried to be sad became happy.

Schooler, Ariely, and Loewenstein (2003) reported that results from both an experiment and a field study suggested that attempts at maximizing happiness can backfire, even in the absence of cognitive load. The authors first examined the impact of effort and monitoring on one's ability to achieve happiness in a laboratory setting and hypothesized that explicitly trying to become happy and monitoring one's continuing hedonic experience would lead to reductions in happiness. To test this, they had participants listen to a piece of hedonically ambiguous music (i.e., Stravinsky's *Rite of Spring*). However, prior to listening, participants were assigned to one of four conditions: (1) simply listen to the music (control); (2) try to be as happy as possible; (3) frequently monitor their happiness using an adjustable scale; (4) both try to be as happy as possible and frequently monitor their happiness. Results indicated that participants who had tried to be happy, who had frequently monitored their happiness, and those who both tried to be happy and frequently monitored their happiness felt worse than individuals in the control condition, suggesting that explicitly trying to be happy and asking oneself "Am I happy?" can impede actually feeling happy.

To further explore this relationship, Schooler and colleagues (2003) conducted a field study during the final week of December 1999 wherein participants were asked to complete a series of questions pertaining to their New Year's Eve plans. Participants were then contacted two months later (March, 2000) to inquire about their actual New Year's Eve experience. Results point to a potentially important mechanism by which the pursuit of happiness may lead to undesirable outcomes, that is, high expectations. Individuals who had put the most effort into preparing for their celebrations and expected to have the biggest, most extravagant parties were the most disappointed afterwards. Alternatively, those who had curbed their expectations and expected to have a small celebration or, none at all, did not face such disappointment. Building on this, Mauss and colleagues (2011) theorized that individuals who greatly value happiness often set very high standards for its achievement. These seemingly unattainable expectations can result in feelings of disappointment, which in turn paradoxically lead to decreases in happiness. They found that when respondents' life stress was low, overall wellbeing was worse the more they valued happiness. They further tested this hypothesis via an experiment in which participants were randomly assigned to a valuing happiness or control condition. Compared to the control group, individuals who had been induced to value happiness (by reading about its benefits) felt less happy in a positive setting (watching a happy video) but not in a negative setting (watching a sad video). This effect was mediated by participants' disappointment regarding their emotional experience. In sum, these results suggest that valuing happiness can paradoxically result in unhappiness, especially when happiness is thought to be easily attainable and expectations are high.

A number of findings have since substantiated these results. For instance, research has shown that highly valuing happiness is correlated with, and even causes, greater feelings of loneliness (Mauss et al., 2012). Extreme valuing of happiness has also been found to be associated with greater symptoms and diagnosis of major depressive disorder (Ford, Shallcross, Mauss, Floerke, & Gruber, 2014), and risk for, diagnosis of, and illness-course for bipolar disorder (Ford, Mauss, & Gruber, 2015). In a sample of college students, Tamir and Ford (2012) found that participants' preferences for seeking happiness in contexts in which it is unlikely to be useful (e.g., confrontational social situations) were associated with decreased psychological wellbeing and adaptive functioning (i.e., interpersonal support and college grade point average). Similarly, Kim and Maglio (2018) found not only that seeking happiness leads to less happiness and feelings that time is limited, they also found that viewing the pursuit of happiness as effortful and time-consuming leads to the perception that time is scarce, ultimately reducing happiness.

16.4 Cultural Valuations of Happiness

These studies suggest that the more individuals value, seek, and pursue happiness, the less likely they are to actually feel happy. Yet, much of this research has been conducted in the United States, thus calling into question the generalizability of such findings. It is possible that the paradoxical effects of seeking happiness may be specific to Western cultural contexts. Several scholars have argued that results from Western cultures should not be generalized to other cultures before indigenous theoretical and empirical investigations have occurred (e.g., Joshanloo, 2013). This is important, as there is considerable variation in the extent to which people value happiness both within and between cultures (Eid & Diener, 2001). Recognizing this, Ford and colleagues (2014) note that studying the pursuit of happiness as a within-culture factor, particularly within North America, is not a substitute for cross-cultural investigation. Indeed, when one begins to examine the pursuit of happiness through an alternative cultural lens, it becomes clear that happiness is not always highly pursued. For instance, individuals in some Eastern societies may be hesitant to seek happiness because doing so is believed to have a number of negative and even immoral connotations (Heine, Lehman, Markus, & Kitayama, 1999; Uchida & Kitayama, 2009). In Islamic cultures, expressing happiness is often regarded as tempting fate, calling forth the evil eye, and facilitating a path to sin; individuals who express happiness can be regarded as somewhat frivolous or irresponsible (Joshanloo & Weijers, 2014). Such beliefs can cause the pursuit of happiness to be shunned. Further, ways in which happiness is both pursued and defined seems to differ across cultures (Uchida, Norasakkunkit, & Kitayama, 2004).

Scholars have suggested that happiness is most likely universal when it is considered as a state of mind; however, its meaning is ultimately tied to cultural context (Pflug, 2009; Tov & Diener, 2007). Lomas' (2016, 2018) recent work on "untranslatable" words highlights cultural differences in the construction of happiness and wellbeing. At the same time, he notes that although most languages have a translative equivalent for happiness, cross-culturally "happiness is a complex, polyvalent term, encompassing a multitude of positive feelings" (p. 548). The terms used in many languages to describe the construct of happiness reflect a spectrum of nuanced aspects of happiness valued in respective cultures. By becoming familiar with these broader, alternative ways of construing happiness and wellbeing, Lomas suggests we can enrich our own experiences of happiness.

Other approaches to examining cross-cultural differences in happiness consider how societies define the self (Joshanloo, 2014). Cultures differ in the extent to which they endorse individualistic versus collectivistic values (Triandis, 1995), resulting in conceptualizations of the self as falling along a continuum of independent to interdependent (Markus & Kitayama, 1991). As outlined by Oyserman, Coon, and Kemmelmeier (2002), in more individualistic societies, such as the United States, wherein the self is viewed as primarily independent, key concerns include maintaining a positive sense of self, promoting personal success, and expressing one's unique attributes. In contrast, in more collectivistic cultures such as China, wherein the self is viewed as more interdependent, greater value is placed on maintaining harmonious relationships, carrying out social roles, and making sacrifices for the collective good. Societies that are highly individualistic often cultivate a construal of the self that is seen as unique, autonomous, and separate from others (De Leersnyder, Kim, & Mesquita, 2015; Haberstroh, Oyserman, Schwarz, Kühnen, & Ji, 2002; Wirtz & Chiu, 2008), whereas highly collectivistic cultures foster a construal of the self that is seen as connected, related, and less differentiated from others. Contrasting meanings of and attitudes towards happiness emerge from these differences in cultural orientations (i.e., individualism vs. collectivism) and models of the self (i.e., independent vs. interdependent).

In many North American and Western European cultural contexts, happiness is viewed as an emotional state contingent upon personal achievement and the maximization of positive personal attributes (Uchida et al., 2004). When forming perceptions of happiness, individuals in these societies emphasize autonomous agency and self-enhancement, as well as the gratification of personal needs and desires (Lu & Gilmour, 2004; Uchida & Ogihara, 2012). Thus, it is not surprising that personal accomplishment (Emmons, 1986) and self-esteem (Yuki, Sato, Takemura, & Oishi, 2013) are key predictors of happiness in individualistic cultures. Alternatively, many Middle Eastern and East Asian cultures define happiness in terms of interpersonal connectedness and belonging (Lambert D'raven & Pasha-Zaidi, 2014a; Uchida & Oishi, 2016). Perceptions of happiness in these societies emphasize the fulfillment of role obligations, maintaining social harmony, and promoting collective prosperity (Lu & Gilmour, 2006). Key predictors of happiness in such cultures include social support (Suhail & Chaudhry, 2004) and relational harmony (Kwan, Bond, & Singelis, 1997). Further, the important role that spirituality and religion plays in forming notions of happiness in many interdependent cultures cannot be understated, as such belief systems are instrumental in shaping individuals' understanding and experience of happiness (Abdel-Khalek, 2007; Joshanloo, 2014).

While social connection is a key feature of happiness for members of collectivistic cultures, it is not limited to such societies. In fact, interpersonal relationships are considered a universal ingredient of happiness (Diener, 2013, Delle Fave, Brdar, Freire, Vella-Brodrick, & Wissing, 2011) and are an essential component of Westerners' happiness as well (Diener & Seligman, 2002). As Uchida and Ogihara (2012) note, although Western societies prize an independent self, individuals in these societies still actively pursue, engage in, and value interpersonal relationships. Nonetheless, many Westerners still tend to emphasize personal achievement over social relationships when forming ideas of happiness, even though interpersonal connection is a necessary condition for happiness (Diener & Oishi, 2005). Individualistic notions of happiness that heavily emphasize personal outcomes have been criticized for being excessively self-focused (Joshanloo, 2014). Placing such a strong focus on personal outcomes and achievement can impair social connection (Park & Crocker, 2005). Research supports the notion that people who strive for more individualistic, self-focused forms of happiness experience decreased social connection and as a result, negative consequences. For example, in the United States greater valuing of happiness (in this context, construed in terms of achievement of personal goals) predicted greater loneliness (Mauss et al., 2012). Findings such as these suggest that an overemphasis on the pursuit of happiness through personal gains necessarily equates to reduced attention being paid to maintaining close, personal relationships, ultimately resulting in greater disconnection, loneliness, and unhappiness.

Cross-cultural investigations have also examined differences in the definition and manner of pursuing happiness and how these differences produce different outcomes. A study that collected data from university students in the United States, Germany, Russia, and East Asia found that culturally-shaped definitions of happiness and thus, differences in routes to pursuing happiness, did indeed help to explain differences in whether pursuing happiness was associated with negative outcomes (Ford et al., 2015). In Russia and East Asia, collectivistic cultures where happiness is defined in socially engaged terms, the motivation to pursue happiness was positively correlated with wellbeing. Yet, in the individualistic culture of the United States, where happiness is defined in terms of personal outcomes, the motivation to pursue happiness was negatively correlated with wellbeing. In Germany, considered to be in the middle of the individualistic-collectivistic continuum, no association was found between the motivation to pursue happiness and wellbeing. It was also found that those who defined happiness in social terms were more likely to have higher wellbeing regardless of how motivated they were to seek happiness and which culture they were from. Such findings support the universal importance of social connection.

16.5 Cultural Shifts and Happiness

Happiness is fundamentally tied to cultural context. Culture, however, is not a static and rigid entity, rather it is fluid, flexible, and dynamic (Matsumoto, Kudoh, & Takeuchi, 1996). Cultures are susceptible to change, and thus, the meanings we ascribe to happiness and the manners in which we pursue happiness can change as well. These considerations are especially relevant in today's world where cross-cultural contact and influence is prominent. Indeed, Uchida and Ogihara (2012) note that a number of Eastern cultures are experiencing a shift towards more individualistic, Western ideas of happiness due to pressures of globalization. Globalization can be defined as "a process through which material and social phenomena generated in one or more parts of the world become part of the lives of people in other parts of the globe" (Prilleltensky, 2012, p. 613). Although globalization can reduce barriers between cultures, the process appears to be biased towards simply making societies more Westernized (Ogihara & Uchida, 2014). In fact, some scholars even refer to globalization as Westernization (e.g., Mehmet, 2001). Berry (2008) argues that globalization is of critical importance when examining cultural change, as it is the starting point for acculturation, "the dual process of cultural and psychological change that takes place as a result of contact between two or more cultural groups and their individual members" (Berry, 2005, p. 698). Globalization and acculturation are powerful forces that reshape cultural landscapes. At the cultural/group level, changes occur in social structure, collective activities, and social climate, while at the psychological/individual level, changes occur in individuals' behavioural repertoires, attitudes, and values (Graves, 1967; Matsudaira, 2006; Sam & Berry, 2010).

It has been suggested that globalization and acculturation, largely tied to the spread of Western values and practices, is responsible for the rise in individualism throughout many traditionally collectivistic cultures, such as Japan (e.g., Toivonen, Norasakkunkit, & Uchida, 2011). Evidence of this phenomenon at the group level comes from Japan's declining average household size, rising divorce rate, growing adoption of school systems designed to encourage student uniqueness, and the upsurge of individual performance-based wage systems (Chiang & Ohtake, 2014; Hamamura, 2012; Ogihara, 2017). Japan is not the only Eastern society experiencing such change. China, the United Arab Emirates (UAE), and many countries in the Middle East and North Africa (MENA) region are examples of societies experiencing shifts in cultural norms primarily attributable to economic transformation fostered by globalization. With increased flow of commodities and services across borders, integration of financial markets, and rapid spread of technology, globalization is stimulating substantial economic growth and development in these parts of the world (Mishkin, 2009; Samimi & Jenatabadi, 2014). On the heels of this is an almost inevitable cultural shift away from collectivism towards individualism (Hofstede, 1980). For instance, research indicates that in China there is a growing adherence to individualistic values (Parker, Haytko, & Hermans, 2009; Sun & Ryder, 2016; Yan, 2010). These transformations have been especially pronounced in Gulf Cooperation Council nations (i.e., UAE, Saudi Arabia, Qatar, Oman, Bahrain, and Kuwait) where globalization and economic development are advancing at blistering speeds (Looney, 2007). Higher levels of individualism have been observed in younger UAE nationals compared to older citizens (Whiteoak, Crawford, & Mapstone, 2006). Combined with increased wealth spurred by rapid economic growth, these shifts toward individualism have a number of implications for happiness.

Seeking to provide an explanation for the sometimes reported positive correlation between national wealth and national aggregated levels of happiness, Ahuvia (2002) proposed that economic growth creates a cultural setting in which individuals make decisions to maximize their happiness rather than fulfill social obligations. He notes "this cultural transformation away from obligation and toward the pursuit of happiness is part of a broader transition away from collectivism and toward individualist cultural values and forms of social organization" (p. 25). This model suggests that economic development releases individuals from previously culturally-sanctioned social obligations, which, while reducing social capital, allows individuals to make decisions that focus more fully on satisfying intrinsic needs including investing energy into more inherently-valued relationships. While Ahuvia's theorizing is compelling, this may not be the whole story.

Ogihara and Uchida (2014) theorized that individualism in Western cultural contexts differs from individualism in traditionally collectivistic cultural contexts. They studied differences between American and Japanese patterns of relationships among individualistic values, happiness, and number of close friends. While individualism in America entails being independent from others but still actively creating interpersonal relationships, Japanese adoption of individualism may be characterized by feeling the need to cut off existing personal relationships in order to achieve independence. Ogihara and Uchida posited that once these relationships have been cut off, Japanese may not possess the appropriate strategies (e.g., engaging in self-disclosure) helpful in creating new interpersonal connections, the end result being a reduction in the number of close relationships and by extension, happiness. Alternatively, such strategies have been cultivated over extended periods of time in Western societies, leaving individuals in these contexts readily equipped with the means to create new relationships. Thus, individualistic values in America need not necessarily be associated with such decreases in the number of close friends and happiness. Results of their study supported this theorizing. In Japan, the number of close friends mediated the negative effect of individualistic values on happiness; that is, those with strong individualistic orientations reported having fewer close friends and resultant lower levels of happiness. This was not the case in the American sample, however, in which the number of close friends people reported did not emerge as a significant mediator of the relationship between a strong inclination towards individualism and lesser happiness.

Amidst cultural shifts towards greater individualism, individual variability still exists in the extent to which people adopt these new values (Berry, 1997). Some individuals may maintain traditional cultural values, while others may deviate from traditional norms (Uchida & Ogihara, 2012). Although some suggest that globalization will eventually give rise to a homogenization of world cultures (Steger, 2013; see also Wilk, 1995), with Eastern societies converging toward Western ones, a more probable outcome will be some degree of change for both cultures entailing the sharing of certain qualities while at the same time the retention of key features of each respective culture (Berry, 2008). Pflug (2009) argues that collectivistic societies that have been subject to Western influences often display a combination of both individualistic and collectivistic values. Supporting this claim, Pflug cites a number of studies that used Taiwanese, Indian, or South African samples. In all of these studies, evidence is provided for how members of each of these cultures uniquely combine Western and Eastern values.

A central feature of globalization is also rising immigration (Shimpi & Zirkel, 2012), which some scholars have suggested influences individualistic Western cultures to become more collectivistic (Lalonde & Cameron, 1993). Supporting this claim are results from survey studies (e.g., Parker et al., 2009), which indicate a rise in collectivistic values among American students. Nonetheless, while globalization does spark change in both cultures such that homogenization is not the most likely scenario, globalization and its related processes tend to affect one culture more than the other (Berry, 1997). Indeed, trends towards collectivism are less salient in Western cultures than are trends towards individualism in Eastern cultures (Lu & Gilmour, 2004).

This age of cultural fusion has important implications for happiness (Lu & Gilmour, 2004). Steele and Lynch (2013) found that over time, the Chinese have increasingly prioritized individualist factors in assessments of their own happiness while collectivist factors, though still present, have become less important. In a qualitative study involving university students from twelve Middle Eastern countries, Lambert D'raven and Pasha-Zaidi (2014b) found that while participants reported primarily pursuing happiness using other/collectivist strategies such as engaging in good deeds and being of service to others, self/individualist strategies such as goal setting and enjoying pleasures were also employed. These findings demonstrate that members of Eastern cultures integrate individualistic components into their conceptions and pursuits of happiness. In sum, it is unclear at this time whether the inclusion of individualistic components will lead to paradoxical effects for Easterners. Values, behaviours, and systems that are adaptive in Western societies may potentially be maladaptive and harmful in Eastern cultures (Lambert, Pasha-Zaidi, Passmore, & York Al-Karam, 2015; Ogihara & Uchida, 2014). Individuals in collectivistic societies who are becoming more individualistic may begin to define happiness in exceedingly more individualistic ways, and as a result may also begin to pursue happiness in less socially engaged ways.

16.6 Repercussions of Societal Valuing of Happiness

The research presented thus far has primarily focused on the negative consequences of valuing happiness at the individual level, that is, on the repercussions that stem from *individuals* setting happiness as a personal goal. However, as Bastian (2013) notes, "it is not only people's own goal pursuits that may have the ironic effect of reducing happiness, but social pressures that arise in contexts where people are collectively focused on the goal of feeling happy" (p. 6). A research programme led by Bastian and colleagues has begun to examine the effects of broad social valuing of certain emotional states over others and the implications this has for individuals' emotional experiences. Emotions are fundamentally social phenomena; they are often experienced and expressed in social settings and understood within cultural contexts (Bastian et al., 2012; Keltner & Haidt, 1999; Parkinson, 1996). Therefore, cultural norms play a critical role in determining individuals' emotional states.

Two common cultural norms associated with happiness are that individuals should seek to (1) maximize positive emotions and (2) minimize negative emotions (McGuirk et al., 2018). These norms are especially salient in Western societies. Although both positive and negative affect surface in conceptualizations of happiness across cultures (Diener, 1984; Lambert, D'raven, & Pasha-Zaidi, 2014a) and although people generally favour positive emotions over negative emotions (Larsen, 2000; Tsai, 2007), cultures still differ in their valuations of these emotional states (Wirtz, Chiu, Diener, & Oishi, 2009). For instance, in Western societies, happiness is based on the incremental model wherein positive emotions and situations are believed to invite additional positive outcomes (Uchida & Ogihara, 2012). An incremental model of happiness motivates individuals to maximize positive affect and avoid negative affect because "negative" emotional states are considered to be a hindrance to happiness. In contrast, dialecticism forms the foundation for many Eastern notions of happiness (Lu & Gilmour, 2004, 2006). Three principles underlie Eastern dialectical thinking (Spencer-Rodgers, Boucher, Mori, Wang, & Peng, 2009). The first is *change*, such that positive and negative emotions are not considered permanent experiences, but rather transitory states that eventually alternate in a recurring fashion. The second principle is *contradiction*, wherein positive and negative emotions are seen as complementary rather than opposite states. Within this dimension positive and negative emotions exist in a harmonious, balanced manner. The last principle, *holism*, asserts that nothing exists in isolation, that all things are interconnected and mutually dependent. Thus, one's current positive state is linked to future negative states (Goetz, Spencer-Rodgers, & Peng, 2008; Ma, Tamir, & Miyamoto, 2018; Peng & Nisbett, 1999).

Under the Western incremental model of happiness, positive emotions are strongly desired and pursued, while negative emotions are devalued and avoided (Uchida & Oishi, 2016; Yoo & Miyamoto, 2018). Alternatively, under the Eastern dialectical model of happiness, both positive and negative emotions are equally valued. Supporting these differences, research has shown that positive and negative affect are correlated inversely in America, but correlated positively in East Asian cultures such as China and Japan (e.g., Bagozzi, Wong, & Yi, 1999; Schimmack, Oishi, & Diener, 2002). One of the reasons why Easterners hold a more balanced valuation of these emotional states is because they recognize negative features of positive emotions and positive features of negative emotions (Joshanloo et al., 2014; Miyamoto, Ma, & Wilken, 2017). For example, in Iran, sadness is often considered a positive state associated with personal insight and reflection (Joshanloo & Weijers, 2014). In line with this are results from studies by Uchida and colleagues. In the first study (Uchida & Kitayama, 2009), Americans and Japanese were asked to describe five features of happiness; these features were then rated as either "positive" or "negative" by research assistants blind to the nationality of the participants. While virtually all (over 98%) of the features that Americans used to describe happiness were rated as positive, only 67% of the features that Japanese used to describe happiness were rated as positive. In a second study (Uchida, 2011), American and Japanese participants rated the validity of features of happiness from an aggregate list gathered from data produced by participants in the first study. Compared to American participants, Japanese participants were more likely to view negative aspects as valid components of happiness. Relatedly, Joshanloo (2014) notes that members of some Eastern cultures view positive emotions as too brief and marginal to be considered a main criterion upon which happiness can be evaluated.

Cultural differences also exist in how positive and negative affect are regulated. For instance, Miyamoto and Ma (2011) reported that after experiencing a pleasant event, East Asians were more likely to dampen their positive emotions than Americans, and that this cultural difference in emotion regulation was mediated by dialectical beliefs about positive emotions (i.e., beliefs that there are negative aspects of positive emotions). Alternatively, Miyamoto, Ma, and Petermann (2014) found that after experiencing an unpleasant event, East Asians were less likely to down-regulate their negative emotions than Americans, a relationship that was mediated by dialectical beliefs about negative emotions (i.e., beliefs about the utility of negative emotions). In sum, evidence exists demonstrating that the dominant cultural mandate in Western societies, fundamentally tied to instrumentalism, is to maximize positive affect and minimize negative affect (Bastian et al., 2012). By contrast, the dominant cultural mandate in Eastern societies, fundamentally tied to dialecticism, is to experience a balance between positive and negative emotions (Miyamoto & Ma, 2011). These cultural rules regarding experiencing emotions are also tied to cultural differences in individualism versus collectivism (Eid & Diener, 2001). For example, Sims and colleagues (2015) found that compared to individuals from collectivistic cultures, individuals from individualistic cultures express a greater desire to maximize positive and minimize negative emotional states and as a result experience fewer mixed affective experiences. That is, persons from individualistic cultures are less likely to experience the good with the bad, and the bad with the good, compared to their collectivistic counterparts.

How do individuals adopt the norms for experiencing emotions prescribed by their culture? Tsai (2007) notes that cultural norms and values, which play a role in shaping the affective states that people ideally want to feel, are socially transmitted. Yoo and Miyamoto (2018) suggest that members internalize their society's emotion norms through repeated exposure to cultural practices, products, and institutions that endorse certain affective states over others. This process begins at a young age, with parents socializing their children in a manner that reflects the desired emotion norms of their culture (Eid & Diener, 2001). Miyamoto and colleagues (2014) suggest that cultural differences in hedonic emotion regulation (i.e., up-regulation of positive affect and down-regulation of negative affect) are expressed in child rearing practices. For example, American parenting practices emphasize promoting children's self-esteem by providing positive feedback, while Chinese parenting practices stress the importance of effective disciplinary strategies (Miller, Wang, Sandel, & Cho, 2002). Further research indicates that when children fail a task, American mothers are more likely to offer positive statements, whereas Chinese mothers are more likely to offer negative statements (Ng, Pomerantz, & Lam, 2007). These parenting strategies are likely to be adopted by children as their own emotion regulation strategy, reflecting the salient cultural norm.

Parental practices are not the only way individuals learn to value certain affective states. Exposure to cultural products is also influential. Written works are one example. Examining the affective content of the top 10 bestselling storybooks for children in the United States and Taiwan, Tsai, Louie, Chen, and Uchida (2007) found that compared to Taiwanese bestsellers, American bestsellers depicted characters that had more excited and wider smiles, and who were more engaged in arousing activities (e.g., running). Content of these storybooks influenced the affective states children ideally wanted to feel. After being exposed to an exciting storybook, children across cultures were 7.6 times more likely to perceive an excited (vs. calm) smile as indicative of greater happiness as those exposed to a calm storybook. In a study examining the affective content of school textbooks, Imada (2012) found that stories in American textbooks highlighted themes of individualism (e.g., achievement) while stories in Japanese textbooks highlighted themes of collectivism (e.g., group harmony). American textbooks had more happy stories than Japanese textbooks (82% vs. 63%), while Japanese textbooks had more sad stories than the American sample (24% vs. 1.4%), striking more of a balance between the two affective states.

Religion is another medium by which individuals learn cultural emotion norms. By their very nature, religious writings, texts, sermons, and paintings prescribe the valuing and pursuit of specific emotional states (Tsai, Miao, & Seppala 2007). For example, a study comparing affective content in classic Buddhist texts (e.g., Dhammapada) to that in classic Christian texts (e.g., Gospel of Matthew) found that high-arousal positive states were promoted more in classic Christian texts than in Buddhist works. This was also found to be true in modern bestselling Buddhist and Christian self-help books. Additionally, modern (but not classic) Buddhist books were found to endorse low-arousal positive states more so than Christian books. Further, when asked directly, practicing Christians and Buddhists differed in their endorsement of affective states they would ideally like to feel. Reflective of the affective content in their respective religious texts, Christians placed greater value on high-arousal positive states and less value on low-arousal positive states than did Buddhists.

In sum, cultural norms for experiencing emotion are socially transmitted. Through repeated exposure to cultural practices, products, and institutions, individuals learn to internalize the emotion norms prescribed by their culture (Tsai, 2007; Yoo & Miyamoto, 2018). Consequently, members of Western societies tend to perceive positive affect as desirable and appropriate and negative affect as undesirable and inappropriate. There is immense societal pressure in the West to feel happy and not sad. This social expectancy, "the felt social pressure to maximize positive emotion and minimize negative emotion" (McGuirk et al., 2018, p. 756) is ubiquitous. As noted in the introduction, happiness has developed into a cultural obsession in Western society. North American popular culture is virtually drowning in daily messages from films, television, podcasts, radios, magazines, and advertising campaigns that stress the importance of happiness, while common emotional experiences such as sadness are rendered as pathological and in need of treatment (Fernández-Rios & Novo, 2012; Horwitz & Wakefield, 2007).

These societal norms so emphatically preached in Western cultures hold a number of implications for emotional functioning. Pressure to feel positive but not negative emotions backfires, with unsanctioned negative emotions being experienced more often and more intensely (Bastian et al., 2012). It is critical that we understand how these social expectancies translate into emotional dysfunction and secondary disturbances (i.e., the process of getting upset about being upset). Bastian (2013) suggests that individuals reflect on themselves negatively when experiencing an emotional state viewed as undesirable; a discrepancy is perceived between what one "should" be feeling and what one is actually feeling. Not only do we hold personal expectations for how we think we should feel, societal expectations also provide powerful reference values. Social expectancies prescribe emotional goals that are difficult to ignore as they are repeatedly reinforced via salient cultural cues denoting the value of happiness and the cost of sadness. Falling prey to this messaging, individuals either explicitly or implicitly feel compelled to strive for these culturally-sanctioned emotional goals. The end result in unambiguous: Failure to achieve happiness is a personal failure (Eid & Diener, 2001) causing negative self-reflection and lower happiness.

Empirical evidence supports this model. Social expectancies to be happy have been found to be a more important predictor of emotional dysfunction and reduced wellbeing than are personal expectancies (Bastian et al., 2012). This finding suggests that even if individuals change their personal expectations regarding their own emotional experiences, they are likely to still experience negative outcomes due to omnipresent social expectancies. Further, negative self-focused thinking was found to mediate the relationship between social expectancies and emotional functioning and wellbeing such that when people experienced negative emotional states that deviated from the desired cultural norm, they reflected negatively on themselves, which in turn led to experiencing more negative emotions and reductions in wellbeing. These effects were found in both Australia and Japan; however, they were especially apparent in Australia, where happiness norms are more highly endorsed. Moreover, social expectancies were also found to lead to secondary disturbances. These are not the only findings that have emerged from Bastian and colleagues' research program. Perceived social pressure not to experience negative emotions has been linked to greater loneliness (Bastian et al., 2015), selective avoidance of negative emotional information (Bastian, Pe, & Kuppens, 2017), and depressive symptomology in daily life (Dejonckheere, Bastian, Fried, Murphy, & Kuppens, 2017).

Surprisingly, Bastian, Kuppens, De Rover, and Diener (2014) found that people are more satisfied with their lives in societies where happiness is highly valued; however, increases in life satisfaction are less pronounced for people who frequently experience negative emotions. The authors posited that experiencing high levels of negative affect may be more problematic than experiencing low levels of positive affect, in that individuals may not ruminate to the same extent about their lack of positive emotions as they would for their experiences of negative emotions. McGuirk and colleagues (2018) found that social expectations to avoid negative affect are positively correlated with increased rumination. They demonstrated that prioritizing positive emotion (such as in Western societal expectancies) increased rumination in response to failure, with rumination mediating the relationship between societal expectancies to not be sad and reduced wellbeing.

These findings highlight the role that social norms play in individuals' emotional functioning. Instead of increasing happiness, norms to maximize positive affect and minimize negative affect paradoxically reduce happiness and negatively impact downstream wellbeing outcomes. While these social expectancies are especially salient in Western cultures, they are also emerging in places like Japan. As noted, cultures are subject to change, and these social expectancies are likely to become more prevalent in Eastern cultures as well, particularly with the increasingly worldwide popularity of Western films and music (e.g., Pharrell Williams' international hit song, "Happy"). These influences may not only increase social expectancies in non-Western cultures, they may also compromise the emotional fit between an individual's emotional patterns and the normative emotional patterns historically present in these cultures, all of which can diminish happiness and overall wellbeing (e.g., De Leersnyder, Mesquita, Kim, Eom, & Choi, 2014; Yoo & Miyamoto, 2018).

16.7 Social Determinants of Happiness

Messages promoting materialistic values (a focus on wealth, possessions, image, and status) as a pathway to happiness are embedded within Western culture. Unfortunately, such messages are also among the ideological exports of Western nations (Delhey, 2010). In their recent examination of World Gallup Poll results from 2005 through 2015, Diener, Diener, Choi, and Oishi (2018) suggest that low life satisfaction for citizens of some countries may be attributable to desiring the material goods and possessions they perceive to be an indicator of "the good life" in wealthier nations. Yet, valuing wealth and financial success is inherently incompatible with valuing social relationships, community, and spirituality, values which are highly predictive of enhanced happiness and wellbeing (Kasser, 2016). Increasing national levels of materialism over time have been found to be indicative of decreasing national levels of citizens' wellbeing in Norway (Hellevik, 2003) and the United States (Twenge et al., 2010). Accumulating material wealth tends to make people less generous, both with their money and time (Piff, Kraus, Côté, Cheng, & Keltner, 2010), ultimately resulting in greater self-focus, more isolation, and less happiness.

On a national level, however, a complex relationship exists between the wealth of a nation and its happiness and life satisfaction. While in some countries, such as The Netherlands, Italy, and Denmark, an increase in economic growth has been accompanied by an increase in national happiness and life satisfaction (Hagerty & Veenhoven, 2003; Stevenson & Wolfers, 2008), in other countries (e.g., United States, Germany, Indonesia) this is not the case (Easterlin, McVey, Switek, Sawangfa, & Zweig, 2010; Rahayu, 2016). Why would this be so? A growing body of research suggests that income inequality could be the answer to this question. Using longitudinal data from 34 countries, Oishi and Kesebir (2015) demonstrated that when increases in GDP per capita were accompanied by growing income inequality (e.g., Austria, Portugal, Belgium, El Salvador), temporal changes in average national life satisfaction were not associated with rising GDP. Yet, when increases in GDP per capita did not result in greater income inequality, national increases in life satisfaction corresponded to increases in GDP. This pattern also emerged in American data over a 37-year period (Oishi, Kesebir, & Diener, 2011). On average, Americans were less happy in years with greater national income inequality than in years without.

In the United States (Oishi et al., 2011) and in a sample of 30 European countries (Delhey & Dragolov, 2014), lower levels of general trust, perceived fairness, and state-anxiety mediated the negative relationship between income inequality and happiness. That is, greater national income inequality led to a decline in citizens' overall levels of trust and an enhancement of feelings of unfairness and anxiety; these negative cognitive views and emotions resulted in plummeting levels of happiness and life satisfaction. Distrust was found to be the primary mechanism leading to decreased happiness in more affluent countries, whereas anxiety was the primary mechanism in less affluent countries. Taken together, these research findings suggest that "the key to a happy nation might be economic growth that is accompanied by relatively equal redistribution of national wealth among citizens" (Uchida & Oishi, 2016, p. 132).

Citizens living in countries with more progressive taxation (i.e., a higher tax rate for higher income brackets) are happier than citizens living in countries with less progressive taxation (Oishi, Schimmack, & Diener, 2012). This link between more progressive taxation and greater levels of happiness is spurred by citizens' greater satisfaction with public goods (e.g., education, public transportation). Gandelman, Piani, and Ferre (2012) reported that satisfaction with access to and quality of public goods was a significant predictor of happiness and life satisfaction for citizens of Uruguay.

Social capital (i.e., honesty, trust, freedom of choice and control) is an important contributor to happiness in both affluent and less affluent nations (Sarracino, 2013). Sarracino also found that social capital has a stronger effect on happiness in high-income countries (e.g., Saudi Arabia, Switzerland, Finland; see Hsu, Chang, Chong, & An, 2016 regarding social trust as predictor of happiness in Taiwan) than in low-income countries (e.g., Bangladesh, Uganda, Nigeria). Nonetheless, Bartolini, Mikucka, and Sarracino (2017) argue that "even in the most extreme cases—such as transition countries [e.g., Estonia, Hungary, Bulgaria, Poland]—where material concerns are pivotal" the trends of a link between social trust and happiness and life satisfaction are, in the medium-term (over four to six years), strongly and significantly related (p. 88). In congruence with these findings, the 2018 World Happiness report states that the happiest countries (i.e., Finland, Norway, Denmark) have high values of income *along with* high levels of generosity, freedom, social support, and social trust (Helliwell, Layard, & Sachs, 2018).

Tying this research together is Ott's (2010a, b, 2011) work on quality of governance as a determinant of nations' happiness. Ott proposed that good governance may be a universal condition of happiness, and provided evidence that independent of culture, the technical quality of a country's government (its perceived effectiveness, ability to maintain regulations, enforcement of justified laws, and control of corruption) is significantly predictive of citizens' happiness (overall $r = 0.75$ in a sample of 127 nations). This association emerged in Western cultures ($r = 0.70$), the Middle East ($r = 0.71$), Africa ($r = 0.52$), and in Asia ($r = 0.73$). Helliwell, Huang, Grover, and Wang (2018) recently corroborated Ott's findings using data covering 157 countries from 2005–2012: Greater life satisfaction was reported in countries with better governance quality. It has been suggested that social trust is the foundation of both good governance and wellbeing (Bjørnskov, 2006). This relationship also holds true at the municipal level. For example, in the Iranian city of Tehran, a sense of security evidenced a strong, significant relationship with life satisfaction (Kazemi, Sajjadi, Kaleji, & Razavian, 2017).

There are a number of social determinants of happiness at the city and neighbourhood level (Florida, Mellander, & Rentfrow, 2013). For example, education plays a central role in the happiness of cities as it can afford residents enhanced opportunities and resources with which to better their lives. Unemployment and housing values also play significant roles. Areas with lower levels of unemployment are happier. Surprisingly, happiness is higher in cities where housing costs are less affordable. At first glance this is perplexing. However, Florida and colleagues explain that higher housing prices are (generally) an indicator of higher quality amenities and greater access to public goods, which in turn are associated with greater happiness and life satisfaction. Leyden, Goldberg, and Michelbach (2011) examined key factors shaping happiness in ten cities (i.e., Milan, New York, Paris, Toronto, Seoul, London, Berlin, Tokyo, Stockholm, and Beijing). Results revealed that those who felt that their city offered plenty of job opportunities and who believed that their city provided many opportunities to volunteer were happier. Individuals who felt that they could trust their city government and who believed it did a good job of addressing citizens' concerns and requests also reported higher levels of happiness. Those who believed their city was a good place to raise children felt the same. When examining place and built environment variables, access to culture and leisure facilities (e.g., museums, concert halls, movie theaters), convenient public transportation, and libraries were all linked to happiness. Leyden and colleagues suggest that these aspects of the built environment help to promote social connection, which in turn, bolsters happiness.

Similarly, Goldberg, Leyden, and Scotto (2012) found that the happiness of city residents is linked to their ratings of both place (e.g., ratings of how beautiful they think their city is, how easy it is to gain access to amenities such as parks and movie theatres) and performance (e.g., ratings of the quality of a city's schools, services for the disadvantaged, safety) variables, which have both direct and indirect effects on citizens' happiness through social connection and health. Building on this research, Hogan and colleagues (2016) examined how the importance of these variables varies across the lifespan. They found that the happiness of younger residents is more affected by place variables, whereas the happiness of older residents is more affected by performance variables.

Easy access to quality urban green spaces and public parks is critical for city residents' happiness and overall wellbeing (see review by Capaldi, Passmore, Nisbet, Zelenski, & Dopko, 2015). For example, demographic studies have consistently found that living in a neighbourhood with more green space is associated with greater mental health (e.g., de Vries, Verheij, Groenewegen, & Spreeuwenberg, 2003; Maas et al., 2009; Van den Berg, Maas, Verheij, & Groenewegen, 2010; White, Alcock, Wheeler, & Depledge, 2013) and life satisfaction (White et al., 2013). Neighbourhood green space is also associated with enhanced social trust, security, and social connections (e.g., Kuo, 2003; Kuo, Sullivan, Coley, & Brunson, 1998; Sommer, 2003; Sullivan, Kuo, & Depooter, 2004). On a broader level, Cloutier, Larsen, and Jambeck (2014) provide evidence that more sustainable cities might be happier ones, and in a review article examining planning for healthy communities, Pfeiffer and Cloutier (2016) recommend providing residents access to open and natural green space and incorporating design features that ensure personal security and features that allow for social interaction in order to boost individuals' happiness.

16.8 Conclusion

The aim of this chapter was to integrate and review the extant research on the consequences of individual and societal valuing of happiness. At the individual level, this research highlights that *being* happy results in drastically different outcomes than does *striving to be* happy. Although being happy results in numerous beneficial outcomes, outcomes of striving for happiness seem to be the opposite. Directly, intently, and relentlessly pursuing happiness paradoxically leads to reductions in happiness itself, as well as to a host of other negative outcomes such as increased loneliness, depressive symptomology, and wellbeing. However, the vast bulk of research evidencing this effect has been conducted in the United States. As a result, it is not known whether these negative outcomes are specific to Western cultures.

To address this question we highlighted the role that culture plays in shaping ideas of happiness. We noted how in individualistic cultures, happiness is often viewed as an emotional state that is contingent on personal achievement. Alternatively, in Eastern cultures, happiness is typically defined in terms of interpersonal connection. Flowing from these differing conceptualizations of happiness are differing pathways to pursuing happiness. Given that Westerners usually define happiness in a relatively self-focused manner, individuals in Western cultural contexts typically pursue happiness via less socially engaged ways than do Easterners. This is problematic: Interpersonal connection is considered to be a universal ingredient of happiness. As Chris Peterson, one of the founding fathers of positive psychology often said: "Other people matter". Moreover, connection is the essence of broader wellbeing and meaning in life (Baumeister & Vohs, 2002). Yet, many Eastern societies may be experiencing a shift towards Western ideas of happiness, as the export of Western popular culture and ideologies is rapidly following on the heels of economic globalization. Consequently, members of traditionally collectivistic cultures may increasingly incorporate individualistic elements into their definitions and pursuits of happiness. Further research is needed in this area to examine if the incorporation of these features will lead to negative outcomes in these cultural contexts.

With regard to consequences of the societal valuing of happiness, we reviewed emotion norms that exist in Western and Eastern cultures and how these norms are socially propagated. Whereas Westerners generally value seeking positive affect and avoiding negative affect, Easterners seek to experience more of a balance between these emotions. These cultural mandates are socially transmitted through cultural practices, products, and institutions and internalized by members of a given culture. Unbalanced Western emotion norms, wherein negative emotions are largely avoided, place an immense pressure on individuals to be happy. This social expectancy adversely affects wellbeing, ironically leading to an increase in negative emotions and a decrease in overall mental health. Although such a "you should feel happy" social expectancy is especially prevalent in Western cultures, Japanese are beginning to report feeling similar pressure to not feel sad. With increasing exposure to Western popular culture, it is possible that these social expectancies will appear in other Eastern cultures. Time, and further research, will tell.

As a collective, global society, we must acknowledge that we cannot simply tell people to "be happy". We must recognize that happiness has both individual and social determinants. In the last section of the chapter, we examined a number of key social determinants of happiness at various levels of society. We examined how the endorsement of materialistic values is detrimental to individual and social wellbeing. We briefly reviewed the complex relationship between countries' economic growth and citizens' happiness and life satisfaction. To avoid the Easterlin paradox, wherein economic growth is not accompanied by growth in happiness, income equality, progressive taxation, social capital, and good governance must also be present. Social determinants of happiness at the city and neighborhood level were highlighted, such as education, access to amenities, low levels of unemployment, and in particular, access to quality urban green spaces. All of these are vital conditions for human happiness that communally we must strive to institute in our neighbourhoods, cities, and countries.

In summary, emerging lines of research indicate that pursuing happiness can be detrimental to individuals' wellbeing. How then can we reap the diverse benefits—more fulfilling and stable relationships, enhanced physical health and longevity, even greater career success—that happiness brings? We posit that this is possible by defining and pursuing happiness in a socially-engaged manner. Regardless of culture, people who define happiness in social terms and who employ social strategies for improving happiness (e.g., volunteering, spending time with loved ones, engaging in charitable acts) have greater happiness, life satisfaction, and overall wellbeing (Aknin et al., 2013; Ford & Mauss, 2014; Ford et al., 2015; McMahan Ryu, & Choi, 2014; Rohrer, Richter, Brümmer, Wagner, & Schmukle, 2018; Wiwad & Aknin, 2017). These findings highlight that not all happiness pursuits are equal; the direct route, least of all. Questions of this sort will become more important as the spread of happiness research, as well as its prioritization by governments in societies across the Middle East region, intensifies. This, coupled with greater globalization (Westernization), will provide various flashpoints for research, policy, and practice considerations in the region that will ideally protect and promote regional cultures, as well as integrate the science of wellbeing in striving towards the greater good. By furthering our understanding of the repercussions of individual and societal valuing of happiness, we can advocate for and implement individual behaviours and social policies that will ultimately enhance our collective wellbeing.

References

Abdel-Khalek, A. M. (2007). Religiosity, happiness, health, and psychopathology in a probability sample of Muslim adolescents. *Mental Health, Religion & Culture, 10,* 571–583.

Action for Happiness. (2010). Retrieved from http://www.actionforhappiness.org.

Ahuvia, A. C. (2002). Individualism/collectivism and cultures of happiness: A theoretical conjecture on the relationship between consumption, culture and subjective wellbeing at the national level. *Journal of Happiness Studies, 3,* 23–36.

Aknin, L. B., Leigh, C. P., Dunn, E. W., Helliwell, J. F., Burns, J., Biswas-Diener, R., … Norton, M. I. (2013). Prosocial spending and wellbeing: Cross-cultural evidence for a psychological universal. *Journal of Personality and Social Psychology, 104,* 635–652.

Bagozzi, R. P., Wong, N., & Yi, Y. (1999). The role of culture and gender in the relationship between positive and negative affect. *Cognition and Emotion, 13,* 641–672.

Bartolini, S., Mikucka, M., & Sarracino, F. (2017). Money, trust and happiness in transition countries: Evidence from time series. *Social Indicators Research, 130,* 87–106.

Bastian, B. (2013). Normative influences on secondary disturbance: The role of social expectancies. *Australian Psychologist, 48,* 85–93.
Bastian, B., Kuppens, P., De Roover, K., & Diener, E. (2014). Is valuing positive emotion associated with life satisfaction? *Emotion, 14,* 639–645.
Bastian, B., Kuppens, P., Hornsey, M. J., Park, J., Koval, P., & Uchida, Y. (2012). Feeling bad about being sad: The role of social expectancies in amplifying negative mood. *Emotion, 12,* 69–80.
Bastian, B., Koval, P., Erbas, Y., Houben, M., Pe, M., & Kuppens, P. (2015). Sad and alone: Social expectancies for experiencing negative emotions are linked to feelings of loneliness. *Social Psychological and Personality Science, 6,* 496–503.
Bastian, B., Pe, M. L., & Kuppens, P. (2017). Perceived social pressure not to experience negative emotion is linked to selective attention for negative information. *Cognition and Emotion, 31,* 261–268.
Baumeister, R. F., & Vohs, K. D. (2002). The pursuit of meaningfulness in life. In C. R. Snyder & S. J. Lopez (Eds.), *Handbook of positive psychology* (pp. 608–618). Oxford, UK: Oxford University Press.
Berry, J. W. (1997). Immigration, acculturation, and adaptation. *Applied Psychology: An International Review, 46,* 5–68.
Berry, J. W. (2005). Acculturation: Living successfully in two cultures. *International Journal of Intercultural Relations, 29,* 697–712.
Berry, J. W. (2008). Globalisation and acculturation. *International Journal of Intercultural Relations, 32,* 328–336.
Bjørnskov, C. (2006). The multiple facets of social capital. *European Journal of Political Economy, 22,* 22–40.
Brülde, B. (2007). Happiness theories of the good life. *Journal of Happiness Studies, 8,* 15–49.
Burgoon, J. K., Guerrero, L. K., & Floyd, K. (2016). *Nonverbal communication*. New York, NY: Routledge.
Capaldi, C. A., Passmore, H.-A., Nisbet, E. K., Zelenski, J. M., & Dopko, R. L. (2015). Flourishing in nature: A review of the benefits of connecting with nature and its application as a wellbeing intervention. *International Journal of Wellbeing, 5,* 1–16.
Chiang, H.-Y., & Ohtake, F. (2014). Performance-pay and the gender wage gap in Japan. *Journal of the Japanese and International Economies, 34,* 71–88.
Chida, Y., & Steptoe, A. (2008). Positive psychological wellbeing and mortality: A quantitative review of prospective observational studies. *Psychosomatic Medicine, 70,* 741–756.
Cloutier, S., Larson, L., & Jambeck, J. (2014). Are sustainable cities "happy" cities? Associations between sustainable development and human wellbeing in urban areas of the United States. *Environment, Development and Sustainability, 16,* 633–647.
Dejonckheere, E., Bastian, B., Fried, E. I., Murphy, S. C., & Kuppens, P. (2017). Perceiving social pressure not to feel negative predicts depressive symptoms in daily life. *Depression and Anxiety, 34,* 836–844.
De Leersnyder, J., Kim, H., & Mesquita, B. (2015). Feeling right is feeling good: Psychological wellbeing and emotional fit with culture in autonomy-versus relatedness-promoting situations. *Frontiers in Psychology, 6,* 630.
De Leersnyder, J., Mesquita, B., Kim, H., Eom, K., & Choi, H. (2014). Emotional fit with culture: A predictor of individual differences in relational wellbeing. *Emotion, 14,* 241–245.
Delhey, J. (2010). From materialist to post-materialist happiness? National affluence and determinants of life satisfaction in cross-national perspective. *Social Indicators Research, 97,* 65–84.
Delhey, J., & Dragolov, G. (2014). Why inequality makes Europeans less happy: The role of distrust, status anxiety, and perceived conflict. *European Sociological Review, 30,* 151–165.
Delle Fave, A., Brdar, I., Freire, T., Vella-Brodrick, D., & Wissing, M. P. (2011). The eudaimonic and hedonic components of happiness: Qualitative and quantitative findings. *Social Indicators Research, 100,* 185–207.

De Neve, J.-E., Diener, E., Tay, L., & Xuereb, C. (2013). The objective benefits of subjective wellbeing. In J. Helliwell, R. Layard, & J. Sachs (Eds.), *World Happiness Report 2013* (pp. 54–79). New York, NY: UN Sustainable Development Solutions Network.

De Vos, M. (2012). The unbearable lightness of happiness policy. In P. Booth (Ed.), *... and the pursuit of happiness* (pp. 181–204). London: The Institute of Economic Affairs.

de Vries, S., Verheij, R. A., Groenewegen, P. P., & Spreeuwenberg, P. (2003). Natural environments—Healthy environments? An exploratory analysis of the relationship between greenspace and health. *Environment and Planning A, 35,* 1717–1731.

Diener, E. (1984). Subjective wellbeing. *Psychological Bulletin, 95,* 542–575.

Diener, E. (2000). Subjective wellbeing: The science of happiness and a proposal for a national index. *American Psychologist, 55,* 34–43.

Diener, E. (2013). The remarkable changes in the science of subjective wellbeing. *Perspective on Psychological Science, 8,* 663–666.

Diener, E., & Chan, M. (2011). Happy people live longer: Subjective wellbeing contributes to health and longevity. *Applied Psychology: Health and Wellbeing, 3,* 1–43.

Diener, E., Diener, C., Choi, H., & Oishi, S. (2018). Revisiting "Most people are happy"—and discovering when they are not. *Perspectives on Psychological Science, 13,* 166–170.

Diener, E., Heintzelman, S. J., Kushlev, K., Tay, L., Wirtz, D., Lutes, L. D., & Oishi, S. (2017). Findings all psychologists should know from the new science on subjective wellbeing. *Canadian Psychology, 58,* 87–104.

Diener, E., & Oishi, S. (2005). The nonobvious social psychology of happiness. *Psychological Inquiry, 16,* 162–167.

Diener, E., Oishi, S., & Lucas, R. E. (2015). National accounts of subjective wellbeing. *American Psychologist, 70,* 234–242.

Diener, E., Sapyta, J. J., & Suh, E. (1998). Subjective wellbeing is essential to wellbeing. *Psychological Inquiry, 9,* 33–37.

Diener, E., & Seligman, M. E. (2002). Very happy people. *Psychological Science, 13,* 81–84.

Dolan, P., & Metcalfe, R. (2012). Measuring subjective wellbeing: Recommendations on measures for use by national governments. *Journal of Social Policy, 41,* 409–427.

Easterlin, R. A., McVey, L. A., Switek, M., Sawangfa, O., & Zweig, J. S. (2010). The happiness-income paradox revisited. *Proceedings of the National Academy of Sciences of the United States of America, 107,* 22463–22468.

Eid, M., & Diener, E. (2001). Norms for experiencing emotions in different cultures: Inter- and intranational differences. *Journal of Personality and Social Psychology, 81,* 869–885.

Emmons, R. A. (1986). Personal strivings: An approach to personality and subjective wellbeing. *Journal of Personality and Social Psychology, 51,* 1058–1068.

Fernández-Rios, L., & Novo, M. (2012). Positive psychology: Zeigeist (or spirit of the times) or ignorance (or disinformation) of history? *International Journal of Clinical and Health Psychology, 12,* 333–344.

Florida, R., Mellander, C., & Rentfrow, P. J. (2013). The happiness of cities. *Regional Studies, 47,* 613–627.

Ford, B. Q., Dmitrieva, J. O., Heller, D., Chentsova-Dutton, Y., Grossmann, I., Tamir, M., ... Mauss, I. B. (2015). Culture shapes whether the pursuit of happiness predicts higher or lower wellbeing. *Journal of Experimental Psychology: General, 144,* 1053–1062.

Ford, B. Q., & Mauss, I. B. (2014). The paradoxical effects of pursuing positive emotion: When and why wanting to feel happy backfires. In J. Gruber & J. Moskowitz (Eds.), *The dark and light sides of positive emotion* (pp. 363–381). New York, NY: Oxford University Press.

Ford, B. Q., Mauss, I. B., & Gruber, J. (2015). Valuing happiness is associated with bipolar disorder. *Emotion, 15,* 211–212.

Ford, B. Q., Shallcross, A. J., Mauss, I. B., Floerke, V. A., & Gruber, J. (2014). Desperately seeking happiness: Valuing happiness is associated with symptoms and diagnosis of depression. *Journal of Social and Clinical Psychology, 33,* 890–905.

Freedman, J. (1978). *Happy people: What happiness is, who has it, and why*. New York, NY: Harcourt Brace Jovanovich.

Gandelman, N., Piani, G., & Ferre, Z. (2012). Neighborhood determinants of quality of life. *Journal of Happiness Studies, 13,* 547–563.

Ghosh, S. (2016, January 22). Happiness is overused in ads, says Coke's creative boss. *Campaign*. Retrieved from https://www.campaignlive.co.uk/article/happiness-overused-ads-says-cokes-creative-boss/1380527.

Goetz, J. L., Spencer-Rodgers, J., & Peng, K. (2008). Dialectical emotions: How cultural epistemologies influence the experience and regulation of emotional complexity. In R. M. Sorrentino & S. Yamaguchi (Eds.), *Handbook of motivation and cognition across cultures* (pp. 517–538). Amsterdam: Elsevier.

Goldberg, A., Leyden, K. M., & Scotto, T. J. (2012). Untangling what makes cities liveable: Happiness in five cities. *Proceedings of the Institute of Civil Engineers: Urban Design and Planning, 165,* 127–136.

Graves, T. D. (1967). Psychological acculturation in a tri-ethnic community. *Southwestern Journal of Anthropology, 23,* 337–350.

Haberstroh, S., Oyserman, D., Schwarz, N., Kühnen, U., & Ji, L.-J. (2002). Is the interdependent self more sensitive to question context than the independent self? Self-construal and the observation of conversational norms. *Journal of Experimental Social Psychology, 38,* 323–329.

Hagerty, M. R., & Veenhoven, R. (2003). Wealth and happiness revisited: Growing national income does go with greater happiness. *Social Indictors Research, 64,* 1–27.

Hamamura, T. (2012). Are cultures becoming individualistic? A cross-temporal comparison of individualism-collectivism in the United States and Japan. *Personality and Social Psychology Review, 16,* 3–24.

Happiness Alliance. (2010). Retrieved from http://www.happycounts.org/about.html.

Harper, F. D., Guilbault, M., Tucker, T., & Austin, T. (2007). Happiness as a goal of counselling: Cross-cultural implications. *International Journal for the Advancement of Counselling, 29,* 123–136.

Heine, S. J., Lehman, D. R., Markus, H. R., & Kitayama, S. (1999). Is there a universal need for positive self-regard? *Psychological Review, 106,* 766–794.

Held, B. S. (2002). The tyranny of the positive attitude in America: Observation and speculation. *Journal of Clinical Psychology, 58,* 965–991.

Hellevik, O. (2003). Economy, values, and happiness in Norway. *Journal of Happiness Studies, 4,* 243–283.

Helliwell, J., Huang, H., Grover, S., & Wang, S. (2018). Empirical linkages between good governance and national wellbeing. *Journal of Comparative Economics, Advance online publication*. https://doi.org/10.1016/j.jce.2018.01.004.

Helliwell, J., Layard, R., & Sachs, J. (2018). *World Happiness Report 2018*. New York, NY: Sustainable Development Solutions Network.

Hofstede, G. (1980). *Culture's consequences: International differences in work-related values*. Beverly Hills, CA: Sage.

Hogan, M. J., Leyden, K. M., Conway, R., Goldberg, A., Walsh, D., & McKenna-Plumley, P. (2016). Happiness and health across the lifespan in five major cities: The impact of place and government performance. *Social Science and Medicine, 162,* 168–176.

Horwitz, A. V., & Wakefield, J. C. (2007). *The loss of sadness*. New York, NY: Oxford University Press.

Hsu, H.-C., Chang, W.-C., Chong, Y.-S., & An, J. S. (2016). Happiness and social determinants across age cohorts in Taiwan. *Journal of Health Psychology, 21,* 1828–1839.

Imada, T. (2012). Cultural narratives of individualism and collectivism: A content analysis of textbook stories in the United States and Japan. *Journal of Cross-Cultural Psychology, 43,* 576–591.

Joshanloo, M. (2013). A comparison of Western and Islamic conceptions of happiness. *Journal of Happiness Studies, 14,* 1857–1874.

Joshanloo, M. (2014). Eastern conceptualizations of happiness: Fundamental differences with Western views. *Journal of Happiness Studies, 15,* 475–493.

Joshanloo, M., Lepshokova, Z. K., Panyusheva, T., Natalia, A., Poon, W. C., Yeung, V. W. L., … Tsukamoto, S. (2014). Cross-cultural validation of fear of happiness scale across 14 national groups. *Journal of Cross-Cultural Psychology, 45,* 246–264.

Joshanloo, M., & Weijers, D. (2014). Aversion to happiness across cultures: A review of where and why people are averse to happiness. *Journal of Happiness Studies, 15,* 717–735.

Kasser, T. (2016). Materialistic values and goals. *Annual Review of Psychology, 67,* 489–514.

Kazemi, M., Sajjadi, J., Kaleji, L. K., & Razavian, M. T. (2017). Environmental and social determinants of life satisfaction in Tehran: A perception study. *Journal of Environmental Management and Tourism, 8,* 1325–1333.

Keltner, D., & Haidt, J. (1999). Social functions of emotions at four levels of analysis. *Cognition and Emotion, 13,* 505–521.

Kim, A., & Maglio, S. J. (2018). Vanishing time in the pursuit of happiness. *Psychonomic Bulletin & Review, 25*(4), 1337–1342.

Kuo, F. E. (2003). Social aspects of urban forestry: The role of arboriculture in a healthy social ecology. *Journal of Arboriculture, 29,* 148–155.

Kuo, F. E., Sullivan, W. C., Coley, R. L., & Brunson, L. (1998). Fertile ground for community: Inner-city neighborhood common spaces. *American Journal of Community Psychology, 26,* 823–851.

Kwan, V. S. Y., Bond, M. H., & Singelis, T. M. (1997). Pancultural explanations for life satisfaction: Adding relationship harmony to self-esteem. *Journal of Personality and Social Psychology, 73,* 1038–1051.

Lalonde, R. N., & Cameron, J. E. (1993). An intergroup perspective on immigration acculturation with a focus on collective strategies. *International Journal of Psychology, 28,* 57–74.

Lambert, L., Pasha-Zaidi, N., Passmore, H.-A., & York Al-Karam, C. (2015). Developing an indigenous positive psychology in the United Arab Emirates. *Middle East Journal of Positive Psychology, 1,* 1–23.

Lambert D'raven, L., & Pasha-Zaidi, N. (2014a). Happiness in the United Arab Emirates: Conceptualisations of happiness among Emirati and other Arab students. *International Journal of Happiness and Development, 2,* 1–21.

Lambert D'raven, L., & Pasha-Zaidi, N. (2014b). Happiness strategies among Arab university students in the United Arab Emirates. *The Journal of Happiness and Wellbeing, 2,* 1–15.

Larsen, R. J. (2000). Toward a science of mood regulation. *Psychological Inquiry, 11,* 129–141.

Leyden, K. M., Goldberg, A., & Michelbach, P. (2011). Understanding the pursuit of happiness in ten major cities. *Urban Affairs Review, 47,* 861–888.

Lomas, T. (2016). Towards a positive cross-cultural lexicography: Enriching our emotional landscape through 216 'untranslatable' words pertaining to wellbeing. *Journal of Positive Psychology, 11,* 546–558.

Lomas, T. (2018). *Translating happiness: A cross-cultural lexicon of wellbeing*. Cambridge: MIT Press.

Looney, R. (2007). The Arab world's uncomfortable experience with globalization. *The Middle East Journal, 61,* 341–345.

Lu, L., & Gilmour, R. (2004). Culture and conceptions of happiness: Individual oriented and social oriented SWB. *Journal of Happiness Studies, 5,* 269–291.

Lu, L., & Gilmour, R. (2006). Individual-oriented and socially oriented cultural conceptions of subjective wellbeing: Conceptual analysis and scale development. *Asian Journal of Social Psychology, 9,* 36–49.

Lyubomirsky, S. (2013). *The myths of happiness: What should make you happy, but doesn't, what shouldn't make you happy, but does*. New York, NY: Penguin Press.

Ma, X., Tamir, M., & Miyamoto, Y. (2018). A socio-cultural instrumental approach to emotion regulation: Culture and the regulation of positive emotions. *Emotion, 18,* 138–152.

Maas, J., Verheij, R. A., de Vries, S., Spreeuwenberg, P., Schellevis, F. G., & Groenewegen, P. P. (2009). Morbidity is related to a green living environment. *Journal of Epidemiology and Community Health, 63,* 967–973.

Markus, H. R., & Kitayama, S. (1991). Culture and the self: Implications for cognition, emotion, and motivation. *Psychological Review, 98,* 224–253.

Matsudaira, T. (2006). Measures of psychological acculturation: A review. *Transcultural Psychiatry, 43,* 462–487.

Matsumoto, D., Kudoh, T., & Takeuchi, S. (1996). Changing patterns of individualism and collectivism in the United States and Japan. *Culture & Psychology, 2,* 77–107.

Mauss, I. B., Savino, N. S., Anderson, C. L., Weisbuch, M., Tamir, M., & Laudenslager, M. L. (2012). The pursuit of happiness can be lonely. *Emotion, 12,* 908–912.

Mauss, I. B., Tamir, M., Anderson, C. L., & Savino, N. S. (2011). Can seeking happiness make people unhappy? Paradoxical effects of valuing happiness. *Emotion, 11,* 807–815.

McGuirk, L., Kuppens, P., Kingston, R., & Bastian, B. (2018). Does a culture of happiness increase rumination over failure? *Emotion, 18,* 755–764.

McMahan, E. A., Ryu, S., & Choi, I. (2014). Lay conceptions of wellbeing among undergraduate students from the United States and South Korea: Culture-level differences and correlates. *Social Indicators Research, 119,* 321–339.

Mehmet, O. (2001). Globalization as westernization: A post-colonial theory of global exploitation. In B. N. Ghosh (Ed.), *Contemporary issues in development economics* (pp. 211–223). New York, NY: Routledge.

Miller, P. J., Wang, S.-H., Sandel, T., & Cho, G. E. (2002). Self-esteem as folk theory: A comparison of European American and Taiwanese mothers' beliefs. *Parenting: Science and Practice, 2,* 209–239.

Mishkin, F. S. (2009). Globalization and financial development. *Journal of Development Economics, 89,* 164–169.

Miyamoto, Y., & Ma, X. (2011). Dampening or savouring positive emotions: A dialectical cultural script guides emotion regulation. *Emotion, 11,* 1346–1357.

Miyamoto, Y., Ma, X., & Petermann, A. G. (2014). Cultural differences in hedonic emotion regulation after a negative event. *Emotion, 14,* 804–815.

Miyamoto, Y., Ma, X., & Wilken, B. (2017). Cultural variation in pro-positive versus balanced systems of emotions. *Current Opinion in Behavioral Sciences, 15,* 27–32.

Myers, D. G., & Diener, E. (2018). The scientific pursuit of happiness. *Perspectives on Psychological Science, 13,* 218–225.

Ng, F. F.-Y., Pomerantz, E. M., & Lam, S.-F. (2007). European American and Chinese parents' responses to children's success and failure: Implications for children's responses. *Developmental Psychology, 43,* 1239–1255.

Ogihara, Y. (2017). Temporal changes in individualism and their ramification in Japan: Rising individualism and conflicts with persisting collectivism. *Frontiers in Psychology, 8,* 695.

Ogihara, Y., & Uchida, Y. (2014). Does individualism bring happiness? Negative effects of individualism on interpersonal relationships and happiness. *Frontiers in Psychology, 5,* 135.

Oishi, S., & Kesebir, S. (2015). Income inequality explains why economic growth does not always translate to an increase in happiness. *Psychological Science, 26,* 1630–1638.

Oishi, S., Kesebir, S., & Diener, E. (2011). Income inequality and happiness. *Psychological Science, 22,* 1095–1100.

Oishi, S., Schimmack, U., & Diener, E. (2012). Progressive taxation and the subjective wellbeing of nations. *Psychological Science, 23,* 86–92.

Ott, J. C. (2010a). Good governance and happiness in nations: Technical quality precedes democracy and quality beats size. *Journal of Happiness Studies, 11,* 353–368.

Ott, J. C. (2010b). Greater happiness for a greater number: Some non-controversial options for governments. *Journal of Happiness Studies, 11,* 631–647.

Ott, J. C. (2011). Government and happiness in 130 nations: Good governance fosters higher level and more equality of happiness. *Social Indicators Research, 102,* 3–22.

Oyserman, D., Coon, H. M., & Kemmelmeier, M. (2002). Rethinking individualism and collectivism: Evaluation of theoretical assumptions and meta-analyses. *Psychological Bulletin, 128,* 3–72.

Park, L. E., & Crocker, J. (2005). Interpersonal consequences of seeking self-esteem. *Personality and Social Psychology Bulletin, 31,* 1587–1598.

Parker, R. S., Haytko, D. L., & Hermans, C. M. (2009). Individualism and collectivism: Reconsidering old assumptions. *Journal of International Business Research, 8,* 127–139.

Parkinson, B. (1996). Emotions are social. *British Journal of Psychology, 87,* 663–684.

Parks, A. C., Schueller, S. M., & Tasimi, A. (2013). Increasing happiness in the general population: Empirically supported self-help? In S. David, I. Boniwell, & A. C. Ayers (Eds.), *Oxford handbook of happiness* (pp. 962–977). Oxford, UK: Oxford University Press.

Peng, K., & Nisbett, R. E. (1999). Culture, dialectics, and reasoning about contradiction. *American Psychologist, 54,* 741–754.

Pfeiffer, D., & Cloutier, S. (2016). Planning for happy neighborhoods. *Journal of the American Planning Association, 82,* 267–279.

Pflug, J. (2009). Folk theories of happiness: A cross-cultural comparison of conceptions of happiness in Germany and South Africa. *Social Indicators Research, 92,* 551–563.

Piff, P. K., Kraus, M. W., Côté, S., Cheng, B. H., & Keltner, D. (2010). Having less, giving more: The influence of social class on prosocial behavior. *Journal of Personality and Social Psychology, 99,* 771–784.

Prilleltensky, I. (2012). The what, why, who, and how of globalization: What is psychology to do? *Journal of Social Issues, 68,* 612–629.

Rahayu, T. P. (2016). The determinants of happiness in Indonesia. *Mediterranean Journal of Social Sciences, 7,* 393–404.

Rohrer, J. M., Richter, D., Brümmer, M., Wagner, G. G., & Schmukle, S. C. (2018). Successfully striving for happiness: Socially engaged pursuits predict increases in life satisfaction. *Psychological Science, 29,* 1291–1298.

Sam, D. L., & Berry, J. W. (2010). Acculturation: When individuals and groups of different cultural backgrounds meet. *Perspectives on Psychological Science, 5,* 472–481.

Samimi, P., & Jenatabadi, H. S. (2014). Globalization and economic growth: Empirical evidence on the role of complementarities. *PLoS ONE, 9,* e87824.

Sarracino, F. (2013). Determinants of subjective wellbeing in high and low income countries: Do happiness equations differ across countries? *The Journal of Socio-Economics, 42,* 51–66.

Savage, J. (2009, February 21). A design for life. *The Guardian*. Retrieved from https://www.theguardian.com/artanddesign/2009/feb/21/smiley-face-design-history.

Schimmack, U., Oishi, S., & Diener, E. (2002). Cultural influences on the relation between pleasant emotions and unpleasant emotions: Asian dialectic philosophies or individualism-collectivism? *Cognition and Emotion, 16,* 705–719.

Schooler, J. W., Ariely, D., & Loewenstein, G. (2003). The pursuit and assessment of happiness can be self-defeating. In J. Carrillo & I. Brocas (Eds.), *The psychology of economic decisions* (pp. 41–70). Oxford, UK: Oxford University Press.

Shimpi, P. M., & Zirkel, S. (2012). One hundred and fifty years of "the Chinese question": An intergroup relations perspective on immigration and globalization. *Journal of Social Issues, 68,* 534–558.

Sims, T., Tsai, J. L., Jiang, D., Wang, Y., Fung, H. H., & Zhang, X. (2015). Wanting to maximize the positive and minimize the negative: Implications for mixed affective experience in American and Chinese contexts. *Journal of Personality and Social Psychology, 109,* 292–315.

Sommer, R. (2003). Trees and human identity. In S. Clayton & S. Opotow (Eds.), *Identity and the natural environment: The psychological significance of nature* (pp. 179–204). Cambridge, MA: MIT Press.

Spencer-Rodgers, J., Boucher, H. C., Mori, S. C., Wang, L., & Peng, K. (2009). The dialectical self-concept: Contradiction, change, and holism in East Asian cultures. *Personality and Social Psychology Bulletin, 35,* 29–44.

Stamp, J. (2013, March 13). Who really invented the smiley face? *Smithsonian*. Retrieved from https://www.smithsonianmag.com/arts-culture/who-really-invented-the-smiley-face-2058483/.

Steele, L. G., & Lynch, S. M. (2013). The pursuit of happiness in China: Individualism, collectivism, and subjective wellbeing during China's economic and social transformation. *Social Indicators Research, 114,* 441–451.

Steger, M. B. (2013). *Globalization: A very short introduction*. Oxford, UK: Oxford University Press.

Stevenson, B., & Wolfers, J. (2008). *Economic growth and subjective wellbeing: Reassessing the Easterlin paradox (Brookings Papers on Economic Activity)*. Washington, DC: The Brookings Institution.

Suhail, K., & Chaudhry, H. R. (2004). Predictors of subjective wellbeing in an eastern Muslim culture. *Journal of Social and Clinical Psychology, 23,* 359–376.

Suissa, J. (2008). Lessons from a new science? On teaching happiness in schools. *Journal of Philosophy of Education, 42,* 575–590.

Sullivan, W. C., Kuo, F. E., & Depooter, S. F. (2004). The fruit of urban nature: Vital neighborhood space. *Environment and Behavior, 36,* 678–700.

Sun, J., & Ryder, A. G. (2016). The Chinese experience of rapid modernization: Sociocultural changes, psychological consequences? *Frontiers in Psychology, 7,* 477.

Tamir, M., & Ford, B. Q. (2012). Should people pursue feelings that feel good or feelings that do good? Emotional Preferences and wellbeing. *Emotion, 12,* 1061–1070.

Toivonen, T., Norasakkunkit, V., & Uchida, Y. (2011). Unable to conform, unwilling to rebel? Youth, culture, and motivation in a globalizing Japan. *Frontiers in Cultural Psychology, 2,* 207.

Tov, W., & Diener, E. (2007). Culture and subjective wellbeing. In S. Kitayama & D. Cohen (Eds.), *Handbook of cultural psychology* (pp. 691–713). New York, NY: Guilford.

Triandis, H. C. (1995). *Individualism and collectivism*. Boulder, CO: Westview Press.

Tsai, J. L. (2007). Ideal affect: Cultural causes and behavioral consequences. *Perspectives on Psychological Science, 2,* 242–259.

Tsai, J. L., Louie, J., Chen, E. E., & Uchida, Y. (2007). Learning what feelings to desire: Socialization of ideal affect through children's storybooks. *Personality and Social Psychology Bulletin, 33,* 17–30.

Tsai, J. L., Miao, F. F., & Seppala, E. (2007). Good feelings in Christianity and Buddhism: Religious differences in ideal affect. *Personality and Social Psychology Bulletin, 33,* 409–421.

Twenge, J. M., Gentile, B., DeWall, C. N., Ma, D., Lacefield, K., & Schurtz, D. R. (2010). Birth cohort increases in psychopathology among young Americans, 1938–2007: A cross-temporal meta-analysis of the MMPI. *Clinical Psychology Review, 30,* 145–154.

Uchida, Y. (2011). A holistic view of happiness: Belief in the negative side of happiness is more prevalent in Japan than in the United States. *Psychologia, 53,* 236–245.

Uchida, Y., & Kitayama, S. (2009). Happiness and unhappiness in East and West: Themes and variations. *Emotion, 9,* 441–456.

Uchida, Y., & Ogihara, Y. (2012). Personal or interpersonal construal of happiness: A cultural psychological perspective. *International Journal of Wellbeing, 2,* 354–369.

Uchida, Y., & Oishi, S. (2016). The happiness of individuals and the collective. *Japanese Psychological Research, 58,* 125–141.

Uchida, Y., Norasakkunkit, V., & Kitayama, S. (2004). Cultural constructions of happiness: Theory and evidence. *Journal of Happiness Studies, 5,* 223–239.

United Nations. (2011). *Happiness: Towards a holistic approach to development*. Retrieved from http://www.un.org/ga/search/view_doc.asp?symbol=A/RES/65/309.

United Nations. (2012). *International day of happiness*. Retrieved from http://www.un.org/ga/search/view_doc.asp?symbol=A/RES/66/281.

Van den Berg, A. E., Maas, J., Verheij, R. A., & Groenewegen, P. P. (2010). Green space as a buffer between stressful life events and health. *Social Science and Medicine, 70,* 1203–1210.

Walsh, L. C., Boehm, J. K., & Lyubomirsky, S. (2018). Does happiness promote career success? Revisiting the evidence. *Journal of Career Assessment, 26,* 199–219.

Wegner, D. M. (1994). Ironic processes of mental control. *Psychological Review, 101,* 34–52.
Wegner, D. M., Erber, R., & Zanakos, S. (1993). Ironic processes in the mental control of mood and mood-related thought. *Journal of Personality and Social Psychology, 65,* 1093–1104.
White, M. P., Alcock, I., Wheeler, B. W., & Depledge, M. H. (2013). Would you be happier living in a greener urban area? A fixed-effects analysis of panel data. *Psychological Science, 24,* 920–928.
Whiteoak, J. W., Crawford, N. G., & Mapstone, R. H. (2006). Impact of gender and generational differences in work values and attitudes in an Arab culture. *Thunderbird International Business Review, 48,* 77–91.
Wilk, R. (1995). Learning to be local in Belize: Global structures of common difference. In D. Miller (Ed.), *Worlds apart: Modernity through the prism of the local* (pp. 110–133). London, UK: Routledge.
Wirtz, D., & Chiu, C. (2008). Perspectives on the self in the East and West: Searching for the "subdued" ego. In H. Wayment & J. Bauer (Eds.), *Transcending self-interest: Psychological explorations of the quiet ego*. Washington, DC: American Psychological Association.
Wirtz, D., Chiu, C., Diener, E., & Oishi, S. (2009). What constitutes a good life? Cultural differences in the role of positive and negative affect in subjective wellbeing. *Journal of Personality, 77,* 1167–1196.
Wiwad, D., & Aknin, L. B. (2017). Motives matter: The emotional consequences of recalled self- and other-focused prosocial acts. *Motivation and Emotion, 41,* 730–740.
Yan, Y. (2010). The Chinese path to individualization. *The British Journal of Sociology, 61,* 489–512.
Yoo, J., & Miyamoto, Y. (2018). Cultural fit of emotions and health implications: A psychosocial resources model. *Social and Personality Psychology Compass, 12,* e12372.
Yuki, M., Sato, K., Takemura, K., & Oishi, S. (2013). Social ecology moderates the association between self-esteem and happiness. *Journal of Experimental Social Psychology, 49,* 741–746.

Chapter 17
Concluding Thoughts on the Development of a Middle East/North Africa Positive Psychology

Louise Lambert and Nausheen Pasha-Zaidi

Abstract From education, health and business to public policy and infrastructure, an agenda for building the positives, and not merely reducing the negatives, has now been set across the MENA region. We are confident that researchers, policymakers and practitioners will get on board along with organizations, educational institutions, ministries, non-profits, and other stakeholders to ask big, bold questions that add, challenge and enrich what we love and know to be true about the region. Yet, questions, challenges and many unknowns remain; thus, we end this book with the practical in mind and set forth some future directions and closing thoughts.

17.1 Introduction

In this book, we cover a variety of topics of interest to positive psychology in the MENA region. These include policy initiatives and ideas for wellbeing that emerge from and reflect the goals of government entities and private sectors. We address how positive psychology is making its mark in educational systems and work environments. We also highlight the trends and challenges of doing research in the region, consider the ways in which culture and religion shape the lived experiences of "positivity", and provide ideas for the application of positive psychology principles. We add some final thoughts for researchers, policymakers, and practitioners to get on board with the positive psychology agenda that is already in place in the hopes of making it more relevant and real for the people of the region.

L. Lambert (✉)
United Arab Emirates University, Al Ain, UAE
e-mail: ltlamber@yahoo.com

N. Pasha-Zaidi
Houston Community College, University of Houston-Downtown, Houston, TX, USA
e-mail: nausheenpasha@outlook.com

L. Lambert and N. Pasha-Zaidi (eds.), *Positive Psychology in the Middle East/North Africa*, https://doi.org/10.1007/978-3-030-13921-6_17

17.2 The Role of Regional Government in Wellbeing

Achieving wellbeing has always been a priority of governments; however, it has never been articulated as an end-state. Instead, it was considered the accomplishment of a remediation or minimization of factors known to hinder life satisfaction and wellbeing. Enforcing mandatory school attendance, instituting helmet laws, and requiring childhood immunizations are examples of such policies devised with the aim to free people from the burdens of illness, illiteracy, and accidents. Yet, as most governments meet the basics of security and survival and have implemented systems and structures to support a good life, a new standard has emerged, that of instituting wellbeing as an explicit, direct, measurable policy goal (Diener & Biswas-Diener, 2019). Consequently, governments play a leading role in driving wellbeing as an input of policy and not a mere incidental—or accidental—output. This is a new frontier and trial for governance worldwide. Thanks in part to an emerging science of wellbeing, it is also now possible.

Research in a variety of domains shows that governments can do a lot to boost wellbeing and that many universal contributors exist across countries. For example, strengthening relationships (Helliwell & Wang, 2012; Ngamaba & Soni, 2018), offering entrepreneurial opportunities and the means for self-employment (Binder & Coad, 2013; Hessels, Arampatzi, van der Zwan, & Burger, 2018), and high quality education (Blanchflower & Oswald, 2004) contribute immensely to wellbeing. Additionally, living in, or close to urban centers that have good cultural, recreational, educational and healthcare amenities and services (Miyazaki, Saeki, Yada, & Ikegami, 2018; Wang & Wang, 2016) also makes a difference. More personally, being married (Naess, Blekesaune, & Jakobsson, 2015), giving to charity (Aknin et al., 2013; Dunn, Aknin, & Norton, 2014), experiencing positive affect (Franke, Huebner, & Hills, 2017; Hagenauer, Gläser-Zikuda, & Moschner, 2018), reporting a state of good health (Kööts-Ausmees & Realo, 2015; Ngamaba & Soni, 2018) and being satisfied with one's living standards (i.e., price, location, noise, size of dwelling) (Azimi & Esmaeilzadeh, 2017; Zhang, Zhang, & Hudson, 2018) are other examples. Policies at the municipal, federal or emirate level are imperative to develop and ensure that these aspects of life are possible and equally attainable.

The ability to ensure these building blocks are in place rests on good governance, a non-negotiable factor in the development of greater wellbeing (Helliwell, Huang, Grover, & Wang, 2018). Individuals are happier under good governance as services are transparent, efficient, and equally available to all, and do not involve or require corrupt practises. Individuals are also happier for what good governance allows them to accomplish in life. Entrepreneurial activity and access to necessary funds, a stable and good family life through policies that allow state-sponsored day care and parental leave, and low-cost or free high quality education are examples of such practices. Good governance directly impacts people's lives on a daily basis, and allows them to develop a meaningful, interesting, successful and joyful life that maintains human dignity and social cohesion. National accounts of wellbeing, on which suitable wellbeing policies can be derived, are increasingly being developed.

These further allow the contributors and outcomes of wellbeing to be tracked over time (Diener, Oishi, & Lucas, 2015).

17.3 Teaching Wellbeing in the Region

Wellbeing is not only an outcome of good governance; it can also be a direct input. Policies and accompanying programs, structures, and processes which aim to deliberately boost wellbeing are now being offered in schools, workplaces and communities and include the development of character strengths or positive psychology interventions (e.g., Lambert, 2017; Lambert, Passmore, & Joshanloo, 2018; Lambert, Passmore, Scull, Al Sabah, & Hussain, 2018), as well as organizational programs designed to increase workplace engagement, the use of character strengths at work, workplace wellbeing, as well as certification schemes for wellbeing-compliant companies. These programs can be mandated, offered by governments themselves, or outsourced to agencies on their behalf.

This book has reviewed much evidence showing that the skills for wellbeing can indeed be taught and the gains can be maintained over time. What is usually of greatest concern is whether the skills for wellbeing can be taught in the MENA region. While few positive psychology intervention (PPI) programs exist regionally, two empirically validated studies serve as examples. Recently completed in the UAE was a PPI study conducted in Dubai (Lambert, Passmore, & Joshanloo, 2018). This 14-week PPI program was delivered within the context of an existing university psychology class with largely Muslim students from 39 different nations. This program included the delivery of positive psychology instruction, including weekly interventions such as the gratitude letter, Best Possible Self activity, self-compassion, mindfulness, and savoring as examples. Relative to a control group and at three months post intervention, students participating in the happiness group realized sustainable gains in hedonic and eudaimonic wellbeing, as well as lower levels of fear around happiness. Boosts in life satisfaction and net-positive affect were also evidenced at follow-up.

A second study in Kuwait (Lambert et al., 2018) delivered weekly 15 min happiness interventions to almost 1000 university and secondary students over the course of one semester. This was a pilot study to demonstrate the feasibility and effectiveness of an ongoing two-year program. Sites included Kuwait's national university and several public schools. Teachers were trained to use the program, then delivered all the instruction with little disruption to the school day. Relative to a control group and at post-follow-up, university students reported greater eudaimonic wellbeing, while secondary students achieved greater gains in hedonic wellbeing. Interviews after the program revealed that teachers also experienced greater satisfaction at work, noting that they enjoyed the children more, had less stressful days, fewer intentions to leave their jobs, and that these benefits spilled over to their personal home lives. The program was officially recognized as an integral part of the "New Kuwait 2035" national strategy and adopted by Kuwait's Ministry of Education for use in all the nation's schools. Both studies demonstrate that PPI programs do work regionally, although long-term effects remain to be seen.

17.4 The Impact of Cultural Context

Recent reviews illustrate that the dissemination of PPIs and positive psychology is growing worldwide (Hendriks et al., 2018a; Kim, Doiron, Warren, & Donaldson, 2018). In fact, Hendriks et al., (2018b) reported that one third of PPI studies globally are non-Western, with many of these adapted to cultural contexts (see Al Ghalib & Salim, 2018 as an example). Yet, there continue to be programs that merely replicate Western originating PPIs and/or blindly disseminate positive psychology content that contain individualistic and democratic values not generally acknowledged or applicable in other cultural contexts (Arnett, 2008; Bermant, Talwar, & Rozin, 2011; Christopher & Hickinbottom, 2008; Joshanloo, 2013). Working in Islamic cultures, it is important to bear in mind that the expression of happiness is commonly thought to call forth what is known as the evil eye, or seen as a means to ridicule or flout the power of God, thus inviting the possibility of negative ramifications in one's life. Further, openly demonstrating too much happiness can make people appear immature, foolish or as though they are merely seeking attention. Knowing this, Lambert, Passmore, and Joshanloo (2018) ended their UAE study asking what might be the unforeseen consequences on culture, given that the content of their wellbeing classes focused on dispelling many beliefs about the fear and fragility of happiness. As these beliefs are rooted in cultural and religious belief, is it ethical and moral to challenge them, even if wellbeing increases as a result?

One solution is to introduce PPIs in ways that are more culturally-congruent. Diener and Biswas-Diener (2019) refer to the "tall poppy syndrome" whereby recipients of character strength interventions, for example, may be more open to strategies that are promoted as a means to contribute to society rather than as ways to appear unique and stand out, both of which are more reflective of individualistic value systems. Further, many PPIs are self-focused (versus other-focused) and work to strengthen aspects of the self, such as self-efficacy, self-regulation, self-confidence, self-compassion, and self-identity. The value placed on improving the individual self as opposed to the self in relation to others may have consequences for traditionally collectivist cultures. However, it is also important to bear in mind that many cultures fall at different points on the individualist—collectivist continuum. Even among collectivist cultures, differences exist. For example, in a study of academic resilience variables, Pasha-Zaidi, Afari, Sevi, Urganci, and Durham (2018) found cultural differences in self-efficacy, task value (the value that students place upon the academic tasks they are required to perform) and self-regulation among university students in the UAE, Turkey, and the United States. Although Turkey and the UAE are more similar to each other than to the United States based on Hofstede's Cultural Dimensions (Fig. 17.1), there were nonetheless differences in the ways in which the academic resilience variables were manifested in each context. Although task value and self-efficacy were positively correlated in each of the three contexts, only self-efficacy was a significant predictor of self-regulation in the UAE and neither task value nor self-efficacy were related to self-regulation behaviors in Turkey.

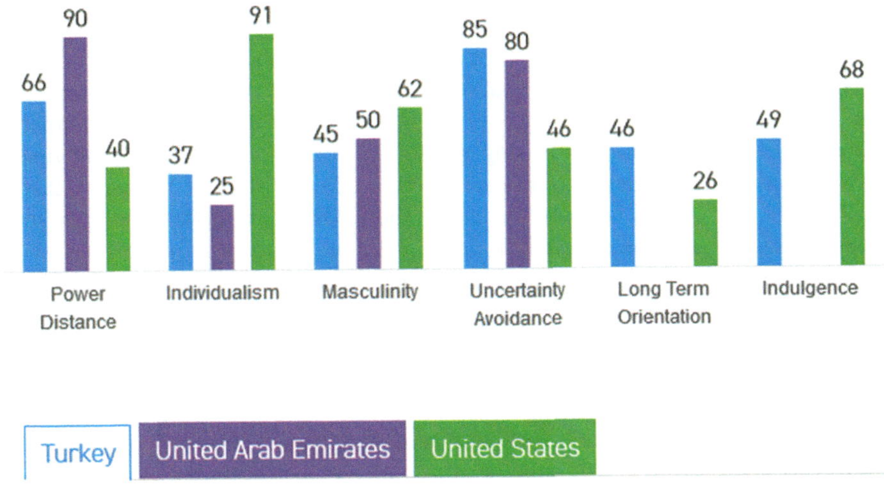

Fig. 17.1 Comparison of Turkey, UAE, and US on Hofstede's cultural dimensions (Hofstede's Insights: Country comparison, https://www.hofstede-insights.com/country-comparison/turkey,the-united-arab-emirates,the-usa/)

Individualistic tendencies are also more common in younger adults as well as those living in urban societies. Thus, PPIs that reflect the values of the culture must take into account a variety of variables that are specific to the society in which they are implemented. Current studies are focusing on this question (Lambert, Karabchuk, Joshanloo, Al Rasbi, & Cody, in preparation), but the fact that most (positive) psychology practitioners in the GCC are Western is concerning as they are often the last to notice the philosophical assumptions that their theoretical models carry (Schuilenberg et al., 2016).

Many constructs also hold little relevance in the region. The PERMA model (Seligman, 2011), which posits five pathways to wellbeing (positive emotion, engagement, relationships, meaning and accomplishment) is an established framework in the positive psychology literature. However, in a PPI program conducted by the first author with an Emirati group of women, engagement was found to be the least understood and relatable to the audience, echoing previous research (Lambert D'raven & Pasha-Zaidi, 2016). As engagement involves participation in activities such as sports, music, arts, and other recreational pursuits, female participants were hard-pressed to create such a life for themselves due to gender norms limiting their ability to engage in such activities. Many were prohibited from participating in musical pursuits as it is considered by some families to be un-Islamic, and music was further prohibited in their university hostel accommodations. The restrictions on female participation in such leisurely pursuits, thus, limited their ability to engage in activities that would promote a state of flow (Csikszentmihalyi, 1990), which is the ultimate reward of the pathway of engagement. Instead, the pathways of meaning and relationships served as the central focus of such programming as these were already aligned with the cultural values and behaviors of the participants.

National context and socio-political settings also matter. A recent study (Lambert, Karabchuk, & Joshanloo, forthcoming) of Gallup data on over 17,000 participants in the UAE revealed some surprising results. For example, while unemployment has been shown to detract from life satisfaction (Calvo, Mair, & Sarkisian, 2015; Wulfgramm, 2014), this was not the case in the UAE as it is buffered by generous economic safety nets. The study also found that despite evidence showing that greater personal freedoms influence life satisfaction across many countries (Crescioni, Baumeister, Ainsworth, Ent, & Lambert, 2016; Inglehart, Foa, Peterson, & Welzel, 2008; Ngamaba & Soni, 2018; Verme, 2009; Welzel & Inglehart, 2010), this was again not the case in the UAE. It is imperative, therefore, to look at the contributors to happiness and wellbeing in non-Western nations and to challenge what is known to be true in other areas of the world and presented as universal phenomena in the literature.

17.5 The Need for a More Balanced Positive Psychology

Whether in psychology, medicine, political science, or biology, theories and models are regularly contested. Gruman, Lumley and Gonzalez-Morales (2018) recently identified ongoing challenges to positive psychology, some of which are being addressed, while others have yet to be rectified. Positive psychology was developed as the antidote to the overwhelmingly negative focus of traditional psychology where distress and disorder were the only aspects of life worth examining. Yet, the extremeness of that bent is also mirrored in positive psychology; meant to rebalance the field towards both positive and negative, it often appears to have merely shifted the pendulum the other way. Efforts to counter the rise of overly positive outlooks and what has been called "smiling fascism" can be found in the shift towards Positive Psychology 2.0 (Lomas, 2016; Wong, 2011), the integration of both the positive and the negative and corresponding theories and treatment models that incorporate both the good and the bad in life. This new phase of positive psychology is helping to rebalance the field of psychology overall, but at present, the bulk of enquiry and practise remains firmly centered on the positive and not on its integration with the negative.

Gruman et al. (2018) further contend that the negative consequences of the positives need to be examined as there is an assumption that just because something is positive, it must be good. For example, a number of recent opinion pieces contest the importance of "grit" (Duckworth & Eskreis-Winkler, 2015), the persistence used by individuals in the face of challenge. Critics have pointed out that this character strength is dispositional, that is, dependent on the individual, but fails to consider the sociopolitical contexts in which it is expected to develop (Syed, Santos, Yoo, & Juang, 2018). To suggest that minorities simply work harder and develop more persistence, tenacity and resilience, is to overlook systemic discrimination and structural inequality that no amount of additional effort will help to overcome. Focusing merely on developing positive aspects of one's character—versus advocating for systemic changes—espouses and entrenches the privileged view that positive psychology has been trying hard to dispel.

Further, not all positive concepts result in positive outcomes. For example, very high levels of optimism can impair coping or at best, be ineffective and contribute nothing in the face of illness (Coifman, Flynn, & Pinto, 2016; Hurt et al., 2014; Schofield et al., 2004; Veenhoven, 2008), despite popular prescriptions saying otherwise. Positive psychology interventions may also be contraindicated in some cases. For example, suggesting that a recently widowed Syrian refugee be grateful is insulting at best and can lead to greater harm. Research has shown that harm may emerge when the fit between the person, intervention, timing, culture and context is not right (Nelson & Lyubomirsky, 2014; Sergeant & Mongrain, 2011).

17.6 The State of Science in the Region

While the science of wellbeing is more advanced in the West, it is still nascent in the region, as is science and psychology overall. In their meta-analysis of global PPI studies, Hendriks et al. (2018a) noted that most Western PPI studies consistently show small to moderate effect sizes on both wellbeing and ill-being; yet, non-Western studies consistently oversell the results of PPI efficacy by three to five times! The authors identify two reasons for such stunning results. First, the methodologies in non-Western studies tend to show less scientific rigour—a problem with the regional state of science overall, which produces inconsistent or incorrect results. Also, in contexts where there are few existing psychological services to begin with, almost anything can work. Thus, intervention success may simply be due to the fact that participants receive attention of any kind. Indeed, many participants of the programs undertaken by the first author reported that it was the first time they were able to talk about happiness (and unhappiness) and acquire skills to deal with their overall emotional state, something not generally taught in schools or within most families.

Another reason for such exaggeration may have to do with overinflated participant responses, a common limitation of survey work in a region where few people feel comfortable stating that they are unhappy or even moderately so, especially in light of the government's repeated announcements to become the happiest nation in the world. Anything short of being perfectly happy may be perceived as being disloyal to the cause. A recent research experiment undertaken by the first author had to be abandoned for this reason as pre-test measures showed highly inflated, extraordinary subjective wellbeing scores, which left no possible room for improvement given the proposed intervention. The cultural importance of saving face (Feghali, 1997) may also have played a part. A recent analysis of pilot data on Islamic religiosity conducted by the second author showed a similar trend, with self-reports of religiosity among participants surveyed in the UAE and Turkey being strongly skewed towards the higher end. Thus, the norms of communication in the region may also affect participants' responses.

In attempting to understand the nuances of experience in the Middle East, it is imperative to remind ourselves of our positioning in the research process. One of the challenges for scientific enquiry is the lack of indigenous knowledge among Western researchers who conduct studies in the region. We all have inherent biases. Researchers who do not belong to the group being studied may find it difficult to make sense of the behaviors and attitudes of their participants, whereas members of the group may have an easier time identifying root causes and implications. However, as the language of scientific discourse is predominantly English, this may limit the ability of residents in the MENA region to engage in the research process, and to communicate effectively to ensure that cultural nuances are captured. As a proponent of participatory research, the second author often enlists the help of members of the cultural group being studied to review and adapt measurement tools, translate and back-translate survey instruments, gather data, and analyse results. Such practices enable local communities to be involved in the research process and go a long way in promoting buy-in from groups that have been traditionally marginalized or from those who may be wary of foreign influence.

Among many Westerners, even those in academic circles, the Middle East and its diverse population is often viewed as a monolithic "Other". To combat the negative stereotypes of the region, it is necessary to get local communities involved. This would boost the state of science in the region as improvements to methodology and research design may result from greater interaction between researchers and the communities they study. In turn, more accurate data would be disseminated, thus allowing for better decision-making among stakeholders within governmental and non-governmental entities. Participatory research may also help dispel the suspicions that many in the region hold about researchers and what they do with the collected data. As Islamophobia is an insidious threat for contemporary Muslims, Western researchers, who are unknown in the region or who do not employ participatory strategies, may experience greater challenges. Thus, building trust and utilizing the strengths of the people in the region would make scientific pursuits more mutually enriching and pave the way for improving scientific practices as well.

17.7 Promoting the Science of Happiness and Wellbeing

"Happiness" as a term is too narrow to be of much use and promotes the idea that one must be smiling, joyful, positive and optimistic at all times; a tall order for most people trying to parent, graduate, work, make money, exercise, attain goals, as well as love and be loved. The failure to communicate and promote the broader notion of wellbeing that includes meaning, belonging, friendship, health, character, etc., and its consequences in the workplace were recently studied. Omar (2018) explored this topic in the UAE showing that immediately after the announcement of its Minister of Happiness and Wellbeing, a significant number of job titles were changed on

LinkedIn, whereby “Happiness experts” emerged in several industries, all without corresponding changes to educational or professional qualifications. Many of these were largely irrelevant and appeared to add little to the jobs themselves. Happiness experts appeared in real estate, accounting, and cosmetology centers. While this was part of the national learning curve in the development of greater “happiness” and now “wellbeing”, this failure nevertheless set the movement back very early on.

As a result, unwarranted claims of expertise continue to proliferate in academia, health care, and education by professionals who cannot name a single theory, model or concept in the field and do not rely on, or offer empirical evidence to support their interventions. The global and regional happiness industry needs regulation. The potential for harm is high given that regional audiences in particular are unsuspecting, undiscerning, and may lack knowledge about psychology in general. A solution would be to suggest that positive psychology practitioners take training in such areas of psychology; yet, this too, has been overshadowed by an element of marketing, profit and disregard for the psychology profession, from which positive psychology stems. Lomas and Ivtzan (2016) offer a broad critique and recommendations for professionalizing the area of positive psychology, especially in light of the large numbers of “MAPPsters”—graduates of Masters in Applied Positive Psychology programs. Broadly appealing, such programs do not require students to have an undergraduate degree in psychology. Claims abound that such programs may not be very arduous given the absence of prerequisites and a lack of required hypothesis testing in their Master’s level research projects. Such programs produce unaccredited practitioners and not researchers, scientists, or licensed psychologists, who are legislated as well as mandated to have training in ethics and supervised practice of over 1500 h. Gruman et al. (2018) charge that such commercially driven programs are divorced from psychology, which helps to explain some of the hostility from the field of psychology overall. Structuring the field of positive psychology will require a simultaneous clean-up of the psychology profession as well, which regionally, suffers from a lack of professional accreditation, practise standards, supervision, ethical protocols, as well as licensing and disciplinary bodies (Hands, 2017; Schuilenberg et al., 2016). This lack of oversight is worrying as legislation and regulation exist for a reason, i.e., the protection of the client (even if it is focused on the positive), fidelity of the profession, and safeguards against liability for the professional.

17.8 Moving Forward

Moving forward, science and the happiness industry must work together to develop programs that are evidence-based and culturally relevant. After all, positive psychology is *psychology*—the empirical investigation of human behavior, emotions, perceptions, and cognitive processes. Treating an investigation of the positive as seriously as we do the negative is the way forward, and this relies on the scientific method just as it does in any other science. Although the field of psychology itself continues to be dominated by quantitative methods, which are still considered more "scientific" and "objective" in mainstream academic circles, this should not limit researchers working in the Middle East to utilize other research designs. Exploring culture-bound knowledge and understandings of social and individual wellbeing (Donaldson, Dollwet, & Rao, 2015; Kim et al., 2018) may require qualitative or mixed method approaches. These have been integral to anthropological and sociological studies and deserve to be more welcomed in the halls of psychology. Relying on both rigorous qualitative and quantitative methods can be helpful in developing a regional positive psychology that is relevant, responsive, reflective and useful for the region.

A clear benefit of positive psychology is that it is still a new field, particularly so in the region, which means there is ample room for researchers and practitioners to ask, develop, and test big, bold hypotheses. Additionally, the notion of generalizability, the value that is placed on purely quantitative methods, has taken a hit in the discipline due to criticisms noting the dominance of Western populations in large scale studies. Given that much of the historical research and theories in psychology are based on data from American college students or reflect the values of European males, how generalizable are these findings really?

With respect to the MENA region, which has the highest concentration of Muslims in any area (DeSilver & Masci, 2017), it is perhaps time that more effort is placed in building an indigenous Islamic positive psychology. The roots of psychological enquiry are not new in the region; psychological constructs were being contemplated by Muslim thinkers such as Al-Ghazali, Ibn Sina, and Al-Tabari during the Islamic Golden Age, which lasted from approximately 750 AD to 1250 AD (Haque, 2004). Badrī (1979) called for the development of an Islamic psychology for Muslims a few decades ago; more recently others (Abu Raiya, 2012; Rothman & Coyle, 2018; Skinner, 2010) have begun advocating for the same. Currently, much of the work has focused on clinical and counseling applications (Abu-Raiya, 2015; Ansari, 2002; Hamjah & Akhir, 2014; Haque & Keshavarzi, 2012; York Al-Karam, 2018) or on the philosophical conceptualizations of the mind and personality (Haque & Mohamed, 2009; Ivry, 2008). Utilizing Islamic perspectives to create an indigenous positive psychology would certainly be a useful endeavor and may be more applicable for creating a relevant science of wellbeing in the region.

17.9 Conclusion

Mainstream psychology, education, healthcare, organizational and human resource work, policy development and many other fields have focused on malfunction, disease, distress, and other sore spots needing attention for so long that opportunities, strengths, talents, genius, positive emotion and goodness had all been forgotten. This is the main gift positive psychology has given the world; a language of human possibility, the tools to investigate such opportunities, and strategies to create and amplify such prospects. Despite the field's limitations and early struggles, this gift is worthy of investment and praise. We hope that readers will take home this message and incorporate the "positive" into their new worldview of what is possible for the region and advocate for its inclusion in policy, research, education, and practice.

This book was developed with the fundamental conviction of the goodness, talent, ingenuity, creativity, and courage of the people of the MENA region. Governments, like those of the UAE and others, are wholeheartedly stepping up to the challenge; it is not lip service. We fully anticipate the bright lights across the region to champion the movement and urge their respective governments to set forth an agenda where wellbeing—that is, a life of dignity, respect, love, joy, safety, interest, hope and meaning—is possible and a central concern for everyone. A good life encompasses all these factors and more. Isn't that a goal worth striving for—for us, our families, communities, science and society as a whole?

References

Abu-Raiya, H. (2012). Toward a systematic Qura'nic theory of personality. *Mental Health, Religion & Culture, 15*(3), 217–233.

Abu-Raiya, H. (2015). Working with religious Muslim clients: A dynamic, Qura'nic-based model of psychotherapy. *Spirituality in Clinical Practice, 2*(2), 120–133.

Aknin, L. B., Barrington-Leigh, C. P., Dunn, E. W., Helliwell, J. F., Burns, J., Biswas-Diener, R., … Norton, M. I. (2013). Prosocial spending and well-being: Cross-cultural evidence for a psychological universal. *Journal of Personality and Social Psychology, 104*(4), 635–652.

Al-Ghalib, S. J., & Salim, A. Y. (2018). A mindfulness based intervention to enhance university student wellbeing in Saudi Arabia. *Middle East Journal of Positive Psychology, 4*(1), 142–157.

Ansari, Z. (2002). Islamic psychology. In R. P. Olson (Ed.), *Religious theories of personality and psychotherapy: East meets West* (pp. 325–357). New York, NY, USA: Haworth Press.

Arnett, J. J. (2008). The neglected 95%: Why American psychology needs to become less American. *American Psychologist, 63*(7), 602–614.

Azimi, N., & Esmaeilzadeh, Y. (2017). Assessing the relationship between house types and residential satisfaction in Tabriz. *Iran. International Journal of Urban Sciences, 21*(2), 185–203.

Badrī, M. (1979). *The dilemma of Muslim psychologists*. London, UK: MWH London.

Bermant, G., Talwar, C., & Rozin, P. (2011). To celebrate positive psychology and extend its horizons. In K. M. Sheldon, T. B. Kashdan, & M. F. Steger (Eds.), *Designing positive psychology: Taking stock and moving forward* (pp. 430–438). Oxford, UK: Oxford University Press.

Binder, M., & Coad, A. (2013). Life satisfaction and self-employment: A matching approach. *Small Business Economics, 40*(4), 1009–1033.

Blanchflower, D., & Oswald, A. J. (2004). Well-being over time in Britain and the USA. *Journal of Public Economics, 88*(7), 1359–1386.

Calvo, E., Mair, C. A., & Sarkisian, N. (2015). Individual troubles, shared troubles: The multiplicative effect of individual and country-level unemployment on life satisfaction in 95 nations (1981–2009). *Social Forces, 93*(4), 1625–1653.

Christopher, J., & Hickinbottom, S. (2008). Positive psychology, ethnocentrism, and the disguised ideology of individualism. *Theory & Psychology, 18*(5), 563–589.

Coifman, K. G., Flynn, J. J., & Pinto, L. A. (2016). When context matters: Negative emotions predict psychological health and adjustment. *Motivation and Emotion, 40*(4), 602–624.

Crescioni, A. W., Baumeister, R. F., Ainsworth, S. E., Ent, M., & Lambert, N. M. (2016). Subjective correlates and consequences of belief in free will. *Philosophical Psychology, 29*(1), 41–63.

Csikszentmihalyi, M. (1990). *Flow: The psychology of optimal experience*. New York, NY: Harper-Perennial.

DeSilver, D., & Masci, D. (2017). *World's Muslim population more widespread than you might think*. Pew Research Center. Retrieved from http://www.pewresearch.org/fact-tank/2017/01/31/worlds-muslim-population-more-widespread-than-you-might-think/.

Diener, E., & Biswas-Diener, R. (2019). Well-being interventions to improve societies. In *Global Happiness and Wellbeing Policy Report 2019* (Chapter 6, pp. 95–112). Dubai, UAE: Global Council for Happiness and Wellbeing. Retrieved from https://s3.amazonaws.com/ghwbpr-2019/UAE/GHWPR19.pdf

Diener, E., Oishi, S., & Lucas, R. E. (2015). National accounts of subjective well-being. *American Psychologist, 70*(3), 234–242.

Donaldson, S. I., Dollwet, M., & Rao, M. A. (2015). Happiness, excellence, and optimal human functioning revisited: Examining the peer-reviewed literature linked to positive psychology. *Journal of Positive Psychology, 10*(3), 185–195.

Duckworth, A. L., & Eskreis-Winkler, L. (2015). Grit. In J. D. Wright (Ed.), *International encyclopedia of the social and behavioral sciences* (2nd ed., pp. 397–401). Oxford, UK: Elsevier.

Dunn, E. W., Aknin, L. B., & Norton, M. I. (2014). Prosocial spending and happiness: Using money to benefit others pays off. *Current Directions in Psychological Science, 23,* 41–47.

Feghali, E. (1997). Arab cultural communication patterns. *International Journal of Intercultural Relations, 21*(3), 345–378.

Franke, K. B., Huebner, E. S., & Hills, K. J. (2017). Cross-sectional and prospective associations between positive emotions and general life satisfaction in adolescents. *Journal of Happiness Studies, 18*(4), 1075–1093.

Gruman, J. A., Lumley, M. N., & Gonzalez-Morales, M. G. (2018). Incorporating balance: Challenges and opportunities for positive psychology. *Canadian Psychology/Psychologie Canadienne, 59*(1), 54–64.

Hagenauer, G., Gläser-Zikuda, M., & Moschner, B. (2018). University students' emotions, life-satisfaction and study commitment: A self-determination theoretical perspective. *Journal of Further and Higher Education, 42*(6), 808–826.

Hamjah, S. H., & Akhir, N. S. M. (2014). Islamic approach in counseling. *Journal of Religion and Health, 53,* 279–289.

Hands, J. (2017). Views on wellbeing research, policy and practice: An interview with Dr. Joanne Hands. *Middle East Journal of Positive Psychology, 3*(1), 24–27.

Haque, A. (2004). Psychology from Islamic perspective: Contributions of early Muslim scholars and challenges to contemporary Muslim psychologists. *Journal of Religion and Health, 43*(4), 357–377.

Haque, A., & Keshavarzi, H. (2012). Integrating indigenous healing methods in therapy: Muslim beliefs and practices. *International Journal of Culture and Mental Health, 7*(3), 297–314.

Haque, A., & Mohamed, Y. (Eds.). (2009). *Psychology of personality: Islamic perspectives*. Kuala Lumpur, Malaysia: Cengage Learning Asia.

Helliwell, J. F., & Wang, S. (2012). The state of world happiness. In J. F. Helliwell, R., Layard & J. Sachs (Eds.), *World Happiness Report* (pp. 10–57). New York, NY: The Earth Institute, Columbia University.

Helliwell, J. F., Huang, H., Grover, S., & Wang, S. (2018). Empirical linkages between good governance and national well-being. *Journal of Comparative Economics*, https://doi.org/10.1016/j.jce.2018.01.004.

Hendriks, T., Schotanus-Dijkstra, M., Hassankhan, A, Graafsma, T., Bohlmeijer, E., & de Jong, J. (2018a). The efficacy of positive psychology interventions from non-Western countries: A systematic review and meta-analysis. *International Journal of Wellbeing, 8*(1), 71–98.

Hendriks, T., Warren, M. A., Schotanus-Dijkstra, M., Hassankhan, A., Graafsma, T., Bohlmeijer, E., & de Jong, J. (2018b). How WEIRD are positive psychology interventions? A bibliometric analysis of randomized controlled trials on the science of well-being. *The Journal of Positive Psychology*, 1–13.

Hessels, J., Arampatzi, E., van der Zwan, P., & Burger, M. (2018). Life satisfaction and self-employment in different types of occupations. *Applied Economic Letters, 25*(11), 734–740.

Hurt, C. S., Burn, D. J., Hindle, J., Samuel, M., Wilson, K., & Brown, R. G. (2014). Thinking positively about chronic illness: An exploration of optimism, illness perceptions and well-being in patients with Parkinson's disease. *British Journal of Health Psychology, 19*(2), 363–379.

Inglehart, R., Foa, R., Peterson, C., & Welzel, C. (2008). Development, freedom and rising happiness: A global perspective 1981–2006. *Perspectives on Psychological Science, 3*(4), 264–285.

Ivry, A. (2008). Arabic and Islamic psychology and philosophy of mind. *Stanford Encyclopedia of Philosophy.* Retrieved from https://plato.stanford.edu/entries/arabic-islamic-mind/.

Joshanloo, M. (2013). The influence of fear of happiness beliefs on responses to the satisfaction with life scale. *Personality and Individual Differences, 54*(5), 647–651.

Kim, H., Doiron, K., Warren, M. A., & Donaldson, S. I. (2018). The international landscape of positive psychology research: A systematic review. *International Journal of Wellbeing, 8*(1), 50–70.

Kööts-Ausmees, L., & Realo, A. (2015). The association between life satisfaction and self-reported health status in Europe. *European Journal of Personality, 29,* 647–657.

Lambert, L. (2017). *Developing character strengths at university (For a GCC audience). The facilitator's manual.* Amazon Publishing. Retrieved from http://a.co/2sxBX3M.

Lambert D'raven, L., & Pasha-Zaidi, N. (2016). Using the PERMA model in the United Arab Emirates. *Social Indicators Research, 125*(3), 905–933.

Lambert, L., Karabchuk, T., & Joshanloo, M. (under review). *Paradoxes of life satisfaction predictors in a wealthy society: Empirical analysis of the United Arab Emirates Gallup data.*

Lambert, L., Passmore, H.-A., & Joshanloo, M. (2018). A positive psychology intervention program in a culturally-diverse university: Boosting happiness and reducing fear. *Journal of Happiness Studies*, https://doi.org/10.1007/s10902-018-9993-z.

Lambert, L., Karabchuk, T., Joshanloo, M., Al Rasbi, Z., & Cody, B. (in preparation). *Using positive psychology interventions in the United Arab Emirates: Boosting wellbeing but, changing what else?*

Lambert, L., Passmore, H.-A., Scull, N., Al Sabah, I., & Hussain, R. (2018). Wellbeing matters in Kuwait: The Alnowair's Bareec education initiative. *Social Indicators Research*, https://doi.org/10.1007/s11205-018-1987-z.

Lomas, T. (2016). Positive psychology—The second wave. *The Psychologist, 29,* 536–539.

Lomas, T., & Ivtzan, I. (2016). Professionalising positive psychology: Developing guidelines for training and regulation. *International Journal of Wellbeing, 6*(3), 96–112.

Miyazaki, G., Saeki, D., Yada, N., & Ikegami, T. (2018). The effects of living in urban environments on residents' life satisfaction: Findings from two online surveys using a multifaceted urban living environment scale. *The Japanese Journal of Psychology, 89*(1), 50–60.

Naess, S., Blekesaune, M., & Jakobsson, N. (2015). Marital transitions and life satisfaction: Evidence from longitudinal data from Norway. *Acta Sociologica, 58*(1), 63–78.

Nelson, S. K., & Lyubomirsky, S. (2014). Finding happiness: Tailoring positive activities for optimal well-being benefits. In M. Tugade, M. Shiota, & L. Kirby (Eds.), *Handbook of positive emotions* (pp. 275–293). New York, NY: Guilford.

Ngamaba, K. H., & Soni, D. (2018). Are happiness and life satisfaction different across religious groups? Exploring determinants of happiness and life satisfaction. *Journal of Religion and Health, 57*(6), 2118–2139.

Omar, O. (2018). Signing up for happiness: An exploratory study of workforce changes in the UAE market in response to the National Program for Happiness and Wellbeing. *Middle East Journal of Positive Psychology, 4*(1), 80–101.

Pasha-Zaidi, N., Afari, E., Sevi, B., Urganci, B., & Durham, J. (2018). Responsibility of learning: A cross-cultural examination of the relationship of grit, motivational belief and self-regulation among college students in the US, UAE and Turkey. *Learning Environments Research*, 1–18. https://doi.org/10.1007/s10984-018-9268-y.

Rothman, A., & Coyle, A. (2018). Toward a framework for Islamic psychology and psychotherapy: An Islamic model of the soul. *Journal of Religion and Health, 57*(5), 1–14.

Schofield, P., Ball, D., Smith, J. G., Borland, R., O'Brien, P., … Joseph, D. (2004). Optimism and survival in lung carcinoma patients. *Cancer, 100*(6), 1276–1282.

Schuilenberg, S., Warren, M. A., Crookes, A., Al Serkal, A., Donaldson, S. I., & McBride, D. (2016). Professional psychology associations in the GCC: Positive institutions whose time has come. *Middle East Journal of Positive Psychology, 2*(1), 61–78.

Seligman, M. E. P. (2011). *Flourish: A visionary new understanding of happiness and well-being*. New York, NY: Free Press.

Sergeant, S., & Mongrain, M. (2011). Are positive psychology exercises helpful for people with depressive personality styles? *The Journal of Positive Psychology, 6*(4), 260–272.

Skinner, R. (2010). An Islamic approach to psychology and mental health. *Mental Health, Religion & Culture, 13*(6), 547–551.

Syed, M., Santos, C., Yoo, H. C., & Juang, L. P. (2018). Invisibility of racial/ethnic minorities in developmental science: Implications for research and institutional practices. *American Psychologist, 73*(6), 812–826.

Veenhoven, R. J. (2008). Healthy happiness: Effects of happiness on physical health and the consequences for preventive health care. *Journal of Happiness Studies, 9*(3), 449–469.

Verme, P. (2009). Happiness, freedom and control. *Journal of Economic Behavior & Organization, 71,* 146–161.

Wang, F., & Wang, D. (2016). Geography of urban life satisfaction: An empirical study of Beijing. *Travel Behaviour and Society, 5,* 14–22.

Welzel, C., & Inglehart, R. (2010). Agency, values, and well-being: A human development model. *Social Indicators Research, 97,* 43–63.

Wong, P. T. P. (2011). Positive psychology 2.0: Towards a balanced interactive model of the good life. *Canadian Psychology/Psychologie canadienne, 52*(2), 69–81.

Wulfgramm, M. (2014). Life satisfaction effects of unemployment in Europe: The moderating influence of labour market policy. *Journal of European Social Policy, 24*(3), 258–272.

York Al-Karam, C. (2018). *Islamically integrated psychotherapy: Uniting faith and professional practice*. West Conshohocken, PA: Templeton Press.

Zhang, F., Zhang, C., & Hudson, J. (2018). Housing conditions and life satisfaction in urban China. *Cities, 81,* 31–44.

9783030139209